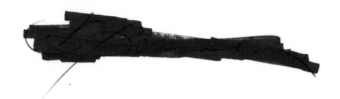

DISEASES OF THE SINUSES

DISEASES OF THE SINUSES

A Comprehensive Textbook of Diagnosis and Treatment

Edited by

M. ERIC GERSHWIN, MD
and **GARY A. INCAUDO, MD**

Division of Rheumatology, Allergy,
and Clinical Immunology
University of California at Davis, CA

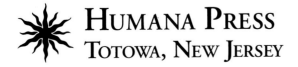
HUMANA PRESS
TOTOWA, NEW JERSEY

DEDICATIONS

For my mother and father, who gave me love and the love of learning
M.E.G.

and

In memory of Eva Sefcik, whose love and inspiration still lives
G.A.I.

© 1996 Humana Press Inc.
999 Riverview Drive, Suite 208
Totowa, New Jersey 07512

For additional copies, pricing for bulk purchases, and/or information about other Humana titles, contact Humana at the above address or at any of the following numbers: Tel.: 201-256-1699; Fax: 201-256-8341; E-mail: humana@interramp.com

This publication is printed on acid-free paper. ∞
ANSI Z39.48-1984 (American National Standards Institute) Permanence of Paper for Printed Library Materials.

Photocopy Authorization Policy:
Authorization to photocopy items for internal or personal use, or the internal or personal use of specific clients, is granted by Humana Press Inc., provided that the base fee of US $5.00 per copy, plus US $00.25 per page, is paid directly to the Copyright Clearance Center at 222 Rosewood Drive, Danvers, MA 01923. For those organizations that have been granted a photocopy license from the CCC, a separate system of payment has been arranged and is acceptable to Humana Press Inc. The fee code for users of the Transactional Reporting Service is: [0-89603-317-1/96 $5.00 + $00.25].

Printed in the United States of America.   10 9 8 7 6 5 4 3 2 1

Library of Congress Cataloging-in-Publication Data

Diseases of the sinuses : a comprehensive textbook of diagnosis and
    treatment / edited by M. Eric Gershwin and Gary A. Incaudo.
        p.   cm.
    Includes index.
    ISBN 0-89603-317-1 (alk. paper)
    1. Paranasal sinuses—Diseases. I. Gershwin, M. Eric, 1946–   .
II. Incaudo, Gary A.
    [DNLM: 1. Sinusitis—diagnosis. 2. Sinusitis—surgery. WV 345
D611 1996]
RF421.D55 1996
616.2'12—dc20
DNLM/DLC
for Library of Congress   95-39511
                                                              CIP

PREFACE

To many physicians, the study of sinus disease reflects a discipline only slightly less interesting than a Johnson and Johnson gauze pad, a pursuit followed by dilettanti and eccentric professors. To others, it represents a subsection of an undefined discipline that crosses barriers of internal medicine, pediatrics, allergy, chest disease, and otolaryngology. To patients, sinus problems are synonymous with headaches and a chronic source of morbidity. Yet few physicians have been prepared, until recently, to do much more than prescribe antibiotics, intranasal steroids, antihistamines, and commiserate for the misery involved. Fortunately, this picture shows significant signs of impending remission. The disciplines of clinical immunology, allergy, and otolaryngology have made enormous strides of late, as have improvements in imaging and microbiology. It is our goal in *Diseases of the Sinuses* to bring to the practicing physician many of the newer concepts that can be applied in a beneficial way to patients.

Throughout most medical centers, sinus problems are one of the most common health care complaints. However, the diagnosis and treatment of sinus disease has been hampered by limited training in medical schools. Additionally, there is no uniform understanding among experts on how to approach this problem effectively. Attempts to organize a consensus of opinion on sinus disease diagnosis and treatment have gathered momentum, and are now being discussed in scattered journal reviews. It is thus now widely recognized that sinus dysfunction is a multifactorial process with multiple influences on treatment outcome. The authors of this text, *Diseases of the Sinuses*, established subspecialists and surgeons from various parts of the world, offer their special insights and broad experience in every area associated with the diagnosis and treatment of nasal and paranasal sinus pathology.

The comprehensive nature of this text will appeal to a wide range of physicians including generalists, otolaryngologists, and allergists. Family physicians, internists, pediatricians, and allergists will each profit from having a single source that provides an in-depth review of topics pertaining to sinus diseases. The otolaryngologist will benefit from having a single text that provides a detailed discussion of the many ancillary medical problems that influence sinus function and, therefore, surgical outcome. We hope that all readers will enjoy the international choice of authors whose topics have been purposely allowed to overlap in an effort to provide the broadest possible scope of information. We expect *Diseases of the Sinuses* to serve as the foundation of an ever-stronger ongoing effort to combat sinus disease.

As with any book, there may be errors and omissions. We have attempted to eliminate these insofar as possible. The flaws that remain in this text are ours alone, and we welcome correspondence from our colleagues and patients in full confidence it will prove constructive toward the next edition some years hence.

ACKNOWLEDGMENTS

This book would not have been possible without the enthusiasm and dedication of our administrative coordinator Theresa Andreozzi. Not only did Theresa manage to organize and help edit the book, but more importantly she managed to work with our contributors, and our deadlines, without offending anyone. The editors owe her a debt of gratitude. Finally, we have always been, and continue to be, appreciative, for the support and encouragement of our publisher, Tom Lanigan Sr.

M. Eric Gershwin
Gary A. Incaudo

CONTENTS

CONTRIBUTORS

MARK L. BENSON, MD, *Department of Neuroradiology, Johns Hopkins Hospital, Baltimore, MD*

CHRISTOPHER CHANG, MD, PHD, *Division of Rheumatology, Allergy, and Clinical Immunology, University of California, Davis, CA*

PETER CLEMENT, MD, PHD, *ENT Department, Academisch Ziekenhuis, Vrije Universiteit Brussel, Brussels, Belgium*

DEAN M. CLERICO, MD, *Department of Otorhinolaryngology, Head and Neck Surgery, University of Pennsylvania Medical Center, Philadelphia, PA*

PHILIP COLE, MD, FRCSC, *Department of Otolaryngology, University of Toronto, Canada; The Gage Research Institute, Toronto, Canada*

VINCENT L. CUMBERWORTH, MB, CHB, BSC, FRCS, *Senior ENT Registrar, Royal Hospitals, NHS Trust, London*

THOMAS CUPPS, MD, *Division of Rheumatology, Immunology, and Allergy, Georgetown University Medical Center, Washington, DC*

TERENCE M. DAVIDSON, MD, *Department of Otorhinolaryngology, Head and Neck Surgery, University of California, San Diego, CA*

WILLIAM K. DOLEN, MD, *Department of Allergy–Immunology, The Medical College of Georgia, Augusta, GA*

HOWARD M. DRUCE, MD, *Therapeutic Research, Hoffmann La Roche Inc. Nutley, NJ; Department of Internal Medicine, University of Medicine and Dentistry of New Jersey, New Jersey Medical School, Newark, NJ*

M. ERIC GERSHWIN, MD, *Division of Rheumatology, Allergy, and Clinical Immunology, University of California, Davis, CA*

ANDRZEJ ROMAN HALAMA, MD, PHD, *ENT Department, Academisch Ziekenhuis, Vrije Universiteit Brussel, Brussels, Belgium*

GEORGES M. HALPERN, MD, *Division of Rheumatology, Allergy, and Clinical Immunology, University of California, Davis, CA*

MICHAEL HAWKE, MD, FRCSC, *Department of Otolaryngology, University of Toronto, Canada*

DAVID HENICK, MD, *Department of Otorhinolaryngology, Head and Neck Surgery, University of Pennsylvania Medical Center, Philadelphia, PA*

DAVID J. HOWARD, FRCS, FRCSED, *Institute of Laryngology and Otology, London*

GARY A. INCAUDO, MD, *Division of Rheumatology, Allergy, and Clinical Immunology, University of California, Davis, CA*

MICHAEL A. KALINER, MD, *Institute for Asthma and Allergy, Washington Hospital Center, Washington, DC*

KATHERINE A. KENDALL, MD, *Department of Otolaryngology, University of California Davis Medical Center, Sacramento, CA*

DAVID W. KENNEDY, MD, *Department of Otolarhinolaryngology, Head and Neck Surgery, University of Pennsylvania Medical Center, Philadelphia, PA*

MICHAEL J. LIGHT, MD, *Department of Pediatric Pulmonology, University of California, San Diego, CA*

VALERIE J. LUND, MS, FRCS, FRCSED, *University College, London Medical School, Institute of Laryngology and Otology, London*

RODNEY P. LUSK, MD, *St. Louis Children's Hospital at Washington University School of Medicine, St. Louis, MO*

IAN S. MACKAY, FRCS, *ENT Surgeon, Royal Brompton and Charing Cross Hospitals, London*

RICHARD B. MOSS, MD, *Division of Allergy, Immunology and Respiratory Medicine, Stanford University Medical Center, Palo Alto, CA*

CLAIRE MURPHY, PHD, *San Diego State University and University of California, San Diego, CA*

STANLEY NAGUWA, MD, *Division of Rheumatology, Allergy, and Clinical Immunology, University of California, Davis, CA*

HAROLD S. NOVEY, MD, *Division of Basic and Clinical Immunology, University of California, Irvine, CA*

PATRICK J. OLIVERIO, MD, *Department of Neuroradiology, Johns Hopkins Hospital, Baltimore, MD*

ZDENEK PELIKAN, MD, PhD, *Department of Allergology and Immunology, Institute Medical Science "De Klokkenberg," Breda, The Netherlands*

ROGER PEYNEGRE, MD, *Department of Otolaryngology, Head and Neck Surgery, University Mondor Paris XII, Paris-Creteil, France*

JILL RAZANI, MA, *Doctoral Program in Clinical Psychology, San Diego State University and University of California, San Diego, CA*

MARK A. RICHARDSON, MD, *Department of Otolaryngology, Head and Neck Surgery, Johns Hopkins University, Baltimore, MD*

RENATO ROITHMANN, MD, *Department of Otolaryngology, University of Toronto, Canada; The Gage Research Institute, Toronto, Canada*

PIERRE ROUVIER, MD, *Department of Otolaryngology, Head and Neck Surgery, Jean Imbert Hospital, Arles, France*

JOHN C. SELNER, MD, *Allergy Respiratory Institute of Colorado, Denver, CO*

CRAIG W. SENDERS, MD, *Department of Otolaryngology, University of California Davis Medical Center, Davis, CA*

GUY A. SETTIPANE, MD, *Brown University of Medicine and Division of Allergy/Immunology, Department of Medicine, Rhode Island Hospital, Providence, RI*

RUSSELL A. SETTIPANE, MD, *Division of Allergy/Immunology, Department of Medicine, Rhode Island Hospital, Providence, RI*

SHELDON C. SIEGEL, MD, *UCLA School of Medicine and Allergy Medical Clinic, Los Angeles, CA*

ELLEN R. WALD, MD, *Department of Pediatrics and Otolaryngology, University of Pittsburgh School of Medicine; Division of Pediatric Infectious Diseases, Children's Hospital of Pittsburgh, PA*

MICHEL R. WAYOFF, MD, *Department of ORL and Cervico-Facial Surgery, Central Hospital, Medical University, Nancy, France*

IAN WITTERICK, MD, FRCSC, *Department of Otolaryngology, Mount Sinai Hospital, Toronto, Ontario, Canada*

L. GRETCHEN WOODING, MD, *Department of Internal Medicine, Division of Rheumatology, Allergy, and Clinical Immunology, University of California, Davis, CA*

STEVEN H. YOSHIDA, PhD, *Department of Food Science and Technology, University of California, Davis, CA*

S. JAMES ZINREICH, MD, *Department of Neuroradiology, Johns Hopkins Hospital, Baltimore, MD*

PART I ANATOMY AND PHYSIOLOGY

1 Anatomy and Anatomical Variations of the Paranasal Sinuses

Influence on Sinus Dysfunction

Roger Peynegre, MD and Pierre Rouvier, MD

CONTENTS

INTRODUCTION

The anatomy of the sinuses has been previously investigated in many studies. Without going back to the earliest reported works of the ancient Greeks and Romans, let us mention some of the more recent, well-known investigators, such as Boyer, and others who were active during the late nineteenth century: Zuckerkandl *(1),* Sieur *(2),* Jacob *(2),* Mouret *(3–5),* Onodi *(6),* Grünwald *(7),* and Killian *(8,9),* who made detailed studies on the formation and structure of the most complex structures in the sinuses: the ethmoidal labyrinth, or the structures of the middle meatus. Unfortunately, these authors gave different names to the same anatomical structures, and sometimes the same name was given to different structures. Consequently, it is sometimes less difficult to recognize structures in the labyrinth of ethmoidal cells than in that of the different terms and definitions. Undoubtedly, a revised, unified system of terminology is necessary. However, habits and surgical practice

From: *Diseases of the Sinuses* (M. E. Gershwin and G. A. Incaudo, eds.), ©1996 Humana Press Inc., Totowa, NJ.

have given rise to definitions that are somewhat inexact, but have entered the scientific jargon through usage. The recent enthusiasm for endoscopic surgery of the nasal cavities and sinuses as a result of studies by Messerklinger *(10),* and later Stammberger *(11),* Kennedy et al. *(12),* Buiter *(13,14),* Friedrich *(15,16),* Wigand *(17),* Rouvier et al. *(18–20),* and so forth, the precise description and accurate detail provided by endoscopy, and also advances in modern imaging techniques have revived interest in the anatomy of the sinuses.

Research by Terrier *(21)* and Agrifolio et al. *(22)* and the Swiss school of Lausanne has conferred value on a systematic description of the ethmoid sinus, the keystone in the sinus system. Such a systematic classification is not solely of academic interest because development of CT-scan imaging techniques has conferred practical value on it. It also corresponds to a clinical reality, since diagnostic value results from knowledge of lesional extent. Solely anterior or solely posterior involvement in relation to the septal partition of the middle concha is a finding that suggests suppurated sinusitis. Anterior and posterior compartment involvement support the diagnosis of nasal polyposis if lesions are bilateral.

Endoscopy also makes it possible to describe a new anatomical reality. From a surgical standpoint and based on abnormal tissue findings, it is perhaps impossible to identify every cell, but each cell group can be found. Nevertheless, the recognition of some key anatomical landmarks continues to be the fundamental approach in preventing iatrogenic events.

THE RHINOSINUS UNIT

The Embryological Unit: the Olfactory Placode and Its Development

In adults, the relative autonomy that the different paranasal air sinuses appear to enjoy is only an apparent one; in fact, all the air-filled cavities of the face are connected to each other, in particular as a result of their embryological origin. Development of the nasosinus cavities in a cranial direction occurs at the same time as growth of the palate downward, facial cranium anteriorly, and cerebral cranium above (frontonasal process). The entire system of sinuses arises from the lateral wall of the primitive choanae. At this level, approximately at midterm of fetal development, three ectodermal elevations appear: one is inferior (maxilloturbinate) and gives rise to the inferior concha; another is superior (ethmoidal-turbinate) and will produce the superior and middle conchae; and the last is anterior (nasoturbinate) and forms the agger nasi. It is between the first two outlines, in the primitive middle meatus, that at about the 13th wk of development, an evagination of the lateral wall of the nasal fossa produces a blind diverticulum: the infundibulum whose colonization of adjacent bones will form the different sinuses *(23)*.

THE EMBRYONIC INFUNDIBULUM (FIG. 1)

This gives rise to the entire anterior sinus complex. All craniofacial structures, at first made of cartilage, and then of bone, that are adjacent to the infundibular region, can be subject to penetration by the process of evagination and then erosion; the maxillary bone, frontal bone, ethmoidal conchae, and nasoturbinate bone (agger nasi) will be invaded and filled with air from the ethmoidal cells: the ethmoido-maxillary, ethmoido-frontal, ethmoido-bullar, ethmoido-uncinate, and ethmoido-aggarian cells, respectively. This colonization produces

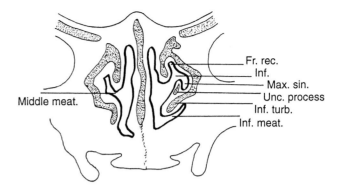

Fig. 1. Drawing of a 64-mm human embryo section through the developing nasal cavity. Fr. rec., frontal recess; Inf., infundibulum; Max. sin., maxillary sinus; Unc. process, uncinate process; Inf. turb., inferior turbinate; Inf. meat., inferior meatus; Middle meat., middle meatus.

irregular, somewhat extensive offshoots, sometimes invading "foreign areas," such as the palate, floor or roof of the orbit, and so on.

THE MAXILLARY SINUS

This appears first, at about the 10th wk; it thus is present at birth, although very small, dominated by an ethmoidal mass twice as large. This explains its secondary role in infection in infants, with mainly ethmoidal involvement. It retains its rounded shape even after the eruption of the deciduous teeth, which has little impact on its development. It is with retraction of the facial cranium and especially the eruption of the permanent teeth starting at age 6 that the maxillary sinus gradually assumes its pyramidal shape to attain its definitive size between 15 and 18 yr of age. In spite of some cases of asymmetrical development (1.5%), it generally is symmetrical, but rare, unilateral agenesis can occur, just as certain types of more or less complete partitioning.

THE FRONTAL SINUS AND ANTERIOR ETHMOID

These arise from the infundibulum on which the outlines of four swellings are impressed. The upper extremity becomes individualized at the 13th wk in the form of the frontal recess or processus frontalis; a terminal infundibular cell will continue the frontal recess above and will form the frontal sinus; the others by colonizing the anterior ethmoid will give rise to cell groups of the bulla ethmoidalis, the uncinate-ungueal region, and the middle concha, but can also colonize the frontal bone to create the frontal bullae next to it. Colonization of the frontal

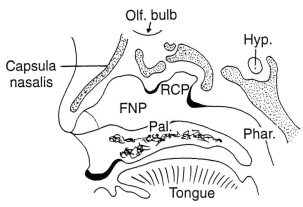

Fig. 2. Sagittal section of a fetal head showing the origin of the sphenoidal sinus. FNP, primitive nasal cavity; RCP, recessus copularis posterior; PAL, palatal process; Hyp., pituitary gland; Olf. bulb., olfactory bulb.; Phar., pharynx.

sinus only begins during the first year of life and progresses slowly to become identifiable only at about 12 yr of age; generally, asymmetrical development occurs, but unilateral or bilateral agenesis may also occur (10%).

THE POSTERIOR ETHMOID AND THE SPHENOIDAL SINUS (FIG. 2)

These also are derived from the ethmoid, but not from the infundibulum; it is later than for the anterior ethmoid, at about the third month, behind the maxilloturbinate bud in the embryonic superior meatus that three cells appear, which will colonize the posterior ethmoid. The most recessed of these cells, known as Onodi cells, come into contact with the anterior wall of a cavity hollowed out in the thickness of the sphenoidal bone that is the sphenoidal sinus; the latter is not, however, directly part of the ethmoidal bone, but rather an offshoot of the furthest part of the primitive nares: the posterior recessus capsularis. This apparently independent and primitive development (after the first year of life) of the sphenoidal sinus could perhaps explain the relative autonomy of sphenoidal disorders.

The Anatomical Unit

NASOSINUSAL STRUCTURAL ORGANIZATION (FIG. 3)

This is contained entirely in the frontomaxillary-malar bony mass, which is very often involved in facial injuries. The sinus and orbital cavities form a cellular structure that is relatively fragile, but protected by the craniofacial bony covering and its bony reinforcements located in the middle one-third of the face (Lefort's pillars) in the frontal band

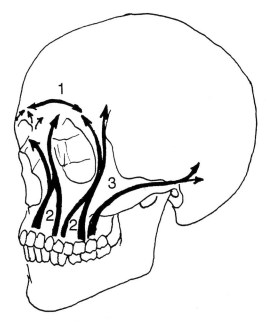

Fig. 3. Functional structure of skull. (1) Frontal reinforcement, (2) frontal-nasal pillar, (3) zygomatic arch pillar.

and in the base of the skull. This structural unit accounts for involvement of the entire system of sinuses in maxillofacial injuries.

VASCULARIZATION

Vascularization of the sinuses is largely supplied from two sources *(24)*. The nasal mucosal vasculature consists of branches of the sphenopalatine artery and the anterior and posterior ethmoidal arteries. The osseous vasculature consists of branches of vessels running from tissues surrounding the sinus. Four main arteries provide the vascularization of the sinuses. The anterior ethmoidal artery arises from the ophthalmic artery. It enters through the anterior ethmoidal foramen of the ethmoid bone into the anterior cranial fossa, via the cribiform plate into the nasal cavity. It branches into the anterior part of the nasal cavity at the lateral and medial walls. The posterior ethmoidal artery arises from the ophthalmic artery, a branch of the internal carotid artery. It sends branches into the dura mater of the brain and into the adjacent part of the nasal fossa. The sphenopalatine artery is a branch of the maxillary artery passing from the pteryogopalatine fossa through the sphenopalatine foramen. It ramifies into posterior septal branches and lateral posterior nasal arteries. These arteries supply the posterior lateral and medial walls of the nasal cavity. The infraorbital artery arises from the maxillary artery and passes through the infraorbital groove and canal. It sends branches to the mucosa of the maxillary sinus.

Veins drain into the facial vein, sphenopalatine vein, pterygomaxillary plexus, subcutaneous veins, orbital and intracranial cavernous system.

Lymph flows into the lymphatic vessels of the nasal fossa and the meninges.

INNERVATION

The medial and lateral posterior nasal nerves, branches of the maxillary division (V2) of the trigeminal nerve, supply sensation to the sinus mucosa. They enter the nasal fossa through the sphenopalatine foramen. These branches carry parasympathetic and sympathetic nerve fibers as well as afferent fibers. The anterior and posterior ethmoidal nerves, branches of the ophthalmic nerve (V1), provide sensory innervation to the mucosa of the frontal, ethmoidal, and sphenoidal sinuses. Branches of the trigeminal nerve supply additional afferent fibers through the surrounding structures from ostia of the sinuses.

Histological Unit

As the interface between the outside environment and the internal medium, and thus the point of initial contact between the body and inspired air and inhaled particles, the mucosal lining of the sinuses is continuous with the nasal, tubotympanic and tracheobronchial mucosa. It is comprised of:

> A respiratory epithelial lining as in the nasal mucosa, but without tubo-acinar glands; it consists mainly of a very thin basement membrane, but whose intact structure is of vital importance, ciliated columnar cells whose cilia ensure mucociliary transport by their coordinated (metachronal) movement toward the natural ostium along an unchanging pathway, and scarce goblet cells, which secrete mucus required for effective ciliary sweeping movement;
> The lamina propria, which is very thin, but can thicken considerably during inflammation; and
> Vascularization that is fragile and confined to a subepithelial network of exchange; it forms a capillary bed below the basement membrane, consisting of fenestrated vessels, which perform fluid transfers between the circulation and the lamina propria.

THE ETHMOIDAL SINUS AS THE CORNERSTONE OF THE SINUS SYSTEM

The Ethmoidal Cast

Each ethmoidal mass has a covering, referred to as the ethmoidal cast by Guerrier and Rouvier *(25)*. It has six faces and contains the ethmoidal cells, which open into the nasal cavity.

THE MEDIAL ASPECT (FIG. 4A,B)

The medial aspect is referred to as the turbinate plate by Mouret *(3–5)*. It is continuous with the orbital process of the palatine bone posteriorly and with the frontal process of the maxilla anteriorly. It is crossed by the insertion of the middle turbinate bone. The middle nasal concha is attached anteriorly, 5 mm from the upper wall of the nasal cavity, and extending backward to demarcate the lamina cribrosa. Posteriorly, the middle concha inserts at about 15 mm from the upper wall passing below the sphenopalatine foramen. The insertion of the middle turbinate bone divides the medial aspect of the ethmoidal labyrinth into two parts.

The anterior and inferior part can be investigated by lifting the middle turbinate medially upward. It corresponds to the middle meatus. The most anterior projection is the agger nasi, a bony crest. It begins at the anterior insertion of the middle turbinate and continues into the ascending ramus of the superior maxilla at the upper extremity of Terrier's preturbinate fold. It runs downward toward the inferior turbinate. It has a variable degree of development. If extensive, it can be situated between the lacrimal duct laterally and the nasal fossa medially. The lateral wall of the middle meatus has two projections: the uncinate process and the ethmoidal bulla, which are rudimentary and inverted turbinates.

The Uncinate Process. The uncinate process is a thin, sagittally oriented lamella that runs from the roof of the ethmoid bone. The anterosuperior portion lies in a slightly frontal plane. The upper portion of the uncinate process may attach to the roof of the ethmoid bone or gradually taper off anteriorly. It may also run medially and fuse with the middle turbinate. In such cases, the frontal sinus and the frontal recess open into the ethmoidal infundibulum. When the uncinate process inserts laterally on the lamina papyracea, the frontal sinus drains into the middle meatus medial to the infundibulum.

Below, the uncinate process lies parallel to the anterior surface of the bulla ethmoidalis. It joins the

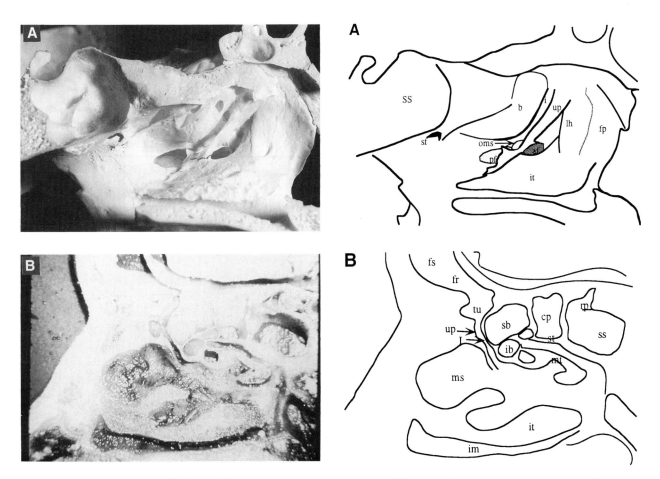

Fig. 4. (A) Lateral nasal wall. The middle turbinate has been resected. SS, sphenoidal sinus; b, bulla; i, infundibulum; up, uncinate process; lh, lacrimal hump; fp, frontal process of the maxilla; sf, sphenopalatine foramen; pf, posterior fontanelle; af, anterior fontanelle; oms, orifice of maxillary sin; it, inferior turbinate. (B) Anatomic sagittal section showing the frontal sinus, the frontal recess, the terminal uncinate cell, and the infundibulum. fs, frontal sinus; fr, frontal recess; tu, terminal uncinate cell; up, uncinate process; sb, supra bullar cell; ib, intrabullar cell; cp, central posterior cell; rp, remote posterior cell; ss, sphenoidal sinus; ms, maxillary sinus; it, inferior turbinate; mt, middle turbinate; st, superior turbinate; im, inferior meatus.

bulla posteriorly and laterally. At its posterior end, thin bony spicules attach the uncinate process to the lamina perpendicularis of the palatine bone and to the ethmoidal process of the inferior turbinate.

These prolongations delimit four bony defects or fontanelles, which are covered with dense connective tissue and the mucosa of the maxillary sinus and the nasal fossa. The anterior and superior fontanelle is the ostium of the maxillary sinus. It lies at the junction of the vertical and horizontal portions of the uncinate process.

The Ethmoidal Bulla. The second landmark is the ethmoidal bulla. It is a fundamental point of reference in ethmoidectomy. Between the bulla and the agger nasi lies the upper part of the posterior border of the vertical portion of the uncinate pro-

cess, which limits the infundibulum. The term infundibulum is not specific. Previously, different interpretations have been given to this term. In modern endoscopic studies, Buiter *(13,14)* applies this term to the deep groove forming the anterior part of the hiatus semilunaris. The definition retained in the international anatomic nomenclature is that it is the lower part of the uncinate groove and the hiatus semilunaris is its opening. Austrian anatomists use it to refer to a cleft-like space in the lateral wall of the nasal fossa, belonging to the anterior ethmoid. It comprises all the air-filled structures between the uncinate process and the orbit.

The uncinate process and the bulla determine small grooves. The uncinate groove, uncinate bullar groove, or infundibulum, lies above and

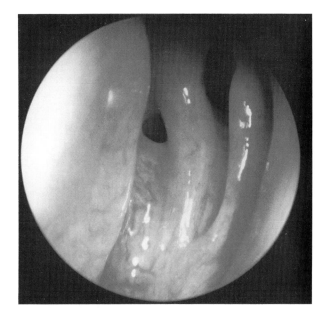 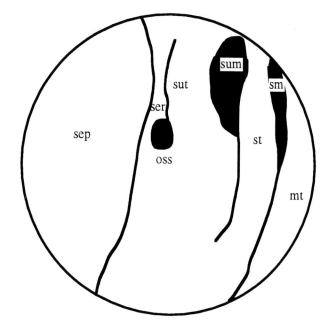

Fig. 5. Superior meatus and sphenoethmoidal recess, left nasal cavity. oss, ostium of sphenoidal sinus; sut, supreme turbinate; st, superior turbinate; mt, middle turbinate; ser, sphenoethmoidal recess; sum, supreme meatus; sm, superior meatus.

behind the uncinate process. The bullar groove, retrobullar groove, or superior semilunar hiatus, or bullar sinus is located behind the ethmoidal bulla.

A third groove is formed by the anterosuperior attachment of the middle turbinate to the lateral side. Referred to as the recessus meatus medii by Mihalkovics *(26),* or the recessus frontalis by Killian *(8,9),* it is termed the meatal groove by Terrier *(21).* The uncinate bullar and meatal grooves form what Terrier calls the "bullar rundabout." The endoscopic aspect observed with a 70° lens endoscope has led Terrier to call it the "tristar of the grooves." According to this author, it is not only a restricted anatomical structure, but also an overall functional complex, including all the anterior sinuses and their ostia: the frontal sinus, anterior ethmoid, and maxillary sinus draining into the middle meatus.

The posterosuperior part consists of the turbinate plate only. It can be demarcated by the outline of the superior turbinates. The superior meatus lies below the superior turbinate. Above, Santorini's turbinate or the supreme turbinate was reported in 52% of Agrifolio et al.'s cases *(22).* It sometimes limits the upper border of a supreme meatus, where the ostium of an ethmoidal posterior cell is found in 57% of cases. Between the superior turbinate and septum lies the sphenoethmoidal recess, which Terrier *(21)* calls the juxta-septal meatus or septal meatus. The sphenoethmoidal recess contains the

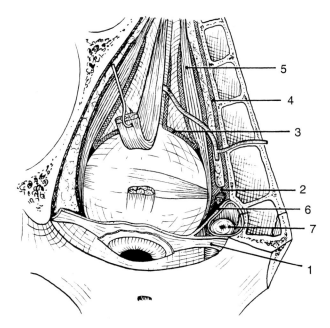

Fig. 6. (1) Medial canthal ligament, (2) medial attachment of suspensory ligament, (3) fascia bulbi, (4) periorbita, (5) medial rectus muscle, (6) reflected tendon of medial palpabral ligament; (7) lacrimal sac. Drawing by Q. P. Wang.

sphenoid ostium, which is the most posterior orifice and is the one closest to the septum. (Fig. 5).

THE LATERAL OR ORBITAL SIDE (FIG. 6)

Three portions can be described. The anterior one-fourth or lacrimal fourth is narrow and deli-

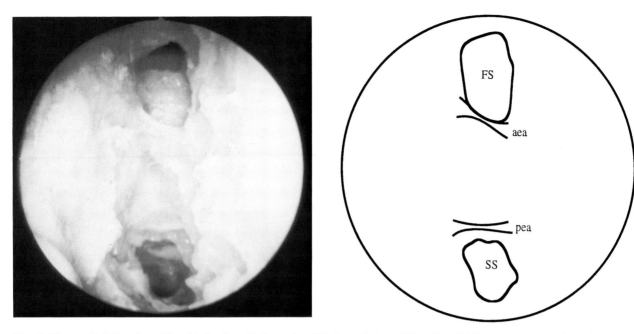

Fig. 7. The roof of the ethmoid and left ethmoidal arteries. FS, frontal sinus; SS, sphenoidal sinus; aea, anterior ethmoidal artery; pea, posterior ethmoidal artery.

cate. It is bounded anteriorly by the lacrimal bone, a small bony membrane that borders the lacrimal groove, and the fossa for the lacrimal sac and the nasolacrimal duct. A fracture of the posterior edge at the level of the lacrimal bone can injure the lacrimal duct during uncinatectomy. The two middle fourths are often paper-thin. They bound the ethmoid from the orbit. The real borderline is in fact the periorbita (periosteum of the orbit). There is a loose connection between the bones and the periorbit, except at the level of the anterior and posterior ethmoidal foramina and the insertion of the canthal tendons on the posterior lacrimal crest. Three structures are in close contact, and adverse events can occur if the orbital wall is penetrated: the internal rectus muscle, flat, elongated, and low-inserted, the origin of the anterior ethmoidal artery for which retraction of the proximal end can cause an intraorbital hematoma in case of injury and intraorbital retraction, and the fat, which fills the orbital voids. The posterior one-fourth presents a very delicate relation: the optic canal and the optic nerve, which can protrude into the last ethmoid-sphenoidal cell.

Basal Cranial Aspect

The superior ethmoidal cells open upward. The frontal bone forms the roof of this structure.

Posterior Two-Thirds. The underlying ethmoidal cells make an impression on the posterior two-thirds. This bony plate is extended by the roof of the sphenoid posteriorly and the floor of the frontal sinus anteriorly. These two anatomical structures are important reference points in ethmoidectomy. The medial part is very oblique inferiorly and medially. It extends into the turbinate plate and the middle turbinate, which are also significant reference points in ethmoidectomy.

Two bony projections lie underneath (Fig. 7). Anteriorly, the anterior ethmoidal artery is oblique anteriorly and medially. This artery runs in a bony canal (Fig. 8) just below the roof of the ethmoid, usually at the foot of the bulla lamella or 1 or 2 mm posteriorly. This is a basic reference structure in ethmoidectomy. In 40% of cases, this canal exhibits bony dehiscences that can result in a partially or completely open canal. These dehiscences can differ from one side to the other. Posteriorly, the posterior ethmoidal artery (Fig. 7) runs in a transverse bony canal. Here, the bony plate is usually hard and strong. However, it can present many bony rarefactions and even dehiscences *(27)* observed in 14% of cases (Fig. 9), mainly anteriorly in the medial part of the roof of the ethmoid, behind the anterior ethmoidal artery. The most critical area of the entire ethmoid is where the ethmoidal anterior

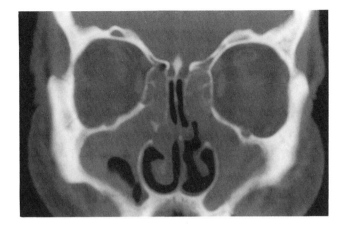
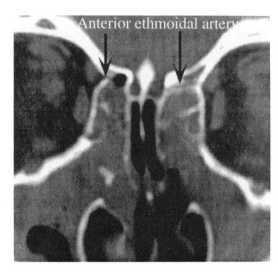

Fig. 8. CT view. Frontal section.

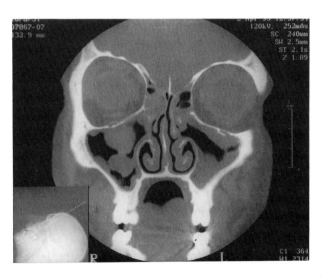
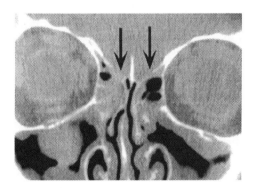

Fig. 9. This CT scan demonstrates the thin medial wall of the ethmoidal roof (arrow). Coronal CT section.

artery enters the anterior cranial fossa through the lateral lamella of the lamina cribrosa. At this point, the lateral lamella is only one-tenth as strong as the roof of the ethmoid and presents the area of least resistance. This occurs where the frontal bone joins the lateral lamella of the lamina cribrosa. This junction forms the lateral border of the olfactory fossa. Here, the roof of the ethmoid may be somewhat above the lamina cribrosa. The cribriform plate lies 4–7 mm below the roof of the ethmoid in 70% of patients, and 12–16 mm lower than the roof in 18%. It is important for the ENT surgeon to keep in mind the height, width, and shape of the roof of the ethmoid observed on CT scan in relation to the height of the cribriform plate during a surgical procedure.

The entire bony plate is covered by the dura mater, which is firmly attached to the lamina cribrosa medially, especially where the anterior ethmoidal artery, its branches, and the olfactory filaments pass through the cribriform plate. Higher up, the olfactory bulb lies medial and the frontal lobe lateral to it.

The Anterior One-Third. The floor of the frontal sinus lies somewhat spread out on the anterior ethmoid, whose cells form bony swellings or bulla around the superior orifice of the frontonasal duct.

THE MAXILLARY ASPECT

This is divided into two parts by the maxillary canal. The anterior one-third is adjacent to the agger nasi and the uncinate groove, between the lacrimal duct laterally and the nasal fossa medially. The posterior two-thirds form the borderline between the maxillary sinus inferiorly, and the posterior ethmoid and bulla superiorly.

CONTACT WITH THE LACRIMAL BONE ANTERIORLY

The anterior side is divided by the anterior lacrimal crest on which the medial palpebral ligament inserts. The anterior portion consists of strong, thick bone: the frontal process of the maxilla (Fig. 6). The periosteum is closely adherent to the bone, making it difficult to detach. It contains blood vessels and is in contact with the skin of the medial canthus.

The posterior part is adjacent to the lacrimal groove. The lacrimal bone is a thin, papery bone, forming the medial wall of the orbit and covered by a weak sticky layer of the periorbita. Lower down, it continues with the nasolacrimal duct, which opens into the nasal cavity at the entry of the middle meatus in an area that enables the operator to perform endonasal dacryocystorhinostomy. This groove forms the deep wall of the lacrimal sac compartment that is closed posteriorly by the reflected tendon of the medial palpebral ligament, and lined with connective tissue of the orbital septum, and anteriorly by the tendon of the medial palpebral ligament.

CONTACT WITH THE SPHENOIDAL BONE POSTERIORLY

The lateral three-fourths are comprised of the anterior side of the body of the sphenoid. The medial fourth forms the sphenoethmoidal recess. Morphology of the wall varies depending on the degree of pneumatization of the ethmoid sinus.

The Basal Lamellae

The ethmoidal sinus contains several cells of very different shape and size depending on the extent of air filling the ethmoidal cavity. The number of cells also depends on the development of septa in the interturbinate meatus. Overall, ethmoidal cells are smaller and more numerous anteriorly, and there are larger and fewer cells posteriorly.

Several authors, e.g., Seydel *(28)*, Zuckerkandl *(1)*, Mouret *(3–5)*, and, more recently, Terrier *(21)*, have proposed a precise system of classification. Each turbinate arises from the medial plate of the ethmoid and from the lamina papyracea via a bony sheet. Each turbinate consists of two parts: the

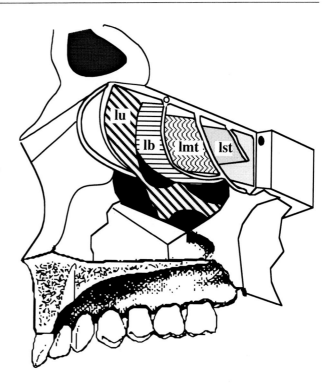

Fig. 10. Basal lamellae and cellular space. lu, lamella of the uncinate process; lb, lamella of the bulla; lmt, lamella of the middle turbinate; lst, lamella of the superior turbinate.

medial part is rolled up and is visible inside the nasal cavity and the lateral part is a bony septum.

Known as basal or ground lamella, these thin lamellae descend into the ethmoid, forming septa that divide the cellular group. These basal lamellae are relative constant anatomical findings, despite the extensive deformations they undergo in response to the degree of pneumatization. The basal lamella of the uncinate process, bulla, middle turbinate, superior turbinate, and occasionally the supreme turbinate can be seen in an anteroposterior view (Figs. 10–13).

THE BASAL LAMELLA OF THE MIDDLE TURBINATE BONE

The basal lamella of the middle turbinate forms the border between the anterior ethmoid and the posterior ethmoid. It consists of two parts: the anterior portion lies almost in a frontal plane. It fastens the middle third of the middle turbinate to the lamella papyracea. The posterior half of the basal lamella lies almost in a horizontal plane. It attaches the posterior third of the middle turbinate to the lamina papyracea and the medial side of the maxillary sinus. The frontal plane of the anterior

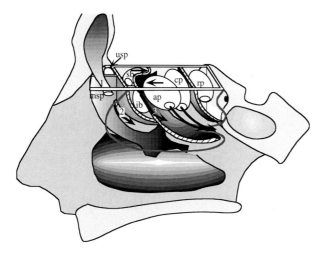

Fig. 11. usp, uncinate space; msp, meatal space; 1, meatal groove; 2, uncinate groove; 3, bullar groove; sb, suprabullar cell; ib, intrabullar cell; ap, advanced posterior cell; cp, central posterior cell; rp, remote posterior cell.

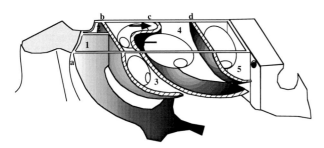

Fig. 12. Basal lamellae and cellular space modified after G. Terrier. (1) Meatal space; (2) uncinate space; (3) bullar space; (4) central posterior space; (5) remote posterior space; (a) Basal lamella of the uncinate process; (b) Basal lamella of the bulla; (c) Basal lamella of the middle turbinate; (d) Basal lamella of the superior turbinate.

portion can be altered by well-inflated anterior ethmoidal cells, especially the suprabullar cell, which, in extreme cases, may extend to the anterior wall of the sphenoid sinus. Conversely, the posterior ethmoidal cells can greatly displace the ground lamella anteriorly. Such a deformation can cause the ground lamella to bulge dorsally in its lateral midsection and anteriorly in its medial midsection. They often impart an S-shaped aspect to the vertical portion of the ground lamella. However, a number of variations can provide a highly variable appearance for the ground lamella of the middle turbinate. Such variations may make intraoperative identification and interpretation of preoperative CT scans extremely difficult.

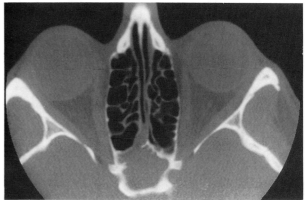

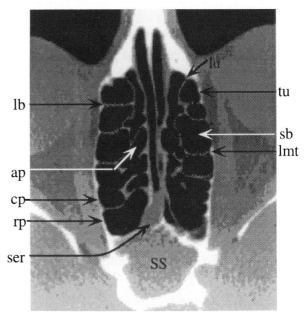

Fig. 13. Axial CT section, a few millimeters below the lamina cribrosa. It shows a sphenoidal sinusitis. tu, terminal uncinate cell; ib, intrabullar cell; ap, advanced posterior cell; cp, central posterior cell; rp, remote posterior cell; ser, sphenoethmoidal recess; lu, lamella of the uncinate process; lb, lamella of the bulla; lmt, lamella of the middle turbinate; SS, sphenoidal sinus.

BASAL LAMELLA OF THE BULLA

The basal lamella of the bulla lies in a more anterior position as a frontally oriented plate. It forms the border between the bullar space posteriorly and the prebullar space anteriorly. Upward, the basal lamella of the bulla can reach the roof of the ethmoid. It thus forms the posterior wall of the frontal recess. The intraethmoidal course of the anterior ethmoid artery generally is on the same level as this lamella. The latter may be vestigial or completely missing. In this case, there is direct communication between the frontal recess and a pneumatized space referred to as the sinus lateralis or lateral sinus by Grünwald *(7)*, and is located above and behind the bulla.

THE BASAL LAMELLA OF THE UNCINATE PROCESS

The basal lamella of the uncinate process divides the meatal space medially from the uncinate space laterally. The uncinate space contains the group of the uncinate cells. The meatal space contains the meatal cells—particularly, the anterior ethmoidal cell. The basal lamella of the uncinate process constitutes the wall separating the superior uncinate cell or Boyer's cell and the anterior meatal cell. The frontal sinus is more commonly formed from the anterior meatal cell and sometimes from Boyer's cell. These facts are of fundamental importance in endoscopic surgery of the ethmoid. Resection of the uppermost portion of the uncinate process enlarges the opening of the frontal sinus and creates a pathway between the two cavities. Resection of the "beak" of the bulla between anterior and posterior meatal cell, including the orifice of the meatal cell, enlarged the passage even more.

THE BASAL LAMELLA OF THE SUPERIOR TURBINATE

The basal lamella of the superior turbinate or of the supreme turbinate may or may not extend to the lamina papyracea. The basal lamella of the middle turbinate anteriorly and the basal lamella of the superior turbinate posteriorly determine the central posterior space. Between the basal lamella of the superior turbinate and the posterior wall of the ethmoid lies the remote posterior space, which contains the remote posterior cell.

Classification and Arrangement of Ethmoidal Cells (Figs. 13–15)

THE ANTERIOR ETHMOID

It comprises three cellular systems: the bullar system and the prebullar system that is divided into two systems, the uncinate and meatal systems.

The Bullar System. The bullar system consists of the group of intrabullar cells and the group of suprabullar cells (Figs. 16 and 17A,B). They all drain into the bullar groove. The bullar lies between the basal lamella of the bulla anteriorly and the basal lamella of the middle turbinate posteriorly. The intrabullar cell is contained within the ethmoidal bulla. It consists of one to four cells. Some cells which appear to belong to the bullar group, but drain into either the uncibullar groove or the supe-

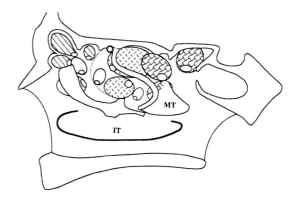

Fig. 14. Arrangement of the ethmoidal cells. ⊘, Bullar cells; ⊘, meatal cells; ⊘, uncinate cells; ⊘, posterior cells.

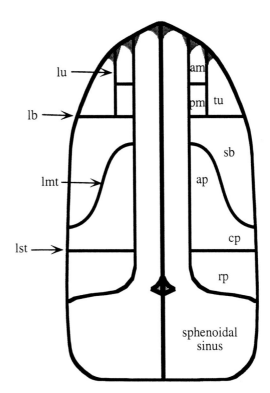

Fig. 15. Basic structures of the ethmoid according to G. Terrier. Ethmoidal cells: tu, terminal uncinate cell; am, anterior meatal cell; pm, posterior meatal cell; sb, suprabullar cell; ap, advanced posterior cell; cp, central posterior cell; rp, remote posterior cell. Basal lamellae: lu, lamella of the uncinate process; lb, lamella of the bulla; lmt, lamella of the middle turbinate; lst, lamella of the superior turbinate.

rior meatus, are not bullar cells. This is true for the posterior uncinate cell, which drains into the uncinate groove or the cell at the base of the bulla, which may be a central posterior cell and opens into the superior meatus.

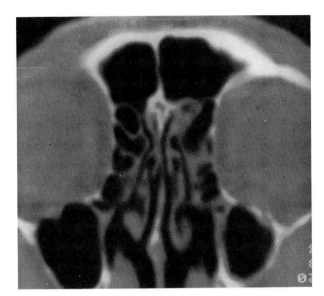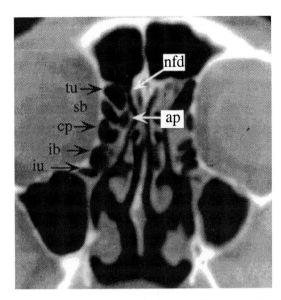

Fig. 16. CT scan semifrontal section. tu, terminal uncinate cell; iu, inferior uncinate cell; sb, suprabullar cell; ib, intrabullar cell; ap, advanced posterior cell; cp, central posterior cell; nfd, nasofrontal duct.

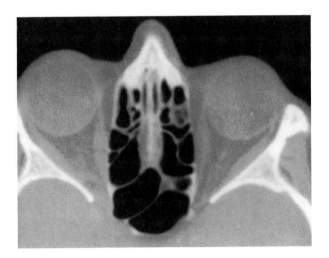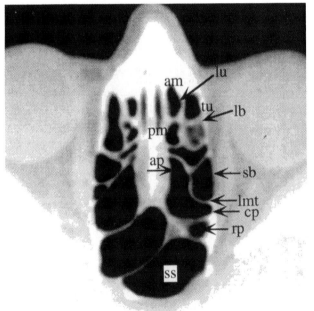

Fig. 17. (A) Axial CT scan, upper section. tu, terminal uncinate cell; pu, posterior uncinate cell; am, anterior meatal cell; pm, posterior meatal cell; sb, suprabullar cell; ib, intrabullar cell; ap, advanced posterior cell; cp, central posterior cell; lu, lamella of the uncinate process; lb, lamella of the bulla; lmt, lamella of the middle turbinate; ss, sphenoidal sinus.

The suprabullar cell lies at the top of the bullar system. It spreads laterally and posteriorly. Sometimes, it lies parallel to the posterior ethmoidal cell and may reach the sphenoidal sinus. This significant posteriorly extension produces an S-shaped deformity in the basal lamella of the middle turbinate. The basal lamella lies in a frontal plane

inferiorly. As it ascends, it twists superiorly and posteriorly and becomes almost sagittal. This S-shaped lamella is an important radiological landmark on the CT scan (Fig. 17A).

Occasionally, the suprabullar cell may extend anteriorly and form an impression on the frontal sinus. It may even form a posterolateral bulla

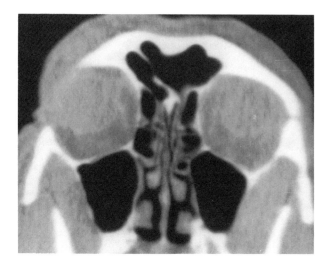

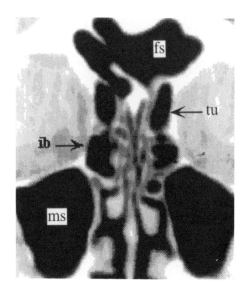

Fig. 17. (B) CT scan frontal section. fs, frontal sinus; ms, maxillary sinus; ib, intrabullar cell; tu, terminal uncinate cell.

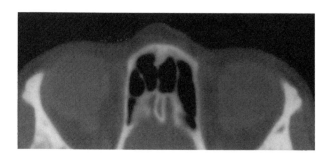

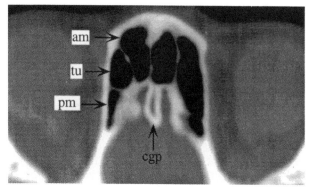

Fig. 18. Axial CT scan, upper section, anterior ethmoid. am, anterior meatal cell; tu, terminal uncinate cell; pm, posterior meatal cell; cgp, crita galli process.

in the posterior wall of the frontal sinus. However, the term "suprabullar cell" is discussed by Stammberger *(11)*, who does not consider the term "cell" to be appropriate for this space. This author considers that it is only a cleft between the roof of the ethmoid, the ground lamella, and the bulla. This space is also designated by Grünwald *(7)* as the sinus lateralis and by Hajek *(29,30)* as the recessus suprabullaris. If well pneumatized, and whether or not the basal lamella of the bulla extends the roof of the ethmoid partially, the sinus lateralis may continue anteriorly into the frontal recess.

The Prebullar System. It lies in front of the basal lamella of the bulla. It is separated into two groups of cells by the basal lamella of the uncinate process, which runs here in a sagittal plane. The uncinate group

of cells lies laterally. The meatal group of cells lies medially (Figs. 11–13, 15, 17A, 18–21) *(31,32)*.

The Prebullar System: The Uncinate Cell Group. Four cells can be identified. They all drain into the uncinate groove.

The terminal uncinate cell is the uppermost. It extends the uncinate groove and sometimes opens like a funnel. For that reason, Boyer refers to it as the infundibulum *(33)*.

This cell may project superiorly and form the frontal sinus. Sometimes it may only pneumatize the frontal bone partially, forming an external frontal bulla. This superior uncinate cell lies just medially to the lacrimal bone and the orbit, so it has been called the ethmoido-orbital cell by Mouret *(3–5)* and Grünwald *(7)*. The basal lamella of the unci-

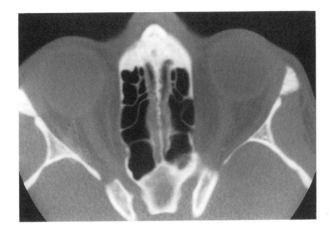

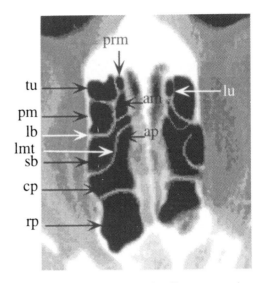

Fig. 19. Axial CT scan, upper section. tu, terminal uncinate cell; am, anterior meatal cell; prm, premeatal cell; pm, posterior meatal cell; sb, suprabullar cell; ap, advanced posterior cell; cp, central posterior cell; rp, remote posterior cell; lu, lamella of the uncinate process; lb, lamella of the bulla; lmt, lamella of the middle turbinate.

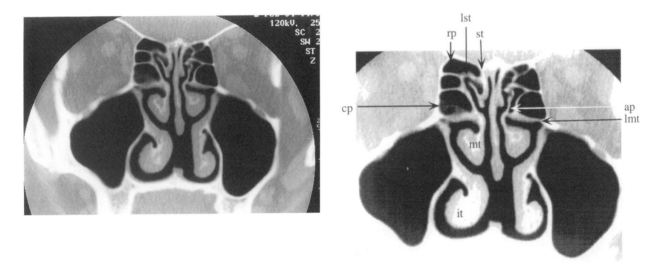

Fig. 20. Coronal CT scan, posterior section. ap, advanced posterior cell; cp, central posterior cell; rp, remote posterior cell; lmt, lamella of the middle turbinate; lst, lamella of the superior turbinate.

nate process borders the terminal uncinate cell medially and separates it from the ostium of the meatal anterior cell. Resection of the upper part of the uncinate process unites the two orifices and enlarges the frontal aperture.

The anterior uncinate cell or agger nasi cell is not a constant finding, observed in 52% of cases reported by Agrifolio et al. *(22).* It covers to some extent the frontal process of the maxilla displacing the insertion of the uncinate process anteriorly.

Sometimes, it pneumatizes this structure. Usually, it drains into the uncinate groove. Occasionally, it opens directly into the nasal cavity just behind the bulge of the nasolacrimal duct.

The posterior uncinate cell is not a constant finding (25%). It lies in front of the basal lamella of the bulla. It drains anteriorly through the posterior surface of the uncinate groove.

The inferior uncinate cell also may or may not be present (15%). It can extend between the roof of the

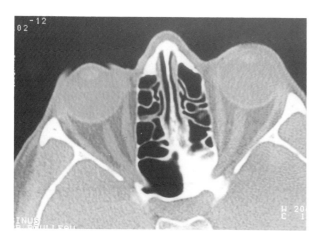 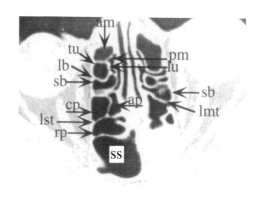

Fig. 21. Axial CT section exploring the upper part of the ethmoid bone. tu, terminal uncinate cell; am, anterior meatal cell; pm, posterior meatal cell; sb, suprabullar cell; ap, advanced posterior cell; cp, central posterior cell; rp, remote posterior cell; lu, lamella of the uncinate process; lb, lamella of the bulla; lmt, lamella of the middle turbinate; lst, lamella of the superior turbinate; ss, sphenoidal sinus.

maxillary sinus and the orbital plate of the maxilla. It is then called a Haller's cell (Fig. 16). Usually, the inferior uncinate cell drains into the uncinate groove, above and behind the ostium of the maxillary sinus.

The Prebullar System: The Meatal Cells. Three cells can be differentiated: the premeatal, anterior meatal, and posterior meatal cells.

The premeatal cell is found in 72% of cases by Agrifolio et al. *(22).* It can sometimes be present in double and rarely triple form. It is located behind the anterosuperior attachment of the middle turbinate. Its development varies and sometimes may be reduced to simply an outpocketing. It can produce an impression on the floor of the frontal sinus or even form a frontal bulla.

According to the majority of authors, the anterior meatal cell gives rise to the frontal sinus.

The posterior meatal cell is found in 82% of cases *(22).* It often protrudes into the posterior part of the frontal sinus or forms a frontal projection. The anterior ethmoidal artery is found at the junction of its posterior wall and the roof of the ethmoid in 95% of cases, most commonly in the thickness of the partitioning root of the bulla. This cell is an important surgical reference point because it is less concealed than the anterior meatal cell by the upper part of the uncinate process. Its identification together with that of the anterior ethmoidal artery serves to locate a perilous area for the surgeon because of the fragile

bony wall. All of the meatal cells drain into the meatal groove.

THE POSTERIOR ETHMOID SYSTEM

The posterior ethmoid system includes two groups of cells. (Figs. 11–13, 15, 17A, 20, and 21) *(31,32).*

The Superior or Central Group of Cells. The superior group lies between the basal lamella of the middle turbinate and the basal lamella of the superior turbinate. It contains the advanced posterior cell and the central posterior cell. The advanced posterior cell lies behind the basal lamella of the middle turbinate. Sometimes it extends anteriorly and medially, and participates in twisting of the ground lamella of the middle turbinate. It drains into the anterosuperior part of the superior meatus.

The central posterior cell usually is located at the level of the intrabullar cell. Sometimes it reaches the roof of the ethmoid, and then projects between the advanced and the remote posterior cell. It opens into the superior meatus behind the advanced cell.

The Supreme Group of Cells. The supreme group of cells lies behind the basal lamella of the superior turbinate. Usually it includes the only remote posterior cell. This cell drains into the supreme meatus. However, it may open into the superior meatus and thus should be considered as part of the superior group. When located in an upper position, the remote posterior cell is called Onodi cell or what Onodi refers to as the sphenoethmoidal cell *(6)*. Less commonly, the central posterior cell or exceptionally the suprabullar cell may reach the sphenoid, and constitute a pseudoremote posterior cell. Onodi cell is an important landmark in ethmoidectomy in the surgeon's approach to the sphenoidal sinus. Its lateral wall may reach the optic canal, which projects into its lumen and is highly vulnerable. These cells can be in intimate relationship to the optic nerve, which may project onto the lateral wall of an Onodi cell. The internal carotid artery may also appear prominently on the lateral wall of the posterior ethmoidal cells. After perforation of the basal lamella of the middle turbinate, dissection should not be carried out posterolaterally along the orbital wall to locate the sphenoidal sinus behind the posterior wall of Onodi cell. This is the point where the optic nerve might be encountered and (unintentionally) injured.

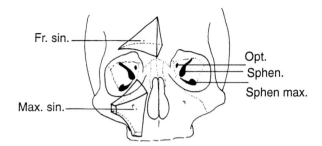

Fig. 22. Maxillary sinus and frontal sinus, shape and location. Fr. sin, frontal sinus; Max. sin, maxillary sinus; Opt., optic canal; Sphen., superior orbital fissure; Sphen. max, inferior orbital fissure.

FUNCTIONAL UNITS AND PATHOPHYSIOLOGICAL CONSEQUENCES

The functional sinus units are based on the arrangement of ethmoidal cells, the basal lamella, and the drainage pathways of the sinus into which the sinus orifices open. Two main sinus units can be described. They are separated by the ground lamella of the middle turbinate. The anterior sinus system consists of the maxillary sinus, the frontal sinus with the meatal group, and the anterior ethmoid. The anterior ethmoid is made up of the uncinate group and the bulla cells. All these cells, except for the bulla cells, drain into the unci-bullar groove (or uncinate groove or infundibulums) whose definition is listed above. The bulla open into the bullar groove (Fig. 14). The posterior sinus unit and its variations comprise the posterior ethmoid and the superior meatus, the sphenoidal sinus, and the juxtaseptal meatus.

The Anterior Sinusal System

THE MAXILLARY SINUS

This is the largest of the sinus cavities and is probably the one most frequently involved in sinus disorders because it participates in the respiratory system, and is similarly subject to the same infectious and inflammatory processes, and because it is in close contact with the superior dental arch. Located in the body of the upper maxillary, it thus assumes a quadrangular pyramid shape with an

endonasal medial base and a lateral zygomatic apex (Fig. 22). Classically, it is described as having four walls: an anterior jugal wall, a superior orbital wall, a posterior infratemporal wall, and an inferior wall, which is the floor of the sinus.

None of these aspects can by itself claim to be of greatest surgical significance because all of these structures can be variously involved in surgical procedures that are both numerous and varied: anterior approach of the jugal aspect by sublabial route, endonasal approach to the medial aspect, posterior approach to the subtemporal fossa, approach to the floor of the maxillary sinus in radiculodental disorders, or in corrective surgery for maxillofacial dysmorphism, approach to the upper facial area in the treatment of trauma to the floor of the orbit, and so forth.

Each of these walls has its own importance in various surgical procedures. Three walls actually form an aspect of approach to the sinus cavity: the anterior (jugal), medial (endonasal), and the superior (orbital) walls. The other two walls, i.e., posterior and inferior, can only be accessed from within the sinus cavity.

The medial side is formed by the intersinus nasal septum which projects onto the lower half of the nasal fossa among:

1. The lacrimal duct in front, which forms an anterior barrier;
2. The vertical plate of the palatine bone—a thick, resistant posterior structure that protects the descending palatine artery and the anterior palatine nerve, located in the posterior palatine duct and that goes to the palatine fibromucosa. It contains the sphenopalatine foramen above, which allows passage for the sphenopalatine

artery and which approximately locates the posterosuperior angle of the medial wall;

3. Above the lateral mass of the ethmoid; and
4. Below the palatine process of the maxilla and of the palatine bone, which form the floor of the nasal fossa and which are indeed located above the floor of the sinus.

On the endonasal medial side, this aspect is blocked by the insertion of the inferior concha delimiting the middle meatus above and the inferior meatus below.

The middle meatus has also been described above, and we will not repeat its description. The inferior meatus consists of a bony wall with no dehiscences that protrudes into the sinus cavity and presents a fragile area in the middle of the inferior turbinate insertion, a preferred site of puncture via the inferior meatal route. The bony lacrimal duct empties into the inferior meatus at the highest point of insertion of the inferior concha. However, the mucosal duct can descend quite low into the meatal wall, sometimes as far as the floor of the sinus, and hence is highly vulnerable to trauma (sometimes unintentional) in the approach to this sinus via inferior meatotomy. This "lower down" location of the floor of the sinus with relation to the floor of the nasal fossa makes it possible to understand why an inferior meatotomy, even extended widely, has scarcely any chance of being useful in draining the sinus; in addition, the mucociliary sweep, which is invariably directed toward the main ostium in the middle meatus, makes it inoperative and limits the value of inferior meatotomy to approaches and procedures on the endosinus.

On the endosinus lateral side, this aspects presents a fossa called the Vilar Fiol's fossa lying just below the floor of the orbit and behind the lacrimonasal duct. It is bordered below by an outline (Terrier's ledge) and has an orifice that has a highly variable shape, the sinus orifice of the maxillary duct.

Behind this fossa, the area of ethmoidal-maxillary contact, oblique below and inward, gradually widens rearward, between the orbit outside, the nasal fossa inside, and the sphenopalatine foramen, behind. This is the area for trepantation of the posterior ethmoid sinus described by De Lima *(34)*.

The Anterior Wall. This is the wall for the classical sublabial approach to the sinus (Caldwell). It is limited by the inferior border of the orbit above, by the alveolar arch and teeth going from the first canine to the first molar below, by the maxillomalar support laterally, and by the piriform orifice and canine pillar medially. On the jugal side, this aspect is blocked by the cul-de-sac of the vestibule, which separates it into two parts: a superior segment, which connects with the cheek, and a ginigivobuccal inferior segment, which is continuous with the gengival periosteum. This wall is indeed a thin fossa at its center and becomes thicker peripherally, bordered by the suborbital foramen above, and crossed in its thickness by suborbital nerve branches to teeth, including an anterior branch extending to the canine teeth, a middle branch to the first and second premolars, and a posterior branch, which continues to the molar teeth. From this arrangement, it becomes apparent that a wide approach to this wall with major bone destruction will produce insensitivity of all canine and premolar and molar teeth. Conversely, a minimum approach, as in puncturing a sinus, or a minimal approach not exceeding 1 cm, situated right in the central depressed area of this face will conserve innervation to these teeth and also the posterior nerve, so that only the middle dental nerve, not always present, will be sacrificed.

It is covered by thick periosteum, which must be spared during trepanation of the sinus, doubled with a layer of muscle and a thick layer of skin.

On the endosinus side, this wall, which is almost flat and has no projections, becomes gradually narrower laterally as it comes to join the apex of the pyramidal-shaped sinus in the zygomatic fossa. Medially, at the level of the canine pillar, with the outline of the lacrimal duct, it can form a sinus diverticulum that is difficult to access surgically. Last, below, its extent depends on the height of the alveolar support, which is not very extensive in patients who have lost their teeth.

The Superior Wall. This orbital wall, which is noticeable because its fragility, is probably the most vulnerable. On the orbital side, it forms the greatest part of the floor of the orbit, triangular-shaped and delimited in front by the sphenomaxillary fissure, which separates it frankly from the posterior face, continuing medially with no clear demarcation with the medial wall of the orbit, and which is opposite the lateral wall of the ethmoid and the unguis (*see* p. 8). It is crossed from back to front by the suborbital groove and then duct, which contains the suborbital pedicle accentuating its fragility at this level. It is lined by the periorbital sheath, which separates it from the content of the orbit. At this level, the periorbital sheath protects the inferior oblique muscle and the inferior rectus muscle of the eye, which are commonly involved in fractures of the floor of the orbit.

On the sinus side, it protrudes into the sinus cavity; the suborbital nerve makes an imprint on it in its anterior half. It is attached to the medial wall in the area of ethmoidal-maxillary contact (*see* section on Contact with the Lacrimal Bone Anteriorly).

Floor of the Sinus. The floor of the sinus is really an inferior face that has an original aspect because of its relation to the teeth. The relations between sinus and teeth are such that it is possible to see the floor of the sinus bristling with dental roots whose clinical significance in disease is readily apparent. In fact, it is an anteroposterior groove that progresses with age. As the eruption and development of the teeth progress, the size of the maxillary sinus increases with the descent of the floor of the sinus. When the permanent teeth have erupted, this sinus is now of full size, and the floor of the sinus is almost constantly located 15 mm from the neck of the teeth. When there is loss of upper teeth, the sinus does not increase in size, and its floor becomes thin and flattened.

Alterations in the size of this sinus are also determined by facial growth with a large maxillary sinus in retrognanthia, which may involve the malar bone, palate, and so on, whereas in short faces, this sinus is small with dental apexes very high up, almost in the floor of the nasal fossa. Thus, the size of the sinus can vary between a volume of 5 and 20 cm^3.

The Infratemporal Posterior Wall (Fig. 23). Designated by the term maxillary tuberosity, this wall is regularly concave at the level of the maxillary tuberosity in all directions and has almost no projections. It is a thick wall and continues with the infratemporal fossa. It is thus through it that certain structures that it contains can be accessed: the internal maxillary artery or the maxillary nerve, which is higher up, or structures in the pterygopalatine fossa, the sphenopalatine ganglion, and the nerve of the pterygoid canal. This is the wall most readily accessible with endoscopy.

Drainage of the Maxillary Sinus. The maxillary sinus drains via the maxillary duct, which is 6–8 mm in length, depending on the width of the uncinate process and the size of the bulla. It opens

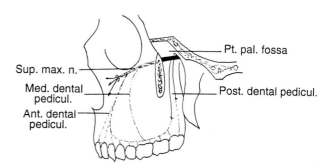

Fig. 23. Infratemporal fossa, V2—Dental nerves. Sup. max. n., superior maxillary nerve; Med. dental pedicul., medial dental pediculous; Ant. dental pedicul., anterior dental pediculous; Pt. pal. fossa, pterygopalatine fossa; Post. dental pedicul., posterior dental pediculous.

on one side into the sinus at the level of fossa. On the nasal side, it opens into the groove of the infundibulum.

THE FRONTAL SINUS

"The frontal sinus is only a large ethmoidal cell (Watson-Williams, cited in Terracol *[35]*), which has developed within the thickness of the frontal bone." This ethmoido-frontal anatomical unit, which has a common embryological development, accounts for disorders that can involve both structures and often combined surgical procedures.

Located at the junction of the squamous portion of the temporal bone and the horizontal part of the frontal bone on either side of the midline, the frontal sinuses, which have highly variable dimensions and are almost always asymmetrical, have an overall triangular pyramid shape whose apex lies above a cutaneous anterior wall, a cerebromeningeal posterior wall, a medial septum between the sinuses, and a nasoorbital base (Fig. 22).

The Anterior Cutaneous Side. Toward the Cutaneous Lining, this side extends anteriorly toward the forehead within a (surgical) triangular compartment, demarcated:

> Below, by the supraorbital margin, which has a notch for the supraorbital vascular bundle and the sensory branch of the supraorbital nerve going to the frontal sinus;
> Laterally, by an oblique line leading from the middle of the supraorbital arch below to the midline above, 2 or 3 cm from the root of the nose; and
> Medially, by the midline.

The highly variable shape and size of the frontal sinuses should be emphasized, which are difficult to locate during surgery and can only be achieved by using a forehead-plate radiological incidence with installation of metal markers on the midline and in the wrinkles of the forehead.

The bony plane is covered with thick skin, which contains the eyebrow below, is lined with muscle, and especially with very resistant, easily detachable periosteum, which is widely used in surgical procedures.

Toward the Sinus Cavity, this wall is smooth, concave posteriorly, and is covered with a thin mucosa. Extensive pneumatization can expand the eyebrow arch, the glabella, and extend the anterior wall very high up into the squamous part of the frontal bone, sometimes up to the hairline; conversely, a small sinus barely occupies the vertical part of the frontal bone and can only be approached through the orbit.

The Posterior, Cerebromeningeal Side. This is a plate of thin, compact bone (1–2 mm), whose upper part is vertical and gradually curves downward and posteriorly, where it then is almost horizontal.

Toward the Endocranial Cavity, the two vertical segments join at the midline to form the internal frontal crest on which the falx cerebri inserts; the two horizontal segments are separated by a notch that houses the two cribriform plates separated by the crista galli. This horizontal part of the frontal sinus continues posteriorly with the roof of the ethmoidal cast and like it lies in a plane supra-adjacent to the cribriform plate (*see* section on Basal Cranial Aspect).

This side is in contact with the frontal lobe from which it is separated by the dura mater that can easily be detached, enabling the operator to obtain extradural access to the roof of the ethmoidal sinus from above.

Toward the Sinus Cavity, the posterior wall is regularly convex below and anteriorly lies relatively close to the anterior wall depending on the size of the sinus, and is covered with a thin, little-vascularized mucosa. It joins the floor of the sinus at an acute angle, unless an ethmoidal air cell invades this area (posterior bulla) and rounds off this angle, creating a vertical, plane, or convex segment.

The Medial Side, Frontal Septum. Separating the two sinuses, thin and lying in a sagittal direction, rarely dehiscent, it is always in the midline below, but very commonly is deflected upward by the protruding aspect of one of the sinuses; it can

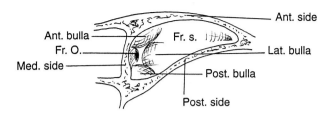

Fig. 24. Nasoethmoidal floor. Ant. bulla, anterior bulla; Fr. O., Frontal ostium; Fr. s., frontal sinus; Ant. side, anterior side; Lat. bulla, lateral bulla; Post. bulla, posterior bulla; Post. side, posterior side; Med. side, medial side (septum).

become horizontal, with one sinus covering the other one.

The Inferior Side, Orbitonasal Floor (Fig. 24). The base of the pyramidal-shaped frontal sinus lies on the orbit on the outer side and on the nasal cavity on the inner side, and has two segments: one is lateral, orbital, and the other is medial, nasoethmoidal.

The floor of the orbit is comprised of thin bone, which thus collapses easily and plays a major part in the spread of some disorders, i.e., sinusitis, mucocele, tumors, and so forth, toward the orbit.

Toward the Orbital Cavity, the floor is lined with very resistant periosteum, which can be readily detached from the roof of the orbit; it is closely adherent to the upper margin as well as the remainder of the orbital circumference before it is reflected in the orbital septum, arranging for orifices on the inside to allow passage of the supraorbital vasculonervous bundle in a notch of the bony margin, and the internal and external frontal bundle more on the inside. This periosteum forms a solid aponeurotic sac that protects its content enveloped within a homogeneous layer of adipose tissue; the floor of the sinus in its outer aspect is immediately in contact with the levator palpebrae superioris and especially the superior oblique muscles. The body of the latter changes direction by sliding onto a fibrous ring (a reflecting pulley) lodged in a bony fossa (trochlear fossa) located 5 mm behind the superior orbital margin, on the internal orbital process of the frontal bone, above the unguis. At this level, the periosteal orbital sac, which is closely adherent to the bone, must be very carefully dissected to make certain that the pulley holding the superior oblique muscle is in proper position at the end of the surgical procedure.

Toward the Sinus Cavity, the floor of the sinus is regularly convex above and inward, and extends more or less laterally above the orbital cavity depending on the size of the sinus; in cases of extensive development of the frontal sinus, it can occupy the entire dome of the orbit and extend up to the external orbital process on the outside.

The nasoethmoidal floor is located below on the opposite side of the orbital segment between the latter on the outside and the septum between the sinuses on the inside, thus forming a depression commonly referred to as the frontal recess in which the frontonasal duct opens 8–10 mm outside of the septum between the sinuses. The anterior edge of this recess, oblique below and behind, consists of a very thick bony mass of the nasal spinous process of the frontal bone fused to the bones of the nose and to the frontal process of the maxilla. Antero-posterior widening of the frontal recess can only occur at the expense of this anterior edge by abrading the bony outline. The posterior edge, oblique below and in front, not very thick, and thus much more fragile, overhangs the lateral mass of the ethmoid and the cribriform plate behind.

This schematic arrangement is commonly altered by the protrusion of anterior ethmoidal cells on the floor of the sinus forming one or more "frontal bullae" (Fig. 25):

> This posterior bulla situated at the back of the frontonasal duct is common because it is formed by the often extensive posterior meatal cell (meatic system) or more rarely by the suprabullar cell (bullar system);
> The anterior bulla is formed by expansion of the premeatal cell (meatic system), forming a protrusion in front of the frontonasal duct in the anterior wall of the sinus; and
> Outside the frontonasal duct, situated between the opening of this duct and the pars orbitalis of the sinus floor, the external frontal bulla is formed by the terminal uncinate cell (unciform system).

All these bulla narrow the outlet of the frontonasal duct; during surgery on the frontal sinus, they have to be resected and the cavities joined together to enlarge the opening into the frontal sinus and prevent stenosis.

THE ANTERIOR ETHMOID AND THE MIDDLE MEATUS

The presence of the turbinates and the corresponding meatal grooves makes the lateral wall of the nasal cavity irregular. At first sight, the

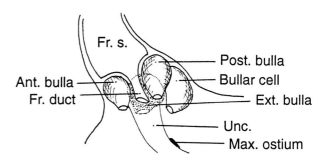

Fig. 25. Frontal bullae. Fr. s., frontal sinus; Ant. bulla, anterior bulla (premeatal cell); Fr. duct, frontonasal duct; Ext. bulla, exterior bulla (terminal uncinate cell); Post. bulla, posterior bulla (postmeatal cell); Unc., uncinate cell; Max. ostium, maxillary ostium.

endoscopist observes two main structures: the inferior and middle turbinate with their respective meatuses.

The middle turbinate inserts directly onto the base of the skull at the lateral edge of the lamina papyracea. The only free vertical segment of the turbinate can be seen from the medial side. The head of the turbinate is free. It overlies the entrance of the meatus partially. The insertion of the turbinate to the lateral wall narrows to form a neck (Fig. 26).

Laterally, the neck of the middle turbinate continues in the fold of the uncinate process. This narrow passage, referred to as the middle premeatal fissure by Terrier (21), is limited by the head of the turbinate medially and by the uncinate process laterally (Fig. 27). A preturbinate fold runs downward from the neck of the middle turbinate to the inferior turbinate. It corresponds to the anterior insertion of the uncinate process on the ascending process of the maxilla behind the outline of the lacrimal canal called the "lacrimal hump" by Rouvier et al. (18,19). When the uncinate process is expanded by an agger nasi cell (Fig. 28), this fold forms a furrow that is important in endoscopic surgery. In the anterior-to-posterior operative technique for ethmoidectomy, the first step involves the opening of the ethmoidal infundibulum by resecting the uncinate process. A curved knife blade is inserted into the uncinate process, along this furrow in a plane parallel to the medial wall of the orbit. The middle meatus is bordered by the inferior and the middle turbinate. The pathway to the middle meatus through the premeatal fissure leads to the bulla.

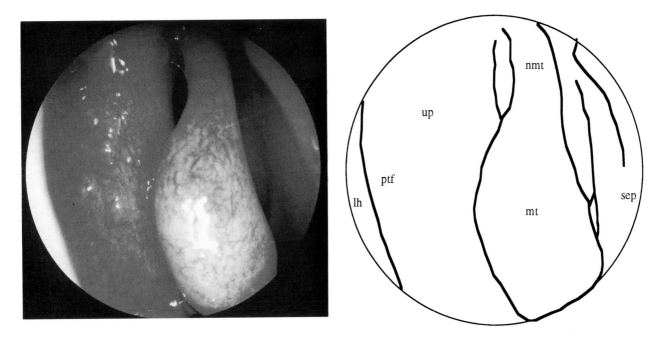

Fig. 26. Right nasal cavity, the head of the middle turbinate. nmt, neck of the middle turbinate; mt, middle turbinate; up, uncinate process; ptf, preturbinal fold; lh, lacrimal hump.

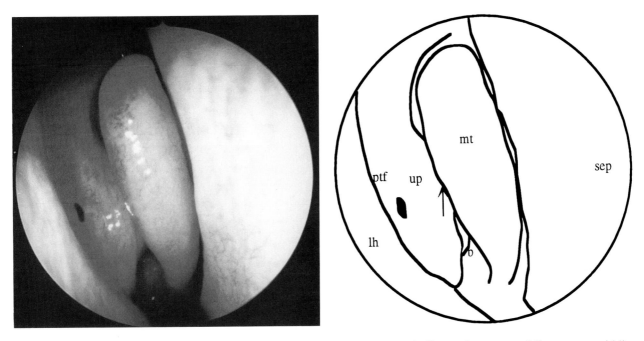

Fig. 27. The uncinate process and the head of the middle turbinate. The arrow indicates the premeatal fissure. mt, middle turbinate; up, uncinate process; ptf, preturbinal fold; lh, lacrimal hump; b, bulla; sep, septum.

The bulla appears between the uncinate process laterally and the middle turbinate medially. Terrier *(21)* described the important system of grooves, which he called the "bulla roundabout." It is defined as the confluence of three grooves: the uncinate groove lying laterally between the bulla and the uncinate process, the meatal groove lying antero-superiorly between the uncinate process and the middle turbinate, and finally the bullar groove lying superomedially between the bulla and the middle

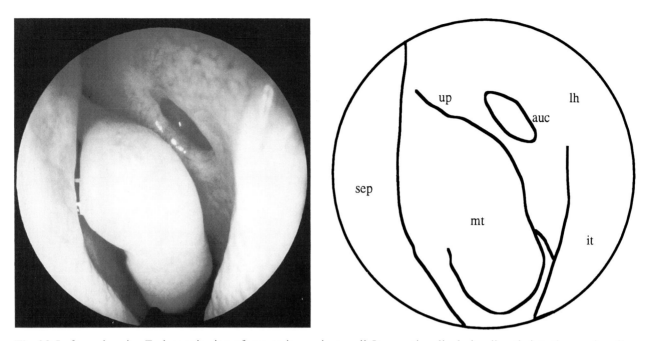

Fig. 28. Left nasal cavity. Endoscopic view of an anterior uncinate cell. It exceptionally drains directly into the nasal cavity. up, uncinate process; lh, lacrimal hump; sep, septum; mt, medial turbinate; it, inferior turbinate; auc, orifice of the anterior uncinate cell.

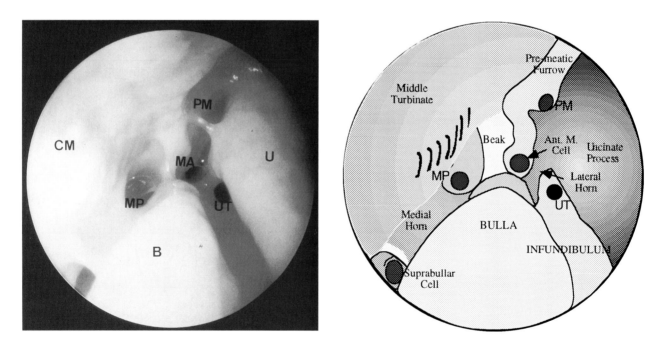

Fig. 29. "Bullar roundabout and tristar of the grooves," left nasal cavity. MP, posterior meatal cell; PM, premeatal cell; UT, terminal uncinate cell.

turbinate. With the 70° lens, the junction of theses grooves has a characteristic appearance called the "tristar of the grooves" by Terrier *(21)* (Fig. 29).

The uncinate cells and the maxillary sinus open into the uncinate groove. It is difficult to see the

maxillary ostium, hidden on the floor of the ethmoidal infundibulum behind the junction of the vertical and the horizontal part of the uncinate process (Fig. 30). The meatal cells drain into the meatal groove. At the superior end of the ethmoid bulla, a

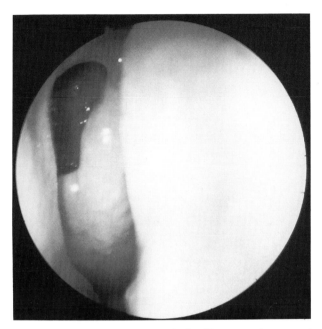 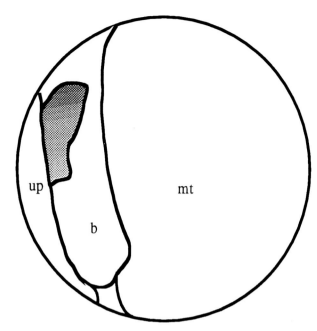

Fig. 30. Right nasal fossa. The bulla (b) appears between the middle turbinate (mt) medially and the uncinate process (up) laterally.

thin septum separates the anterior meatal orifice, which is the opening of the frontal sinus, and the posterior meatal orifice, which is the opening of the posterior meatal cell (Fig. 29). At the superior end of the uncinate groove, a septum that is the lamella of the uncinate process separates the posterior meatal orifice from the orifice of the terminal uncinate cell. The bullar groove and the uncinate groove join to form the "main drainage channel" running as far as the choanae over the posterior end of the uncinate process and the posterior end of the inferior turbinate.

Posterior Sinus System

The posterior ethmoid and the sphenoid sinuses fall under the heading of posterior sinuses, whose basic structural unit is explained by its extrainfundibular embryological origin and thus by posterior drainage, above the middle concha. This anatomical unit accounts for isolated disorders that occur less commonly than with the anterior sinus system.

THE POSTERIOR ETHMOID AND THE SUPERIOR MEATUS

The superior turbinate and sometimes a supreme turbinate (Santorini's turbinate) and a second supreme turbinate (Zuckerkandl's turbinate) can be found. They limit the superior meatuses (Fig. 5). The posterior ethmoid cells open into the superior meatuses.

THE SPHENOIDAL SINUS

The sphenoidal sinus is generally double, very often asymmetrical and of various sizes (36) depending on the degree of pneumatization; its multiple morphology is such that it appears more logical to describe a single large sphenoidal sinus. Expanded into the sphenoid bone, in the craniofacial center, it has six sides: four endocranial sides, i.e., the superior, two lateral, and accessorily the posterior side protrude into the cranial cavity and account for the symptoms manifest in infectious or tumoral disorders; and two sides, the anterior and inferior, overhang the nasal cavity and nasopharynx, enabling access to the sinus.

Toward the Endocranial Cavity. The upper side or roof takes part in the formation of the anterior and middle floors of the base of the skull, and lies in direct contact, from front to back, with the olfactory strips located in the two grooves carved out of the sphenoidal jugum, further on with the optic chiasma in the chiasmic groove, and finally, with the hypophysis corresponding to the sella turcica and its content. The latter relation is probably the most important from a surgical standpoint, because it enables transsphenoidal access to the hypophysis.

Each lateral side contains two parts, the cranial part behind and the orbital one in front; the fact that this bony wall is very thin exposes two very impor-

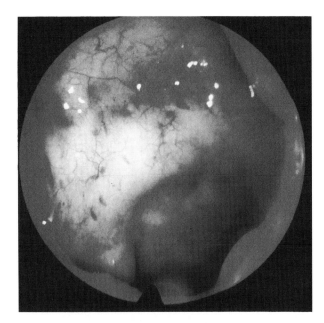
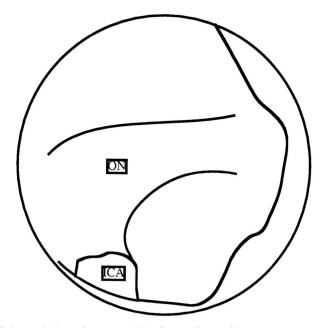

Fig. 31. Surgical endoscopic view of a right sphenoid sinus. ON, optic nerve; ICA, internal carotid artery.

tant structures, the internal carotid artery and the optic nerve (Fig. 31), all the more immediate when the sinus is very pneumatized. Posteriorly, the cranial portion of this wall, oblique below and on the outside, is in contact with the cavernous sinus (Fig. 32) and its content. It is here that the internal carotid artery (Figs. 31 and 33) makes an impression on the bone, especially in front in its "genu" in the curve from which it continues upward. Nerves in the sphenoidal fissure, which arise from the petrous portion of the temporal bone, form a less immediate relation: the sixth cranial nerve, lodged in the cavernous sinus, is closest, whereas the third and fourth cranial nerves and the ophthalmic branch of the fifth nerve, like the maxillary nerves, lodged in the lateral wall of the cavernous sinus, are further away. In front, the orbital portion of this wall demarcates on the inside the most recessed part of the orbital cone. Here it comes into contact, above, with the optic canal lying between the two roots of the lesser wing of the sphenoid; the optic canal crosses the angle of union of the anterior, superior, and lateral walls where it makes an imprint. The content of the optic canal, i.e., the optic nerve and ophthalmic artery, without a doubt form the closest and most vulnerable relation of this lateral wall of the sphenoidal sinus. Lower, below the optic canal, between the greater and lesser wings of the sphenoid, the lateral wall demarcates the sphenoidal fissure on the inside; at this level of the wall of

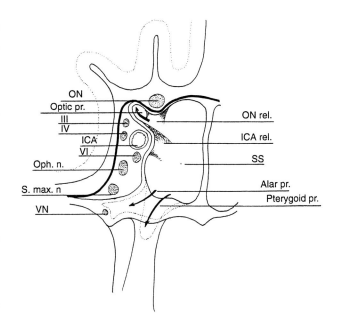

Fig. 32. Sphenoidal sinus. ON, optic nerve; Optic pr., optic prolongation; ICA, internal carotid artery; ICA rel., internal carotid relief; Oph. n., ophthalmic nerve; S. max. n., superior maxillary nerve; VN, vidian nerve; ON rel., optic nerve relief; SS, sphenoidal sinus; Alar pr., alar prolongation; Pterygoid pr., Pterygoid prolongation.

the sinus, the thicker and more solid Zinn's ring inserts, crossed by the oculomotor nerve, and the nasal and sympathetic nerves, which are less vulnerable.

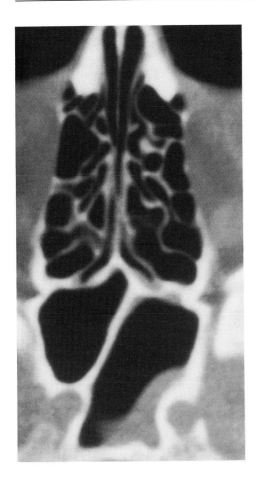

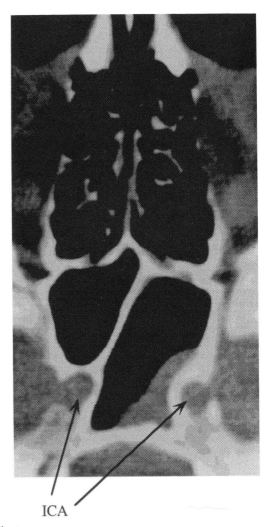

ICA

Fig. 33. ICA internal carotid artery.

The posterior side generally is separated from the posterior floor of the base of the skull by a thick plate of spongy bone, 5–20 mm thick, and it is only in cases of extensive pneumatization (*see* Toward the Sinus Cavity *later*), that the sinus can come into contact with the basilar arterial trunk and its bifurcation into the posterior vertebral arteries, the pons and the fourth cranial nerve.

Toward Nasopharyngeal Side. The inferior side or floor forms the dome of the choanae (posterior nares) and the rhinopharynx, which follows it; here the bone is relatively thick, reinforced by the ala of the ptyergoid and vomer. Anteriorly, the union of the anterior and inferior walls forms an obtuse, soft angle, more or less pronounced, described by Terrier (21) as the "choanal arcade"; this outline which demarcates the border between the nasal cavity in front and the rhinopharynx

behind, forms a very important landmark on the anterior wall.

The anterior side is the wall of endoscopic and surgical approach. This anterior aspect of the body of the sphenoid, connected to the perpendicular plate of the ethmoid in the midline and to the lateral masses on each side, forms a free, vertical corridor above each nasal cavity, on either side of the septum. These three septal, nasal, and ethmoidal segments account for the three possible approaches to the sinus: transseptal approach in the midline, transethmoidal, laterally, and per ostal endonasal direct approach between the two. The septal median segment is very thick, and access requires especially laborious abrading after resection of the septum. Conversely, the thickness of the anterior wall decreases laterally where the ethmoid forms the backing; here it can become very thin depending on penumatization of the sphenoid through Onodi's ethmoido-sphenoidal buffer cell.

It thus is easy to collapse following posterior ethmoidal eccentration. The intermediate segment, which is free in the nasal cavity, is the sphenoethmoidal recess, also called the juxtaseptal meatus by Terrier *(21)*, we will describe later (cf. The Septal Meatus *later*). It is here, near the septum and almost at midheight, that the sphenoidal ostium is located, which is wide in dry bone, but narrows to 2–3 mm in diameter from coverage with the mucosa, and it can be accessed by endonasal approach and widened laterally and below to perform a sphenoidotomy.

Toward the Sinus Cavity. The sphenoid indeed consists of compartments divided into two right and left cavities by a thin septum between the sinuses, but is never dehiscent and rarely in a median sagittal direction. Variations in the arrangement of this septum, such as those of pneumatization, are such that average dimensions are of no value; endoscopic investigation of the sphenoidal sinus cannot be planned without precise CT scanning and knowledge of the more or less obvious structures that project into the sinus cavity.

In the upper wall, the arch corresponding to the hypophyseal compartment can always be recognized; in front of it, the roof of the sphenoidal sinus is in continuity with the roof of the ethmoidal sinus, and so is a useful landmark in ethmoidal evisceration performed from back to front beginning with the sphenoidal sinus, when all other landmarks are difficult to recognize.

On the lateral side, the optic canal forms an impression within the cavity, where it can be recognized by its location in the angle uniting the anterior, superior, and lateral surfaces, and by the direction of its outline medially and posteriorly. If pneumatization is extensive, this canal may be sometimes very prominent, and its wall may be dehiscent. Use caution in performing endosinus procedures here! Just back of the optic canal, the outline of the carotid artery becomes visible, mainly marked ahead, but in very well-pneumatized sinuses, the entire pathway of the carotid artery may project into the sinus cavity.

The sinus cavity is never regular in shape, but rather has a tortuous and variable arrangement, depending on the extent of pneumatization, which may induce prolongations and recesses in neighboring bones: the lesser or greater wings of the sphenoid, palatine bone, and pterygoid and basilar process. This makes the neighboring structures highly vulnerable. Pneumatization within the lesser wing and the anterior clinoid process (optic prolongation) can isolate the optic canal in all its aspects; pneumatization of the greater wing (alar prolongation) often associated with pneumatization within the root of the pterygoid process can work its way in between the middle cranial fossa at the top and the pterygopalatine fossa below, and come into contact with the foramen rotundum in front, which passes the maxillary nerve, and the foramen ovale behind, which passes the maxillary nerve. Pneumatization may extend along the orbit (orbital prolongation), within the posterior ethmoid system and the orbital process of the palatine bone; this anterior extension exposes the optic nerve even more in the orbital cone. Pneumatization downward posteriorly within the basilar process of the occipital bone (basilar prolongation) makes the sphenoid sinus lie adjacent to the basilar artery and the cerebral pons.

THE SEPTAL MEATUS

The sphenoid sinus opens into the sphenoethmoid recess. The sphenoethmoidal recess, also referred to as the "juxtaseptal meatus" or the "septal meatus" by Terrier *(21)*, lies between the supreme turbinate and the septum (Figs. 5 and 34). It is located above the choana and the sphenopalatine artery. The choana is limited laterally by the medial plate of the pterygoid process, medially by the posterior border of the septum, superiorly by the body of the sphenoid and by the posterior edge of the wings of the vomer, and inferiorly by the horizontal plate of the palatine bone, which coincides with the posterior limit of the floor of the nasal cavity. The sphenopalatine artery passes through the sphenopalatine foramen, which lies 10–12 mm in front of the choanal arcade, above the posterior end of the middle turbinate, which must be resected for an easier approach. The sphenopalatine artery anatomoses with the lateral posterior nasal arteries and posterior septal branches. When middle meatotomy or ethmoidectomy is performed, bleeding can occur from the area of the posterior end of the middle turbinate because of its proximity to the sphenopalatine foramen. Inferiorly, the nasopalatine artery runs along the choanal arch toward the septum. Bleeding may occur when sphenoidotomy is extended widely inferiorly.

Superiorly, the ostium of the sphenoid is the most posterior orifice and the one closest to the septum. It

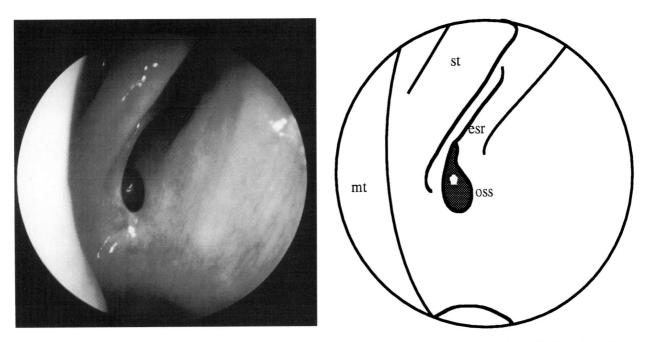

Fig. 34. Right nasal cavity, ethmoidosphenoidal recess and ostium of sphenoid sinus. oss, ostium of sphenoidal sinus; st, superior turbinate; mt, middle turbinate; esr, ethmoidosphenoidal recess.

has a variable shape: circular or especially in a vertical fissure. Secretions from the sphenoidal sinus pass through the ostium into the sphenoethmoidal recess.

THE POSTERIOR DRAINAGE PATHWAYS

A second route of mucociliary transport combines the secretions of the posterior ethmoidal cells and the sphenoidal sinus. These secretions mix in the sphenoethmoidal recess. Then they pass above and behind the eustachian tube and are transported toward the nasopharynx.

Infundibulo-Meatal Dysfunction

The source of infundibulo-meatal dysfunction can be local (rhinogenic), regional (dental), or systemic (mucosal disease). However, drainage of mucus and ventilation are the two most important factors in the maintenance of normal physiology of the paranasal sinus.

Mucus moves toward the primary or natural ostium. If accessory ostium is present in a maxillary sinus or if a nasoantral window is created surgically, usually only minor amounts of mucus are actively transported through the accessory ostia or the nasoantral window. The rest of the mucus usually bypass these ostia and move toward the natural ostium.

Except for the bullar cells, the entire anterior cell sinus system drains into the ethmoidal infundibu-

lum. The frontal sinus, maxillary sinus, and the anterior ethmoid sinus with their drainage pathways comprise an ostiomeatal unit whose components are interconnected.

In this narrow area, the mucosal surfaces are very close to each other. Mucus can be removed more easily, and the sinus more effectively drained because of ciliary sweeping motion in these narrow areas on the layer of mucus from two or more sides. If, however, the opposing mucosal surfaces in this cleft come into contact, drainage and ventilation of the sinus may be seriously impaired because ciliary sweeping motion is immobilized. Consequently, mucus is no longer evacuated. Sometimes pneumatization is extensive to the middle turbinate (Fig. 35). It may be bullous. It can be so extensive as to reach the lateral nasal wall. It compresses the bulla and the uncinate process, and restricts access to the maxillary and frontal sinuses. A paradoxically bent middle turbinate can also narrow the middle meatus and restrict the air flow to the anterior sinuses (Fig. 36).

Ventilation ensures gaseous exchange. Such exchanges through the ostium prevail over exchanges across the mucosa. The ostium generally is quite small, so that any alteration of its size, however minor, can have deleterious consequences. Unfavorable conditions are exacerbated

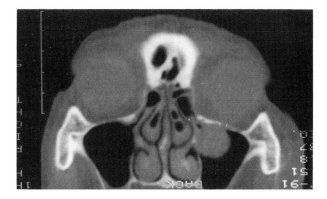
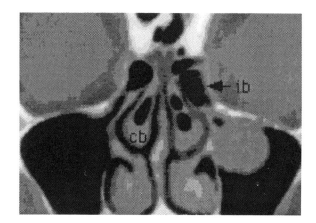

Fig. 35. Concha bullosa (cb) CT view, frontal section.

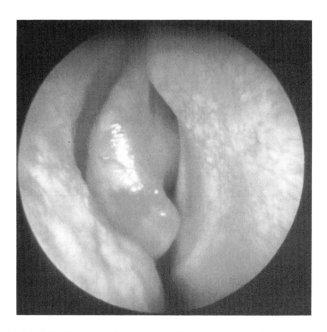
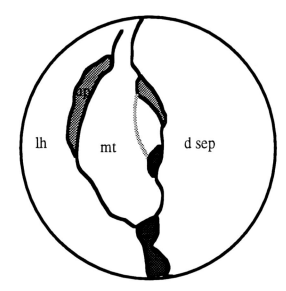

Fig. 36. Right nasal cavity, deviated septum and paradoxically bent middle turbinate. up, uncinate process; lh, lacrimal hump; mt, middle turbinate; d sep, deviated septum.

even more by the fact that this is not simply an ostium, at least for the main sinuses, i.e., frontal and maxillary sinuses, but is indeed a true duct. The frontonasal duct extends the lumen of the frontal sinus into the middle meatus between the lateral side of the middle concha and the uncinate process cells laterally. The maxillonasal duct is a narrow space bordered by the bulla and the uncinate process. It is more or less long and narrow, depending on the height of the unciform process and the descent of the bulla. Up to a certain size, the composition of gases in the sinus depends more on blood flow than on gaseous exchange through the ostium.

If the ostium becomes occluded, PO_2 decreases, but mucocilary sweeping motion remains effective if blood flow is adequate. It subsequently decreases with concomitant reduced blood flow. When edema develops, the ostium quickly becomes blocked because of its small diameter. Edema, hypoxia, decreased ciliary motion, exudate and transudates, and increasing edema form a vicious circle that facilitates possible infection. Suppuration then develops either as a result of the influx of aerobic bacteria that consume large amounts of oxygen and generate free radicals, or by a gradual decrease in PO_2 pressure that makes phagocytosis less effective and allows colonization by anaerobic organisms to occur.

The second local cause of inflammation and infection is dental disease. Chronic periodontitis (desmodontitis), periapical granuloma, and paradontal disease can cause and then maintain chronic inflammation of the mucosa in the maxillary sinus. Such inflammation can spread to the entire mucosa of the sinus. Considering the location of the maxillary ostium at the lower part of the infundibular groove, edema can then progressively involve the infundibular mucosa, and impair drainage and ventilation of nearly the entire anterior cell system.

The location of the nasal cavities with respect to air flow exposes this region to various airborne invasive agents. Any alteration in this area has an impact above. This fragile region of the anterior ethmoid is the site of persistent edema, which causes all disorders confined to the anterior ethmoidal intersection and to so-called anterior sinusitis. Small areas like this may be the underlying cause of serious problems. If mucosal swelling and mucus retention occur in the infundibulum, then ventilation and drainage of the maxillary sinus, as well as that of the anterior ethmoidal cells and the frontal sinus, may become impaired. Secretions from these sinuses are retained. Bacterial growth can then develop on the retained mucus.

The frontal sinus is more rarely involved, but does not escape the consequences of ostiomeatal obstruction. There is a fragile pressure balance maintained by the frontonasal duct and the infundibular groove, both of which are especially narrow. This arrangement promotes effective drainage because mucociliary sweeping motion can act on mucosal surfaces opposite, but the slightest edema will have consequences above.

In conclusion, it can be stated that the development of air cells is highly variable from one person to another, as well as the position of various cells in relation to the base of the skull. The most important sites are: the grooves, which are the source of cell groups and which ensure drainage, and the basal lamellae, which define the cellular groups. These observations are of both therapeutic and diagnostic value. Solely anterior or solely posterior involvement in relation to the septal partition of the middle concha are factors that suggest suppurated sinusitis. Involvement of both the anterior and posterior compartments suggests nasal polyposis if lesions are bilateral. This observation also demonstrates the necessity to resect diseased tissue and to clear off the key areas, such as the maxillary ostium or

anterior ethmoid. The goal of such endoscopic surgery is related to the function of the mucociliary system of clearance. Re-establishment of drainage and ventilation via the natural pathways is usually achieved without the need for direct intervention on these sinuses.

REFERENCES

1. Zuckerkandl E. Normale und pathologische Anatomie der Nasenhöhle und ihrer pneumatischen Anhänge. Wien: Braunmüller, 1893.
2. Sieur C, Jacob O. Recherches anatomiques cliniques et opératoires sur les fosses nasales et leurs sinus. Paris: J Rueff, 1901.
3. Mouret J. Anatomie des cellules ethmoïdales. Revue hebd de Laryng d'Otol et de Rhinol 1898;31:913–924.
4. Mouret J. Le schéma des masses latérales de l'ethmoïde. Revue hebd de Laryng d'Otol et de Rhinol 1922;1:9–22.
5. Mouret J. Rapport du sinus frontal avec les cellules ethmoïdales. Revue hebd de Laryng d'Otol et de Rhinol 1901;22:576–603 and 609–632.
6. Onodi A. Des rapports entre le nerf optique et le sinus sphénoïdal. La cellule ethmoïdale postérieure en particulier. Revue hebd de Laryng d'Otol et de Rhinol 1903; 25:721–740.
7. Grünwald L. Descriptive und topographische Anatomie der Nase und ihrer Nenbenhöhlen. In: Denker A, Kahler O, eds., Handbuch der Hals-Nasen-Ohrenheilkunde. Berlin: Springer, 1925; pp. 1–95.
8. Killian G. Anatomie der Nase menschlicher Embryonen. II. Die ursprüngliche Morphologie der Siebbeingegend. Arch. für Laryngologie und Rhinologie. Wien: Hölder, 1900; pp. 1004–1096.
9. Killian G. Die Nebenhöhlen der Nase in ihren Lagebeziehungen zu den Nachbarorganen. Jena: Fischer, 1903.
10. Messerklinger W. Endoscopy of the Nose. Baltimore, MD: Urban and Schwarzenberger, 1978.
11. Stammberger H. Functional Endoscopic Sinus Surgery. Philadelphia: BC Decker, 1991.
12. Kennedy DW, Zinreich SJ, Johns M. Functional endoscopic surgery. In: Goldman JL, ed., The Principles and Practice of Rhinology. New York: Wiley, 1987; pp. 879–901.
13. Buiter CT. Endoscopy of the Upper Airways. Amsterdam: Excerpta Medica, 1976.
14. Buiter CT. Nasal antrostomy. Rhinology 1988;26:5–18.
15. Friedrich JP, Terrier G. Chirurgie endoscopique de la sinusite par voie endonasale. Med et Hyg 1983;41: 3722–3726.
16. Friedrich JP, Terrier G. La chirurgie sinusale maxillaire endoscopique par voie endonasale. Problèmes actuels d'ORL 1984;7:187–189.
17. Wigand ME, Steiner W, Jaumann MP. Endonasal sinus surgery with endoscopical control: from radical operation to rehabilitation of the mucosa. Endoscopy 1978;10: 225–260.
18. Rouvier P, El Khoury J. Dacryocystorhinostomy by endonasal approach: 95 cases. Acta Otorhinolaryngologica Belgica 1992;46;401–404.

19. Rouvier P, Vaille G, Garcia C, Teppa H, Freche C, Lerault PR. La dacryocsytorhinostomie par voie endonasale. Ann Oto-Layngol 1981;98:49–53.

20. Freche Ch, Rouvier P, Peynegre R, Fombeur JP, Jakobowicz M, Lerault PR. L'Endoscopie Diagnostique et Thérapeutique en ORL. Paris: Arnette, 1989.

21. Terrier G. Rhinosinusal Endoscopy. Diagnosis and Surgery. Milano, Italy: Zambon, 1991.

22. Agrifolio A, Terrier G, Duvoisin B. Etude anatomique et endoscopique de l'ethmoïde antérieur. Ann Oto-Laryng Paris 1990;107:249–258.

23. Hamilton WJ, Boyd JD, Mossman HW. Human Embryology, 4th ed. London: William and Wilkins, 1978; 300–304.

24. Frick H, Leonhardt H, Starck D. Human Anatomy. New York: Thieme, 1991.

25. Guerrier Y, Rouvier P. Anatomie des sinus. EMC Oto-Rhino-Laryngologie, 4th ed. folder 20266 p. A10. 4.13.02. Paris: Editions Techniques Edit.

26. Mihalkovicks V. Anatomie und entwicklungsgeschichte der Nase und ihrer Nebenhöhlen. In: Heymann P., ed., Handbuch der Laryngologie und Rhinologie. Wien: A. Hölder, 1899; pp. 1–86.

27. Toshio O. Bony defects and dehiscences of the roof of the ethmoid cells. Rhinology 1981;19, 4:195–207.

28. Seydel O. Ueber die Nasenhöhlen der höheren Säugethiere und des Menschen. Morphologisches Jahrbuch 1891;17:44–99.

29. Hajek M. Indikation der verschiedenen Behandlungs und operationsmethoden bei den entzündlichen Erkrankungen der Nebenhöhlen der Nase. Z Hals Nas Ohrenheilk 1923;4:511–522.

30. Hajek M. Siebbeinzellen und Keilbeinhöhle. In: Denker A, Kahler O, eds., Handbuch der HNO-Heilkunde. Berlin: Springer, 1925; pp. 846–898.

31. Ferrie JC, Azais O, Vandermarcq P, Klossek JM, Drouineau J, Gasquet C. Exploration tomodensitométrique de l'ethmoïde et du méat moyen; radio-anatomie (incidence axiale) et variation anatomique. J Radiol 1991;72,10:477–487.

32. Ferrie JC, Azais O, Vandermarcq P, Klossek JM, Gasquet C. Exploration tomodensitométrique de l'ethmoïde et du méat moyen; radio-anatomie (incidence coronale). J Radiol 1991;72, 8-9:429–436.

33. Boyer A. Traité Complet d'Anatomie, Book 1, 2nd and 4th ed., Ed. Migneret, 1803–1815.

34. Bouche J. The De lima operation. Ann Otolaryngol 1979;96:450,451.

35. Terracol J, Ardouin P. Anatomie des fosses nasales et des cavités annexes. Maloine (Paris) 1965, p. 213.

36. Rice DH, Schaeffer SD. Endoscopic Paranasal Sinus Surgery. New York: Raven, 1988.

2

Physiology of the Nose
and Paranasal Sinuses

Philip Cole, MD, FRCSC

Contents

SPECIAL FEATURES

Introduction

Comparative studies demonstrate the existence of nasal structures and of paranasal sinuses that are common to a wide range of animal species. By contrast with many animals, human olfactory and turbinate structures and functions are vestigial (Figs. 1–3) *(1)*, but human paranasal sinuses are relatively well developed. Obviously useful and important functions of olfaction and respiratory air processing can be attributed to the nose, but despite many thoughtful speculations, conclusive evidence of functional importance of the paranasal sinuses has yet to be found.

The existence of paranasal sinuses may be unexplained, but their susceptibility to disease is a common source of misery for patients and a focus of attention for clinicians. Similar diseases have been found in animals. Sinus diseases are prevalent in both acute and chronic form, and, in most cases, they are closely associated with nasal disorders. Indeed, as a common example, paranasal sinus

involvement has been demonstrated by imaging studies in a large proportion of patients suffering from coryza *(2)*. It is unlikely that other inflammatory "sinus diseases" are confined to sinus cavities, and usually the term rhinosinusitis is more descriptive.

In addition to frequently mistaken self-diagnoses, sinus diseases are common globally (33 million cases/yr in the US—National Center for Health Statistics), they are distressing to the sufferer, and progression to vital structures in their proximity can lead to serious complications, but the relatively benign course of acute rhinosinusitis encourages neglect in many cases. In other cases, its severity, chronicity, and extension to associated air passages and air-containing cavities with attendant complications add a major contribution to the heavy morbidity burden of respiratory diseases—a burden that is most heavily weighted against the very young, the old, and the underprivileged throughout the world. The incidence and lethal complications of respiratory diseases are many times greater in underdeveloped than in developed countries.

Economic consequences of nasal and sinus diseases are substantial. In addition to an incalculable number of cases, it has been estimated that in

From: *Diseases of the Sinuses* (M. E. Gershwin and G. A. Incaudo, eds.), ©1996 Humana Press Inc., Totowa, NJ.

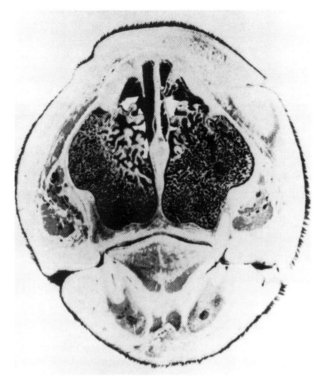

Fig. 1. Coronal section of the nasal cavity of a seal demonstrating enormous turbinate structure. (Reprinted with permission from Negus *[1]*.)

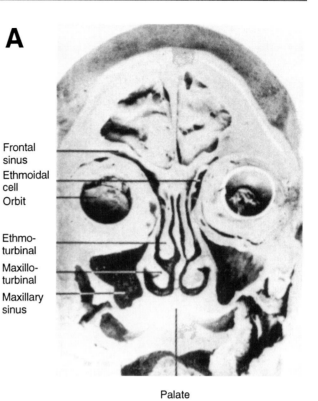

Fig. 2. Comparative anatomical studies of maxilloturbinate turbinates, saggital and coronal views. Note simplicity of human turbinate structure. (Reprinted with permission from Negus *[1]*.)

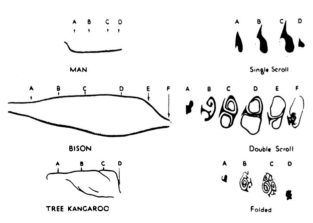

the US alone, they lead to the loss of at least 200 million days of employment annually. More than $5 billion are spent on medication and much of it is symptomatic, as advertising and the shelves of drug stores affirm. Doctor visits, together with diagnostic and surgical measures, add many millions of

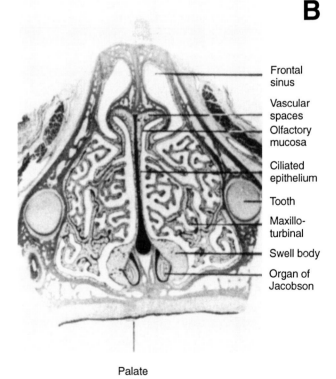

Fig. 3. Coronal nasal sections comparing turbinates of humans **(A)** and domestic cat **(B)**. The nasal olfactory area of the cats also exceeds that of humans. (Reprinted with permission from Negus *[1]*.)

dollars more to the economic burden of rhino-sinusitis *(3)*.

This chapter is concerned mainly with applied physiology of the human nose and paranasal sinuses, and important features of the region that are discussed in detail in other chapters of this book receive only brief reference here.

Nasal and Sinus Mucosa

Apart from the mouth, pharynx, and terminal pulmonary air passages, patency of the respiratory airways and air-containing cul-de-sacs in continuity with them is maintained by relatively inflexible cartilage and by bone. Hygiene and health of these patent passages and cavities are preserved by a specialized ciliated epithelium and a mucociliary defense mechanism, which they share in continuity. They also share ubiquitous respiratory tract diseases that are modified by characteristic features of the passages and cavities, and, in addition, several diseases are unique to particular sites. Furthermore, failure of defense mechanisms of the upper airways can provide a gateway that allows infectious diseases to enter and disseminate to other regions of the body.

Ciliated columnar epithelium that lines the nose and sinuses is bounded by squamous epithelium of the anterior nose and the pharynx, respectively. In both newborn and laryngectomized subjects, ciliated epithelium occupies a greater proportion of the anterior nose than in other subjects, which suggests that squamous metaplasia of ciliated epithelium is a response to the trauma of environmental exposures.

The area of the luminal surface of the columnar epithelium that lines the remainder of the nose and the sinuses is greatly expanded by 200–300 microvilli/cell that enhance the potential for exchanges between epithelial cells and the nasal lumen. A large proportion of these columnar cells also bear cilia, several hundred/cell, which beat 1000×/min in sequence with those of neighboring ciliated cells. The mechanisms underlying this orderly metachronous activity are unexplained.

When the mucociliary mechanism is functioning normally, the cilia beat in a serous periciliary fluid of low viscosity. This fluid is deep enough to avoid entanglement of cilia with discontinuous islands of viscoelastic mucus that float on its surface. Yet it is not so deep as to prevent tips of the beating cilia from propelling the mucus along well-

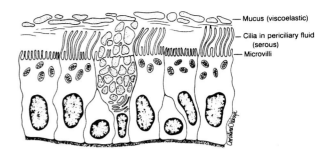

Fig. 4. Mucociliary transport. (Reprinted with permission from Cole *[4]*, p. 24.)

established tracks to the pharynx, where it is swallowed (Fig. 4) *(4)*. The floating masses of mucus contain entrapped and dissolved contaminants from inspired ambient air, and along their course to the pharynx they sweep up cellular debris, microorganisms, and other detritus from the serous surface. It has been estimated that the mucus and its contents cross epithelial cells at a rate of 6–10 cells/s *(5)*, but clearance studies demonstrate that although the mucociliary transport rate averages about 6 mm/min, it is subject to wide variation and it differs also between different sites. Seromucinous glands and epithelial goblet cells secrete the thin pericellular fluid and the thick viscoelastic mucus *(6)*.

In addition to physical removal of microorganisms and other noxious materials by mucociliary transport, an important line of defense is provided by the surface fluids that contain macrophages, basophils and mast cells, leukocytes, eosinophils, and antibacterial/antiviral substances that include immunoglobulins, lactoferrin, lysozymes, and interferons. These cells and substances discourage microbial colonization and enhance the protective properties of the nasal and sinus mucosa that guard against infection.

Cytoplasm of the cilia contains clearly patterned ultrastructural elements whose function is concerned with flexion and extension of ciliary beating *(7)*. Abnormalities of these ultrastructures can result in dyskinesias, which are inherited in some cases as primary disorders (Kartagener's, Young's, and other less clearly defined autosomal recessive inherited syndromes). Abnormalities of the cilia and their ultrastructure are not confined to the nasal mucosa, they are widely distributed, and have been demonstrated in peripheral respiratory epithelium and in other ciliated cells. Abnormalities of the ciliary bodies are found also as accompaniments of mucosal injury (infective and other forms of irritation). They consist of cytoplasmic extrusions in the form of blebs and outgrowths of the ciliary membrane. Aberrant cilia are commonly found also in electron microscope studies of biopsy specimens obtained from apparently healthy subjects. Except in the rare cases of Kartagener's or even more rare Young's and other less well-defined inherited syndromes, the physiological and clinical significance of the many observed ciliary anomalies is unknown.

In health, variations are wide, but abnormalities of metachronal ciliary beat and of secretions and barriers in the course of mucociliary flow can lead to pathological consequences. Ciliary beat frequency and mucus transport rate vary substantially, they are not closely correlated, and each can be modified by quantities and qualities of seromucinous secretions. Cystic fibrosis (mucoviscidosis) is an example of inherited disease of abnormal exocrine secretion, and, more commonly, allergens, infections, and irritants also alter the quantity and the chemical and physical properties of nasal secretion, which can result in impairment of mucociliary function.

Mucociliary function is remarkably resistant to climatic extremes, to moderate concentrations of the majority of environmental air pollutants (including tobacco smoke), to particulate loading, to wide variations in pH, and to most prescription nasal medications. However, some preservatives (e.g., benzalkonium chloride) are harmful (8), and medications containing them should be avoided. Hypotonic and detergent aqueous solutions injure cilia, and desiccation of the mucosa is disastrous to them. Rhinovirus can destroy not only cilia, but also epithelial cells; their junctions loosen, and they may become detached from the basement membrane. As a consequence, impairment of defensive function leaves the mucosa vulnerable to both spreading and secondary infection. Full recovery of mucociliary function following such infection may require several weeks.

Normal mucociliary function provides a first line of defense. It is of fundamental importance to health of the airways and associated recesses, but the narrow middle meatal cleft, which provides the main exit for mucociliary flow from the sinuses to the nasal cavities, is susceptible to obstruction. In this ostiomeatal complex, mucosal swelling, polyps, or thickened secretions that result from common nasal

inflammatory conditions can create a vicious cycle in which pathological changes become irreversible without therapeutic intervention. Occlusion of an ostial orifice, directly or more remotely by obstruction elsewhere within the narrow confines of the middle meatus, is a primary cause of inflammatory sinus disease. Anterior ethmoid cells are common sites of disease, and ethmoiditis is usually associated with an obstructed infundibulum (9,10). (See also Sinus Air Flow later in this chapter.)

The Nasal Airways

Although mouth or tracheostomal breathing can sustain life indefinitely, the parallel nasal cavities provide preferred breathing passages that are supplemented by the oral airway under demanding conditions of exercise or of severe nasal obstruction, but exclusive oral breathing is rare (11). Patients can become firmly habituated to "mouth" (oronasal) breathing, and it can persist despite relief of obstruction.

Thermal and water vapor pressure gradients favoring exchanges between inspiratory air and mucosa are much greater at respiratory portals than elsewhere in the air passages. The portal airway meets major demands in cleansing, heating, and moistening 15 kg of ambient air that is required for pulmonary ventilation of human adults every 24 h. The spontaneously positioned labial orifice enables the mouth to process ambient air effectively (12) in the short term, but continuous secretion and repeated redistribution of saliva (or the oral intake of other aqueous fluid) are necessary to prevent localized drying of mucosa, and to maintain both oral conditioning of ambient air and oropharyngeal comfort. The nose is better equipped than the mouth to meet long-term air-conditioning demands, since, by contrast with salivation, supply of moisture is continuous and its wide distribution over the nasal mucosa is aided by the mucociliary mechanism. Moreover, as will be discussed later in this chapter, the mouth is less effective than the nose in recovering moisture (and heat) from the 15 kg/d of expiratory air.

Nevertheless, although exclusive nasal breathing may be preferable, it is clearly less than essential. It is readily abandoned during exercise when inspiratory air-conditioning demands are great, and it is abandoned also during speech and in other less exacting circumstances, such as surprise and preoccupation. Chronic "mouth" breathing can lead not only to oral and pharyngeal discomfort and to gingivitis, but there is much evidence to support the view that it can lead also to abnormalities of facial growth and dentition.

Nasal Air-Flow Sensation

Nasal symptoms are very common, but patients' subjective assessments of nasal dyspneas are not closely correlated with objective findings *(13)*. Indeed, physiological nasal air-flow resistive changes resulting from exercise, from recovery following exercise, from postural effects, and from the nasal cycle, although frequent and substantial, are seldom noticed, nor is it unusual for gross structural abnormalities to be found on clinical and rhinomanometric examination of patients without complaints of nasal airway obstruction. On the other hand, neither is it unusual for complaints of obstruction to be unsupported by clinical and objective findings. Sensory interpretations of nasal patency are influenced not only by ambient and pathophysiological conditions, but also by psychological factors.

A prominent feature of nasal inspiratory air flow is a sensation of chill within the nasal cavities. Its degree and penetration, which can extend to the pharynx and beyond, are dependent on ambient air conditions of temperature and humidity and on flow velocity. The sensation is absent in expiration, and it is consistent with thermal demands of the air stream. In addition to thermal sensation, auditory sensation accompanies nasal air flow. Its intensity is directly related to air-flow velocity and its consequent flow disturbance, it is present in both inspiratory and expiratory phases, and its presence is a source of great reassurance to parents of sleeping infants. Similar thermal and auditory sensations accompany oral breathing.

In addition to cool air and deep nasal inspiration, several aromatic substances, notably l-menthol, enhance the sensations of chill, air flow, and nasal patency *(13)*. By contrast, ambient air with a heavy concentration of tobacco smoke can produce a sensation of nasal stuffiness. Objective measurements of nasal air-flow resistances have demonstrated, however, that in healthy subjects, despite the nasal sensations, patency is unaffected by these exposures.

l-Menthol also induces a sensation of chill in the oral mucosa and the skin (menthol lozenges and after-shave preparations). This menthol isomer is thought to exert its enhanced sensory effects by altering calcium transport in neural tissues *(13)*, but mechanisms of the sensation of nasal stuffiness induced by tobacco smoke have not been elucidated. Specific nerve endings for temperature or flow detection have not been identified in nasal mucosa, but nonmyelinated sensory nerve fibers with plexiform endings have been demonstrated terminating in the lamina propria and between epithelial cells *(13)*.

In addition to cognition, other sensory neural responses to nasal air flow are widespread. They are reflected in EEG changes *(13)* and may be of importance to mechanics of breathing in both wakefulness and sleep. Breathing cool (fresh!!) air reduces not only the sensation of dyspnea, but also respiratory contractions of thoracic muscles. These effects are enhanced by increased respiratory air flow (deep breaths!!) and diminished by topical nasal anesthesia *(13)*.

NASAL RESISTORS

The Nasal Valve

Nasal resistance to respiratory air flow is of similar magnitude to the sum of the resistances of all the remaining air passages. The major portion of nasal resistance is confined to a narrowed caudal (anterior) segment that is thus the major resistor of the entire respiratory airway system. Beyond the narrowing, the nasal cavum and succeeding airway segments offer comparatively little resistance to inspiratory air flow (Fig. 5) *(14)*. In expiration, the glottis narrows and provides additional resistance to air flow during this phase of breathing (*see* Respiratory Air Processing later in this chapter).

Descriptions of the narrowed nasal segment, termed the nasal valve, can be confused by an unnecessarily extensive terminology that does not simplify understanding of its dimensions or its function *(15)*. The lumen of the valve extends several millimeters beyond the triangular cleft that is evident on rhinoscopic examination of the vestibule. The apex of this triangle is less acute in Negroid than Caucasian noses, thus enabling the inferior turbinate to be examined without instrumentation in such cases. The cleft is the entrance to a dynamic functional segment of the airway, and it is bounded by the caudal edge of the compliant upper lateral cartilage and by a line opposite to it on the comparatively rigid cartilaginous septum. Its

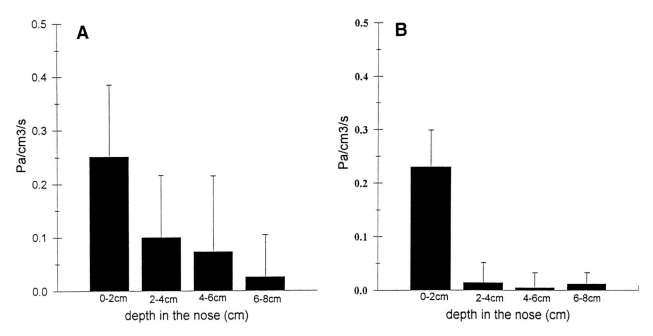

Fig. 5. Distribution of resistance in 2-cm segments of the nasal cavities. The resistance is most marked in the anterior nose. The erectile anterior turbinate portion is reduced, and more caudally situated resistance remains after decongestion. (Reprinted with permission from Hirschberg et al. *[14]*.)

short base lies across the bony nasal floor. It is obliquely situated between horizontal nostril and vertical piriform aperture.

The functional valve extends several millimeters from its triangular entrance to the piriform entrance of the anterior cavum, and it is much shorter and wider ventrally than dorsally. It is bounded laterally by compliant alar tissues and, in the vicinity of the rigid entry to the bony cavum, by erectile tissue at the caudal end of the inferior turbinate. The medial wall of firm septal cartilage supports an extensive body of erectile tissue in its dorsal portion. This mass of septal erectile tissue, although not readily recognizable on rhinoscopic examination, is demonstrated clearly by tomographic imaging and by cadaver studies (*see* Figs. 6–9) *(4,16–18)*. Stability of the compliant alar wall is maintained by resistance to deformation of its tissues and by isometric inspiratory activity of alar muscles. Both oppose inspiratory transmural pressures *(4)*.

The nasal valve is a functional complex of compliant and dynamic tissues. Over a distance of several millimeters, its lumen is regulated by lateral and medial erectile mucosa, modulated by the tone of alar muscles, and stabilized by bone and cartilage. As noted above, it is the major resistor of the respiratory airways, and it performs an essential

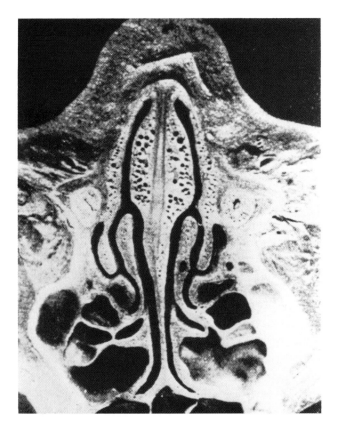

Fig. 6. Injected cadaver material. Extensive accumulations of capacitance vessels that constitute erectile tissues of the septum and lateral nasal walls. This is most marked in the anterior nose. (Reprinted with permission from Wustrow *[7]*.)

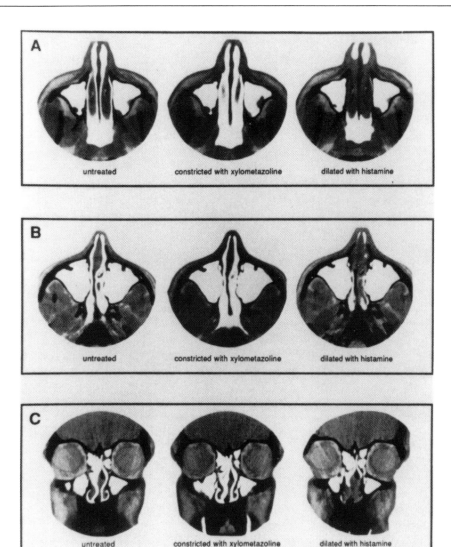

Fig. 7. Computed X-ray axial and coronal tomograms of the nasal cavities. Effects of vasoactive substances. Note both medial (septal body) and lateral erectile tissues in the anterior nose. (Reprinted with permission from Cole et al. *[16]*.)

function in ensuring disruption of laminar flow of the inspiratory air stream (*see* Respiratory Air Processing later in this chapter).

The Nasal Alae

In healthy adult noses, alar movement in response to nasal breathing is insignificant during resting ventilation, but it is often quite marked in young children. Inspiratory nasal alar dilator muscle activity increases with ventilation and opposes transmural pressures. Measurements of alar movement toward the septum induced by inspiratory transmural pressures of exercising adults has been determined by video studies and found to be very small *(4)*, and when exercise is sufficiently

severe, vestibular transmural respiratory pressures are reduced by a switch to oronasal breathing.

EMG studies show alar dilator muscle activity to accompany each nasal inspiration, and the activity varies directly not only with ventilation, but also with nasal resistance, hypoxia, and hypercapnia. It ceases with mouth or tracheostomal breathing *(4)*. As with other upper-airway-stabilizing muscles, alar dilator muscle activity precedes diaphragmatic contraction. The dilator muscles that stabilize the anterior nasal airway also increase its patency in demanding and emotional situations, such as severe exercise, air hunger, anger, and fear.

As the volume of respiratory air flow is maintained through a nasal segment that becomes nar-

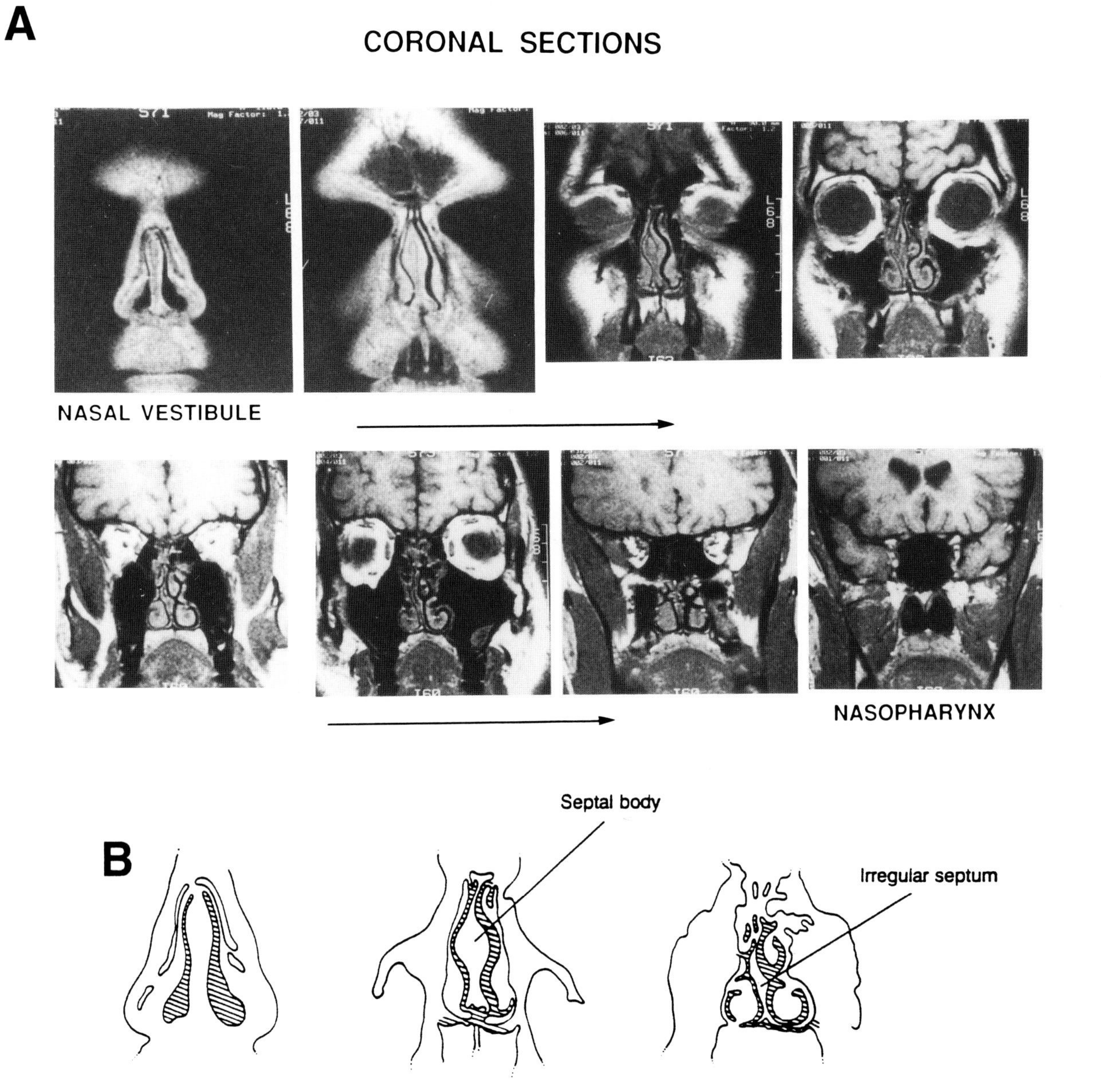

A

CORONAL SECTIONS

NASAL VESTIBULE

NASOPHARYNX

B

Septal body

Irregular septum

Fig. 8. Magnetic resonance imaging of coronal sections of the nasal airways from nostrils to choana. Note septal body and adaptation of airway to septal irregularity. (MRIs from Cole et al. *[18]*. Tracings from Cole *[4]*, p. 27. Reprinted with permission.)

rowed, linear velocity of the air stream increases and elevates transmural pressure, a compressing force, at the site of narrowing (Bernoulli). At a critically elevated inspiratory transmural pressure, the compliant portion of the narrow nasal valve collapses partially or completely, thereby limiting further or occluding the airway *(4)*.

The caudal end of the upper lateral cartilage is free from septal attachment and has a flexible fibrous joint with the lower lateral cartilage. Thus, it is the alar region most disposed to comply with transmural pressures. However, until a critical transmural pressure is achieved, normal alar tissues and dilator muscles provide sufficient rigidity to withstand deformation. Thus, lumen and resistance of the normally functioning valve is little affected by the transmural pressures that are generated by nasal breathing at rest, and, as already noted,

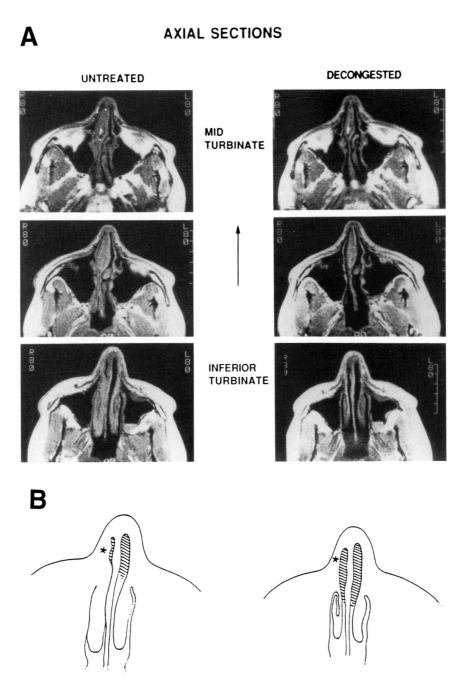

Fig. 9. Magnetic resonance imaging axial views show medial and lateral erectile tissues. Note erectile tissue in valve area caudal to bony inferior turbinate. (MRIs from Cole et al. *[18]*. Tracings from Cole *[4]*, p. 29. Reprinted with permission.)

the switch to oronasal breathing that accompanies exercise reduces the nasal fraction of respiratory air flow and the alar burden of transmural pressure.

Alar dilator muscle weakness increases alar compliance with inspiratory air flow pressures and reduces the critical transmural pressure at which collapse of the valve occurs. Under these condi-

tions, nasal obstruction can result from modest inspiratory air flow, as in cases of Bell's and other facial muscle palsies. The tendency toward alar collapse can be increased also by impairment of normal alar skeletal stiffness or by alar deformity. Such defects are congenital, traumatic, or, more commonly, complications of rhinoplasty *(4)*.

Inspiratory collapse can occur also with normally robust alae and healthy dilator muscles when transmural pressures are elevated by the Bernoulli effect of excessive narrowing in the valve region. Such narrowing can accompany structural abnormalities of the anterior septum, of the alae themselves, of the mucosa, or combinations of these factors.

Wide alar retraction approximately halves airflow resistance of the healthy Caucasian nose. The remaining resistance is reduced even further by the effect of topical decongestants on erectile mucosa of the cavum, mainly in its anterior segment (Fig. 5) *(14)*. By contrast with alar retraction, since the valve is narrow, slight mucosal or skeletal intrusions on the lumen by displacement of its medial and/or lateral wall can result in a substantial decrease in cross-sectional area, and exponential increase in both air-flow resistance and transmural pressure (*see also* Chapter 23).

Nasal obstruction is caused, most commonly, by mucosal swelling that extends into the valve region, and it is exacerbated by structural encroachment on the valve lumen of septal or, more rarely, alar deformity *(4)*. Substantial obstruction can occur with comparatively minor aberrations of this nature, whereas only gross deviations or swelling is obstructive in other parts of the nasal cavities (Figs. 10 and 11) *(19,20)*. However, although an entirely regular midline septum in an adult is not the most common finding, septal irregularity is symptomless in most cases *(4)*.

A predominance of septal deviations in males suggests a traumatic etiology. There is evidence to suggest that they result also, in both sexes, from parturition injuries sustained during rotation of the fetal head in the birth canal and, indeed, they are reported to be less frequent in Caesarean than vaginal births *(4)*.

Rhinomanometry has confirmed benefits of corrective septal surgery in the anterior nasal segment *(21)*. It is reported also that the more demanding corrective surgery of the alar cartilages can restore and, in cosmetic cases, maintain appropriate patency of this region *(21–24)*.

Objective measurements have demonstrated that rapid maxillary expansion, a common orthodontic procedure that enlarges the upper dental arch, widens the piriform aperture and results in a marked and lasting increase in nasal patency *(4)*. This method has been employed as one of the alterna-

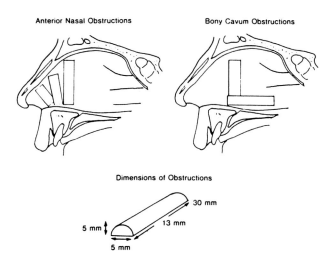

Fig. 10. Septal deviations simulated by means of plastic foam strips of differing thickness, adherent to the septum and sited in the anterior nose and the cavum. (Reprinted with permission from Chaban et al. *[19]*.)

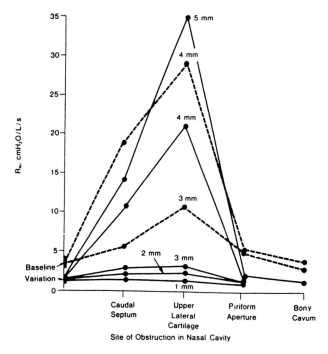

Fig. 11. Resistive effects of simulated septal deviations. This is most marked in the anterior nose. Large simulated deviations and spurs have little resistive effect in the cavum. (Reprinted with permission from Cole *[20]*.)

tives in management of obstructive narrowing in the valve region.

Several different prosthetic devices are available to support the alae in order to maintain or to increase patency of the anterior nose and to improve the comfort of nasal breathing (e.g., Francis dilators). These devices are usually inserted in the nasal vestibule, but a recent innovation (Breathe Right) consists of a spring-loaded plastic strip that adheres to the vestibular skin and opens the valve. Despite undoubted increased patency and ease of breathing, our attempted therapeutic use of these devices to relieve severe snoring and other breathing disorders in sleep has been disappointing.

Erectile Tissue

Erectile tissues of the septum and lateral nasal wall *(4)* achieve particular prominence in the anterior nose (Figs. 6–9). Injection studies of vascular nasal tissues of cadaver material illustrate the manner in which blood content of the capacitance vessels of erectile tissues can regulate airway lumen and air-flow resistance principally in the narrowed valve segment.

In vivo, tomographic imaging, acoustic rhinometry (*see* Chapter 23), and air-flow studies have confirmed the distribution of nasal erectile tissues (Fig. 5) that is demonstrated by cadaver injection studies, and have clearly shown the mucosal volume changes that occur in the spontaneous nasal cycle, and in response to vasoactive substances and to postural stimuli. In addition, imaging studies validate the clinical observation that nasal erectile tissues accommodate to structural irregularities (Fig. 8), and they maintain a remarkably constant airway width of 2–3 mm in the more patent nasal cavum despite marked septal deviations.

Other injection studies of cadaver tissues show nasal erectile tissue as a venous mat 1–5 mm thick *(25)* consisting of accumulations of tortuous, irregular, intercommunicating, valveless venous sinuses. These vessels have a rich sympathetic nerve supply *(26)* and respond by constriction to stimulation of both α-1 and α-2 receptors *(27)*. They terminate in muscular "throttle" veins that possibly regulate venous drainage *(26)*.

The ability of erectile tissues to maintain an adequate nasal airway can be defeated by moderate structural asymmetries at narrowed sites, with resulting intermittent obstruction by cyclic or postural mucosal swelling. More severe skeletal deviation and/or pathological mucosal swelling lead to more persistent obstruction and, as already noted, resistive effects of structural irregularities or mucosal swelling are critical in the valve region where the cross-sectional area is normally restricted *(4)*.

Nasal erectile tissues are not confined to the vascular mucosa of the turbinates. In the congested nose, swelling of erectile tissues covering the bony inferior turbinate is accompanied by swelling of the lateral nasal wall caudal to it. The lateral wall tissues extend several millimeters beyond the bony piriform aperture, and when congested, they intrude on the lumen of the valve. Swelling and shrinking of these tissues, e.g., by topical decongestant, can be detected readily by rhinoscopy and demonstrated clearly by tomography (Fig. 9), acoustic rhinometry, and air-flow studies.

Further substantial intrusions on the valve lumen result from congestion of erectile tissues of the anterior septum (Figs. 6–9). An anterior septal erectile body is well recognized in European rhinological literature, but it is neglected in English language texts. The main mass of septal erectile tissue is located caudal to the middle turbinate and dorsal to the inferior turbinate. It is inconspicuous on rhinoscopic examination, since it is partially masked by the columella and the two sides of the septum cannot be viewed simultaneously.

Tomographic imaging that embraces the anterior nose shows the septal body clearly, but routine sinus tomography does not usually include this region. Although the septal body of erectile tissue is seldom a direct target of therapy, it is interesting to consider the possibility that surgical elevation of anterior septal tissues might inadvertently affect it and contribute to the benefits of septoplasty.

Inflammation brings about a paresis of capacitance vessel tone *(28,29)* that allows these vessels, which constitute the nasal erectile tissues, to fill with blood, most markedly in recumbency. The airways may be narrowed further by other accompaniments of inflammation that include accumulation of extravascular fluid, secretion, transudate, and exudate of fluid and macromolecules through permeable epithelial junctions *(6,30)*, but response to decongestant indicates that a major proportion of the swelling is vascular.

Blood content of capacitance vessels and blood flow through resistance vessels are controlled by vascular tone, and the two systems function independently, but they respond to many stimuli in a similar manner. Vascular tone is influenced by local metabolic and vasoactive substances, by thermal conditions, and by neurotransmission. In addition to adrenergic and cholinergic neurotransmitters, many other substances concerned with neurotrans-

Table 1
Nonadrenergic, Noncholinergic Neuropeptides
and Biochemical Mediators[a]

Neuropeptides	Mediators
Calcitonin gene-related peptide	Adenosine
Galinin	Bradikinin
Gastrin-releasing peptide	Chemotaxins
Neurokinins	Heparin
Neuropeptide Y	Leukotrienes
Peptide histidine isoleucine	Prostaglandins
Somatostatin	Serotinin
Substance P	Trypsin
	Nitric oxide (?)

[a]Nonadrenergic and noncholinergic substances found in reactive nasal mucosa affecting blood vessel tone and permeability and seromucinous secretion.

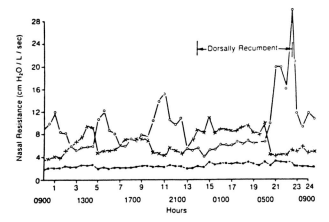

Fig. 12. The nasal cycle demonstrated by nasal air-flow resistances. Amplitude increases in recumbency. Left (x) and right (o) resistances reciprocate. Combined resistances (●) show little change throughout the 24-h period of observation. (Reprinted with permission from Cole *[31]*.)

mission and vasoactivity have been detected in nasal tissues in health and in disease. Several of these substances act also on nasal secretory elements, but, in many cases, their precise functions are unknown. They are listed in Table 1.

The Nasal Cycle

In health, nasal congestion and decongestion alternate over time in each nasal cavity as an apparently spontaneous resistive cycle, and although unilateral resistances can fluctuate between severe obstruction and optimum patency (Fig. 12) *(31,32)*, healthy subjects are usually unaware of the changes. The additional phenomenon of reciprocity of resistances between sides (as one side congests, the opposite side decongests) minimizes alteration of combined resistances of the paired nasal cavities *(4,31,32)* (Fig. 12). Reciprocity is irregular in young children, but when present, as in most adults, stabilization of total nasal resistance might diminish awareness of unilateral resistance changes. The resistive homeostasis of the combined nasal cavities is susceptible to disturbance by structural asymmetry or by inflammatory mucosal disease. Either can result in symptoms owing to obstruction of the airway *(4,33,34)*.

Amplitude and frequency of the resistive nasal cycle are irregular, and the latter parameter is measured in hours (Fig. 12) *(4)*. Minor fluctuations of briefer duration are superimposed on the leisurely progression of the cycle, but reciprocity between sides is fairly consistent and the resulting combined resistance remains fairly stable. Although the constantly changing resistances may not satisfy all

criteria of cyclical activity and may be episodic rather than periodic, the term "nasal cycle" is firmly established and widely known.

This curious cycle has been recognized for several centuries in yoga literature *(35)* where it is cited as a sign of good health. Modification of the cyclical phases by pressures exerted in the axillary region (*see* Posture and Pressure Effects) and by breathing maneuvers plays an important role in the yoga pranayama breathing exercises *(4,35,36)*. The cycle has received attention in Western rhinology literature during the last 100 yr *(37)*.

The nasal cycle is reported to be present in about 80% of the adults in whom it has been sought *(4)*, and its absence may be temporary. It has been found also in children and infants *(4)* in whom, as noted above, frequency and reciprocation between sides are less regular than in adults. A similar resistive cycle has been demonstrated in cats, dogs, pigs, rabbits, and rats, which, like humans, exhibit erectile nasal tissue *(4)*.

In humans, the cycle is amplified in recumbency, but it is otherwise unaffected by sleep, nasal occlusion of short duration, or topical anesthesia, but it is suppressed by tracheostomal breathing and it returns on resumption of the natural airway *(4)*. Since the cycle is a vascular phenomenon, it is abolished temporarily by topical decongestant and, if the decongestant is applied unilaterally, the cycle continues contralaterally *(38)*.

Other cyclical phenomena that demonstrate lateralization synchronous with the nasal cycle have been reported in humans *(4)*. They include electrocortical activity, sweating, pupil size, conjunctival capillary diameter, and even cognitive performance. It seems that the nasal cycle and its modifications *(see next section)* are sensitive indicators of widely distributed neuroautonomic activity that reciprocates between sides of the body. The cycle provides an interesting source of speculation, but does not necessarily perform a functionally useful role in the nose.

Posture and Pressure Effects

Unilateral nasal decongestion results from assumption of contralateral recumbent postures, and to contralateral pressures applied to the body surface in upright subjects, it is accompanied by ipsilateral nasal congestion (Fig. 13) *(39)*. Sweat secretion also responds contralaterally to posture and body surface pressures *(4,39)*, and both nasal and sweat responses appear to be mediated by a similar sympathetic route.

These reciprocal responses of capacitance vessels to pressure stimuli override the spontaneous nasal cycle *(4,39)* whose mucovascular reciprocity they resemble in minimizing change in air-flow resistance of the combined nasal cavities.

As the upper nasal cavity becomes more patent and the lower more resistive on assumption of a lateral recumbent posture, periodic reciprocation of the nasal cycle begins anew if this lateral posture is maintained. However, although reciprocal resistive postural responses occur during brief periods of lateral recumbency, they are temporary, and progression of the cycle does not appear to be affected on return to the dorsal posture.

It seems likely that receptors involved in the nasal vascular pressure reflex are deeply situated, since the response to lateral chest wall pressure that takes place despite local anesthesia of the skin could not be elicited following intercostal nerve block in a single subject who was otherwise consistently responsive. It is of interest to note also that no similar nasal reflex responses were elicited when superficial heat, cold, or painful stimuli were applied unilaterally to the body surface *(4)*.

In standing subjects, amplitude of the cycle is much smaller than in seated or recumbent subjects *(4)*, and it is unaffected by the pressures of weight bearing on one foot or the other. Absence of stimuli

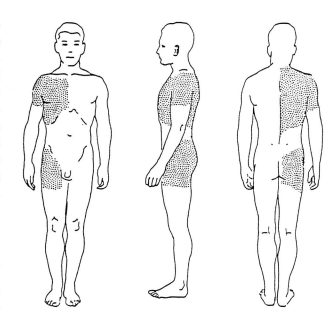

Fig. 13. Topographical anatomy of the pressure points that alter nasal resistance. (Reprinted with permission from Haight and Cole *[39].*)

from gravitational pressures on the trunk region of the body surface or action of the cardiovascular homeostatic reflex of capacitance vessels *(40)* might account for the amplitude differences.

In healthy noses, there is little change in resistance of the combined nasal cavities as a subject assumes dorsal recumbency from an upright position *(28)*, nor are there sleep-related changes of nasal resistance (Miljeteig et al., 1992, unpublished). In recumbency the nasal cycle continues, and vasoactive mucosa of the cyclically decongested side remains little affected. On the congested side, where tone of capacitance vessels is reduced, additional mucosal swelling occurs in response to the increased hydrostatic pressure of recumbency, but the swelling has little effect on resistance of the combined nasal cavities. Even severe unilateral cyclical obstructions that have been noted in recumbent and sleeping subjects do not exert a major effect on total nasal resistance *(41)*.

By contrast, in the presence of nasal mucosal inflammation, as most people are aware, congestion increases on assumption of a recumbent posture *(28,29)*, since capacitance vessel tone is decreased and the vessels respond to postural hydrostatic pressures by increased blood content. Even in the upright patient, as already noted, the nasal cycle is modified by nasal mucosal diseases, and stabilizing reciprocal adjustments are disrupted *(34)*. In the presence of cyclical, postural, or inflammatory mucosal swelling, resistive effects of structural abnormalities are exacerbated and moderate structural obstructions may become evident only under these circumstances.

It has been suggested that the decrease in intranasal pressures that accompanies sniffing may be sufficient, if frequently repeated, to induce distension of capacitance vessels, especially in the presence of inflammation. A vicious cycle, typified by the chronically sniffing patient with nasal obstruction, has been put forward as an example supporting this plausible supposition *(42)*.

Effects of physiological and pathological nasal mucosal swelling in the ostiomeatal complex on the paranasal sinuses are discussed in other sections of this chapter.

AIR FLOW

Nasal Air-Flow Distribution

The distribution of inspiratory and expiratory air flow in human nasal cavities has been studied by many methods. Probably the most definitive results have been obtained by Swift and Proctor (Fig. 14) *(43)*, who used hemi-nasal models obtained as casts from fresh human cadavers. They determined direction and linear velocity of nasal air streams by means of a micro-Pitot device. A transparent plastic sheet substituted for a septum, and a perforation through it enabled the Pitot device to be placed at known nasal sites while air was passed through the model cavity at measured rates.

Figure 14 shows linear flow velocities and directions within the model nasal cavity that are attained by ambient air at a flow approximating resting inspiration. Linear velocity of inspiratory air is markedly greater anteriorly in the region of the nasal valve than elsewhere in the nasal cavity. Indeed, in vivo it is greater than elsewhere in the respiratory passages. The mainstream courses between the inferior and superior turbinates with only minimal flow along the nasal floor and roof. Specialized olfactory mucosa is sheltered from the inspiratory mainstream *(43)* and, thus, avoids exposure to harm from the blast of unmodified ambient air.

Air enters the nose through the horizontal nostril, mainly via its ventral portion. It takes a sharp turn and follows a curved course through the main

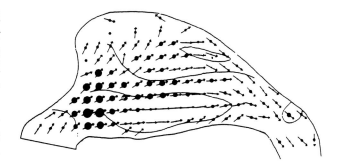

Fig. 14. Direction and velocity of the inspiratory air stream during resting breathing. Size of points indicates velocity, which is greatest in the anterior nose. Main airstream flows between superior and inferior turbinates. (Reprinted with permission from Swift and Proctor *[43]*, p. 80.)

nasal passage to exit to the nasopharynx by the vertical choana, and then takes another sharp turn to the oropharynx. The shape of the nasal vestibular region and its adjustment by alar muscles direct inspiratory air medially to course along the septum where the mainstream proceeds as a ribbon 2–3 mm thick arching between inferior and superior turbinates.

By contrast with the inspiratory air stream, well-conditioned expiratory air is dispersed throughout the nasal cavity. It expels olfactants from the olfactory cleft, and gives up heat and water to nasal mucosa that is cooled by inspired ambient air (*see* Respiratory Air Processing later in this chapter).

Olfactory sniffs, directed by alar positioning, form eddies in the upper nasal cavity *(43)*. Vigorous sniffs assist cilia by propelling mucus toward the nasopharynx, and by dragging mucoelastic secretions from narrow meatal regions and sinus ostia.

Reduction of intranasal pressures by sniffs with partially collapsed alae draws air from the sinuses displacing mucus in proximity with the ostia into the nasal cavity. Snorts dislodge material from the postnasal region to the pharynx, where the nasally produced secretions and their contents are swallowed. Sinus ostia in the middle meatus are sheltered from the nasal mainstream and its noxious contents, but nose blowing, to expel accumulated secretion from the nasal cavities, risks forcing contaminated nasal contents into sinus cavities.

Simulations of nasal airways by models obtained from casts, from tomographic imaging, and generated by computer and the use of water with dyes and particles in place of air have advanced understanding of nasal air flow, but they have not accurately reproduced in vivo flow conditions. In addition to the complex structure of the bony and cartilaginous nasal skeleton, dimensions of the nasal lumen are determined by a dynamic mucovascular lining and, as discussed earlier in this chapter, in the compliant anterior nose by voluntary muscles and transmural respiratory air-flow pressures. Adjustments of the nasal lumen by erectile and alar tissues have not been reproduced in model studies, and normal septal contours, which include the substantial anterior septal body, have been largely ignored. These factors are of importance, since air-flow velocities, pressures, and resistances vary exponentially with cross-sectional areas, and relatively minor dimensional changes, especially in narrowed regions of the nose, can bring about major changes in air-flow parameters. Reproduction of these critical features by model studies has not yet been achieved.

Nasal Air-Flow Characteristics

The mode of distribution of air flow through the nasal cavities and its flow characteristics are crucial to effective cleansing, warming, and moistening, and to recovery processes.

During nasal breathing, ambient air streams converge as they are drawn into the nasal vestibule by inspiratory effort, and convergence promotes laminar flow through the narrow nasal valve (44). Spontaneous positioning of the labial orifice promotes a similar flow pattern during oral inspiration.

If this laminar flow regime persisted through the upper airways where, in many segments, the midstream is several millimeters from the mucosa, an insulating marginal lamina and absence of mixing would impede exchanges of heat, water, and contaminants between air stream and mucosa. Under such conditions, the burden of preparing inspiratory air for gaseous exchanges in the alveoli would fall on bronchial passages of a small cross-section (2-mm diameter in the 4th to 14th subdivisions), where small dimensions and reduced air-flow velocity enable exchanges between air and mucosa to take place under laminar flow conditions. The mucosa of these passages is less well adapted to withstanding hostile environmental exposures than mucosa of the upper air passages.

Fortunately, the unfavorable scenario described above does not prevail during nasal or spontaneous oral breathing. Laminar flow cannot persist beyond the nasal valve (or the labial orifice), except momentarily near the beginning and end of each inspiration. As inspiratory air leaves the narrow valvular region and enters the much larger cross-section of the cavum, its linear velocity, which is as great as 18 m/s in resting subjects, decelerates to 3–4 m/s (43). Deceleration releases kinetic energy ($E = kv^2$ where E = energy, k is a constant, and v represents linear velocity), which is dissipated in the generation of inertial disturbances that disrupt the insulating marginal lamina and promote mixing in the air stream. The disturbances are entrained to the bronchi, and are enhanced en route by frictional forces and irregularities of both lumen and flow velocity (45).

In addition to mass movement of air parallel with the walls of the respiratory passages, disturbances resulting from orifice flow and from frictional forces induce vigorous movement of air particles. As this movement increases with ventilation, the component of air particle velocities perpendicular to the airway walls increases also, and this component determines the effectiveness of exchanges between air stream and mucosa. Therefore, with increasing ventilation, increased disturbances compensate to some degree for decreased transit time through each airway segment, and nonlaminar flow approaches turbulence as disturbances are augmented by increased ventilation.

Respiratory Air Processing

As noted above, effective exchanges between air and mucosa require a disturbed pattern of respiratory air flow. Effectiveness of the exchanges, which include heat, water, and soluble and insoluble ambient air contaminants in both gaseous and particulate form, is dependent on the degree of flow disturbance. Greater penetration of incompletely processed ambient air that accompanies increased ventilation is partially offset, as already described, by increased inertial disturbance, mixing, and mucosal contact.

The nose is the principal site of particle deposition and absorption of soluble gaseous contaminants of inspiratory air. Particulates impinge (46) and are entrapped by surface mucus that is transported to the pharynx by ciliary action and swallowed. A portion of dissolved substances is absorbed into the tissues, and the remainder follows a similar route to that followed by insoluble particulates. Smaller particle size and lesser gaseous solubilities increase penetration of air contaminants.

Table 2
Inspiratory Air Temperature (°C)[a]

	Portal	Pharynx	Subglottis	Trachea	Carina
Nasal breathing	20	31	33	35	36
Tracheostomal breathing	20			30	32

[a]Warming of inspiratory air on its passage to the lungs during resting breathing. Oral inspirations achieve the same temperature at subglottic level as nasal inspirations when lips and mandible are spontaneously positioned. Conditioning of tracheostomal inspirations extend more deeply into the smaller air passages. Respiratory air rapidly achieves and maintains full saturation at all temperatures throughout the air passages.

Cleansing of ambient air and heat and water exchanges are substantial in either nasal or oral breathing passages *(45,47)*. Indeed, they are of similar extent when the mouth and labial orifice are spontaneously positioned, and they extend more deeply into the air passages during tracheostomal breathing (Table 2). However, neither nasal nor oral air conditioning is complete, and disturbed flow and processing continue in the large-diameter airways leading to the lungs. Thermal and aqueous equilibria are approached by the reduced velocity and close contact of the air stream with the enormous mucosal area of the smaller bronchi, and finally, inspiratory air mixes with the large volume of residual air that provides an additional buffer against incomplete conditioning *(47)*. Temperature of the peripheral air passages and of pulmonary blood is unaffected even by great extremes of ambient air temperature *(45,47)*, and thermal damage by these extremes is confined to the proximal airway mucosa.

On expiration, orifice flow, resulting from narrowing of the glottis, ensures disturbed flow, and as a consequence, convective exchanges between air and cooled mucosa bring about partial recovery of heat and water. Recovery takes place mainly in the nasal cavities, where the temperature gradient between expired air and cooled mucosa is greater than elsewhere in the respiratory passages, and the recovery process is much less effective in oral expiration.

Recovery of heat and water has survival value for many animal species in extreme habitats *(45)*, but it is not of great physiological importance to humans except in severely demanding circumstances, such as vigorous physical activities of polar hunters or high-altitude climbers. Complex turbinate structures with relatively large mucosal surface areas are found in several animal species *(1)* living in both Arctic and hot desert conditions,

and these features are related also to body surface insulation and to sweating *(48)*. Well-insulated and nonsweating animals tend to exhibit relatively large turbinate mucosal areas. Turbinate mucosal area of the seal (Fig. 1) exceeds its skin surface area, that of the sheep is similarly extensive, and turbinate area of the domestic cat exceeds that of the human adult *(1)* (Figs. 2 and 3).

As in the thermoregulatory regions of the skin of humans and animals (e.g., rabbits' ears), the vascular system of the nasal mucosa *(26,27)* is rich in arteriovenous shunts. These shunts and their blood flow are concerned with adjustment of skin and nasal mucosal temperature. In circumstances in which it is necessary to lose body heat, elevated blood flow elevates surface temperature. The increased temperature gradient between skin or mucosal surface and adjacent air increases heat (and water) loss. In circumstances in which heat (and water) needs to be retained, blood flow is appropriately decreased, resulting in decreased surface temperature and decreased heat loss. Thus, the nasal mucosa appropriately adjusts retention or release of heat (and water) in expiratory air as it leaves the body.

In humans, recovery approximates 30% in temperate conditions, and it increases to about 50% in Arctic conditions. Losses are much greater during oral or tracheostomal breathing, and also by pyrexial patients whose respiratory water loss may assume clinically important proportions. Recovery percentages are increased or decreased to meet the need for loss or retention of heat, and the ranges of these proportions are greatly extended in animals whose body surface insulation and turbinate mucosal areas are greater than in humans and whose ability to lose heat by sweating is less *(45,47)*.

There is no evidence to support the suggestion that nasal mucosal blood flow adjusts to rapid changes in the temperature of inspired ambient air as might occur as a subject moves from warm indoors to cold outdoors or the reverse. These circumstances are accommodated by extension of inspiratory air conditioning more or less deeply toward the peripheral airways, where an immense reserve of mucosal area is available to meet incompletely satisfied heat and moisture demands *(45)*.

Sinus Air Flow

The paranasal sinuses do not play a significant role in processing respiratory air and, by comparison with the nasal cavities, air flow through them is inconsequential. Sinus ostia in the middle meatus are sheltered from direct exposure to contamination and injury by ambient air. Fluctuations of nasal respiratory air flow pressures at resting ventilation approximate $<\pm100$ Pa (±1.0 cm H_2O) and displace air through patent ostia with each breath. This minute volume is supplemented by diffusion and the pumping effect of pulse wave pressures *(49,50)*. Greater pressures generated by increased ventilation, by nose blowing, and by vigorous sniffs against collapsed alae enhance exchanges of air between nasal and paranasal cavities, and also increase the risk of introducing noxious material.

There is exchange also between the air content of a sinus and its surface fluid by movement of gas molecules along vapor pressure gradients *(49,50)*. In the presence of obstructed ostia, gas diffusion can affect intrasinus pressures and result in a sensation of fullness, discomfort, or even pain.

Benefits of "aeration" of a diseased sinus by surgical creation of an artificial or an enlarged ostium probably result from equilibration of pressures between nasal and paranasal cavities, and improved drainage rather than from increased flow of air. It is of interest to note, however, that despite the creation of an artificial opening into the nose, patterns of mucociliary flow persist within the maxillary sinus, and trails of red cells tracking toward the natural ostium can be seen on sinus endoscopy.

Patency of the ostia is essential to the health of the paranasal sinuses, and the dangers of obstruction in the region of an ostium, e.g., by inflammatory disease of the nose or sinus, have been mentioned earlier in this chapter. Recent investigations have shown that in health, despite marked

physiological congestion of the nasal mucosa, by lateral recumbent postures, sinus ostia remain patent. Experiments with an intubated antrum (Haight and Cole, 1992, unpublished) showed ostial resistance to air flow to increase as a subject assumed ipsilateral recumbency from an upright position, and the resistance was decreased by assumption of the contralateral posture (*see also* Posture and Pressure Effects, earlier in this chapter). However, recording of antral air pressures demonstrated that they reflected freely the respiratory pressures in the nose in all postures, indicating that despite resistive mucosal changes, the maxillary ostium remained patent. It was undetermined whether the site of resistance changes was in the immediate ostial tissues or in adjacent tissues of the middle meatus.

CONCLUSIONS

The Nasal and Paranasal Sinus Cavities

A secretory mucosa and unobstructed mucociliary transport are essential to respiratory and olfactory functions of the nose, and to health of the nasal cavities and the paranasal sinuses. The ostiomeatal complex within the narrow cleft of the middle meatus is susceptible to obstructions of mucociliary flow from the sinuses. Mucosal swelling, polyps, and altered properties of secretion that result from common nasal disorders can impair mucociliary clearance, and sinus disease is a common consequence. Imaging studies have demonstrated that inflammatory nasal disease is frequently accompanied by sinusitis, and the converse has been verified in a large proportion of cases.

Nonlaminar characteristics of inspiratory air flow are induced by the constricted lumen of the nasal valve and entrained through the airways leading to the lungs. These characteristics are of essential physiological importance in that they promote cleansing and conditioning of ambient air, and thereby protect peripheral pulmonary air passages and their terminations from injury by ambient air. In addition, the human nose exhibits vestiges of a process of recovery of heat and water from expiratory air that is much more extensive and of survival value in animal species adapted to extreme environments. The paranasal sinuses do not make a significant contribution to the respiratory air processing that takes place in the nasal cavities.

REFERENCES*

1. Negus VE. The comparative anatomy and physiology of the nose and paranasal sinuses. London: Livingstone, 1958.
2. Gwaltney JM Jr, Phillips D, Miller RD, Riker DK. Computed tomographic study of the common cold. N Engl J Med 1994;330:25–30.
3. Kimmelman CP. The problem of nasal obstruction. Otolaryngol Clin North Am 1989;22(2):253–264.
4. Cole P. The Respiratory Role of the Upper Airways. St. Louis, MO: Mosby-Year Book, 1993; pp. 1–59.
5. Proetz AW. Air currents in the upper respiratory tract and their clinical importance. Ann Otol Rhinol Laryngol 1951;60:439–467.
6. McCaffrey TV. The nose and sinus mucosa and mucous. Curr Opinion Otolaryngol Head Neck Surg 1994;2:10–15.
7. Jorissen M, Cassiman J-J. Relevance of the ciliary ultrastructure in primary and secondary dyskinesia: a review. Am J Rhinol 1991;5(3):91–101.
8. Deitmer T, Scheffler R. The effects of different preparations of nasal decongestants on ciliary beat frequency in vitro. Rhinology 1993;31:151–153.
9. Stammberger H. Endoscopic endonasal surgery—concepts in treatment of recurring rhinosinusitis. Part 1. Anatomic and pathophysiolgic considerations. Otolaryngol Head Neck Surg 1986;94(2)143–147.
10. Messerklinger W. Diagnosis and endoscopic surgery of the nose and its adjoining structures. Acta Otolaryngol (Belg) 1980;34(2):170–176.
11. Cole P. The mouth and throat. In: The Respiratory Role of the Upper Airways. St. Louis, MO: Mosby-Year Book, 1993.
12. Cole P, Forsyth R, Haight JSJ. Respiratory resistance of the oral airway. Am Rev Respir Dis 1982;125:363–365.
13. Cole P. Assessment of the upper airways. In: The Respiratory Role of the Upper Airways. St. Louis, MO: Mosby-Year Book, 1993.
14. Rhinology 1995;33:10–13.
15. Kasperbauer JL, Kern EB. Nasal valve physiology implications in nasal surgery. Otolaryngol Clin North Am 1987;20(4):699–719.
16. Cole P, Haight JSJ, Cooper PW, Kassel EE. A computed tomographic study of nasal mucosa: effects of vasoactive substances. J Otolaryngol 1983;12(1):58.
17. Wustrow F. Schwellkorper am Septum nasi. Z Anat Entwicklung 1951;116:139.
18. Cole P, Haight JSJ, Naito K, Kucharczyk W. Magnetic resonance imaging of the nasal airways. Am J Rhinol 1989;3(2):63.
19. Chaban R, Cole P, Naito K. Simulated septal deviations. Arch Otolaryngol Head Neck Surg 1988;114:413.
20. Cole P, Chaban R, Naito K, Oprysk D. The obstructive nasal septum: effect of simulated deviations on nasal airflow resistance. Arch Otolaryngol Head Neck Surg 1988;114:410.

21. Mertz JS, McCaffrey TV, Kern EB. Objective evaluation of anterior septal surgical reconstruction. Otolaryngol Head Neck Surg 1984;92(3):308–311.
22. Briant TDR. Management of severe septal deformities. J Otolaryngol 1985;14(2):120–124.
23. Sulsenti G, Palma P. The nasal valve area: structure, function, clinics and treatment. Acta Otolaryngol Ital 1989;(Suppl 22):3–25.
24. Adamson P, Smith O, Cole P. The effect of cosmetic rhinoplasty on nasal patency. Laryngoscope 1990;100:357–359.
25. Batson OV. The venous networks of the nasal mucosa. Ann Otol Rhinol Laryngol 1954;63(3):571–580.
26. Cauna N. Blood and nerve supply of the nasal lining. In: Proctor DF, Andersen IB, eds., The Nose: Upper Airway Physiology and the Atmospheric Environment. Amsterdam: Elsevier Biomedical, 1982; pp. 45–69.
27. Bende M. The physiologic importance of the nasal mucosal vascular bed: a review. Am J Rhinol 1990;5:189–191.
28. Rundcrantz H. Postural variations of nasal patency. Acta Otolaryngol (Stockh) 1969;68:435–443.
29. Hasegawa M, Saito Y. Postural variations in nasal resistance and symptomatology in allergic rhinitis. Acta Otolaryngol 1979;88:268–272.
30. Erjefalt I, Persson CGA. Inflammatory passage of plasma macromolecules into airway wall and lumen. Pulmon Pharmacol 1989;2(2):93–102.
31. Cole P, Haight JSJ. Posture and the nasal cycle. Ann Otol Rhinol Laryngol 1986;95:233.
32. Stocksted P. Rhinometric measurements for determination of the nasal cycle. Acta Otolaryngol (Stockh) 1953;(Suppl 109):159–175.
33. Arbour P, Kern EB. Paradoxical nasal obstruction. Can J Otolaryngol 1975;4(2):333–338.
34. Ogura JH, Stocksted P. Rhinomanometry in some rhinologic diseases. Laryngoscope 1958;68:2001–2014.
35. Singh B, Chhina GA. Some reflections on ancient Indian physiology. In: Keswani NH, Manchandra SK, eds., The Science of Medicine and Physiological Concepts in Ancient and Mediaeval India. 26th International Congress of Physiological Sciences, New Delhi, 1974.
36. Shannahoff-Khalsa D. Lateralized rhythms of the central and autonomic nervous systems. Intern J Psychophysiol 1991;11(3):225–251.
37. Kayser R. Die exacta Messung der Luftdurchgangigkeit der Nase. Arch Laryngol Rhinol 1895;3:101–120.
38. Principato JJ, Ozenberger JM. Cyclical changes in nasal resistance. Arch Otolaryngol 1970;91:71–77.
39. Haight JSJ, Cole P. Unilateral nasal resistance and asymmetrical body pressures. J Otolaryngol 1986;Suppl 16:1–31.
40. Rothe CF. Reflex control of veins and vascular capacitance. Physiol Rev 1983;63(4):1281–1342.
41. Hudgel DW, Robertson DW. Nasal resistance during wakefulness and sleep in normal man. Acta Otolaryngol (Stockh) 1984;98:130–135.
42. Brown EA. Measurement of resistance of the nasal passages 1–3. Rev Allerg 1967;21:472–857.

*Several references in this list have been chosen for their own extensive reference lists which may be useful for readers who wish to refer to original work on which this chapter is based.

43. Swift DL, Proctor DF. Access of air to the respiratory tract. In: Brain D, Proctor DF, Reid LM, eds., Respiratory Defense Mechanisms. New York: Marcel Dekker, 1977; pp. 63–93.

44. Swift DL. Physical principles of airflow and transport phenomena influencing air modification. In: Proctor DF, Andersen I, eds., The Nose: Upper Airway Physiology and the Atmospheric Environment. Amsterdam: Elsevier Biomedical, 1982;337–348.

45. Cole P. Cleansing and conditioning. In: The Respiratory Role of the Upper Airways. St. Louis, MO: Mosby-Year Book, 1993.

46. Leopold DA. Pollution: The nose and sinuses. Otolaryngol Head Neck Surg 1992;106:713–719.

47. Cole P. Modification of inspired air. In: Mathew OP, Sant'Ambrogio G, eds., Respiratory Function of the Upper Airway. New York: Marcel Dekker, 1988.

48. Scott JH. Heat regulating function of the nasal mucous membrane. J Laryngol 1953;87:461,462.

49. Aust R, Falck B, Svanholm H. The intrinsic functions of the paranasal sinuses in health and inflammation. Rhinology 1984;22:105–107.

50. Drettner B. The maxillary ostium in sinusitis. Eye, Ear, Nose, Throat Monthly 1966;45:66–70.

3

Human Nasal Host Defense and Sinusitis

Michael A. Kaliner, MD

CONTENTS

INTRODUCTION

Sinusitis is an exceptionally common disorder, affecting an estimated 35 million Americans per year. The development of sinusitis requires both the presence of a virulent pathogen and obstruction of the normal drainage pattern from the sinus cavities. Moreover, the development of chronic or recurrent sinusitis indicates a failure of the local immune system to prevent or effectively combat the infection. Identification of the components of the upper respiratory immune defense system and the possible areas of dysfunction that predispose to sinusitis may be important steps in eventually preventing this common disease.

The nasal and sinus passages are lined by respiratory mucous membranes. Recent studies have identified some of the constituents found in mucus and their roles in human health and disease. However, the local immune system of the respiratory mucosa is largely unknown, and its role in sinusitis is conjectural.

From: *Diseases of the Sinuses* (M. E. Gershwin and G. A. Incaudo, eds.), ©1996 Humana Press Inc., Totowa, NJ.

Nasal secretions include many proteins that serve important functions in local mucosal host-defense. Most of these host-defense molecules are synthesized and secreted by serous cells in the submucous glands, and it appears that the serous cell is the resident antimicrobial cell in mucous membranes. Current data suggest that serous cell secretion is abnormal in patients with recurrent sinusitis and that effective treatment leads to correction of the secretory abnormality along with improvement in sinusitis.

THE HUMAN NASAL MUCOUS MEMBRANE

Mucous membranes are named for their capacity to generate mucus. Respiratory mucous membranes begin at the nasal vestibule, and continue through the nose, pharynx, larynx, trachea, bronchi, and bronchioles. Nasal airway secretions and their constituent proteins derive from epithelial cells (including goblet cells), submucosal glands (including both serous and mucous cells), blood vessels, and secretory cells resident in the mucosa (including plasma cells, mast cells, lymphocytes,

Table 1
Constituents of Human Nasal Secretions[a]

Mucous cell products
    Mucous glycoproteins
Serous cell products
    Lactoferrin
    Lysozyme
    Secretory IgA and secretory component
    Neutral endopeptidase
    Aminopeptidase
    Uric acid
    Peroxidase
    Secretory leukoprotease inhibitor
Plasma proteins
    Albumin
    Immunoglobulins—IgG, IgA (monomeric), IgM, IgE
    Carboxypeptidase N
    Angiotensin-converting enzyme
    Kallikrein
Indeterminate sources:
    Calcitonin gene-related peptide
    Urea
    Substance P

[a]Modified from ref. 30.

and fibroblasts). Respiratory secretions consist of a mixture of mucous glycoproteins, glandular products, and plasma proteins (1) (Table 1). Baseline, resting secretions include the following major proteins: albumin (representing about 15% of total protein), IgG (2–4%), secretory IgA (15%), lactoferrin (2–4%), lysozyme (15–30%), nonsecretory IgA (about 1%), IgM (<1%), secretory leukoprotease inhibitor (10%), and mucous glycoproteins (about 10–15%) (2).

Careful immunohistochemical analysis has shown that plasma proteins, such as albumin and IgG, are found throughout the lamina propria of the mucosa, with an apparent increased concentration at the basement membrane (3). Some albumin can also be found staining submucosal gland lumens and tracking between epithelial cells, presumably being exported toward the airway lumen. By contrast, staining for lysozyme, lactoferrin, and S-IgA is seen exclusively in the serous cells, serous crescents, and ducts of the submucosal cells (4,5). More recently, several enzymes important in metabolizing neuropeptides have also been localized to the serous cells (6). Neutral endopeptidase, which metabolizes substance P and endothelin as well as other neuropeptides, is also found in glands, as well as in the nasal epithelium and in the endot-

helium of small blood vessels. Not only is neutral endopeptidase localized to serous cells, but NEP is also secreted in response to a variety of stimuli.

THE CONSTITUENTS OF HUMAN NASAL SECRETIONS AND THEIR FUNCTIONS

Epithelial Lining Fluid

The secretory blanket consists of two separable layers; the surface mucous (or gel) layer and a deeper aqueous (or serous, periciliary) layer in which the base of the cilia are located. The concept of a two-layered epithelial lining fluid (ELF) is quite old, dating back more than 50 years. In the nose, particles trapped in the surface mucous layer are transported by mucociliary action to the posterior pharynx at the rate of 1 cm/min. The surface mucous blanket is then swallowed and is constantly being replaced, about every 10–20 min under resting conditions. Analysis of lavage proteins indicates that only about 15% of the total protein is attributable to mucous glycoproteins (MGP), although this figure fails to take into account that MGP is at least 80% carbohydrate (7). Thus, the mucous blanket of MGP is secreted constantly, and is constantly removed and replaced. This rapid turnover contributes to the barrier functions of the mucous blanket. Microorganisms and particulate materials are trapped in the mucus and passively removed by these processes. The blanket is selective, since large particles never reach the mucous membrane, whereas smaller molecules do, and are readily absorbed. Thus, the mucous layer is a selective sieve.

The layer on which the mucus floats and in which the cilia beat is the periciliary or serous layer. Based on recently completed experiments, this layer of fluid appears to follow very different kinetics than does the mucous blanket. This periciliary fluid (PCF) contains most of the aqueous proteins listed in Table 1, many of which derive from the serous cells of the submucous glands. The proteins within the PCF partially reconstitute themselves within 10–20 min after repeated lavages, and may require 4–24 h before achieving resting concentrations (8). The anterior portion of the nose is lined by about 100 µL of ELF, whereas each nostril is lined by 800 µL of PCF. The PCF does not turnover quickly, and the stability of this layer of fluid may provide many of the protective functions of secretions in host defense.

Table 2
Molar Concentration of Proteins in Nasal Secretions[a]

	Baseline	Histamine stimulated	Methacholine stimulated
Albumin	0.76 μM	96.6 μM	0.59 μM
IGG	0.22 μM	27.6 μM	0.38 μM

[a]Modified from ref. 8.

Table 3
Roles and Functions of Human Nasal Secretions[a]

Protective functions
    Antioxidant (uric acid)
    Humidification
    Lubrication
    Waterproofing
    Insulation
    Provide proper medium for ciliary actions
Barrier functions
    Macromolecular sieve
    Entrapment of microorganisms and particulates
    Transport and elimination of entrapped materials
Host-defense functions
    Extracellular source of IgA/IgG
    Extracellular site for multiple enzyme actions
    Antimicrobial functions
        Lysozyme
        Lactoferrin
        IgA/IgG
        Rapid deployment of multiple plasma proteins

[a]Modified from ref. 30.

The capacity actually to measure the PCF employing quantitation of secretory and plasma urea levels allows calculation of the actual molar concentrations of proteins in nasal secretions (Table 2). It appears that this two-layered design of the ELF provides a superficial mucous blanket that traps and exports foreign materials away from the mucous membrane and a stable aqueous PCF in which molecules providing important host-defense functions may be concentrated.

Mucous Glycoproteins

Table 1 lists the major proteins and other molecules found in nasal secretions. It is clear that this complex mixture of molecules serves a variety of functions. Our current understanding of the roles and functions of respiratory secretions is summarized in Table 3. Because the mucous membrane has no keratin layer to protect it from various exoge-

nous stresses, mucus provides many of the protective functions of the outer layer of skin. Because of the large size of the MGP molecule (200–400,000 Dalton) and capacity to polymerize extensively into a size greater than 2,000,000 Dalton (7), MGP provides a replaceable, flexible, continuous extracellular surface, coating and protecting the mucous membranes. This gelatinous layer insulates the epithelium, waterproofs it by trapping an aqueous layer beneath it, lubricates the surface, and humidifies the inspired air. Each MGP molecule absorbs water of hydration onto itself, providing a generous source of humidification for inspired air. Temperature transfer through the airway secretions to inspired air is facilitated by the gel-like structure of mucus, which allows for a gradual transfer of heat to inspired air, while protecting the underlying mucosa from excessive cooling.

HOST-DEFENSE FUNCTIONS OF HUMAN RESPIRATORY SECRETIONS

Inspiration of toxic or infectious materials deposits these potential pathogens onto the mucous blanket of the nose. The effectiveness of nasal secretions to neutralize or eliminate potentially harmful pathogens is evident by the relative health that most of us enjoy as an ordinary part of life.

Immunoglobulins

The major specific mediators of host defense in secretions are the immunoglobulins. IgA and IgG are the major immunoglobulins in secretions, and they appear to act quite differently. IgG is a plasma protein that is distributed in the nasal mucosa by microvascular permeability. IgG is found diffusely throughout the mucosa, but in highest concentration near the basement membrane (9). Analysis of IgG-producing plasma cells reveals that about 25% of the plasma cells in the human nasal mucosa produce IgG, whereas the remainder are IgA-producing (9). IgA is produced locally by plasma cells located within 50 μm of submucous glands. The locally produced IgA is dimeric, being joined by a J chain before secretion. Dimeric IgA binds to secretory component produced by serous cells and forms secretory IgA. S-IgA is transported transcellularly through the serous cells into glandular secretions and becomes a glandular secretory product. S-IgA acts primarily by binding microorganisms in the airway lumen and preventing attachment of these potential pathogens to the mucosa.

By contrast, IgG acts primarily in the mucosa itself to limit invasion by microorganisms that reach the epithelium. Although IgG is present in secretions (about 2–4% of total protein in baseline secretions), it is found in a much higher concentration in the tissue fluid itself. IgG levels in secretions are increased up to 125 times by the process of vascular permeability (Table 2). Thus, one could reason that one purpose of acute inflammation is to bathe the mucosa in an IgG-rich secretion.

The nonspecific antimicrobial properties of mucus and the presence of normal amounts of IgG must compensate adequately for the functions of S-IgA, since most IgA-deficient patients are generally asymptomatic, suffering from a normal incidence of infections. By contrast, patients deficient in IgG or unable to synthesize new IgG after exposure to pathogens usually require medical help because of recurring respiratory infections. It therefore appears that the protective functions served in the mucosa by IgG are of greater importance in preventing the development of respiratory infections than is S-IgA.

Lysozyme and Lactoferrin

There are several nonspecific antimicrobial proteins in nasal secretions that have broad-spectrum antimicrobial actions. Lysozyme is a relatively small protein (14,000 Dalton) found in all body secretions. Fleming discovered lysozyme in human nasal secretions while searching for molecules capable of killing bacteria (10). He recognized that lysozyme killed most bacteria found in the air, but only some bacteria that ordinarily reside on the mucosa. Thus, lysozyme, which represents 15–30% of the protein normally found in nasal secretions, effectively prevents mucosal infections from most airborne bacteria. Lysozyme is synthesized and secreted by the serous cell of the submucosal gland.

Lactoferrin is another antimicrobial protein made by serous cells that is both bacteriostatic and bacteriocidal to susceptible bacteria (11). Lactoferrin binds iron, and it is presumably this action that kills bacteria. Lactoferrin constitutes about 2–4% of nasal proteins.

There are multiple specific and nonspecific antimicrobial factors in human plasma. Processes that lead to increased microvascular permeability cause the outpouring of plasma proteins into the nasal mucosa and then into nasal secretions. The increased volume of secretions may lead to clearance of particulate materials, as well as the availability of increased amounts of IgG, albumin (which may nonspecifically bind particulate materials), and other plasma proteins. It has been suggested that this outpouring of plasma proteins might represent the first line of host defense at mucosal surfaces (12).

REGULATION OF HUMAN NASAL SECRETIONS

Adrenergic and Cholinergic Control

After washing the nose to remove existing secretions, the relative amounts of proteins in nasal secretions are remarkably reproducible from patient to patient. However, initial washes reveal remarkable variability, probably reflecting the concentration of ELF over time. The innervation of the nose includes parasympathetic nerves that innervate the glands and vascular bed, sympathetic nerves that innervate the vascular bed, and sensory nerves that originate in the epithelium and arborize to include the vascular beds and glands (13). Parasympathetic nerves are the major motor nerves in the nose. Stimulation of parasympathetic nerves leads to increased secretions, whereas addition of cholinomimetics onto the nasal mucosa or initiation of oral gustatory reflexes also leads to secretions (5,14). Parasympathetic stimulation causes secretions enriched for the glandular proteins (Table 4), although plasma proteins are also included in these secretions.

When the relative amounts of proteins in secretions are determined by dividing the individual protein by the total protein concentration, a figure is generated that has been termed the "protein" percent. Cholinergic stimulation of glandular secretion may change the relative percent of lysozyme in secretions from 15–20 up to 30%; lactoferrin from 2–4% to 8%; and S-IgA from 15 to 25%. The plasma proteins found in glandular secretions do not change. Thus, albumin remains at 15% of total protein and IgG at 2–4%.

Adrenergic stimulation of the mucosa either has no effect on secretions (β adrenergic stimulation) or mildly stimulates glandular secretions (α adrenergic stimulation) (15). The effects of adrenergic stimulation have been studied both in vivo and in vitro with similar findings (15).

Table 4
Nasal Secretory Responses[a]

Protein	Stimulation	Response
Plasma proteins	Parasympathetic	+
Glandular proteins		+++
Ipsilateral	Histamine or allergen challenge	
Plasma proteins		++++
Glandular proteins		+
Contralateral		
Plasma proteins		+
Glandular proteins		+++
Early phase	Upper respiratory infection	
Plasma proteins		++++
Glandular proteins		+
Later stage		
Plasma proteins		+
Glandular proteins		+++

[a]Modified from ref. 30.

Neuropeptides

Sensory nerves contain several associated neuropeptides, including CGRP, GRP, SP, and NKA (16). The distribution of these neuropeptides has been carefully studied in the nasal mucosa by immunohistochemistry. Of the sensory nerves, all have some fibers apparently innervating submucosal glands. However, CGRP and GRP (as well as the parasympathetic neuropeptide VIP) are most evident in regard to glandular innervation (17–19). The presence of neuropeptide receptors was examined in the nasal mucosa by binding 125-I-labeled neuropeptides to their binding sites. It was found that GRP had the most intense binding to glands, whereas both VIP and SP also had gland receptors (20). The capacity of these neuropeptides to cause mucous and serous cell secretion of specific products has been examined in vitro employing human nasal turbinates in short-term culture. GRP and VIP were the most potent stimuli for glandular secretion, although both SP and NKA had some activity as well. These data are summarized in ref. (2).

Bradykinin is a mediator generated by action of the plasma or tissue enzyme kallikrein on the substrate kininogen. Bradykinin has been found in nasal secretions (21) and has its receptors exclusively on blood vessels (22). Topical application onto the mucosa results in secretions rich in vascular proteins and is also associated with increased nasal blood flow (23).

Table 5
Chronic Conditions that Predispose to Sinusitis

Anatomic abnormality
Allergic and nonallergic rhinitis
Cystic fibrosis
Common variable immunoglobulin deficiency
IgG subclass deficiency
IgA deficiency (especially when combined with IgG deficiency)
Ciliary dyskinesia, Kartagener's syndrome, Young's syndrome
Aspirin sensitivity
Acquired Immunodeficiency Syndrome
Bronchiectasis
Rhinitis Medicamentosa
Cocaine abuse
Wegener's granulomatosis

ABNORMALITIES ASSOCIATED WITH SINUSITIS

Secretory Abnormalities

Sinusitis may occur in otherwise normal individuals or the likelihood of developing sinusitis may be increased in association with the conditions listed in Table 5. Appropriate evaluations to exclude these underlying problems are appropriate in subjects with chronic sinusitis or frequently recurring disease. One recent study evaluated the capacity of patients with recurrent sinusitis (two or more episodes for two or more years) to respond appropriately to topical methacholine or histamine challenge, evaluating the constituents of the nasal secretions that resulted (24). Several distinct abnormalities were discovered. Baseline washing of sinusitis patients had an abnormally high concentration of the glandular proteins lysozyme and lactoferrin in relation to total protein, suggesting that glands were being driven to secrete excessively in the chronically inflamed patient. Conversely, these same patients were unable to respond to cholinergic stimulation with a glandular response. The magnitude of the response included blunted secretion of glandular products as well as the passively transported plasma proteins ordinarily seen in glandular secretions. The abnormal secretory response was restricted to cholinergic reactions, since these patients responded normally to histamine stimulation with increased vascular permeability and glandular secretion. Thus, the glands were likely to have been exposed chronically to cholinergic stimu-

Table 6
An Approach to the Treatment of Persistent Sinusitis[a]

Hydration (6–8 glasses of water/d)
Antibiotics for 21 d or longer (rule of thumb: use antibiotic of choice until the patient is well plus 7 d)
Topical long-acting decongestants, bid for 2–3 wk
Nasal douche with saline, employing an ear bulb syringe or Waterpik plus a Grossan adapter
Topical corticosteroids (employing dexacort turbinaire as an example)
    3 Sprays bid for 2 wk
    2 Sprays bid, for 2 wk or longer
    1–2 Sprays bid, until sinusitis is resolved or to prevent recurrence

[a]This approach is used only after unsuccessful treatment of sinusitis with more conventional approaches, such as decongestants and antibiotics, has failed.

lation, and therefore were unable to respond to additional cholinergic stimulation, but were still responsive to histamine-mediated responses. These data suggested the possibility that the glandular abnormality might have contributed to the disease by an inability of affected subjects to produce secretions rich in antimicrobial factors necessary to combat new or recurrent insults.

This suggestion was enhanced by the findings after effective treatment. Most of the patients received therapy as described in Table 6. After resolution of their sinusitis, they were restudied with the same provocations. Not only did the patients improve clinically, but their baseline and stimulated secretory responses also returned to normal.

Another recent investigation indirectly adds support to the concept that nasal secretions help control mucosal infections. In a collaborative study conducted at the University of Pittsburgh, patients were experimentally infected with rhinovirus and nasal secretions collected during the course of ensuing URI (25). Of interest, the initial response was found to consist almost exclusively of increased vascular permeability lasting 2 d into the infection. Secretions thereafter became enriched with glandular proteins as the URI resolved. Our interpretation of these data is that the acute inflammatory response causes the generation of vasoactive amines, such as bradykinin, which cause the vascular response. However, as the initial inflammatory response matures, glandular secretion is stimulated, either by cholinergic or peptidenergic mechanisms. The antimicrobial-enriched secre-

tions combine with local immune responses in the mucosa to clear the infection.

Nasal Mucosal Cellular Immunity

The process of identifying the cells that occupy the human nasal mucosa is just under way (26). In the 200 μm beneath the epithelium in normal individuals, the predominant cell is the lymphocyte. Most of the lymphocytes are CD4+, and there is a predominance of CD4+:CD8+ cells. On average, there are about 168 CD3+ lymphocytes/1000 μm of basement membrane. Of these, 117 are CD4+, and 46 are CD8+. There are also macrophages (16/mm of basement membrane) and plasma cells (27/mm of membrane). About 10 mast cells/mm are also seen, overwhelmingly of the MC_{tc} type. The changes that occur in these populations of cells in patients with acute or chronic sinusitis are currently under investigation. Few publications describe the sinus mucosa, although one electron microscopic examination details a spectrum of changes ranging to extreme squamous metaplasia (27). Another study describes desquamation of columnar cells, squamous metaplasia, and frank exfoliation (28). Basement membrane thickening and mucosal edema were also noted, along with focal infiltration with eosinophils in the areas of greatest damage. About half of the samples stained for the presence of major basic protein, most marked in patients who had concomitant asthma. These findings suggested to the authors that chronic sinusitis resembled some of the findings seen in the airways of asthmatics, and that the eosinophil might be playing a role in chronic sinusitis as well (28).

Evaluation of the Immune Status of Patients with Chronic Sinusitis

One of the main issues facing physicians in practice is when and how to evaluate the immunocompetence of a patient with sinusitis. Patients with occasional sinusitis need not be evaluated beyond the careful examination for anatomical abnormalities and the presence of allergic rhinitis. However, if the patient has either chronic or recurring sinusitis (more than two episodes per year for two or more years [24]), then the evaluation of immunocompetence is warranted. The approach we recommend is to obtain quantitative immunoglobulins and a pre- and postimmunization titer to Pneumovax and Haemophilus influenzae B complex, as well as Tetanus toxoid. These immunizations provide an IgG_2, IgG_1, and IgG_1 recall response, respectively. Thus, rather than measure subclasses of IgG, we recommend a more functional response, actually looking at IgG_1 and IgG_2 responses to relevant antigens. As a side benefit, the patient is immunized to *Streptococcus pneumoniae* and *H. influenzae* as part of the procedure, perhaps increasing their resistance to subsequent infections. This procedure takes into account that many of the *H. influenzae* infections are nonencapsulated and that the *H. influenzae* employed for the antigen preparation is encapsulated.

In addition to measuring antibody responses, a CD4:CD8 ratio can be obtained, as can an erythrocyte sedimentation rate. We routinely measure the time it takes to taste a drop of saccharine placed on the inferior turbinate in order to access ciliary function clinically. Anatomical abnormalities are assessed by anterior rhinoscopy, flexible or rigid rhinoscope, or coronal CT scans. The possible presence of allergic disease is suggested by the history, and confirmed by the physical examination and the responses to prick or intradermal skin tests. Although abnormal cellular immunity can predispose to viral infections, sinusitis is generally associated with abnormal humoral immunity. In fact, common variable immunoglobulin deficiency presents as sinusitis or sinusitis and bronchitis 100% of the time.

SUMMARY AND CONCLUSIONS

Human respiratory secretions serve many critical functions, both protecting the mucosa and providing essential host-defense roles. It appears that the serous cell in the submucosal glands is the source of most of the protective proteins that prevent infections of the mucosa. Although glandular secretions are an essential product of the mucosa, secretions are also derived from the vascular bed as a result of increased vascular permeability. These secretions can be recognized by a relative enrichment with vascular proteins, such as albumin and IgG. Analysis of secretory responses to topical histamine *(3)*, allergen challenge *(29)*, and in the first few days after an experimentally induced upper respiratory tract infection *(25)* reveals that vascular permeability is the underlying mechanism responsible. Thus, in those circumstances in which patients complain most commonly of increased secretions (as during a cold or in response to aller-

gen exposure), it is really increased vascular permeability, and not glandular secretions, that is responsible. The proteins increased in secretions as a consequence of increased vascular permeability include IgG, IgM, IgA, albumin, and many other plasma proteins. These proteins mediate both specific (IgG) and nonspecific (albumin) antimicrobial functions.

The sum results of stimulating nasal secretion are the outpouring of fluids capable of preventing or limiting infections, neutralizing toxic materials that may impact on the secretions, and elimination of particulate materials that are trapped. Most humans have a limited number of viral infections and fleetingly few bacterial infections of their respiratory mucosa, speaking eloquently of the effectiveness of the host-defense mechanisms involved. In patients with recurrent sinusitis, cholinergic responses are abnormal, resulting in the limited capacity to secrete mucus. There are data that the sinus epithelium in patients with chronic sinusitis is infiltrated with eosinophils and that these cells may be involved in the chronic inflammatory nature of the disease. In otherwise normal individuals, we have no knowledge of mucosal defects that might predispose to sinus disease. In fact, we really have an extraordinarily limited fund of knowledge about cellular immunity in the upper respiratory tract, despite the obvious clinical importance of rhinitis and sinusitis.

REFERENCES

1. Kaliner M, Shelhamer JH, Borson B, Nadel J, Patow C, Marom Z. Human respiratory mucus. Am Rev Respir Dis 1986;134:612–621.
2. Raphael GD, Baraniuk JN, Kaliner MA. How the nose runs and why. J Allergy Clin Immunol 1991;87:457–467.
3. Raphael GD, Meredith SD, Baraniuk JN, Druce HM, Banks SM, Kaliner MA. The pathophysiology of rhinitis. II. Assessment of the sources of protein in histamine-induced nasal secretions. Am Rev Respir Dis 1989;139:791–800.
4. Raphael GD, Jeney EV, Baraniuk JN, Kim I, Meredith SD, Kaliner MA. The pathophysiology of rhinitis: lactoferrin and lysozyme in nasal secretions. J Clin Invest 1989;84:1528–1536.
5. Raphael GD, Druce HM, Baraniuk JN, Kaliner MA. Pathophysiology of rhinitis. 1. Assessment of the sources of protein in methacholine-induced nasal secretions. Am Rev Respir Dis 1898;138:413–420.
6. Ohkubo K, Baraniuk J, Hohman RJ, Kaulbach HC, Hausfield JN, Merida M, Kaliner MA. Human nasal mucosal neutral endopeptidase (NEP): location, quantitation and secretion. Am J Respir Cell Mol Biol 1993;9:557–567.

7. Patow CA, Shelhamer J, Marom Z, Logun C, Kaliner M. Analysis of human nasal mucous glycoproteins. Am. J. Otolaryngol. 1984;5:334–343.

8. Kaulbach HC, White MV, Igarashi Y, Hahn BK, Kaliner MA. Estimation of nasal epithelial lining fluid using urea as a marker. J Allergy Clin Immunol 1993;92:457–465.

9. Meredith SD, Raphael GD, Baraniuk JN, Banks SM, Kaliner MA. The pathogenesis of rhinitis. III. The control of IgG secretion. J Allergy Clin Immunol 1989;84:920–930.

10. Fleming A. On a remarkable bacteriolytic element found in tissues and secretions. Proc Royal Soc Lond B Biol Sci 1922;93:306–317.

11. Masson PI, Heremans JF, Dive CH. An iron binding protein common to many external secretions. Clin Chim Act 1966;14:735–739.

12. Persson CGA, Erejefalt I, Alkner U, Baumgarten C, Grieff L, Gustafsson B, Luts A, Pipkorn UM, Sundler F, Svensson C, Wollmer P. Plasma exudation as a first line respiratory mucosal defense. Clin Exp Allergy 1991;21: 17–24.

13. Raphael GD, Meredith SD, Baraniuk JN, Kaliner MA. Nasal reflexes. Am J Rhinol 1988;2:109–116.

14. Raphael GD, Hauptschein-Raphael M, Kaliner M. Gustatory rhinitis: a syndrome of food induced rhinorrhea. J Allergy Clin Immunol 1989;83:110–114.

15. Mullol J, Raphael GD, Lundgren JD, Baraniuk JN, Merida M, Shelhamer JH, Kaliner MA. Comparison of human nasal mucosal secretion *in vivo* and *in vitro*. J Appl Physiol 1992;89:684–693.

16. Baraniuk JN, Kaliner MA. Neuropeptides in the upper and lower respiratory tracts. In: Bierman CW and Lee TH, eds., Immunology and Allergy Clinics of North America, Vol. 10, no. 2. Philadelphia: WB Saunders, 1990; pp. 383–408.

17. Baraniuk JN, Lundgren JD, Goff J, Mullol J, Castellino S, Merida M, Shelhamer JH, Kaliner MA. Calcitonin gene related peptide in human nasal mucosa. J Appl Physiol 1990;258:81–88.

18. Baraniuk JN, Lundgren JD, Goff J, Peden D, Merida M, Shelhamer J, Kaliner M. Gastrin releasing peptide (GRP) in human nasal mucosa. J Clin Invest 1990;85:998–1005.

19. Baraniuk JN, Lundgren JD, Okayama M, Mullol J, Merida M, Shelhamer JH, Kaliner MA. Vasoactive intestinal peptide (VIP) in human nasal mucosa. J Clin Invest 1990;86:825–831.

20. Baraniuk JN, Lundgren JD, Okayama M, Goff J, Mullol J, Merida M, Shelhamer JH, Kaliner MA. Substance P and neurokinin A in human nasal mucosa. Am J Respir Cell Mol Biol 1991;4:228–236.

21. Proud D, Baumgartin CR, Naclerio RM, Ward PE. Kinin metabolism in human nasal secretions during experimentally induced allergic rhinitis. J Immunol 1987;138: 428–434.

22. Baraniuk JN, Lundgren JD, Mizoguchi H, Peden D, Gawin A, Merida M, Shelhamer JH, Kaliner MA. Bradykinin and respiratory mucous membranes: analyses of bradykinin binding site distribution and secretory responses in vitro and in vivo. Am Rev Respir Dis 1990;141:706–714.

23. Holmberg K, Bake B, Pipkorn U, Vascular effects of topically applied bradykinin on the human nasal mucosa. Eur J Pharmacol 1990;175:35–41.

24. Jeney EV, Raphael GD, Meredith SD, Kaliner MA. Abnormal cholinergic responsiveness in the nasal mucosa of patients with recurrent sinusitis. J Allergy Clin Immunol 1990;86:10–18.

25. Igarashi Y, Skoner DP, Doyle WJ, White MV, Fireman P, Kaliner MA. Analysis of nasal secretions during experimental rhinovirus upper respiratory infections. J Allergy Clin Immunol 1993;92:722–732.

26. Igarashi Y, Kaliner MA, Hausfeld JN, Irani AMA, Schwartz LB, White MV. Quantification of inflammatory cells in the nasal mucosa. J Allergy Clin Immunol 1993;91:1082-1093.

27. Ohashi Y, Nakai Y. Functional and morphological pathology of chronic sinusitis mucous membrane. Acta Otolaryngol Suppl 1983;397:11–48.

28. Harlin SL, Ansel DG, Lane SR, Myers J, Kephart GM, Gleich GJ. A clinical and pathologic study of chronic sinusitis: the role of the eosinophil. J Allergy Clin Immunol. 1988;81:867–875.

29. Raphael GD, Igarashi Y, White MV, Kaliner MA. The pathophysiology of rhinitis. V. Sources of protein in allergen-induced nasal secretions. J Allergy Clin Immunol 1991;88:33–42.

30. Kaliner MA. Human nasal respiratory secretions and host defense. Am Rev Resp Dis 1991;144:S52–66.

PART
II IMAGING

4   Imaging Techniques

*Conventional Radiography, Computed Tomography,
Magnetic Resonance, and Ultrasonography
of the Paranasal Sinuses*

Mark L. Benson, MD, *Patrick J. Oliverio,* MD,
and S. James Zinreich, MD

CONTENTS

INTRODUCTION

It is estimated that up to 30 million people suffer from inflammatory sinus disease in the United States *(1)*. Because the physical examination can be nonspecific in these patients, radiologic evaluation has been relied upon for many years in the diagnosis of paranasal sinus pathology. Traditionally, conventional radiography was the modality of choice in the evaluation of the paranasal sinuses. In recent years, however, owing to a change in the therapeutic approach, computed tomography has supplanted conventional radiography as the primary diagnostic modality.

Although most patients are medically treated, medical therapy alone often does not resolve the problem. As a result of an improved understanding of the mucociliary clearance mechanisms in the

nasal cavity and paranasal sinuses, improved endoscopes, and the availability of coronal CT images, functional endoscopic sinus surgery was introduced in the United States in 1984. The surgeon, with the use of endoscopes, can directly visualize the surface mucosa within the nose and ethmoid sinuses. However, given the small area occupied by the ethmoid sinuses and their relationship to critical structures, such as the orbit and the intracranial compartment, the radiographic image is actively used to guide the surgeon's approach and to avoid serious complications.

The objective of this presentation is to: discuss the available imaging modalities and techniques, display radiographic anatomy of the paranasal sinuses and adjacent structures, show the more common anatomic variations, discuss the radiographic appearance of frequently encountered pathologies of the paranasal sinuses, and to review the expected radiographic appearance in postop-

From: *Diseases of the Sinuses* (M. E. Gershwin and G. A. Incaudo, eds.),
©1996 Humana Press Inc., Totowa, NJ.

erative patients as well as the appearance of complications that can occur as a result of therapy.

TECHNIQUES OF EVALUATION

Conventional Radiography

The standard radiographic sinus series consists of four views: lateral view, Caldwell view, Waters view, and submentovertex (SMV or base) view *(2)*. The lateral view demonstrates the frontal, maxillary, and sphenoid sinus. It is obtained 5° off the true lateral position in order to avoid superimposition of the posterior walls of the maxillary sinuses. The Caldwell view displays the frontal sinuses and posterior ethmoid air cells. It is obtained in the posteroanterior (PA) projection with 15° of caudal angulation of the X-ray beam. The Waters view is useful to visualize the maxillary sinuses, anterior ethmoid air cells, and orbital floors. It is obtained in the PA projection with the neck in 33° of extension. The submentovertex view can evaluate the sphenoid sinus as well as the anterior and posterior walls of the frontal sinuses. It is obtained in anteroposterior (AP) projection with the head in 90° of extension.

Even though conventional radiographs can depict the changes of acute sinusitis in the maxillary, frontal, and sphenoid sinuses, they cannot delineate the status of the individual ethmoid air cells or the ostiomeatal unit, nor can they accurately show the extent of inflammatory disease in these patients *(3–7)*.

Computed Tomography (CT)

CT is currently the modality of choice in the evaluation of the paranasal sinuses and adjacent structures *(3–7)*. Its ability to optimally display bone, soft tissue, and air facilitates accurate depiction of anatomy and extent of disease in and around the paranasal sinuses *(3–7)*. Axial imaging is important in the evaluation of trauma and sinus neoplasms. In patients with inflammatory disease, imaging in the coronal plane is preferred as the initial screening technique. The coronal plane optimally displays the ostiomeatal unit, the relationship of the brain and ethmoid roof, and it depicts the relationship of the orbits to the paranasal sinuses *(3–7)*. Coronal images correlate with the surgical approach and, therefore, should be obtained in patients with inflammatory sinus disease who are surgical candidates *(7)*.

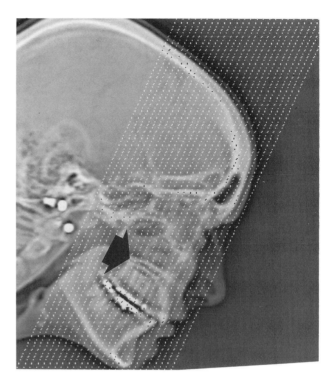

Fig. 1. CT lateral topogram reveals the patients position during the examination. Dotted lines represent scanner gantry angulation, which should be as perpendicular as possible to the hard palate (arrow).

In evaluating the sinuses, the patient is prone with the chin hyperextended on the bed of the CT scanner. The scanner gantry is angled to be as perpendicular as possible to the hard palate (Fig. 1). Scanning is performed from the anterior frontal sinus posteriorly through the sphenoid sinus (Fig. 2). Contiguous 3mm thick images are obtained. The field of view is adjusted to include only the areas of interest. This helps reduce artifact from the teeth and associated metallic restorations, as well as magnifying the small structures of the nasal cavity and adjacent paranasal sinuses *(4)*. Windows are chosen to highlight the air passages, the bony detail, and the soft tissues. Our experience shows that a window width of +2000 Houndsfield Units (HU) with a level of –200 HU is the best starting point. The potentiometers can then be manually manipulated to display optimally the anatomic detail of the uncinate process and ethmoid bulla. This same setting is then used to film the entire study *(3–7)*.

Sagittal reconstructions can be obtained for a morphologic orientation. Various distances and angles can be measured to aid in the passage of instruments during surgery on these views. Axial

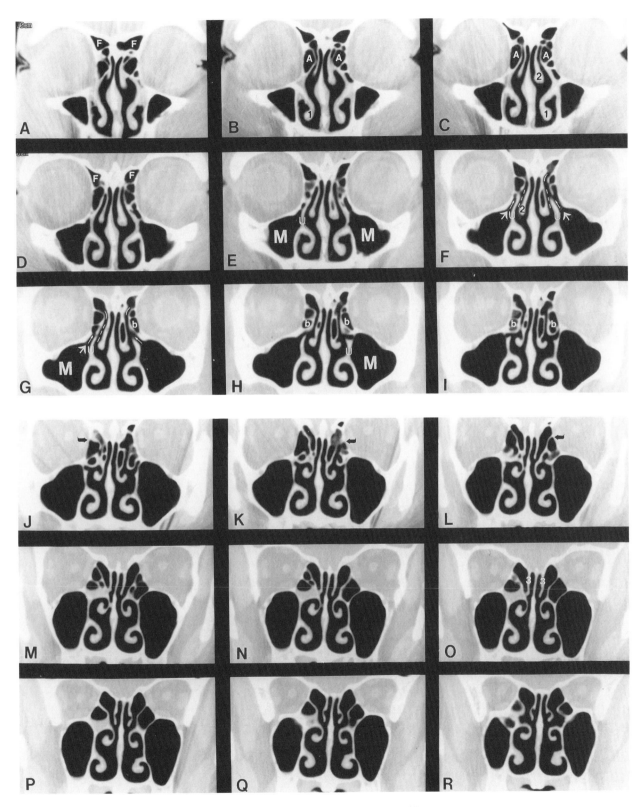

Fig. 2. (A-AA) Coronal CT display of paranasal sinus anatomy. Frontal sinus (F), agger nasi cell (A), ethmoid bulla (b), maxillary sinus (M), basal lamella (black arrow), sphenoid sinus (S), inferior turbinate (1), middle turbinate (2), superior turbinate (3). The anterior ostiomeatal unit is displayed as images F-H: frontal recess (small curved line), middle meatus (dashed line), infundibulum (small arrow), and primary ostium of the maxillary sinus (large white arrow).

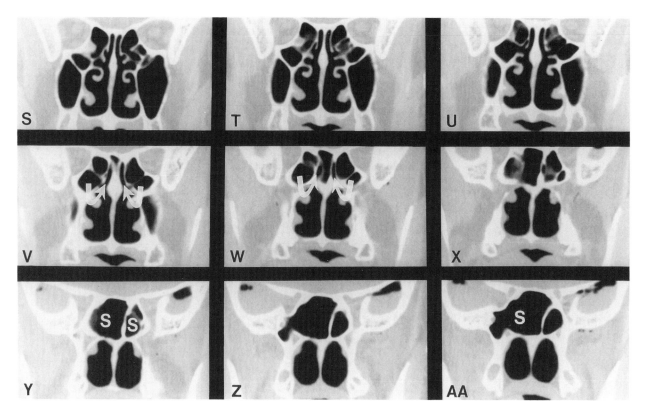

Fig. 2. *(continued)* The sphenoethmoidal recess (curved white arrow) is best demonstrated on images V and W.

reconstructions can be helpful in displaying the position of the internal carotid arteries with respect to the bony margins of the sphenoid sinus.

In patients who cannot tolerate prone positioning (children, patients in advanced age), the "hanging head" technique can be used with the patient in the supine position and the neck maximally extended. A pillow placed under the patients shoulders helps their positioning. The CT gantry is angled to be as perpendicular as possible to the bony palate. It is not always possible to obtain direct coronal images. In patients who are intubated or have tracheostomy sites, it is not technically feasible to position them for coronal scans. Young children, patients with severe cervical arthropathy, and patients who are otherwise debilitated usually will not tolerate the examination. In such patients, thin section, contiguous axial images with coronal reconstructions are performed.

Many authors stress the importance of performing the initial CT scan after a course of treatment with antibiotics and decongestants to eliminate changes of acute sinusitis and to better evaluate the underlying anatomic structures. Several authors

suggest routine pretreatment with a sympathomimetic nasal spray 15 min prior to scanning to reduce nasal congestion *(8)*. This will minimize the mucosal edema and will allow an improved display of the fine bony architecture.

Magnetic Resonance (MR) Imaging

To date, MR imaging in the paranasal sinuses has proven helpful in the evaluation of regional and intracranial complications of inflammatory sinus disease and surgical treatment, detection of neoplastic processes, and an improved display of anatomic relationships between the intra- and extraorbital compartment. The superior soft tissue contrast and the lack of beam hardening artifact define MR imaging as the modality of choice in the evaluation of processes involving the skull base and intracranial compartment. Although MR imaging provides better visualization of soft tissue than CT *(4,5)*, it is not well suited for routine evaluation of the paranasal sinuses. Cortical bone and air yield no MR signal and thus are not depicted on the images. Furthermore, the signal intensity of the mucosal lining during the edematous phase of the nasal cycle is similar to the appearance of mucosal inflammation *(9)*. Although inflammation of the mucosa gives very bright signal intensity on T2 weighted images, neoplastic processes usually are of intermediate increased signal intensity on T2 weighted images.

When evaluating the paranasal sinuses with MR imaging, our standard protocol includes sagittal and axial T1-weighted images (T1WI) and axial T2-weighted images (T2WI). Following the iv administration of Gadolinium-diethylenetriaminepentaacetic acid (DTPA), we obtain axial and coronal T1WI.

Ultrasonography

In the late 1970s and early 1980s, several authors evaluated ultrasonography as a possible adjunct to conventional radiography in the diagnosis of inflammatory sinus disease *(10–13)*. Both A-mode and gray scale B-mode techniques were studied. Although ultrasonography can detect loss of aeration in the maxillary sinus, it cannot reliably visualize the other paranasal sinuses or bony structures, or adequately characterize the underlying pathologic process. With the advent of high-resolution CT scanners coupled with their widespread availability, there now is little clinical utility for ultrasonography in the paranasal sinuses.

NORMAL ANATOMY AND ANATOMIC VARIATIONS

Normal Anatomy

It is essential to the understanding of sinus pathology to be acquainted with the concept that inflammatory sinus disease is largely the result of compromise of the drainage portals (ostiomeatal channels) of the individual sinus cavities. The radiologic representation of the anatomy should stress display of the ostiomeatal channels. These aerated channels provide air flow to and mucociliary clearance from the frontal, maxillary, ethmoid, and sphenoid sinuses *(3–7)*. The term ostiomeatal unit (OMU) refers to the air passages affording communication between the frontal, anterior ethmoid, and maxillary sinuses. The components of the OMU include the ethmoid infundibulum, hiatus semilunaris, middle meatus, and frontal recess *(3–7,14,15)*. It therefore provides communication between the anterior ethmoid sinus and the frontal and maxillary sinuses (Figs. 2 and 3).

An understanding of the anatomy of the lateral nasal wall and its relationship to adjacent struc-

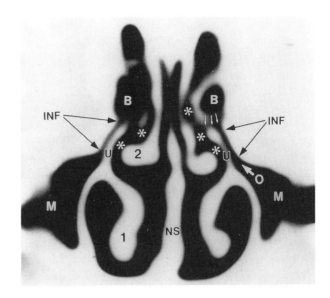

Fig. 3. Normal anatomy of the ostiomeatal unit as seen on CT. The infundibulum (INF) is delimited inferiorly by the maxillary sinus ostium (o), medially by the uncinate process (u), superiorly by the ethmoidal bulla (B), and laterally by the inferomedial orbit. The air space surrounding the ethmoidal bulla inferoposteriorly is the hiatus semilunaris (small arrows). Also identified are the middle meati (*), inferior turbinate (1), middle turbinate (2), maxillary sinuses (M), and nasal septum (NS).

tures is essential *(14,16)*. The lateral nasal wall contains three bulbous projections: the superior, middle, and inferior turbinates (conchae) (Figs. 2 and 3). The turbinates serve to divide the nasal cavity into three distinct air passages: the superior, middle, and inferior meati. The superior meatus drains the posterior ethmoid air cells and, more posteriorly, the sphenoid sinus (via the sphenoethmoidal recess). The middle meatus receives drainage from the frontal sinus (via the nasofrontal recess), maxillary sinus (via the maxillary ostium and subsequently the ethmoidal infundibulum), and the anterior ethmoid air cells (via the ethmoid cell ostia). The inferior meatus receives drainage from the nasolacrimal duct. This structure is usually identifiable on coronal sections. A complete series of thin-section, coronal CT scans of the sinuses is provided in Fig. 2.

On CT scanning, the first coronal images display the outline of the frontal sinuses. The frontal recess is an hourglass-like narrowing between the frontal sinus and the anterior middle meatus through which the frontal sinus drains *(3)*. It is not a tubular structure, as the term nasofrontal duct might imply, and therefore the term recess is preferred. Anterior, lateral, and inferior to the frontal recess is the agger nasi cell, an aerated cavity that represents the most anterior ethmoid air cell. It usually borders the primary ostium/floor of the frontal sinus, and thus, its size may directly influence the patency of the frontal recess and the anterior middle meatus. The frontal recesses are the narrowest anterior air channels and are common sites of inflammation. Their obstruction subsequently results in loss of ventilation and mucociliary clearance of the frontal sinus.

The uncinate process is a superior extension of the lateral nasal wall (medial wall of the maxillary sinus) (3–5). Anteriorly, the uncinate process fuses with the medial wall of the agger nasi cell and the posteromedial wall of the nasolacrimal duct. The uncinate process has a "free" (unattached) superoposterior edge. Laterally, this free edge delimits the infundibulum, and posterior to it is the ethmoid bulla, usually the largest of the anterior ethmoid cells. The ethmoid bulla is enclosed laterally by the lamina papyracea. The gap between the ethmoid bulla and the "free" edge of the uncinate process defines the hiatus semilunaris. Medially, the hiatus semilunaris communicates with the middle meatus, the air space lateral to the middle turbinate (Figs. 2 and 3) (3–5).

Laterally and inferiorly, the hiatus semilunaris communicates with the infundibulum, the air channel between the uncinate process and the inferomedial border of the orbit. The infundibulum serves as the primary drainage pathway from the maxillary sinus (5,6).

The structure medial to the ethmoid bulla and the uncinate process is the middle turbinate. Anteriorly, it attaches to the medial wall of the agger nasi cell and the superior edge of the uncinate process. Superiorly, the middle turbinate adheres to the cribriform plate. As it extends posteriorly, the middle turbinate emits a laterally coursing bony structure, the basal or ground lamella, that fuses with the lamina papyracea just posterior to the ethmoid bulla. In most patients, the posterior wall of the ethmoid bulla is intact, and an air space is usually found between the ground lamella and the ethmoid bulla. This air space, the sinus lateralis, may extend superior to the ethmoid bulla and communicate with the frontal recess. A dehiscence or total absence of the posterior wall of the ethmoid bulla is common and may provide communication between these two usually separated air spaces. The poste-

rior ethmoid sinus consists of air cells between the basal lamella and the sphenoid sinus. The number, shape, and size of these air cells vary significantly from person to person (3,4,6,17).

The sphenoid sinus is the most posterior sinus. It is usually embedded into the clivus and bordered superoposteriorly by the sella turcica. Its ostium is usually in the anterosuperior portion of the anterior sinus wall, and the sinus drains via the sphenoethmoidal recess into the posterior aspect of the superior meatus. The sphenoethmoidal recess lies just lateral to the nasal septum and can sometimes be seen on coronal images, but is best displayed in the sagittal and axial planes (3–5).

The relationship between the aerated portion of the sphenoid sinus and the posterior ethmoid sinus needs to be accurately represented, so the surgeon can avoid operative complications. Usually in the paramedian sagittal plane, the sphenoid sinus is the most superior and posterior air space. More laterally (1–1.5 cm), the sphenoid sinus is located more inferiorly, and the posterior ethmoid air cells become the most superior and posterior air space. This relationship is well demonstrated on axial images. The number and position of the septations of the sphenoid sinus are quite variable. Some of these septations can adhere to the bony wall covering the internal carotid artery, which can frequently penetrate into the sphenoid sinus.

Anatomically, the paranasal sinuses are in close proximity to the anterior cranial fossa, cribriform plate, internal carotid arteries, cavernous sinuses, the orbits and their contents, and the optic nerves as they exit the orbits (18–22). The surgeon must be cautious when maneuvering instrumentation in the posterior direction to avoid inadvertent penetration and drainage of these structures (6,7,19,20).

Anatomic Variants

Even though the nasal anatomy varies significantly from patient to patient, certain anatomic variations are observed more commonly in the general population and appear more frequently with chronic inflammatory disease (3–5,7,23,24). The significance of a particular anatomic variant is determined by its relationship with the major ethmoidal and nasal air passages. The ability of the variant to narrow or obstruct the air passages implies a role in the recurrence of sinusitis. In our experience, the most common variations are as follows (3–5,7,16,24).

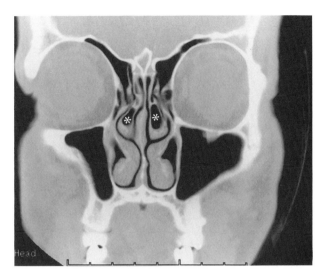

Fig. 4. Direct coronal CT scan shows bilateral conchae bullosa (*). This noninvasive radiologic examination affords a detailed view of the internal architecture of this aerated turbinate.

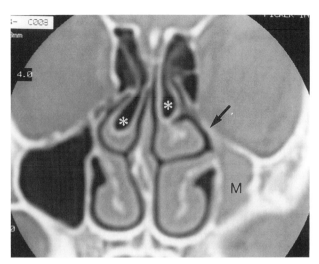

Fig. 5. Direct coronal CT scan shows marked deviation of the bony nasal septum (open white arrow). The OMU pattern of sinusitis is present with inflammatory changes obstructing the middle meati bilaterally (*) with resulting disease in the maxillary and anterior ethmoid sinuses. Air–fluid levels (black arrows) in the maxillary sinuses signify acute sinusitis.

Concha Bullosa

An aerated middle turbinate that may enlarge to obstruct the middle meatus or even the infundibulum. The concha bullosa may be unilateral and/or bilateral. Less frequently, aeration of the superior turbinate may also occur. Aeration of the inferior turbinate is infrequent. The air cavity in a concha bullosa is lined with the same epithelium as the rest of the nasal cavity, and thus these cells can suffer the same inflammatory disorders experienced in the paranasal sinuses (Figs. 4 and 5).

Nasal Septal Deviation
with or without Surgery

This is an asymmetric bowing of the nasal septum that may compress the middle turbinate laterally, narrowing the middle meatus (Figs. 6 and 7). Bony spurs are often associated with septal deviation and this may compromise the OMU.

Paradoxical Middle Turbinate

Here, the middle turbinate has its major curvature projected laterally, whereas in most people, its major curvature is toward the septum, and this can also narrow the middle meatus.

Variation in the Uncinate Process

The course of the "free edge" of the uncinate process has several variations. In most cases, it either extends slightly obliquely toward the nasal septum with the free edge surrounding the infe-

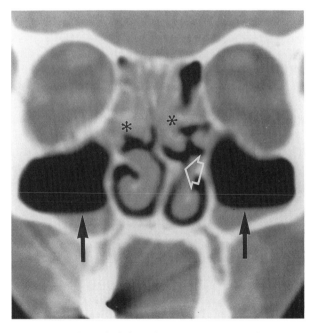

Fig. 6. An atelectatic left uncinate process. The "free edge" of the left uncinate process adheres to the left orbital floor (arrows). Note the resulting opacification of the hypoplastic left maxillary sinus (M). Bilateral conchae bullosa are present (*).

rior/anterior surface of the ethmoid bulla or it extends more medially to the medial surface of the ethmoid bulla (Figs. 2 and 3).

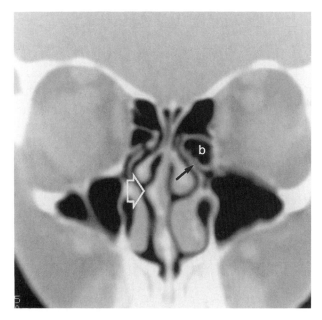

Fig. 7. Prominent left ethmoid bulla (b). This results in narrowing of the left infundibulum (arrow). Also noted is a deviated nasal septum (open white arrow).

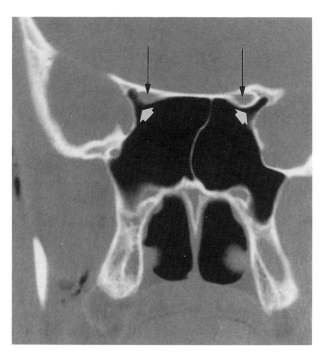

Fig. 8. Extensive pneumatization of the sphenoid sinus. Direct coronal CT shows superolateral pneumatization (white arrows) surrounding much of the optic nerves (black arrows).

Sometimes, the "free edge" of the uncinate is noted to adhere to the orbital floor/inferior aspect of the lamina papyracea. This is referred to as an "atelectatic uncinate process" (Fig. 5). This variant is usually associated with opacification of the ipsilateral maxillary sinus owing to closure of the infundibulum.

If the "free edge" deviates laterally, there can be obstruction of the infundibulum. Less frequently, we have encountered "medial curling" of the uncinate, which will encroach on the middle meatus.

HALLER CELLS

These are ethmoid air cells that extend along the roof of the maxillary sinus. They may contribute to narrowing of the infundibulum.

ONODI CELLS

These are lateral and posterior extensions of the posterior ethmoid air cells. They extend the paranasal sinus cavity to a very close proximity to the optic nerves as they exit the orbits. These "cells" may surround the optic nerve tract and put the nerve at risk during surgery. In our experience, Onodi cells are rare.

PROMINENT ETHMOID BULLA

The largest of the ethmoid air cells, it may enlarge to narrow or obstruct the middle meatus and infundibulum (Fig. 7).

PROMINENT AGGER NASI CELLS

Extensive aeration of these, the most anterior of the ethmoid air cells, can result in obstruction of the frontal recess.

EXTENSIVE PNEUMATIZATION OF THE SPHENOID SINUS

Pneumatization of the sphenoid sinus can extend into the anterior clinoids. This variation may put the optic nerves at increased risk during surgical exploration (Fig. 8).

DEHISCENCE OF THE LAMINA PAPYRACEA

This may be a congenital finding or can be the result of prior facial trauma. In either case, loss of this bony boundary of the paranasal sinuses puts the intraorbital contents at risk, because it is very difficult to differentiate inflamed mucosa from the orbital soft tissues during surgery.

AERATED CRISTA GALLI

Aeration of this normally bony structure can occur. When aerated, these cells may communicate with the frontal recess. Obstruction of this ostium can lead to chronic sinusitis and mucocoele formation.

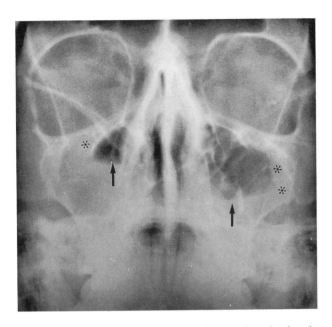

Fig. 9. Acute sinusitis superimposed open chronic sinusitis. Waters view shows air–fluid level in both maxillary sinuses (black arrows) indicative of acute sinusitis. Chronic sinusitis is manifested by bilateral mucoperiosteal thickening (*).

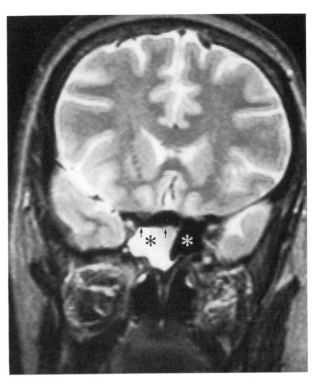

Fig. 10. Acute right sphenoid sinusitis. Coronal T2WI shows hyperintense signal within right side of sphenoid sinus (black *) with associated air–fluid level (small black arrows). Note the normally aerated left sphenoid sinus (white *).

RADIOGRAPHIC APPEARANCES OF SINUS PATHOLOGY

Inflammatory Disease

ACUTE SINUSITIS

Acute sinusitis is usually the result of bacterial superinfection of an obstructed paranasal sinus. The obstruction is often the result of apposition of edematous mucosal surfaces from an antecedent viral upper respiratory tract infection. The edema disrupts the normal mucociliary drainage pattern of the sinus, and obstruction of the sinus ostium results. The accumulation of fluid within the sinus predisposes to a bacterial superinfection. The bacterial pathogens most often responsible include *Streptococcus pneumoniae, Haemophilus influenzae, β Hemolytic streptococcus,* and *Moraxella catarrhalis (25–27).* Acute sinusitis is only rarely the result of a pure viral infection. Acute sinusitis usually only involves a single sinus, with the ethmoid sinus being the most common location *(23,26).* There is an increased risk of regional and intracranial complications with involvement of the frontal, ethmoid , and sphenoid sinuses *(23).*

Radiographically, the hallmark of acute sinusitis is an air–fluid level (Figs. 5, 9, and 10). However, the radiologic findings in acute sinusitis may be nonspecific with smooth or nodular mucosal thickening or complete opacification of the sinus (Fig. 11). On MR imaging, the findings are those of watery secretions with hypointense signal on T1WI and hyperintense signal on T2WI (Fig. 10).

It should be noted that an air–fluid level is not a pathognomonic sign of acute sinusitis. This finding is mimicked by acute blood within the sinus in patients with a history of recent trauma.

CHRONIC SINUSITIS

Chronic sinusitis is diagnosed when the patient has repeated bouts of acute infection or persistent inflammation *(23,26).* The responsible pathogens include *Staphylococcus, Streptococcus, Corynebacteria, Bacteroides, Fusobacteria,* and other anaerobes *(25).* Anaerobes are more commonly involved in chronic sinusitis than in acute sinusitis *(23,28).* The radiographic findings are quite variable (Figs. 9 and 11). Signs suggestive of chronic sinusitis include mucosal thickening or opacification, bone remodeling and thickening owing to

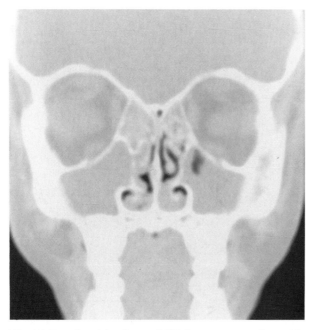

Fig. 11. Pansinusitis. Coronal CT shows near total opacification of maxillary and ethmoid sinuses. This finding can be seen with acute or chronic sinusitis.

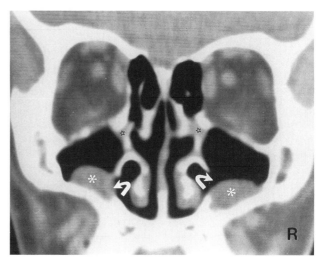

Fig. 12. Infundibular pattern of sinusitis. Coronal CT shows opacification of the infundibulum bilaterally (stars). Mucous retention cysts (*) are present in the maxillary sinuses bilaterally. This patient has previously undergone bilateral nasal antrostomies (curved arrows).

osteitis from adjacent chronic mucosal inflammation, and polyposis *(26,28,29)*. The anterior ethmoid air cells are the most common location involved with chronic sinusitis.

Opacification of the OMU has been found to predispose to the development of sinusitis (Fig. 5). Zinreich et al. found middle meatus opacification in 72% of patients with chronic sinusitis *(6)*. In this study, 65% of these patients had mucoperiosteal thickening of the maxillary sinus *(30)*. All of the patients with frontal sinus inflammatory disease had opacification of the frontoethmoidal recess *(30)*. Frontal sinus opacification involving the OMU without frontal, maxillary, or anterior ethmoid sinus inflammatory disease was rare *(30)*. Yousem et al. found that, when the middle meatus was opacified, there were associated inflammatory changes in the ethmoid sinuses in 82% and in the maxillary sinuses in 84% of patients *(31)*. Bolger et al. found that, when the ethmoid infundibulum was free of disease, the maxillary and frontal sinuses were clear in 77% of patients *(25)*.

Babbel et al. reviewed 500 patients with screening sinus CT scans and defined five recurring patterns of inflammatory sinonasal disease *(32)*. The five anatomic patterns are: infundibular, OMU, sphenoethmoidal recess, sinonasal polyposis, and sporadic or unclassifiable. The infundibular pattern (26% of patients) referred to focal obstruction within the maxillary sinus ostium and ethmoid infundibulum, which was associated with maxillary sinus disease (Fig. 12). The OMU pattern (25% of patients) referred to ipsilateral maxillary, frontal, and anterior ethmoid sinus disease (Fig. 5). This pattern was owing to obstruction of the middle meatus. Sparing of the frontal sinus was sometimes seen owing to the variable location of the nasofrontal duct insertion in the middle meatus. The sphenoethmoidal recess pattern (6% of patients) resulted in sphenoid or posterior ethmoid sinus inflammation resulting from sphenoethmoidal recess obstruction. The sinonasal polyposis pattern (10% of patients) was the result of diffuse nasal and paranasal sinus polyps. Associated radiographic findings included infundibular enlargement, convex (bulging) ethmoid sinus walls, and attenuation of the bony nasal septum and ethmoid trabeculae *(8,32,33)*.

When sinus secretions are acute and of low viscosity, they are of intermediate attenuation on CT images (10–25 HU) (Fig. 5). In the more chronic state, sinus secretions become thickened and concentrated, and the CT attenuation increases with density measurements of 30–60 HU *(34)*.

On MR imaging, the appearance of chronic sinusitis is quite variable because of the changing concentrations of protein and free water protons *(34)*. Initially, the watery secretions appear on MR imaging as hypointense on T1WI and hyperintense on T2WI (Fig. 10) *(34,35)*. According to Som and Curtin, when sinonasal secretions become obstructed, two important physiologic events occur. Namely, the number of glycoprotein-secreting goblet cells in the mucosa increases, and the mucosa resorbs free water. This results in a transition from a thin serous fluid, to a thicker mucus, and ultimately to a desiccated stone-like plug *(34)*. As the protein concentration increases, the signal intensity on T2WI decreases. These charges are presumably owing to crosslinking that occurs between glycoprotein molecules. Som describes four patterns of MR signal intensity that can be seen with chronic sinusitis:

1. Hypointense on T1WI and hyperintense on T2WI with protein concentration <9%;
2. Hyperintense on T1WI and hyperintense on T2WI with total protein concentration increased to 20–25%;
3. Hyperintense on T1WI and hypointense on T2WI with total protein concentration of 25–30%; and
4. Hypointense on T1WI and T2WI with protein concentration >30% and inspissated secretions in an almost solid form *(34,36)*.

A potential pitfall exists on MR imaging of inspissated secretions (i.e., those with protein concentrations over 30%) since the signal voids on T1WI and T2WI may look identical to normally aerated sinuses *(34,35)*.

Certain anatomic variants, as described above, have been implicated as causative factors in the presence of chronic inflammatory disease. Stammberger and Wolfe *(37)* and Lidov and Som *(38)* found that a large concha bullosa can produce signs and symptoms by narrowing the infundibulum. However, Yousem et al. *(31)* found that the presence of a concha bullosa did not increase the risk of sinusitis. This was corroborated by Bolger et al., who found that the presence of a concha bullosa, paradoxical turbinates, Haller cells, and uncinate pneumatization was not significantly more common in patients with chronic sinusitis than in asymptomatic patients *(25)*. Yousem et al. found the presence of nasal septal deviation and a horizontally oriented uncinate process was more common in patients with inflammatory sinusitis *(3)*. Although the presence of these variants may not necessarily predispose to sinusitis, it appears that the size of a given anatomic

variant and its relationship to adjacent structures plays an important role in the development of sinusitis *(17)*.

FUNGAL SINUSITIS

Fungal sinusitis may be suspected clinically when the patient fails to respond to standard antibiotic therapy. Although fungal infection in the paranasal sinuses is uncommon, the fungal pathogens most commonly encountered are *Aspergillus*, *Mucormycosis*, and *Candida* species *(17,39)*. Although *Mucormycosis* and *Aspergillus* are both part of the normal respiratory flora *(23)*, their involvement in the paranasal sinuses can often be differentiated on clinical grounds. *Aspergillus* sinusitis usually occurs in an otherwise healthy patient in a noninvasive, saprophytic form. Allergic fungal sinusitis is usually seen in patients with a history of atopy and/or asthma. There is an association between this entity and marked nasal and sinus polyposis. This process may expand the sinuses bordering the orbits, thus causing proptosis or optic nerve compression *(40)*. The invasive form of *aspergillus* infection can occur in immunocompromised hosts *(23)*. The involvement is much more extensive than that seen in the allergic or saprophytic forms, and deep extension into the mucosa and bone often occurs.

Mucormycosis is caused by various genera *(Rhizopus, Mucor, Absidia)* of the family Mucoraceae. Spores of these organisms are ubiquitous in our environment, and organisms are part of the normal respiratory flora *(41)*. Infection only occurs in immunocompromised hosts, with poorly control diabetics accounting for 50–75% of cases *(42)*.

On imaging (Fig. 13), the presence of an air–fluid level is uncommon. The maxillary and ethmoid sinuses are the most common sites of involvement *(34)*. The imaging findings are quite variable depending on the aggressiveness of the fungus. Nonspecific mucosal thickening or sinus opacification may occur. The allergic form of aspergillus is associated with recurrent sinonasal polyps. With more invasive fungi, sinus opacification with a central mycetoma and associated bony thickening or erosion may occur *(34)*. With both *Mucormycosis* and invasive *Aspergillus*, vascular invasion may occur, which leads to intra- and extracranial thrombosis and infarction.

Several imaging characteristics are suggestive of fungal sinusitis. On CT, a focal hyperdense lesion

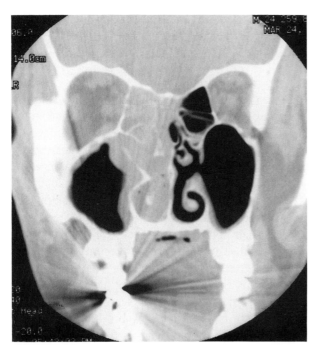

Fig. 13. Aspergillus sinusitis. Coronal CT shows opacification of the right nasal cavity and ethmoid sinus with early erosive changes of the adjacent bony structures.

may be seen with surrounding hypodense mucoid material. On MR imaging, low signal intensity on T1WI and a signal void on T2WI have been found in a high proportion of patients with fungal sinusitis (43). This is thought to be the result of the presence of paramagnetic metals (iron and manganese) (13,43). Even though a similar MR appearance can be seen in chronic bacterial infection owing to desiccated secretions, the decreased signal is not as pronounced as that found with fungal disease (13).

According to Som, two other circumstances can be seen that can suggest the presence of fungal infections (34,35). Soft tissue changes in the sinus with thickened, reactive bone and localized areas of osteomyelitis. Also suggestive of fungal infection is the association of inflammatory sinus disease with involvement of the adjacent nasal fossa and the soft tissues of the cheek. These signs of aggressive infection are atypical for bacterial pathogens (34,35).

ALLERGIC SINUSITIS

Allergic sinusitis occurs in 10% of the population (14). It typically produces a pansinusitis with symmetrical involvement (32). CT often shows a nodular mucosal thickening with thickened turbi-

nates (14). Air fluid levels are rare unless bacterial superinfection occurs (32).

GRANULOMATOUS SINUSITIS

Although many granulomatous diseases can involve the sinonasal cavity, Wegener's granulomatosis and idiopathic midline granuloma are the most commonly encountered.

Wegener's granulomatosis is a necrotizing granulomatous vasculitis of unknown etiology. It may present as a localized or systemic form. The sinonasal region is involved in 64–80% of patients (21). CT endings in sinonasal involvement are often nonspecific, but typically there is a nodular soft tissue Pacification or mucosal thickening with sclerosis of the thicker bones of the involved sinus and destruction of the thinner septa (14). Nasal septal perforation may be one of the first distinguishing features in an otherwise nonspecific chronic inflammatory process (41). The maxillary sinus is the most common sinus involved (14). Sphenoid sinus disease, in particular, can spread to the cavernous sinus, orbital apex, and optic canal.

Idiopathic midline granulomas are a group of diseases that are chronic necrotizing inflammatory disorders, now recognized as being part of the lymphoma spectrum (30). Clinical and radiological manifestations in the paranasal region are similar to Wegener's granulomatosis. The radiographic hallmark is a destructive mass in the nasal septum (14).

Complications of Inflammatory Sinus Disease

MUCOUS RETENTION CYST

This is a small cyst that most commonly occurs in the maxillary sinus floor in patients with a history of previous inflammatory disease. It occurs in 10% of the population. It is the result of inflammatory obstruction of a seromucinous gland within the sinus mucosal lining (14,23). On CT, this will appear as a homogenous, well-circumscribed hypo- to isodense mass (Fig. 12). On MR imaging, it is usually hypointense on T1WI and hyperintense on T2WI.

MUCOCELE

This is a dilated mucus-filled sinus that is lined by mucous membrane. It is the result of a chronically obstructed sinus ostium with resulting enlargement of bony walls owing to mucus secretions filling the sinus cavity (33,34). It is most commonly caused by inflammatory obstruction of the ostium, but can also be secondary to trauma, tumors, or

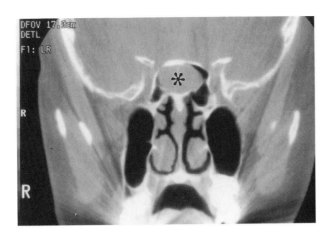

Fig. 14. Posterior ethmoid mucocele. Coronal CT shows a well-defined expansile lesion in the posterior ethmoid sinus (*).

surgical manipulation *(33)*. Sixty-six percent of mucoceles occur in the frontal sinuses with 25 and 10% occurring in the ethmoid and maxillary sinuses, respectively *(23)*. On CT, this will appear as a hypodense, nonenhancing mass that fills and expands the sinus cavity (Fig. 14). On MR imaging, the appearance is variable owing to alterations in protein concentration of the obstructed mucoid secretions. An infected mucocele, a mucopyocele, may demonstrate rim enhancement *(32)*.

INFLAMMATORY POLYPS

Polyps in the paranasal sinuses result from a local upheaval of the sinus mucosa with mucous membrane hyperplasia secondary to chronic inflammation *(32,44)*. Allergic sinusitis often plays a role in the formation of polyps. If large or numerous, polyps can cause local problems because of obstruction of the important ostiomeatal channels, including the sinus ostia. On CT and MR imaging, polyps are often indistinguishable from mucous retention cysts *(44)*.

ORBITAL COMPLICATIONS

About 3% of patients with sinusitis will have some form of orbital involvement, more commonly in children, and orbital manifestations may be the first sign of sinus infection *(16,41)*. Complicated sinusitis is the most common cause of orbital infection with 60–84% of cases attributed to it *(15,18,45)*. The ethmoid sinuses are the most common origin, with frontal, sphenoid, and maxillary sinuses in decreasing order of frequency. The ethmoid and maxillary sinus are present at birth and therefore

are the source in younger children. The frontal sinuses are usually detectable radiographically after 6 yr, but are not usually significant sources of infection until after 10 yr. The sphenoid sinuses likewise develop late and are rarely implicated in the pediatric age group *(16)*.

Most authors recommend obtaining a CT when there is clinical evidence of postseptal infection (i.e., when proptosis and limitation of eye movement are present) or when there is failure to improve with antibiotics *(14,33,46)*. Since the disease can be much more aggressive in the pediatric population, a CT should be considered when there is clinical evidence of preseptal inflammation.

Preseptal orbital edema is a common finding with sinusitis, especially in children. CT reveals diffuse soft tissue density and thickening of the preseptal soft tissues. At this stage, there is swelling and redness of the eyelids, but no proptosis or limitation of eye movement. As infection spreads from the ethmoid sinus to the orbit, there is inflammation of the orbital periosteum. This becomes thickened and elevated, with accumulation of an inflammatory phlegmon. On CT, this appears as an ill-defined, slightly enhancing mass on the sinus and orbital sides of the lamina papyracea. It is limited laterally by the periosteum. However, in more advanced cases, it merges with a thickened and enhancing medial rectus muscle, which is displaced laterally. Subsequently, liquefaction may occur in the subperiosteal compartment to form an abscess. This will be evident on CT as regions of low density, sometimes with an enhancing rim (Fig. 15). The CT finding of low attenuation material surrounded by an enhancing rim suggests the diagnosis of abscess rather than a phlegmon, though the distinction between them can be difficult, given the continuum existing between these two states.

Rare orbital complications of paranasal sinus infection include superior ophthalmic vein (SOV) thrombosis, cavernous sinus thrombosis, and blindness. SOV thrombosis is suspected on CT scans when there is asymmetric enlargement of this vessel (best seen on coronal scans) with relative lack of normal enhancement, though thrombus within the lumen can be hyperdense. MR may demonstrate these changes more accurately. Magnetic resonance angiography (MRA), especially phase-contrast techniques, can establish the presence of SOV thrombosis.

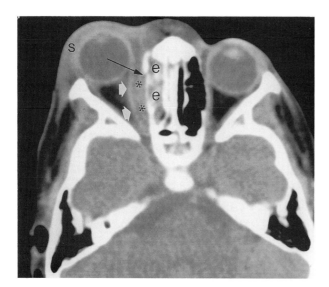

Fig. 15. Subperiosteal orbital abscess in a 9-yr-old. Axial CT shows a subperiosteal abscess (*) as a complication of ethmoid sinusitis (e). The abscess displaces the medial rectus muscle (white arrows). Note the dehiscence of the right lamina papyracea (black arrow). There is associated proptosis and preseptal soft tissue swelling(s) on the right side.

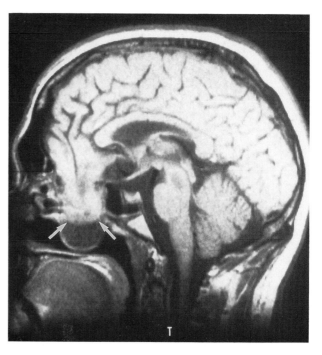

Fig. 16. Basal cephelocele. T1WI sagittal MR image shows a cephelocele (arrows) projecting into the nasal cavity. This should not be mistaken for a neoplastic process.

Cavernous sinus thrombosis will be evident as fullness of the affected side with convexity of the lateral margin of the cavernous sinus, instead of the normal, slightly concave margin. Gadolinium-enhanced, axial, and coronal MR scans would be expected to be more sensitive to the presence of cavernous sinus thrombosis than CT.

Permanent loss of vision is a rare complication of sinusitis, although recent studies report about a 10% incidence in patients with postseptal infection *(15,46)*. Mechanisms for loss of vision may be optic neuritis as a reaction to adjacent infection. Ischemia secondary to thrombophlebitis, arteritis, or pressure on the central retinal artery may also result in blindness.

Benign Neoplasms

There are several soft tissue neoplasms that affect the sinuses, and they are discussed below. However, one should be cognizant of mimics of intrasinus masses. One such example is a herniation of intracranial contents (meninges, CSF, and brain tissue) through a defect in the dura and calvarium-a cephelocele. Basal cepheloceles can invade the sphenoid or ethmoid bones, mimicking a sinonasal mass (Fig. 16) *(47)*. MRI is useful in confirming this diagnosis.

INVERTED PAPILLOMA

Inverted papilloma of the nose and paranasal sinuses is an uncommon tumor, representing <5% of all sinonasal tumors *(48)*. This tumor can be histologically differentiated from other sinonasal tumors by its propensity to invert into the underlying stroma, rather than growing in an exophytic patter *(49,50)*. The inverted papilloma is one of three histologically distinct papillomas—fungiform (50%), inverted (47%), and cylindric cell (3%)—which are known as schneiderian papillomas *(15)*.

Inverted papillomas occur most commonly in males from 40 to 70 yr old, and arise from the lateral nasal wall in the region of the middle meatus and infundibulum. Small lesions will appear as nonspecific polypoid nasal masses. When larger, they are expansile masses that cause bone remodeling. They often have a characteristic appearance on coronal CT, with a soft mass extending from the middle meatus into the maxillary antrum *(51)*. On CT, these tumors are usually well defined, with a moderate heterogenous enhancement. Foci of calcium may be present. With enlargement of tumor, osseus changes are often visualized with the adjacent bony structures becoming thinned, bowed, eroded, or, less commonly, sclerotic (50).

The reported rate of associated malignancy, usually squamous cell carcinoma, is approx 10% (52,53). The presence of adjacent bone destruction should raise this possibility. Inverted papilloma has a strong tendency to recur and requires aggressive resection for a core. CT is important both in diagnosis to display the extent of tumor for resection and in postoperative follow-up for detection of recurrence.

JUVENILE ANGIOFIBROMA

The juvenile angiofibroma is a rare, histologically benign, but locally aggressive, tumor. It occurs almost exclusively in adolescent males. It arises in from the nasopharynx near the pterygopalatine fossa (54). Extension onto the orbit via the inferior orbital fissure and intracranial extension via the pterygoid canal and foramen rotundum are well documented (54,55). Direct extension into the maxillary, sphenoid, and ethmoid sinuses as well as the nasal cavity can occur (54).

On imaging studies, widening of the pterygopalatine fossa is a common and relatively specific sign (56). On CT, the bones are often bowed and remodelled without frank destruction. Because of their highly vascular nature, there is strong and early enhancement on both post-contrast CT and MR imaging with a vascular blush present on angiography. On MR imaging, the mass is of intermediate to low signal intensity on T1WI and intermediate to high signal intensity on T2WI. Multiple flow voids are usually identified.

SCHWANNOMA

Schwannomas are encapsulated tumors that arise from Schwann cells on the surface of nerve fibers. In the sinonasal region, schwannomas usually arise from the ophthalmic and maxillary divisions of the trigeminal nerve and from the autonomic nerves (54). They are slow-growing tumors, and complete excision is curative (10). Although paranasal sinus schwannomas are rare, those that do occur are most common in the ethmoid and maxillary sinuses (54).

On CT, they are usually well-circumscribed homogeneously enhancing masses. On MR imaging, they are often isohypointense on T1WI and hyperintense on T2WI. They typically show moderate enhancement after gadolinium-DTPA administration (54).

Malignant Neoplasms

SQUAMOUS CELL CARCINOMA

Squamous cell carcinoma is the most common malignancy of the sinonasal region, accounting for 50% of cases (57). Approximately 80% of cases arise in the maxillary antrum with 13% occurring in the ethmoid sinuses (57). The frontal and sphenoid sinuses are uncommon primary sites of occurrence. Early symptoms include facial pain, nasal obstruction, and facial swelling. Squamous cell carcinoma is twice as common in men, and 95% occur in patients over the age of 40 yr (58).

Maxillary sinus carcinoma, because of its location, frequently presents with advanced disease with extension into the orbit, pterygopalatine fossa, infratemporal fossa, and adjacent sinuses (54). Orbital involvement occurs in almost two-thirds of patients at the time of presentation (29). Orbital invasion occurs through the orbital floor from the antrum or via the inferior orbital fissure. Lymph node metastasis at the time of initial presentation is uncommon (54).

CT scanning has proven to be helpful in mapping the extent of tumor for surgical planning. On CT, the tumor is usually of homogenous soft tissue density and shows little enhancement with contrast. Areas of necrosis may be present. Aggressive bone destruction, the hallmark of squamous cell carcinoma, is often present. However, early in the course of the disease before bone destruction occurs, the tumor may be indistinguishable from common entities, such as chronic sinusitis and inflammatory polyps. Because of the mild enhancement that occurs, contrast administration with CT is of dubious value in assessing carcinomas in the sinonasal cavity. However, contrast material is often useful in evaluating for intracranial spread (54). One limitation of CT in defining tumor extension is the distinction between tumor and inflammatory reaction within the sinus and adjacent soft tissues, both of which will be soft tissue density. MR imaging has proven to be helpful in this regard. The majority (95%) of sinonasal tumors are highly cellular and are low-to-intermediate signal intensity on T2WI (59). By comparison, the coexistent inflammatory changes often have a high water content and are hyperintense on T2WI. However, more chronic secretions may have varying degrees of T2 shortening (as described above), which can make this distinction between tumor and inflammatory secretions difficult.

The MR appearance of squamous cell carcinoma is often nonspecific, appearing as a homogeneous mass of low-to-intermediate signal intensity on both T1WI and T2WI. The presence of bone destruction is not reliably detected on MR imaging. Another advantage of MR imaging over CT is in the detection of intracranial and intraorbital spread, where gadolinium-DTPA is often helpful.

GLANDULAR TUMORS

This group of tumors arises from either minor salivary glands present in the sinus mucosa or differentiation of stem cells. Approximately 19% of malignant tumors of the sinuses fall into this category (60). The most common entities in this group are: the adenocarcinomas, which tend to occur in the ethmoid sinuses, and adenoid cystic and mucoepidermoid carcinomas, which are more frequent in the maxillary antrum. Many of these tumors are indistinguishable from the more common squamous cell carcinoma on CT and MR. This group of tumors typically remodel bone, in contradistinction to the marked tendency of squamous cell carcinoma to destroy bone. The glandular tumors, as a group, are more likely to exhibit heterogeneous areas on both CT and MR owing to cystic degeneration, mucus secretion, and necrosis (some may be mostly hyperintense on T2 weighted images). Orbital involvement can occur by remodeled bone encroaching on orbital contents or via perineural spread. Adenoid cystic carcinoma, in particular, has a propensity for perineural spread, with the infraorbital nerve acting as a possible conduit to the orbit and orbital apex.

LYMPHOMA

When lymphoma involves the paranasal sinuses, it is usually of the non-Hodgkin type and often is associated with systemic involvement. Lymphoma may account for as much as 8% of paranasal sinus malignancy (60,61). Usually they are found in the maxillary antrum or nasal cavity. These tumors tend to be bulky soft tissue masses that may remodel bone. On CT scanning, they are of homogenous, soft tissue density and enhance moderately. On MR, they are of intermediate signal intensity on all sequences.

ESTHESIONEUROBLASTOMA (OLFACTORY NEUROBLASTOMA)

This is an uncommon tumor arising within the olfactory mucosa in the upper nasal cavity/septum

and the cribriform plate region. About 70% involve the sinuses (26), in particular the ethmoid sinuses. These tumors often present with nasal obstruction or epistaxis (54). On CT, these tumors are of homogenous soft tissue density, sometimes with calcification and strong enhancement. Bone destruction may also be a feature. On MR, the tumor is hypointense on T1WI and hyperintense on T2WI. The tumor is locally aggressive and has a tendency to spread in the submucosa (54). Metastatic involvement of the cervical lymph node chains, as well as more distant sites, often occurs.

OTHER MALIGNANT TUMORS

Extramedullary plasmacytoma represents 2–4% of sinonasal tumors (60,61), and 15% of them present with proptosis (46). CT reveals a homogenous, enhancing mass with bone remodeling. On MR, they are of intermediate signal intensity on all sequences and may show vascular flow voids.

Melanoma occasionally arises in the sinuses. These tumors remodel bone, enhance strongly on CT, and some may exhibit high signal intensity components on T1-weighted images owing to melanin, which is paramagnetic. Various sarcomas (especially rhabdomyosarcoma in the pediatric age group) and metastases (renal, lung, and breast being the most common primary sites) are also encountered in the paranasal sinuses infrequently and appear as aggressive soft tissue masses with variable degrees of bony destruction. Adjacent involvement of the intracranial and intraorbital compartments may occur.

RADIOGRAPHIC EVALUATION OF PATIENTS FOLLOWING FUNCTIONAL ENDOSCOPIC SINUS SURGERY (FESS)

Evaluation Approach

The emphasis of the postoperative evaluation of patients is similar to the preoperative evaluation. Ideally, patients should be followed with coronal CT. Given the fact that a surgical procedure was performed, one must first establish the type and extent of surgery. The emphasis should be on understanding the underlying anatomy as it appears following surgery. Areas that merit close scrutiny are as follows:

1. Frontal recess—the frontal recesses should be identified to determine their patency. Postoperatively, we often find that recurrence of disease is often owing to persistent obstruction in this area. To this end, note should be made of the agger nasi

cell (if it remains), since its persistence may continue to narrow the frontal recess.

2. OMU—note should be made of the extent of the uncintectomy and removal of the ethmoid bulla. The outline of the middle turbinate should be examined to determine whether a middle turbinectomy has been performed. If so, then careful attention should be paid to both the vertical attachment of the middle turbinate to the cribriform plate and the attachment of the basal lamella to the lamina papyracea. Traction applied during the course of middle turbinectomy can inflict damage at these sites.

3. Lamina papyracea—inspection of the entire course of the lamina papyracea should be carried out to evaluate the integrity of this structure. Postoperative dehiscences are commonly found just posterior to the nasolacrimal duct, at the level of the ethmoid bulla and basal lamella attachment.

4. Sphenoid sinus area—the margins of the sphenoid sinus should be evaluated for bony dehiscence and/or cephalocele.

Operative Complications

FESS has become a popular surgical treatment modality in patients with chronic sinusitis that fail medical therapy. The incidence of complications from the procedure is related to the instrumentation, the patient's underlying anatomy, the overall health of the patient, and the extent of disease *(19–22,45,60,61)*.

The field of view available to the surgeon during FESS is quite small, and variant anatomy can make surgical landmarks difficult to identify. The surgeon's view is limited to the surface mucosa; he/she can not see beyond the mucosa directly in view. The presence of various anatomic variants can contribute to surgical complications if not noted prospectively *(20)*. Owing to the need for an accurate surgical road map, all patients scheduled to undergo FESS should have a preoperative coronal CT scan. Scanning in the coronal plane is preferred, since this simulates the surgeon's working plane during endoscopy *(3)*.

Brisk bleeding in the operative field, as well as extensive nasal polyposis, can hinder visibility and predispose the patient to operative complications *(20)*. Standard surgical techniques and microscope-assisted surgery are adjuncts that can be used when the aforementioned problems arise. However, they are fraught with many of the same complications.

In general, complications can be divided into minor and major *(19–21,45,60)*. Minor complications include periorbital emphysema, epistaxis, postoperative nasal synechiae, and tooth pain. Although these all can commonly occur, they are usually self-limited and do not require postoperative radiologic evaluation. Major complications are rarer, but can be severely devastating or fatal *(21)*. Loss of integrity of the lamina papyracea can permit intraorbital fat to herniate into the ethmoid sinuses. Preexisting dehiscence of the lamina papyracea may be the result of prior trauma or erosion from chronic sinus disease. Intraoperative disruption of the lamina papyracea can occur during resection of the middle turbinate if the ground lamella is resected back to its attachment to the lamina papyracea.

Direct damage to the medial rectus muscle, superior oblique muscle, or other orbital contents can occur if there is pre-existing or intraoperative disruption of the lamina papyracea *(61)*. Injuries to the orbital contents may result in postoperative diplopia. The etiology of the diplopia can be from muscle entrapment among bone fragments, direct muscle laceration, or be secondary to nerve injury. Thin-section axial and coronal CT can be of benefit in evaluation of such cases. Clinically, subconjunctival hemorrhage is often associated with extraocular muscle damage *(61)*. If intraorbital and intraocular pressure builds up because of an expanding hematoma or air being forced into the orbit from the nasal cavity (via a dehiscent lamina papyracea), then visual impairment or blindness secondary to ischemia can result *(61)*.

Blindness, temporary or permanent, owing to injury of the optic nerve can occur during posterior ethmoidectomy if the bony limit of the sinus is violated *(19,22,60,61)*. Trauma to the vascular supply to the optic nerve can also result in visual loss.

Massive hemorrhage from direct injury to major vessels can occur. Laceration of the internal carotid artery has been reported and is often a fatal complication *(19,20,22)*. Emergent angiography with balloon occlusion of the lacerated artery has been performed. Patients who report severe postoperative headache, photophobia, or have signs suggesting subarachnoid hemorrhage should have a noncontrast head CT. If subarachnoid blood is found, cerebral angiography is recommended to detect vascular injury *(19,20,45)*.

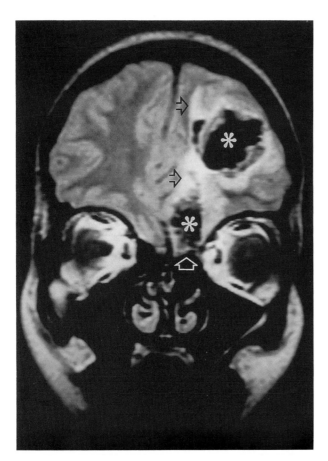

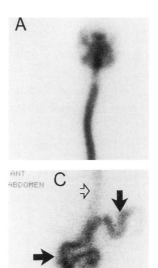

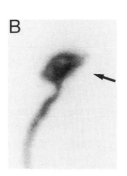

Fig. 18. Post-FESS CSF leak. Indium-111 DTPA CSF study in the **(A)** AP and **(B)** lateral projections shows normal activity in the subarachnoid spaces. No activity is seen within the paranasal sinuses or nasal cavity (thin black arrow). Delayed AP image of the abdomen **(C)** shows abnormal bowel activity owing to swallowed secretions from an occult CSF leakage (thick black arrows). Residual activity within the subarachnoid space (open arrow) is noted.

Fig. 17. Postoperative intracranial hematoma. Coronal T2WI following FESS shows a hypointense hematoma (*) with surrounding hyperintense edema (open black arrows). Note the site of perforation through the cribriform plate (open white arrow).

Injury to the nasolacrimal duct can result during anterior enlargement of the maxillary ostium in the middle meatus. Injury to the membranous portion of the duct may be self-limited and remit by spontaneous fistulization into the middle meatus. Stenosis or total occlusion of the nasolacrimal duct can result from more severe injury *(61)*.

Postoperative cerebrospinal fluid (CSF) leak is another major complication of FESS *(21,22,45,60)*. These leaks occur following inadvertent penetration of the dura. Extension of the injury to involve of the cribriform plate, fovea ethmoidalis, anterior cranial fossa, and the skull base have all been reported (Fig. 17). Secondary nasal encephalocele or deep penetration of the cerebrum can be seen following violation of the cranial vault *(28)*. A CSF leak may not become clinically apparent for up to 2 yr after surgery *(19,20)*. CSF leaks will often

close spontaneously with conservative measures (i.e., lumbar drain) *(19,20)*. However, if they persist, radiologic workup is indicated.

In many institutions, a radionuclide CSF study is utilized as the initial radiologic screening examination in such patients *(62)*. Prior to beginning the study, the otolaryngologist places absorbent pledgets in the nasal cavity. Usually three to four are placed on each side and note is made of their location within the nasal cavity. Subsequent to this, 400–500 µCi of Indium-111 (In-111) labeled DTPA is placed in the subarachnoid space by the neuroradiologist via a cervical or lumbar puncture.

The patient is imaged with a gamma camera at multiple intervals up to 24 h. Any position or activity known to provoke the leak is encouraged. Even though images of the head and neck are obtained, it is unusual actually to see evidence of the leak on these images. Rather, indirect signs of leaking are sought. Images over the abdomen are done to search for activity in the bowel. Such activity indicates that the patient is swallowing CSF as it leaks into the nasal cavity (Fig. 18).

At 24 h, the nasal pledgets are removed and assayed. The results are compared with In-111 activity in a serum sample drawn at the same time. A ratio of pledget activity to serum activity is determined and expressed in terms of counts/g. It is often possible to predict the general area of the leak based on which pledgets show increased activity. If the radionuclide test is positive (directly or indirectly), then a contrast CT cisternogram is done to define the anatomy and to pinpoint the site of leakage.

COMPUTER-ASSISTED SURGERY

A study performed by Kennedy et al. (63) for the American Academy of Otolaryngology and Head and Neck Surgery showed that there is an increasing number of major surgical complications (i.e., death and orbital and intracranial damage) as the number of FESS procedures has increased. Even though CT provides a "road map" for the surgeon, the information that is provided is remote. The surgeon must mentally transfer information from the image to the operative site.

Given the extreme variations in anatomy and the copious amount of intraoperative bleeding that can make landmarks difficult to identify, it is not surprising that inadvertent injuries to the orbital and intracranial compartments occur. There is a need for an objective and interactive correlation of the image data with the actual operative site in the patient. Over the past 5 yr, we have successfully achieved this goal utilizing an ISG Allegro multimodality computer attached to a mechanical sensor (ISG Technologies, Mississauga, Ontario, Canada). Prior to CT scanning, five to ten external markers are placed on the patient's face. These are used to register the data in the computer so that they can be applied to the patient in vivo on the surgical table. With the registration complete and the patient immobilized, the mechanical arm holding a probe can be placed into the nasal cavity. The tip of the probe is the location of the sensor. Axial, coronal, and sagittal reformatted images at the tip of the sensor are generated by the computer and the location of the sensor in the patient is thus provided, and shown by crosshairs on these images.

In this manner, the probe is used to locate specific anatomic structures and avoid penetration of the ethmoid roof and lamina papyracea. It can be used to identify easily the relationship of the sphenoid sinus to the optic nerves and carotid canals. The accuracy of this device has been shown to be approx 2 mm (51).

The limitations of the device are:

1. The need to utilize an additional piece of equipment in the operative field;
2. The unavoidable break in the concentration of the surgeon as he/she operates;
3. The need to utilize general anesthesia in order to ensure that the patient remains still.

We are encouraged by the work of several groups who have attempted to introduce improvements in sensor technology and the computer software that supports the system. In the near future, we expect the use of this technology to become widespread.

REFERENCES

1. Moss A, Parsons V. Current estimates from the National Health Interview Survey, United States—1985. Hyattsville, MD: National Center for Health Statistics, 1986.
2. Som P. Sinonasal cavity. In: Som P, Bergeron P, eds., Head and Neck Imaging. Mosby, St. Louis, MO, 1991; pp. 64–69.
3. Zinreich S. Paranasal sinus imaging. Otolaryngol Head Neck Surg 1990;103(5/2):863–868.
4. Zinreich S. Imaging of chronic sinusitis in adults: X-ray, computed tomography, and magnetic resonance imaging. J Allergy Clin Immunol 1992;90(3/2):445–451.
5. Zinreich S. Imaging of inflammatory sinus disease. Otolaryngol Clin North Am 1993;26(4):535–547.
6. Zinreich S, Abidin M, Kennedy D. Cross-sectional imaging of the nasal cavity and paranasal sinuses. Operative Techniques in Otolaryngol Head Neck Surg 1990;1(2): 93–99.
7. Zinreich S, Kennedy D, Rosenbaum A, Gayler B, Kumar A, Stammberger H. Paranasal sinuses: CT imaging requirements for endoscopic surgery. Radiology 1987; 163(3):769–775.
8. Harnsberger H, Babbel R, Davis W. The major obstructive inflammatory patterns of the sinonasal region seen on screening sinus computed tomography. Semin Ultrasound CT MR 1991;12(6):541–560.
9. Zinreich S, Kennedy D, Kumar A, Rosenbaum A, Arrington J, Johns M. MR imaging of normal nasal cycle: comparison with sinus pathology. JCAT 1988;12(6): 1014–1019.
10. Berger W. Use of A-Mode ultrasound for diagnosis of sinus disease in young children. Ann Allergy 1986; 56:39–43.
11. Landman M. Ultrasound screening for sinus disease. Otolaryngol Head Neck Surg 1986;94(2):157–164.
12. Mabry R. Sinus ultrasound scanning. Otolaryngol Head Neck Surg 1985;93(1):136,137.
13. Pfleiderer A. Ultrasound investigation of the sinuses: a real advance in diagnosis? J Royal Soc Medicine 1985; 78:277,278.

14. Harnsberger H. Imaging for the sinus and nose. In Head and Neck Imaging Handbook. Mosby Yearbook, St. Louis, MO, 1990;387–419.

15. Mafee M. Nonepithelial tumors of the paranasal sinuses and nasal cavity. Role of CT and MR imaging. Radiol Clin North Am 1993;31(1):75–90.

16. Hosemann W. Dissection of the lateral nasal wall in eight steps. In: Wigand ME, ed., Endoscopic Surgery of the Paranasal Sinuses and Anterior Skull Base. Thieme Medical Publishers, New York: 1990; pp. 36–41.

17. Yousem D. Imaging of sinonasal inflammatory disease. Radiology 1993;188(2):303–314.

18. Buus D, Tse D, Farris B. Ophthalmic complications of sinus surgery. Ophthalmology 1990;97:612–619.

19. Hudgins P. Complications of endoscopic sinus surgery—the role of the radiologist in prevention. Radiol Clin North Am 1993;31 (1):21–31.

20. Hudgins P, Browning D, Gallups J. Endoscopic paranasal sinus surgery: radiographic evaluation of severe complications. AJNR 1992;13:1161–1167.

21. Maniglia A. Fatal and major complications secondary to nasal and sinus surgery. Laryngoscope 1989;99:276–283.

22. Maniglia A. Fatal and other major complications of endoscopic sinus surgery. Laryngoscope 1991;101:349–354.

23. Laine F, Smoker W. The ostiomeatal unit and endoscopic surgery: anatomy, variations, and imaging findings in inflammatory diseases. AJR 1992;159(4):849–857.

24. Shankar L, Evans K, Hawke M, Stammberger H. An Atlas of Imaging of the Paranasal Sinuses. Imago, Singapore, 1994, pp. 41–72.

25. Bolger W, Butzin C, Parsons D. Paranasal sinus bony anatomic variations and mucosal abnormalities: CT analysis for endoscopic sinus surgery. Laryngoscope 1991;101(1/1):56–64.

26. Evans F, Sydnor J, Moore W, Moore G. Sinusitis of the maxillary antrum. N Engl J Med 1975;293(15):735–739.

27. Weber A. Inflammatory diseases of the paranasal sinuses and mucoceles. Otolaryngol Clin North Am 1988;21(3):421–437.

28. Kennedy D, Zinreich S, Kumar A, Rosenbaum A, Johns M. Physiologic mucosal changes within the nose and ethmoid sinus: imaging of the nasal cycle by MRI. Laryngoscope 1988;98(9):928–933.

29. Gullane P, Conley J. Carcinoma of the maxillary sinus. A correlation of the clinical course with orbital involvement, pterygoid erosion or pterygopalatine invasion and cervical metastases. J Otolaryngol 1983;12:141–145.

30. Harrison D. Midline destructive granuloma: fact or ficton. Laryngoscope 1987;97:1049–1053.

31. Yousem D, Kennedy D, Rosenberg S. Ostiomeatal complex risk factors for sinusitis: CT evaluation. J Otolaryngol 1991;20(6):419–424.

32. Babbel R, Harnsberger H. Sonkens J, Hunt S. Recurring patterns of inflammatory sinonasal disease demonstrated on screening sinus CT. AJNR 1992;13(3):903–912.

33. Scuderi A, Babbel R, Harnsberger H, Sonkens J. The sporadic pattern of inflammatory sinonasal disease including postsurgical changes. Semin Ultrasound CT MR 1991;12(6):575–591.

34. Som P, Curtin H. Chronic inflammatory sinonasal diseases including fungal infections. The role of imaging. Radiol Clin North Am 1993;31(1):33–44.

35. Som P. Imaging of paranasal sinus fungal disease. Otolaryngol Clin North Am 1993;26(6):983–994.

36. Som P, Bergeron R. Sinonasal cavity. In: Som P, Bergeron R, eds., Head & Neck Imaging. Mosby, St. Louis, MO, 1991; pp. 114–166.

37. Stammberger H, Wolf G. Headaches and sinus disease: the endoscopic approach. Ann Otol Rhinol Laryngol Suppl 1988;134:3–23.

38. Lidov M, Som P. Inflammatory disease involving a concha bullosa (enlarged pneumatized middle nasal turbinate): MR and CT appearance. AJNR 1990;11(5):999–1001.

39. Zinreich S, Kennedy D, Malat J, Curtin H. Epstein J, Huff L, Kumar A, Johns M, Rosenbaum A. Fungal sinusitis: diagnosis with CT and MR imaging. Radiology 1988;169(2):439–444.

40. Moloney J, Badham N, McRae A. The acute orbit, preseptal, periorbital cellulitis, subperiosteal abscess and orbital cellulitis due to sinusitis. J Laryngol Otol 1987;12:1–18.

41. Rohr A, Spector S, Siegel S, Katz R, Rachelefsky G. Correlation between A-mode ultrasound and radiography in the diagnosis of maxillary sinusitis. J Allergy Clin Immunol 1986;78(1/1):58–61.

42. Walters E, Waller P, Hiles D, Michaels R. Acute orbital cellulitis. Arch Ophthalmol 1976;94:785–788.

43. Woodruff W, Vrabec D. Inverted papilloma of the nasal vault and paranasal sinuses: spectrum of CT findings. AJR 1994;162(2):419–423.

44. Babbel R, Harnsberger HR, Nelson B, Sonkens J, Hunt S. Optimization of techniques in screening CT of the sinuses. AJR 1991;157:1093–1098.

45. Stankiewicz J. Complications of endoscopic intranasal ethmoidectomy. Laryngoscope 1987;97:1270–1273.

46. Nelson A, Reed H, Haney P, Varma D, Adams K, Beckett W, Whitley J. Gray-scale (B-Mode) sonography of the maxillary sinus. J Ultrasound Med 1986;5:477–481.

47. Laine FJ, Kuta AJ. Imaging the sphenoid bone and basiocciputi pathologic considerations. Semin Ultra CT MRI 1993;14(3):160–177.

48. Som P, Bergeron R. Sinonasal cavity. In: Som P, Bergeron R, eds., Head and Neck Imaging. Mosby, St. Louis, MO, 1991; pp. 169–224.

49. Chow J, Leonetti J, Mafee M. Epithelial tumors of the paranasal sinuses and nasal cavity. Radiol Clin North Am 1993;31(1):61–73.

50. Lawson W, LeBenger J, Som P, Bernard P, Biller H. Inverted papilloma: an analysis of 87 cases. Laryngoscope 1989;99(11):1117–1124.

51. Zinreich S, Tebo S, Long D, Brem H, Mattox D, Loury M, VanderKolk C, Koch W, Kennedy D, Bryan R. Frameless stereotaxic integration of CT imaging data: accuracy and initial applications. Radiology 1993;188(3):735–742.

52. Fellows D, King D, Conturo T, Bryan R, Merz W, Zinreich S. In vitro evaluation of hypointensity in aspergillus colonies. AJNR 1994;15:1139–1144.

53. Wilbur A, Dobben G, Linder B. Paraorbital tumors and tumor-like conditions: role of CT and MRI. Radiol Clin North Am 1987;25(3):631–646.

54. Hill J, Soboroff B, Applebaum E. Nonsquamous tumors of the nose and paranasal sinuses. Otolaryngol Clin North Am 1986;19(4):723–739.

55. Kimmelman C, Korovin G. Management of paranasal sinus neoplasms invading the orbit. Otolaryngol Clin North Am 1988;21(1):77–91.

56. Som P, Shugar J, Cohen B, Biller H. The nonspecificity of the antral bowing sign in maxillary sinus pathology. J Comput Assist Tomogr 1981;5(3):350–352.

57. Weber A, Stanton A. Malignant tumors of the paranasal sinuses: radiologic, clinical and histopathologic evaluation of 200 cases. Head Neck Surg 1984;6:761–776.

58. Patt B, Manning S. Blindness resulting from orbital complications of sinusitis. Otolaryngol Head Neck Surg 1991;104(6):789–795.

59. Som P. Sinonasal tumors and inflammatory tissues: differentiation with MR. Radiology 1988;167:803.

60. Stankiewicz J. Complications in endoscopic intranasal ethmoidectomy: an update. Laryngoscope 1989; 99:668–670.

61. Neuhaus R. Orbital complications secondary to endoscopic sinus surgery. Ophthalmology 1990;97:1512–1518.

62. Mettler FA, Guiberteau MJ. Cerebrovascular system. In: Mettler FA, Guiberteau MJ, eds., Essentials of Nuclear Medicine Imaging. 3rd ed. Philadelphia: W. B. Saunders, 1991; pp. 73,74.

63. Kennedy D, Shaman P, Hen W, Selman H, Deans D, Lanza D. Complications of ethmoidectomy: a survey of fellows of Otolaryngology-Head & Neck Surgery. Otolaryngol Head Neck Surg. in press.

PART III | CLINICAL DISEASE

5

Microbiology of Acute and Chronic Sinusitis in Children and Adults

Ellen R. Wald, MD

CONTENTS

INTRODUCTION

The microbiology of paranasal sinus infections can be anticipated according to the age of the patient, clinical presentation, and immunocompetency of the host. In acute sinus disease, viral upper respiratory infections frequently precede bacterial superinfection by *Streptococcus pneumoniae, Haemophilus influenzae,* and *Moraxella catarrhalis.* Staphylococci and respiratory anaerobes are common in chronic sinus infection, which may also be caused by exacerbations of infection with the bacterial species that cause acute disease. Enterobacteriacae may be found in patients with nosocomial sinusitis; predisposing causes are prolonged nasogastric and nasotracheal intubation. Finally, fungi may cause chronic disease in immunocompetent hosts or acute infection in immunocompromised patients.

From: *Diseases of the Sinuses* (M. E. Gershwin and G. A. Incaudo, eds.), ©1996 Humana Press Inc., Totowa, NJ.

Sinusitis is a common complication of viral upper respiratory infection and allergic inflammation. Although the paranasal sinuses are believed to be sterile under normal circumstances, the upper respiratory tract—specifically the nose and oral cavity—are heavily colonized with normal flora.

SINUS ASPIRATION

To determine the bacteriology of sinusitis, a sample of sinus secretions must be obtained from one of the paranasal sinuses without contamination by normal respiratory or oral flora. The maxillary sinus is the most accessible of the paranasal sinuses. A transnasal approach affords the easiest and safest route of sinus aspiration in patients. A trocar is passed beneath the inferior nasal turbinate across the lateral nasal wall. However, because the nasal vestibule is so heavily colonized, it is essential to attempt to sterilize the area of the nose beneath the inferior turbinate through which the trocar is passed. If this is not done, contaminating nasal flora isolated in the sinus aspirate may be misconstrued as pathogens. Sterilization can be easily accomplished with a topical solution of 4% cocaine. The advantage of cocaine vs povodine-iodine is that it provides both topical antisepsis and anesthesia, and does not irritate the mucosa. Furthermore, to avoid misinterpretation of culture results, infection is defined as the recovery of a bacterial species in high density, i.e., a colony count of at least 10^4 colony-forming units per milliliter (CFU/mL). This quantitative definition increases the probability that organisms recovered from the maxillary sinus aspirate truly represent *in situ* infection and not contamination. In fact, most sinus aspirates from infected sinuses are associated with colony counts in excess of 10^4 CFU/mL. If quantitative cultures cannot be performed, Gram stain of aspirated specimens affords semiquantitative data. If bacteria are readily apparent on a Gram stain, the approximate bacterial density is 10^5 CFU/mL. The Gram stain is also helpful if bacteria seen on the smear of the specimen fail to grow using standard aerobic culture techniques; anaerobic organisms or other fastidious bacteria should be suspected.

Occasionally a sinus aspirate is insufficient for the diagnosis of a sinus infection. This is especially true in the evaluation of patients with very protracted symptoms in whom fungal sinusitis should be suspected. In this instance, biopsy of the sinus mucosa and both culture and appropriate stains may be required to demonstrate the microbiology.

MICROBIOLOGY OF ACUTE SINUSITIS IN CHILDREN

Despite the substantial prevalence and clinical importance of sinusitis in childhood, there has been relatively limited study of the microbiology of sinusitis in pediatric patients. Using a study design similar to one described by investigators at the University of Virginia *(1)*, we undertook an investigation of the microbiology of acute sinusitis in pediatric patients in 1979 (reported in ref. *2*). Patients were eligible for this study if they were between the ages of 2 and 16 yr, and presented with one of two clinical pictures—onset with either "persistent" or "severe" respiratory symptoms. The majority of subjects presented with "persistent" symptoms, that is, symptoms that lasted more than 10, but <30 d and had not yet begun to improve. A minimal duration of 10 d was used to separate

simple upper respiratory infection (URI) from acute sinusitis, and the maximum duration of 29 d was used to distinguish acute from subacute or chronic sinusitis. The time-course of most simple URIs is 5–7 d. Although a patient with a URI may not be completely asymptomatic by the tenth day, usually their symptoms have peaked in intensity and begun to improve. Therefore, persistence of respiratory symptoms beyond 10 d without improvement suggests the presence of a bacterial complication, i.e., sinusitis. The respiratory symptoms of acute sinusitis consist of nasal discharge of any quality (thick or thin, serous, mucoid, or purulent), daytime cough, or both. A smaller subset of subjects with acute sinusitis presented with "severe" respiratory symptoms. Severity was defined as high fever (temperature of at least 103°F) and purulent (thick, colored, and opaque) nasal discharge. For this presentation, there was no qualifier on duration of symptoms. This clinical dyad is thought to signify sinus infection when contrasted with the course of the usual URI. Most simple URIs begin with clear nasal discharge, which may become purulent after a few days, but then reverts to a clear quality again before finally resolving. If fever is present at all during an uncomplicated URI, it usually occurs at the beginning of the viral syndrome. By the time the nasal discharge becomes purulent, most children with simple URIs are afebrile. Accordingly, the combination of purulent nasal discharge and fever for several days is suggestive of a bacterial complication, i.e., acute sinusitis.

Eligible children with either of these two presentations had sinus radiographs performed. The sinus films were considered to be abnormal if they showed diffuse opacification, mucosal thickening of >4 mm, or an air–fluid level. If the sinus films were abnormal and informed consent was provided by the parent, then a sinus puncture was performed, using a transnasal approach.

When a maxillary sinus aspirate was performed on children presenting with either persistent or severe symptoms and significantly abnormal sinus radiographs, bacteria in high density were recovered from 70% *(3)*. Table 1 shows the bacterial species cultured from 79 sinus aspirates obtained from 50 children in their relative order of prevalence. *S. pneumoniae* was most common, followed closely by *Branhamella catarrhalis* (now known as *M. catarrhalis*), and *H. influenzae*. Both *M. catarrhalis* and *H. influenzae* may be β-lactamase-

of viral infection in cases of bacterial sinusitis might be increased if sinus aspirates were performed earlier in the clinical course of symptoms. Almost certainly, viruses as primary sinus pathogens and copathogens may explain some apparent early antibiotic failures as has been shown for acute otitis media in children (14).

Nosocomial Sinusitis

Patients with nosocomial sinusitis are usually those who require extended periods of intensive care (postoperative patients, burn victims, patients with severe trauma) involving prolonged endotracheal or nasogastric intubation. Nasotracheal intubation provides a substantially higher risk for nosocomial sinusitis than orotracheal intubation (15). Approximately 25% of patients requiring nasotracheal intubation for more than 5 d develop nosocomial sinusitis (16). In contrast to community acquired sinusitis, the usual pathogens are gram-negative enterics (such as *Pseudomonas aeruginosa*, *Klebsiella pneumoniae*, *Enterobacter* species, *Proteus mirabilis*, *Serratia marcescens*) and gram-positive cocci (occasionally *streptococci* and *staphylococci*) (16–20).

MICROBIOLOGY OF CHRONIC SINUS INFECTION IN ADULTS

Bacteriology

The bacteriology of chronic sinus infection is a bit controversial. All of the bacterial pathogens implicated in acute sinusitis occur, but there is a shift in their relative prevalence. By several accounts, the role of *S. aureus* and respiratory anaerobes is increased, whereas the classic pathogens of acute sinusitis diminish (21,22).

In a recent review of the microbial etiology of sinusitis, Gwaltney et al. emphasized that chronic sinus disease represents a repeatedly damaged mucosal lining that has lost its normal state of sterility (12). They emphasized attention to the structural damage and not the "infectious process," and noted that patients with chronic sinus disease may have acute exacerbations with the usual bacterial species that cause acute community acquired sinusitis.

MYCOLOGY

Mycology of Sinus Disease

Fungal sinusitis is being increasingly recognized as a cause of chronic sinusitis in immunocompetent

hosts (23–26). The clinical presentation is similar to that observed in patients with chronic bacterial sinusitis, i.e., persistent nasal congestion and nasal discharge for months to years. Unusual nasal secretions, facial pain, headache, and fever are variably present.

Aspergillus fumigatis is said to be the most common cause of fungal sinusitis in immunocompetent individuals (23). It is a saprophyte of soil, dust, and decaying organic material. The usual portal of entry is the respiratory tract. The organism can colonize the sinuses, external auditory canal, or the tracheobronchial tree. It is not transmitted between patients; sources of infection are endogenous. The disease may take one of four forms: noninvasive, invasive, disseminated, and allergic. The noninvasive type presents as chronic rhinitis and nasal obstruction. If undiagnosed, it may go on to cause invasion. This presentation is similar to an intracranial mass. Fulminant disseminated disease occurs when the organism becomes locally aggressive in immunosuppressed hosts and invades the bloodstream seeding lungs, liver, spleen, bone, and central nervous system. Allergic fungal sinusitis may be caused by *Aspergillus* or other fungal species. It is a chronic sinusitis usually occurring in individuals with asthma or other evidence of atopy. Sinus secretions often contain eosinophils, Charcot Leyden chrystals, and fungal hyphae. The pathogenesis is thought to be a hypersensitivity reaction to the fungal allergen (26).

Other fungal species reported to cause disease in normal hosts include *A. flavus*, *A. niger (27)*, *Sporothrix schenkii (28)*, *Schizophyllum commune (29)*, *Emericella nidulans (30)*, *Pseudoallescheria boydii (31–35)*, *Paecilomyces* sp *(36)*, *Candida* sp *(37)*, *Mucor* sp *(38)*, *Basidobolus haptosporus (39)*, *Stemphyllium mucorsporidium (40)*, *Penicillium melinii (40)*, *Fusarium* sp *(41,42)*, and *Bipolaris* sp *(43)*. Sinusitis has also been caused by dematiacious fungi other than Bipolaris, including *Drechslera hawaiiensis (44)*, *Dreschslera spicifera (45)*, *Alternaria* sp *(46,47)*, *Exserohilum* sp, and *Curvularia lunata (48)*. These fungi are common saprophytes, and infection is acquired by inhalation of fungal spores. Dematiaceous fungi are similar to aspergillus species histologically—septate hyphal organisms. Some reports of aspergillus sinusitis without culture confirmation may actually be cases caused by dematiacious fungi.

SINUSITIS
IN IMMUNOCOMPROMISED PATIENTS

The relative frequency with which various microbiologic species cause acute sinusitis in immunocompromised hosts is unknown. The distribution of pathogens almost certainly depends on the type of immunodeficiency and the time of the infection—during remission or during the active disease state. It is probable that the same bacterial agents and respiratory viruses causing infection in immunocompetent hosts are responsible for infection of the paranasal sinuses in:

1. Patients with cancer or leukemia in remission;
2. Patients with congenital or acquired immunodeficiencies; and
3. Organ transplant recipients more than a few months posttransplant.

Unusual bacterial agents may occur in immunosuppressed patients. A recent report highlighted the occurrence of community acquired *P. aeruginosa* in four patients with advanced human immunodeficiency virus infection *(49)*.

Other bacterial agents that may rarely cause infection are the atypical mycobacteria or nontuberculous mycobacteria *(50)*. The only reported case of maxillary sinusitis caused by *Mycobacterium chelonei* was published in 1981 *(51)*. A 47-yr-old diabetic woman presented with recurrent symptoms of left maxillary congestion. After initial treatment failed, scraping of the sinuses demonstrated acid-fast bacilli in histiocytes and giant cells. *M. chelonei* subsequently grew out of the culture, and the infection responded to treatment with kanamycin and erythromycin for 10 d.

Patients particularly prone to fungal infections of the paranasal sinuses include diabetics, patients with leukemia and solid malignancies who are febrile and neutropenic (most of whom will have received broad-spectrum antimicrobial therapy), patients on high-dose steroid therapy (e.g., for connective tissue disease, transplant recipients), and patients with severe impairment of cell-mediated immunity (transplant recipients, persons with congenital T-cell immunodeficiencies).

The most common cause of fungal sinusitis in immunosuppressed patients is *Aspergillus (23, 52–54)*. Much less commonly, acute or chronic sinusitis may be caused by *Candida* sp or *Mucor* sp; the latter agent most frequently affects diabetic

patients. In addition, *P. boydii (23)*, *Alternaria* sp *(23)*, *Exserohilum* sp, and *Bipolaris* sp have been observed to cause sinusitis in the immunosuppressed *(55)*.

Although protozoan species have not been described as a cause of acute or chronic sinusitis in normal individuals, a case of acute sinusitis caused by *Cryptosporidium* has been reported in a 17-yr-old boy with congenital hypogammaglobulinemia who presented with a 3-wk history of increasingly severe headaches *(56)*. Physical examination showed turbid nasal discharge, friable nasal mucosa, and facial tenderness over the maxillary sinuses. Computed tomography (CT) revealed pansinusitis. The maxillary sinus aspirate contained a moderate number of neutrophils and rare *Cryptosporidium* oocysts. Extensive culturing for other microbiologic species was negative. The patient's headache improved after therapy with oral spiramycin and intravenous 2-difloro-methyl-ornithine-HC1-monohydrate.

An equally rare cause of sinusitis is *Acanthamoeba*, described in a 29-yr-old Haitian man with the acquired immunodeficiency syndrome *(57)*. The patient reported progressive nasal congestion, epistaxis, nasal tenderness, and frontal headaches. CT of the head and sinuses showed soft tissue swelling in the maxillary sinuses and partial opacification of the ethmoid sinuses. Autopsy disclosed abundant edematous, pale yellow mucosa with focal areas of hemorrhage covering all sinus cavities. The histologic examination of the sinuses revealed extensive coagulation necrosis with acute and chronic inflammatory infiltrate and granulomatous reaction; amoebic trophozoites and cysts were present.

Although *Pneumocystis carinii* has not been reported to have been recovered from sinuses, its recent isolation from the middle ear cavity of an immunosuppressed patient suggests that this may also occur *(58)*.

ACKNOWLEDGMENT

The author gratefully acknowledges the secretarial assistance of Donna M. Schuster.

REFERENCES

1. Evans RD Jr, Sydnor JB, Moore WEC, et al. Sinusitis of the maxillary antrum. N Engl J Med 1975;293: 735–739.

2. Wald ER, Milmoe GJ, Bowen AD, Ledesma-Medina J, Salmon N, Bluestone CD. Acute maxillary sinusitis in children. N Engl J Med 1981;304:749–754.

3. Wald ER, Reilly JS, Casselbrant M, et al. Treatment of acute maxillary sinusitis in childhood: A comparative study of amoxicillin and cefaclor. J Pediatr 1984;104:297–302.

4. Rodriguez RS, De La Torre C, Sanchez C, et al. Bacteriology and treatment of acute maxillary sinusitis in children: A comparative study of erythromycin-sulfisoxazole and amoxicillin. Abstracts of the Interscience Conference of Antimicrobial Agents and Chemotherapy (328) Los Angeles, CA, 1988.

5. Wald ER, Byers C, Guerra N, Casselbrant M, Beste D. Subacute sinusitis in children. J Pediatr 1989;115:28–32.

6. Brook I. Bacteriologic features of chronic sinusitis in children. JAMA 1981;246:967–969.

7. Muntz HR, Lusk RP. Bacteriology of the ethmoid bullae in children with chronic sinusitis. Arch Otolaryngol Head Neck Surg 1991;117:179–181.

8. Tinkleman DG, Silk HJ. Clinical and bacteriologic features of chronic sinusitis in children. Am J Dis Child 1989;143:938–941.

9. Shapiro ED, Milmoe GJ, Wald ER, Rodnan JB, Bowen AD. Bacteriology of the maxillary sinuses in patients with cystic fibrosis. J Infect Dis 1982;146:589–593.

10. Friedman R, Ackerman W, Wald E, Casselbrant M, Friday G, Fireman P. Asthma and bacterial sinusitis in children. J Allergy Clin Immunol 1984;74:185–189.

11. Goldenhersh MJ, Rachelefsky GS, Dudley J, et al. The bacteriology of chronic maxillary sinusitis in children with respiratory allergy. J Allergy Clin Immunol 1990;85:1030–1039.

12. Gwaltney JM Jr, Scheld WM, Sande MA, Sydnor A. The microbial etiology and antimicrobial therapy of adults with acute community acquired sinusitis: A fifteen year experience at the University of Virginia and review of other selected studies. J Allergy Clin Immunol 1992;90S:457–461.

13. Wald ER, Chiponis D, Ledesma-Medina J. Comparative effectiveness of amoxicillin and amoxicillin-clavulanate potassium in acute paranasal sinus infection in children: a double blind, placebo-controlled trial. Pediatrics 1986;77:795–800.

14. Chonmaitree T, Owen MJ, Patel JA, Hedgpeth D, Horlick D, Howie VM. Effect of viral respiratory tract infection on outcome of acute otitis media. J Pediatr 1992;120:856–862.

15. Bach A, Boehrer H, Schmidt H, Geiss HK. Nosocomial sinusitis in ventilated patients. Nasotracheal versus oratracheal intubation. Anaesthesia 1992;47:335–339.

16. O'Reilly MJ, Reddick EJ, Black W, et al. Sepsis from sinusitis in nasotracheally intubated patients: A diagnostic dilemma. Am J Surg 1984;147:601–604.

17. Arens JF, LeJeune FE Jr, Webre DR. Maxillary sinusitis, a complication of nasotracheal intubation. Anesthesiology 1974;40:415,416.

18. Caplan ES, Hoyt NJ. Nosocomial sinusitis. JAMA 1982;247:639–641.

19. Kronberg FG, Goodwin WJ. Sinusitis in intensive care unit patients. Laryngoscope 1985;95:936–938.

20. Miner JD, Elliott CL, Johnson CW, et al. Nosocomial sinusitis. Indiana Med 1988;81:684–686.

21. Frederick J, Braude AI. Anaerobic infection of the paranasal sinuses. N Engl J Med 1974;290:135–137.

22. Karma P, Jokipii L, Sipila P, Luotonen J, Jokipii AMM. Bacteria in chronic maxillary sinusitis. Arch Otolaryngol 1979;105:386–390.

23. Morgan MA, Wilson WR, Neil HB III, Roberts GD. Fungal sinusitis in healthy and immunocompromised individuals. Am J Clin Pathol 1984;82:597–601.

24. Washburn RG, Kennedy DW, Gegley MG, Henderson DK, Bennett JE. Chronic fungal sinusitis in apparently normal hosts. Medicine 1988;67:231–247.

25. Lawson W, Blitzer A. Fungal infections of the nose and paranasal sinuses. Part I. Otolaryngol Clin North Am 1993;26:1007–1035.

26. Lawson W, Blitzer A. Fungal infections of the nose and paranasal sinuses. Part II. Otolaryngol Clin North Am 1993;26:1037–1068.

27. Jahrsdoerfer RA, Ejercito VS, Johns MME, et al. Aspergillosis of the nose and paranasal sinuses. Am J Otolaryngol 1979;1:6–14.

28. Agger WA, Caplan RH, Maki DG. Ocular sporotrichosis mimicking mucormycosis in a diabetic. Ann Ophthalmol 1978;10:767–771.

29. Kern ME, Uecker FA. Maxillary sinus infection caused by the Homobasidiomycetous fungus Schizophylumm commune. J Clin Microbiol 1986;123:1001–1005.

30. Mitchell RG, Chaplin AJ, MacKenzie DWR. Emericella nidulans in a maxillary sinus fungal mass. J Med Vet Myc 1987;25:339–341.

31. Bloom SM, Warner RRP, Weitzman I. Maxillary sinusitis: Isolation of Scedosporium (Monosporium) apiospermum, anamorph of Petriellidium (Allescheria) boydii. Mt Sinai J Med 1982;49:492–494.

32. Watters GW, Milford CA. Isolated sphenoid sinusitis due to Pseudoallescheria boydii. J Laryngology Otol 1993;107:344–346.

33. Stamm MA, Frable MA. Invasive sinusitis due to Pseudoallescheria boydii in an immunocompetent host. South Med J 1992;85:439–440.

34. Travis LB, Roberts GD, Wilson WR. Clinical significance of Pseudoallescheria boydii: A review of 10 years' experience. Mayo Clin Proc 1985;60:531–537.

35. Winn RE, Ramsey PD, McDonald JC, Dunlop KJ. Maxillary sinusitis from Pseudoallescheria boydii. Efficacy of surgical therapy. Arch Otolaryngol 1983;109:123–125.

36. Rockhill RC, Klein MD. Paecilomyces lilacinus as the cause of chronic maxillary sinusitis. J Clin Microbiol 1980;11:737–739.

37. Iwamoto H, Katsura M, Fujimaki T. Mycosis of the maxillary sinuses. Laryngoscope 1972;92:903–909.

38. Henderson LT, Robbins T, Weitzner S, et al. Benign Mucor colonization (fungus ball) associated with chronic sinusitis. South Med J 1988;81:846–850.

39. Dworzack DL, Pollack AS, Hodges GR, et al. Zygomycosis of the maxillary sinus and palate caused by Basidiobolus haptosporus. Arch Intern Med 1978;138:1274–1276.

40. Bassiouny A, Maher A, Bucci TJ, et al. Noninvasive antromycosis (diagnosis and treatment). J Laryngol Otol 1982;96:215–228.

41. Wickern GM. Fusarium allergic fungal sinusitis. J Allergy Clin Immunol 1993;92:624,625.

42. Kurien M, Anandi V, Raman R, Brahmadathan KN. Maxillary sinus fusariosis in immunocompetent hosts. J Laryngol Otol 1992;102:733–736.

43. Adam RD, Paquin ML, Petersen EA, et al. Phaeohyphomycosis caused by the fungal genera *Bipolaris* and *Exserohilum*. Medicine 1986;65:203–217.

44. Young CN, Swart JG, Ackermann D, Davidge-Pitts K. Nasal obstruction and bone erosion caused by *Dreschslera hawaiiensis*. J Laryngol Otol 1978;92:137–143.

45. Sobol SM, Love RG, Stutman HR, Pysher TJ. Phaeohyphomycosis of the maxilloethmoid sinus caused by *Drechslera spicifera*: A new fungal pathogen. Laryngoscope 1984;95:620–627.

46. Azar P, Acquavella JV, Smith RS. Keratomycosis due to an *Alternaria* species. Am J Ophthalmol 1975;79:881,882.

47. Shugar MA, Montgomery WW, Hyslop NE Jr. *Alternaria* sinusitis. Ann Otol 1981;90:251–254.

48. Zieske LA, Kopke RD, Hamill R. Dematiaceons fungal sinusitis. Otolaryngol Head Neck Surg 1991;105:567–577.

49. O'Donnell JG, Sorbello AF, Condoluci DV, Burnish MJ. Sinusitis due to *Pseudomonas aeruginosa* in patients with human immunodeficiency virus infection. Clin Infect Dis 1993;16:404–406.

50. Berlinger NT. Sinusitis in immunodeficient and immunosuppressed patients. Laryngoscope 1985;95:29–33.

51. Eron LJ, Huckins C, Park CH, et al. *Mycobacterium chelonei* infects the maxillary sinus: A rare case. Virginia Med 1981;108:335–338.

52. Kavanaugh KT, Parham DM, Hughes WT, Chanin LR. Fungal sinusitis in immunocompromised children with neoplasms. Ann Otol Rhinol Laryngol 1991;100:331–336.

53. McGill TJ, Simpson G, Healy GB. Fulminant aspergillosis of the nose and paranasal sinuses: A new clinical entity. Laryngoscope 1980;90:748–754.

54. Schubert MM, Peterson DE, Meyers JD, et al. Head and neck aspergillosis in patients undergoing bone marrow transplantation. Cancer 1986;57:1092–1096.

55. Douer D, Goldschmied-Reouven A, Segev S, Ben-Basset I. Human exserohilum and bipolaris infections: Report of *Exserohilum* nasal infection in a neutropenic patient with acute leukemia and review of the literature. J Med Vet Mycol 1987;25:235–241.

56. Davis JJ, Heymen MR. Cryptosporidiosis and sinusitis in an immunodeficient adolescent. J Infect Dis 1988;158:649.

57. Gonzalez M, Gould E, Dickinson G, et al. Acquired immunodeficiency syndrome associated with Acanthamoeba infection and other opportunistic organisms. Arch Pathol Lab Med 1986;110:749–751.

58. Gherman CR, Ward RR, Bassis ML. *Pneumocystis carinii* otitis media and mastoiditis as the initial manifestation of the acquired immunodeficiency syndrome. Am J Med 1988;85:250–252.

6 The Role of Allergy in Sinus Disease

Children and Adults

Zdenek Pelikan, MD, PHD

SINUS DISEASE—BASIC FACTS

Definition

The disease of paranasal sinuses, so-called sinusitis, can be classified according to various criteria and divided in various subtypes, being already discussed in other chapters of this book. However, the classification of sinus disease according to the clinical course, acute vs chronic, as well as to the localization of sinus disease concerning the particular sinuses seems to be an important issue with respect to the allergy.

Acute sinusitis may almost exclusively be the result of bacterial or viral infections, and allergy may rarely play a causal role in this form of sinus disease. The acute sinusitis is a common disorder both in children and in adults (1–8).

Chronic sinusitis, especially chronic maxillary sinusitis (CMS), is a common disorder in adults and sometimes in older children (1,2,6–12).

The structure and function of paranasal sinuses have already been established (1,2,6,10,13–19), as well as the diagnosis and treatment of sinusitis (1,2,7,10,20–33). However, most of these studies reflect the role of bacterial and/or viral infections in the pathogenesis of the chronic sinusitis (2,3,7–12,34–37). The association of sinusitis with rhinitis has already been confirmed (1,2,6,7,10,12,15,18,28,30,36,38–44).

The ethiologic role of allergy, and of nasal allergy in particular, in some form of sinus disease, and the involvement of hypersensitivity mechanisms leading to the "sinusitis" or "sinus response," have already been discussed in the literature (1,7,11,15,37,39–56). The use of the term "sinusitis" for a disorder caused by an immunologic process does not appear to be fully suitable. It would be better to designate this disorder as "sinus

From: *Diseases of the Sinuses* (M. E. Gershwin and G. A. Incaudo, eds.),
©1996 Humana Press Inc., Totowa, NJ.

response," "allergic sinusopathy," or "allergic sinus disease" *(56)*.

However, few data are available to illustrate the direct causal relationship of hypersensitivity mechanisms appearing primarily in the nasal mucosa that lead to the secondary response in the mucosal membrane of the sinuses. Our studies, results of which will be presented and discussed later in this chapter, are probably the only ones on this topic *(53–59)*.

With respect to the localization of particular kinds of paranasal sinuses, such as maxillary, frontal, sphenoid, and ethmoidal (anterior and posterior), sinus disease related to allergy may appear most commonly in the maxillary sinuses, sporadically in the frontal sinuses, and has not been reported in the sphenoid or ethmoid sinuses *(45,53,54,56)*. However, some investigators presume that the disease of the maxillary and frontal sinuses, especially that of the bacterial and viral ethiology, is almost always accompanied, if not preceded, by the disease of the ipsilateral anterior ethmoid region, since all three sinus types communicate into middle meatus, which is also called "ostiomeatal complex" *(23–25,60)*. Nevertheless, similar participation of the ethmoid sinuses in the disease of the maxillary and frontal sinuses owing to the hypersensitivity mechanism(s) has not yet been confirmed.

Basic Forms of Sinus Disease Resulting from the Allergy Mechanism

Two basic forms of the sinus disease or so-called sinusopathy, in which hypersensitivity mechanism(s) (allergy reaction) may play the principal causal role, may be recognized: (1) the primary and (2) the secondary (induced) form *(53–57)*.

In the primary form, the antigen–antibody interaction with subsequent steps takes place primarily in the mucosal membrane of the particular sinuses. The primary form of sinus disease can be elicited by the inhalant allergens, which may pass the nasal mucosal barrier and the mucosal filter without initiating any hypersensitivity reaction in the nasal mucosa. The allergen, after passing the nasal mucosal barrier, may be trapped directly into the appropriate sinus, where it interacts with the local antibodies or sensitized T-lymphocytes in the sinus mucosa, a process that is then followed by the subsequent steps, resulting in the primary sinus response, without any accompanying nasal

response. Such a mechanism previously has been proposed by Slavin and colleagues *(1,6,40)*. The primary form can also be caused by the food antigens, which had been digested and then transported through the bloodstream into the sinus mucosa, where they interact with the local antibodies or sensitized T-lymphocytes.

In the secondary form, the inhalant allergens, penetrating into the nasal mucosa from outside, or food antigens, having been delivered to the nasal mucosa from the gut by the bloodstream, interact with the antibody or sensitized T-lymphocytes primarily in the nasal mucosa *(56)*. This primary antigen–antibody interaction in the nasal mucosa leads to the development of the primary nasal mucosa response, which then induces the secondary response of the particular sinuses and/or sinus mucosa *(56)*. The secondary form of the sinus response owing to the hypersensitivity mechanism occurs much more frequently than the primary form *(55,56)*. According to our data, the ratio of the primary vs secondary form of the allergic sinus disease may be approx 1:350 *(55)*.

Sinus–Nose Relationship

The relationship between the nose and sinuses, especially maxillary sinuses, has been well established *(1,2,8,10–12,18,36,37,39–43,45–48,50,51,60–69)*.

In some patients, the CMS has been referred to as a complication of perennial allergic rhinitis. This conclusion has, however, been drawn either from the clinical observation or from the epidemiologic follow-up studies *(12,39,52,61)*.

Interestingly, there are many similarities in the anatomic, physiologic, and pathologic characteristics of the nasal mucosa and mucosal membrane of the paranasal sinuses, especially the maxillary sinuses *(1,2,4–6,12,15–18,35,38,39,46,51,60)*, which are discussed in other chapters of this book. However, these similarities have led some authors to report about one type of the mucosal membrane, both in the nose and in the paranasal sinuses, with only little distinction *(15,18)*.

ANATOMICAL ASPECTS

The ethmoidal sinuses can be divided into three topographical groups, an anterior, middle, and posterior group. The anterior ethmoidal sinuses open into the hiatus semilunaris in the middle meatus, either separately or together with the frontal sinus. The middle ethmoidal sinuses, the bulla ethmoidalis being one of them, open into the middle meatus, between the middle and inferior conchae, just above the uncinate process. The posterior ethmoidal sinuses open into the superior meatus, between the superior and middle conchae, or exceptionally into the sphenoethmoidal recess *(2,4,6,15,18,19,25,38,60,62,70)*.

The frontal sinus opens either through the frontonasal duct directly into the infundibulum in the middle meatus, or it opens into the hiatus semilunaris *(2,4,6,15,18,19,25,38,60,62,70)*. The sphenoidal sinus opens anteriorly into the sphenoethmoidal recess, just above the superior concha *(19,70)*. The maxillary sinus communicates with the nasal cavity through the ostium, a large anatomical opening into the middle meatus, filled in by a series of small bones, which, along with the overlying mucosal membrane, form an anatomical and also functional valve, partly closing the definitive opening, already reduced by the small bones *(2,4,6,15,18,19,25,38,60,62,70)*.

PHYSIOLOGICAL ASPECTS

The maxillary sinus is the only sinus of which the opening and drainage are regulated by the anatomical and functional valve, called ostium, acting also as a protective mechanism, whereas the lumens of the other paranasal sinuses remain continuously open *(37,46,61,62)*. Despite this unique property of having the ostium, the maxillary sinus is involved in the allergic disorders of the upper airways more frequently than the other paranasal sinuses, either as a secondary and accompanying target of the nasal allergy or as a primary location of the hypersensitivity mechanism *(55,56)*. The ostium plays a pivotal role for the maxillary sinus and its mucosal membrane by regulating the drainage of secretions and gas exchange, which is its primary function *(1,2,6,15,18,35, 38,39,46,51)*.

Several factors may disturb the draining function of the ostia, resulting in the retention of secretions in the maxillary sinuses, such as:

1. The swelling of the nasal mucosa, leading to the limited patency of the ostia;
2. The reduced transport capacity of the sinus secretions owing to the abnormalities of the cilia, including not only the quantitative reduction of the cilia and retardation of the ciliar movement, but also the insufficient coordination of the ciliar movement of various areas; and

3. The overproduction of the secretions in the maxillary sinuses leading to the retention of the secretions in the sinus owing to the overloaded drainage capacity *(1,2,6,15,18,25,33,37,39,44–47,50,62)*.

The cross-sectional area of the ostium is also the primary determinant of the gas exchange in the human sinuses *(16,17)*. Another factor influencing the gas exchange in the sinuses is the nasal air flow *(16,17)*. The sinus cavity air exchanges are twice as fast during the nasal breathing than during the oral breathing *(17)*.

Usually, not only does the increase in the edema of the nasal mucosal membrane lead to the mechanical oppression and occlusion of the maxillary ostium from outside by the surrounding nasal mucosa tissue, but also the edema of the nasal mucosa extends to the margin of the ostium and its membranous parts. In this manner, the edematic ostium is no longer able to execute its drainage function sufficiently. Moreover, the edematic ostium disturbs and inhibits the optimal drainage of the sinus. All these changes then lead to the partial or full closing of the sinus, resulting in accumulation of the mucus, gases, and soft tissue mass *(53–58)*.

However, sporadically a paradoxical effect of the increased edema of the nasal mucosa on the maxillary ostium has been observed (unpublished data). The increased edema of the nasal mucosa, especially of the area located anterior to the maxillary ostium, has retracted and stretched the partially closed ostium outward, and in this manner, the orifice became enlarged, resulting finally in the improved drainage *(55)*.

PATHOLOGICAL ASPECTS (THE MECHANISM[S] OF SINUS DISEASE RESULTING FROM ALLERGY)

The hypersensitivity mechanism(s), which means the antigen–antibody or the sensitized T-lymphocytes–antigen interaction with particular subsequent steps, occurring in the nasal mucosa, may lead to various symptoms *(39,64–67)*. Nasal obstruction caused by swelling of the nasal mucosa is, however, one of the most important of these symptoms *(1,10,64–69)*. The edema of the nasal mucosa leads to an edematic obstruction of the paranasal sinus orifice (in the case of the maxillary sinuses, the edematic obstruction of the nasal ostia) and to the decreased ciliary action and increased mucus production in the paranasal sinuses. The whole process then results in the accumulation of the mucus and gas in the sinuses, with the subsequent:

1. Thickening of the mucosal membrane in the sinuses owing to the edema and/or topical infiltration;
2. A decrease in aeration;
3. An increase in opacification, and sometimes the formation of an increased fluid level and soft tissue mass in maxillary sinuses *(1,2,6,9,14,15,16, 25–27,31–33,39,42,43,46,47,50,54–60,71)*.

Another mechanism that can be involved in the development of sinus disease resulting from allergy has been suggested by Slavin et al. *(16,37,39,40)*. These authors have postulated that some foreign particles, e.g., antigen, can escape the filtering mechanisms of the nose and can then be directly trapped into the mucus and mucosal membrane of the sinuses. In such a case, it might be possible that an antigen would also pass the nasal barrier, would be trapped in the paranasal, e.g., maxillary sinuses, and cause there an antigen–antibody interaction with subsequent release of mediators and other steps, topically in the mucosal membrane of the paranasal (maxillary) sinuses. Under such circumstances, the sinus response will be a primary event, without any preceding nasal mucosa response *(56)*.

HYPERSENSITIVITY (ALLERGY) MECHANISMS AND NONSPECIFIC HYPERREACTIVITY

The Basic Schedule of an Allergic Reaction

The antigen–antibody or antigen-sensitized T-lymphocyte interaction leads to the changes on and in the particular immunocompetent or target cells (which can be changed, damaged, or stimulated for secretion of various compounds), resulting in the synthesis and/or activation of the already preformed mediators, followed by their subsequent release. The released mediators act then either directly or indirectly through their effects on other cell types and/or on the various effector organs, such as smooth muscles, mucosal glands, epithelial cells, monocellular secretory units (e.g., goblet cells), endothelial cells, capillary network, various types of receptors, neurovegetative synopses, and a variety of other cell types (Fig. 1). The combined response of the effector organs results in a variety of clinical symptoms, topical, systemic, or whole body, representing the particular allergic disorder.

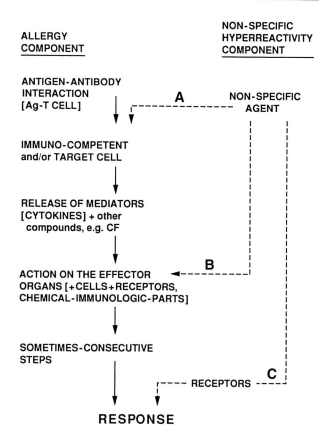

Fig. 1. Basic schedule of the allergy component and the nonspecific hyperreactivity component.

The combined response of the effector organs usually has two parts, a topical part, located on and in the appropriate organ, and a central part, being located in the system and/or in the blood *(46,65,66,72–82)*.

The hypersensitivity (allergic) reaction may be seasonal or nonseasonal (perennial), depending on the kind of allergen(s) involved.

The Basic Types of the Hypersensitivity (Allergic) Reaction

The hypersensitivity reactions can be divided into four basic types (Fig. 2) as proposed by Coombs and Gell *(82)*.

Type I = immediate hypersensitivity (IgE-mediated);
Type II = cytotoxic hypersensitivity (IgG, IgM-mediated);
Type III = late hypersensitivity (IgG-, IgM-complex-mediated); and
Type IV = delayed hypersensitivity (T-cell-mediated).

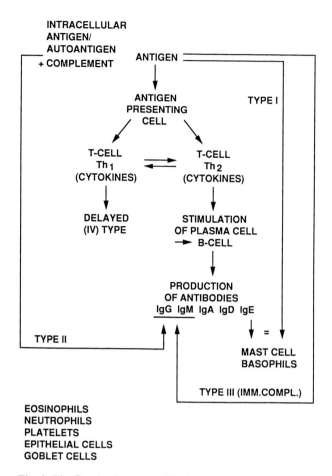

Fig. 2. The four basic types of the hypersensitivity (allergy) mechanism.

The original Coombs and Gell classification *(82)* was later revised by Shearer and Huston *(73)* as follows: Type I = mast cell-mediated: (1) IgE-dependent (anaphylactic), (2) IgE-independent (anaphylactoid); Type II = antibody-mediated (non-IgE):

1. Opsonization;
2. Complement lysis;
3. Antibody-dependent cellular cytotoxicity (ADCC);
4. Stimulating; and
5. Blocking;

Type III = immune complex; and Type IV = cell-mediated:

1. CD4$^+$ T-cell;
2. CD8$^+$ T-cell; and
3. Natural killer (NK) cell.

TYPE I ALLERGY (IMMEDIATE HYPERSENSITIVITY)

This type of reaction occurs usually within seconds to minutes after the antigen–antibody interac-

tion. Specific antibodies usually of the IgE class bound to the surface of the mast cells (in the tissues) or basophils (in the bloodstream) interact with the extrinsic antigens with the aforementioned consequences *(65,66,73,74,79,82)*.

Recently, evidence has been provided for a possible additional role of antibodies of other classes, e.g., IgG, IgA-secretory, and IgM, in this type of hypersensitivity, then called IgE-independent subtype or IgE-low reactors. The cell types participating in the type I allergy include mast cells, basophils, eosinophils, neutrophils, epithelial cells, and endothelial cells. A variety of mediators, chemotactic factors, adhesive glycoproteins, cytokines, and other compounds may participate in the type I hypersensitivity, such as histamine, prostaglandins, leukotrienes, chemotactic factors for eosinophils (ECF-A), neutrophils (NCF-A), platelet-activating factors (PAF), cytokines (e.g., IL-4, TNF-α), adhesive glycoproteins (e.g., ICAM-1, ELAM-1, VCAM-1), and various other compounds.

The type I hypersensitivity may also be divided into two subtypes with respect to the participation of the genetic factors and predisposition: (1) atopic subtype, where predisposition can be transferred genetically; and (2) anaphylactic subtype, where genetic factors do not play any substantial role *(65,66,73,74,79,82)*.

The type I (immediate) hypersensitivity is very common and can be involved in a variety of disorders, such as anaphylactic shock, bronchial asthma, allergic rhinitis, urticaria, atopic eczema, allergic conjunctivitis, secretory otitis media, chronic sinusitis, insect venom allergy, various forms of food allergy, and some forms of drug hypersensitivity *(65,66,73,74,79,82)*.

TYPE II ALLERGY (CYTOTOXIC HYPERSENSITIVITY)

This type of hypersensitivity occurs within a period of minutes to hours. The antigen bound to the surface of the carrier cell or located intracellulary (e.g., tissue antigen) interacts with the circulating antibodies. The antibodies, presumed to be of IgG, IgM, or to a lesser degree of IgA classes may be directed against the structural antigens of the carrier cells or against the antigens from other sources, attached to the surface of the carrier cells. The carrier cell, after the antigen–antibody interaction, may then be phagocytized after adhesion to a phagocyte, may be lysed by activation of the complement cascade or may be destroyed by the "killer" cells, e.g., NK or large lymphocytes. The antibodies are directed against the antigens on the surface of the target cells, such as erythrocytes, neutrophils, platelets, and epithelial cells of glandular or mucosal surfaces, or against the antigens on the tissues, such as basement membranes *(73,79,81,82)*. The sensitizing antigens in these cases can be natural cell-surface antigens, modified cell-surface antigens, or haptens attached to the cell surface *(73,79,81,82)*.

The cytotoxic hypersensitivity can be involved in such disorders as autoimmune hemolytic anemia, some forms of leukocytopenia and thrombocytopenia, hemolytic diseases of newborns, some forms of agranulocytosis, thrombocytopenic purpura, blood transfusion reactions, some kinds of serum sickness, rhesus incompatibility, connective tissue diseases, autoimmune reactions (Hashimoto's thyroiditis, Goodpasture's Syndrome, some forms of nephritis, and glomerulonephritis), and some forms of drug hypersensitivity *(73,79,81,82)*.

Type III Allergy (Arthus Phenomenon, Late Hypersensitivity, Immune Complex-Mediated Hypersensitivity)

This type of reaction occurs 4–12 h after the antigen–antibody interaction and usually lasts for several hours. The circulating antibodies of the IgG and/or IgM classes, being presumed to play a major role, interact with circulating antigens in the bloodstream or in the vascular wall, and in this way form the immune complexes. The immune complexes then activate the complement system cascade, especially C3a, C5a, C5b, C6, and C7, with subsequent activation of the blood-clotting mechanisms, liberation of kinin system components, release of lysosomal enzymes, vascular permeability factors, and other factors from the neutrophils and release of vasoactive amines, lysosomal enzymes, and other factors from the platelets, and activation of the eosinophils. Recently, evidence has been provided for participation of some cytokines, such as IL-1, tumor necrosis factor (TNF) ($\alpha + \beta$), and IL-8, in this mechanism *(64–66,73,75,78,79, 81,82)*. The forming of immune complexes leads to the complex inflammatory reactions resulting in the tissue damage.

The type III reaction may take place either locally or systemically, which depends on the place of entry of the antigen and on the volume ratio of the antigen and the antibody. The complexes

formed at the equivalence of antigen and antibody or in a moderate antigen excess are of the most effective size (medium to larger) for the activation of the complement, are less soluble, and also have the most prolonged residence in the circulation. The complexes formed in an excess of either antigen or antibody are small and soluble, and are deposited within a short period of time in various tissues *(64–66,73,75,78,79,81,82)*.

The larger complexes become trapped, particularly on the basement membrane and in the blood vessels, where they are deposited on the internal elastic lamina.

The localization of the immune complexes in the particular tissue depends on a variety of factors, such as the size of the complexes and their solubility, blood-flow turbulence, the ionic charge, and other factors *(73,78)*. This type of hypersensitivity can be involved in various disorders, such as extrinsic allergic alveolitis (hypersensitivity pneumonitis, organic dust disease), e.g., farmer's lung, pigeon breeder's lung, mushroom worker's lung, allergic bronchopulmonary aspergillosis, vasculitis, lupus erythematosus, rheumatic disorders, and some forms of glomerulonephritis *(73,75,78)*.

Recently, evidence has been provided for an involvement of this type of hypersensitivity also in some forms of allergic bronchial asthma, allergic rhinitis, atopic eczema, urticaria, and reactions to foods and drugs *(64–66,73,75,78,79,81,82)*.

Type IV Allergy (Delayed-Type Hypersensitivity, Cell-Mediated Reactions)

This type of reaction occurs later than 24 h after the antigen–T-cell interaction, usually between 24 and 72 h, and lasts for several days. In this type of hypersensitivity, the antigen, either alone or presented by an antigen-presenting cell (APC), interacts with the activated antigen–specific (sensitized) T-lymphocyte, usually of the helper T-cell subset (CD4$^+$8$^-$ T-cells, especially the Th1-subset) and/or of the cytotoxic T-cell subset (CD8$^+$4$^-$ T-cells), including the NK T-cell subset (CD56, CD45, CD11a, CD16). These cells are able to produce and then release a variety of factors, called lymphokines, a group consisting of interleukines (IL-2 to IL-5, IL-9, IL-10), TNF-β, macrophage-colony stimulating factor (M-CSF), granulocyte-monocyte-colony stimulating factor (GM-CSF), interferon-gamma (IFN-γ), and lymphotoxines, acting then through various pathways and cells on the other systems, effector organs, and target cells, resulting in an immunologic tissue injury and appearance of the clinical manifestation of the delayed hypersensitivity (79,80). There is no doubt about the pivotal role of the activated (sensitized) T-lymphocyte in the cell-mediated ("delayed") hypersensitivity mechanism *(64–66,73,76,77,79–82)*.

The delayed hypersensitivity may be involved in a variety of states and disorders, such as tuberculine reaction (Mantoux test); contact dermatitis and contact eczema; immune surveillance against the tumor cells, as well as various infection (bacterial and viral) agents; allograft (homograft) reactions; reactions against autologous tissues (autoimmune diseases); some human demyelinating and neuromuscular diseases (e.g., allergic encephalomyelitis, multiple sclerosis, Guillain-Barre syndrome), polymyositis, dermatomyositis, inflammatory bowel and liver diseases, including ulcerative colitis and Crohn's disease, pernicious anemia, primary bilary cirrhosis, chronic active hepatitis, and hepatitis B virus (HBV); gluten-sensitive enteropathy; endocrine disorders, such as thyroiditis, Addison's disease, and Graves' disease; infertility; some forms of diabetes mellitus; rheumatic disorders (e.g., lupus erythematosus, rheumatoid arthritis); sarcoidosis; acquired immune deficiency syndrome (AIDS); fungal infections (e.g., coccidioidomyosis, candidiasis); and malignancy (Hodgkin's disease, cancer) *(73,76,77,79–82)*.

Recently, evidence has been provided for the participation of delayed hypersensitivity mechanism(s) also in the allergic bronchial asthma, allergic rhinitis and rhinitis combined with secretory otitis media, sinusitis, migraine, and various adverse reactions to foods, urticaria, atopic eczema, conjunctivitis, and general malaise complaints *(64–66,73,76,77,79–82)*.

Nonspecific Hyperreactivity

In addition to the particular types of the allergic reaction (hypersensitivity mechanisms), there is another very important mechanism, the so-called nonspecific hyperreactivity. This mechanism can lead to a similar spectrum of symptoms as that caused by an immunologic mechanism (Type I hypersensitivity), with some minor differences, but that is not initiated by the antigen–antibody interaction. The nonspecific agents, mainly small molecular chemical compounds, physical factors (temperature differences, vapors, smoke), or

mechanical factors (nonorganic dusts, sand, and so forth), either:

1. Influence the immunocompetent or target cell directly, causing a nonspecific release of mediators, or indirectly, e.g., through the stimulation of the mucosal sensory nerves and/or a variety of mucosal receptors, resulting in the activation and release of various neuropeptides, which then affect the immunocompetent cells;
2. Act via the stimulation of mediator precursors, first leading to stimulation of the mediator production, which then acts directly on the effector organs, and second leading to the feedback inhibition of these mediators or immunocompetent cells; or
3. Act on the effector organs directly, thus causing the clinical effects (Fig. 1) *(63,66,83–89)*.

The nonspecific hyperreactivity can exist in addition to the particular type of allergic reaction in the same patient. Both the components (allergy and nonspecific hyperreactivity), owing to the different mechanisms, may participate in the patient's complaints, however, to various degrees and ratios. They are, however, fully independent and can exist beside one another in the same organ of the patient, but neither can be regarded as a necessary condition for the other *(63,66,84–89)*.

THE BASIC TYPES OF THE NASAL RESPONSE AND THE NONSPECIFIC HYPERREACTIVITY

Patients with nasal allergy, being challenged with an inhalant allergen during the nasal provocation tests (NPT), may develop different types of nasal response, such as immediate (early) nasal response (INR/ENR), late nasal response (LNR), or delayed nasal response (DYNR) (Table 1) *(63–65,66,69,87,90–92)*.

Detection of the Particular Types of Nasal Response

The definite confirmation of the existence of the particular types of nasal response (immediate, late, delayed) owing to a certain allergen, and their participation in the nasal complaints of the individual patient, can only be provided by NPT (challenge) with allergen *(63–65,66,69,87,90–93)*. The most important aspect of the provocation test is the com-

Table 1
Time-Course of the Particular Clinical Types
of Nasal Response to Allergen Challenge

	Onset	Maximum	Resolving
INR	<10	20–45	<90–120 min
LNR	4–6	6–10	<24 h
DYNR	24–30	30–40	<60 h

References: *63–67,90–92,96–116,127,153,160–165,171,224.*

parison of the objective parameters and subjective complaints, before and repeatedly after the challenge with a particular allergen (or nonspecific agent) *(65,66,68,87,93).*

The NPT can be supplemented by a recording of various in vivo as well as in vitro diagnostic parameters and functions, such as clinical symptoms (pulse rate, blood pressure, body temperature), other organs' functions (tympanometry, conjunctival appearance, X-ray or echography of sinuses, lung functions, and so on) or other parameters (nasal biopsy, biochemical, cytologic, and immunologic investigation of the nasal secretions and nasal mucosa, estimation of mediators, immunoglobulins, and other compounds in nasal secretions and/or serum, and physical and chemical properties of nasal secretions, such as consistency, pH, viscosity, and so forth) *(53–59,63–67,69,90–118).*

The nasal response to allergen challenge can be recorded and assessed by various methods and techniques. There are two basic methods: (1) recording of the subjective complaints (obstruction, hypersecretion, sneezing, itching) by means of a score; and (2) recording of the objective parameters related to the changed resistance to inspired air in the nose resulting from the increased nasal obstruction caused by the swelling of the nasal mucosa and hypersecretion, both of them owing to the antigen–antibody interaction or to the direct effects of nonspecific agents *(66,87,88,100).*

Recording of the subjective complaint score only is no longer acceptable because of the high degree of standard deviation, irregular occurrence of the complaints, personal influence, and lack of the reliable quantification *(66,87,88,100).* Recording of the objective parameters, such as nasal airway resistance (NAR), using air-flow and/or air-pressure or their derivatives (air passage and conductance [reciprocal value of nasal airway resistance R_N]), by means of which the nasal

mucosa response can be assessed, deserves preference *(66,93).*

These techniques can be divided into four groups:

1. Nasal peak-flow measurement;
2. Plethysmography;
3. Rhinomanometry (anterior, posterior, combined and/or modified techniques, used either in an active or passive manner); and
4. Nonrhinomanometry techniques, e.g., recording of the nasal blood flow using Doppler velocimetry, the [133]Xenon washout method, or acoustic rhinometry *(56,64,66,68,69,87,90–93,95,98,100,119–124).*

We use the "balloon method," one of the combined rhinomanometry techniques (recording of the NPG = nasopharynx-nostril-pressure gradients, expressed in cm of H_2O), described in detail elsewhere as a standard method *(56,64,66,68,69,87,88).* The passive anterior rhinomanometry is used by us for children, whereas the volume/flow as well as the volume-pressure diagram (active posterior rhinomanometry and active anterior rhinomanometry) are used by us for research purposes or as an arbitrary test.

The basic schedule of NPT is as follows *(56,64,66,68,69,87,88):*

1. "Initial test" or baseline—the NPG values are recorded at 0, 5, and 10 min;
2. "Control values"—after a 3-min application of the control solution (phosphate-buffered saline [PBS], Coca's solution), the values are recorded at 0, 5, and 10 min. If no significant changes in the NPG control values with respect to the initial NPG values appear, the test may be continued; and
3. After an allergen challenge (usually for 3 min), the postchallenge NPG values are recorded at 0, 5, 10, 20, 30, 45, 60, 90, and 120 min, and then every hour up to the 11th (12th) hour and, if necessary (the response has not resolved or a delayed response is expected), every hour on the second and the third day, respectively. A control challenge with control solution is performed in the same way on another day and the NPG parameters are recorded for the same period of time as those after the allergen challenge.

The protection tests, performed at our department as a part of the routine diagnostic procedure, are the nasal challenges carried out after the pretreatment with the particular drug *(63,65,66, 90–92,100,104,105,108,109,113,114,125,126).*

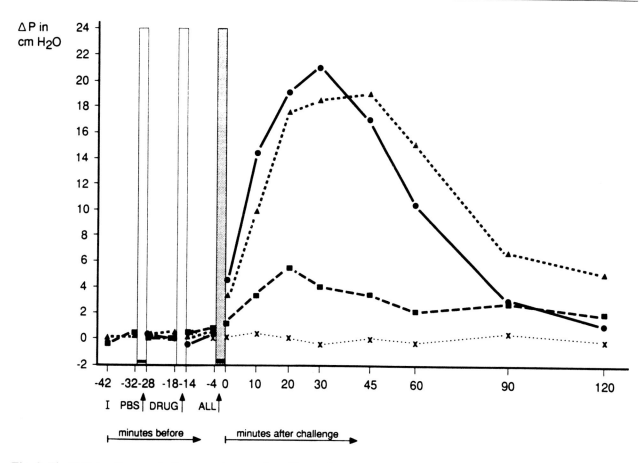

Fig. 3. The INR to allergen challenge and protective effects of DSCG and BUD. The mean nasopharynx-nostril-pressure gradient (NPG) values recorded after the non-pretreated and the pretreated allergen challenges and phosphate-buffered saline (PBS) control NPG values in 24 patients developing 24 positive INR. I, Initial values; PBS, control challenge; ALL, allergen challenge. ●———●, Nonpretreated INR ($n = 24$); ■ – – – ■, INR pretreated with DSCG ($n = 24$); ▲ _ _ _ ▲, INR pretreated with BUD ($n = 24$); X · · · · · · X, PBS control challenge ($n = 24$).

INR/ENR

INR/ENR owing to the immediate hypersensitivity mechanisms (Type I allergy) represents the most common form of the allergic component involved in the allergic rhinitis. The INR has been frequently studied from several points of view, and it is the most commonly described type of nasal response in the literature *(68,69,88)*.

OCCURRENCE

In 81% of the patients with allergic rhinitis, the INR to one or more allergens has been recorded *(69,88)*. The few data in the literature concerning the occurrence of INR somewhat vary for several reasons. The diagnostic procedure, including nasal challenge with allergens, is not performed routinely in all clinics where the patients with allergic rhinitis are examined. The epidemiologic studies were carried out according to different protocols, in differ-

ent groups of patients with allergic rhinitis, and finally, the criteria of evaluation and definition of the basic types of nasal response to allergen and those to nonspecific agents vary. The author's not yet published data, concerning the 785 patients with rhinitis complaints visiting our department during a 3-yr period (1988–1990), indicate that the immediate nasal response may occur in 43% of these patients *(127)*.

CLINICAL FEATURES, CHARACTERISTICS, AND FORMS

The clinical course of the INR, recorded by rhinomanometry, is as follows: onset within 10 min, maximum within 20–45 min, and resolving within 60–90 min after the allergen challenge (Table 1, Figs. 3 and 4) *(65,68,69,88,90)*.

The INR occurs in two forms, either as an "isolated immediate/early nasal response" (IINR) or in a combination with one of the nonimmediate

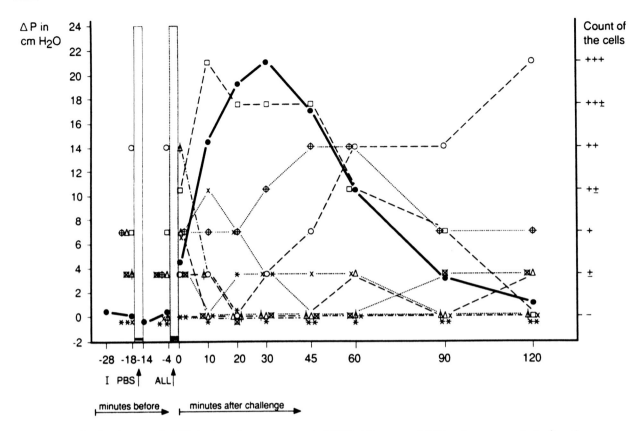

Fig. 4. Cytologic changes in NS during the nonpretreated INR. The mean NPG values recorded after the nonpretreated allergen challenges in 24 patients developing 24 positive INR. The mean changes in the counts of the particular cell types in the NS were calculated from 24 positive INR. I, Initial values; PBS, control challenge; ALL, allergen challenge. ●————●, Nonpretreated INR (*n* = 24); □———□, eosinophils; △ _ _ _ △, basophils; ⩙. _ . _ . _ . ⩙, mast cells; ○ - - - ○, neutrophils; X · · · · · X, goblet cells; ⊠· · · · · · ·⊠, lymphocytes; ⊕· · · · · · · ⊕, epithelial cells; * · · · · · · · · *, plasma cells; * · - · - · - *, monocytes.

responses, the late nasal response, or the delayed nasal response, where the immediate response appears first (within 2 h), and then after a symptom-free period of 3–7 h, or 22–28 h, the late respectively delayed response occurs. These responses were called "dual late response" (DLNR) or "dual delayed response" (DDYNR) in the past, with respect to a presumption that such a combined response (DLNR or DDYNR) should be a compact reaction consisting of two phases *(90–92)*.

However, regarding our recent data concerning the pharmacologic modulation of asthmatic responses to allergen challenge, as well as preliminary data concerning the dual nasal responses, the existence of DLNR as well as DDYNR as a compact reaction of two phases should be doubted *(127–129)*.

It seems that the so-called dual response is in reality an appearance of two independent responses, INR and LNR or DNR, owing to different mechanisms,

which have both been activated by chance by the same allergen at the same time. In this way, both the mechanisms have been developed independently, one beside the other, however, simulating a two-phase reaction on the side projection *(127,128)*.

The INR is usually accompanied by various nasal complaints, nasal obstruction, hypersecretion, sneezing, and itching, appearing to different degrees in the individual patient. The nasal complaints observed during the INR differ from those accompanying the LNR as well as the DYNR (Table 2) *(65,66,68,69,88,90)*.

DETECTION OF INR

The definite confirmation of the existence of the immediate nasal response can only be provided by the NPT with allergen *(65,68,69,88,90)*. In the case of INR, the postchallenge NPG parameters may usually be recorded up to 90–120 min, at least *(65,68,88,90)*.

Table 2
**A Survey of Nasal Complaints Accompanying
the Particular Types of Nasal Response**

Nasal complaints	Nasal response		
	INR	LNR	DYNR
Obstruction	++	+++	+++
Hypersecretion	+++	+	±
Sneezing	+++	+	−
Itching	+++	±	−

−, absent; ±, very slight; +, slight; ++, moderate; +++, severe.
References: *63–67,90–92,96–116,127,153,160–165,171,224.*

THE ASSOCIATION OF INR
WITH OTHER DIAGNOSTIC PARAMETERS

The INR may be associated with other in vivo and in vitro diagnostic parameters, to different degrees, as is summarized in Tables 3 and 4 *(63,65,66,68,69,88,90,127).*

1. The positive disease history to the same allergen was found in 66% of the INR. This correlation was found to be statistically doubtful ($p \leq 0.05$). No significant differences were found with respect to the particular allergens *(63,65,88,127).*

2. Anterior and posterior rhinoscopy and/or nasoscopy: In almost all patients developing the INR, the changed aspect of the nasal mucosa has been found, either a pronounced hyperemia (±32%) or a violaceous aspect (±68%) of the nasal mucosa accompanied by a slight mucosal edema, especially on the middle and inferior turbinate and partly also on the septum. Also, abundant secretions of the serous–mucinous composition and of a watery consistency may be found in these patients. No other changes, like mucosal hemorrhages, have been recorded on the mucosal membrane in patients developing the INR *(63,66,90).*

3. Skin tests: The immediate skin response (ISR) to the same allergen as that causing the INR was found in approx 68% (58–77%) of the INR cases. This relationship was found to be statistically doubtful ($p \leq 0.05$). The following division of the ISR sizes has been found: a slight grade (+) in 15%; a medium grade (++) in 18%; a high grade (+++) in 23%; and a very high grade (++++) in 9%. No significant differences were found with respect to the particular allergens *(63,66,68, 88,90,127).*

4. The concentration of the total IgE antibodies in the serum (PRIST) was found to be significantly increased (>500 IU/mL) in 7–17% of the INR cases, but it was found to be slightly increased (300–500 IU/mL) in 12–14% of the INR cases *(63,65,66,69,88,90,127).*

5. The specific IgE antibodies in the serum (RAST, CAP) to the same allergen as those causing the INR were found to be significantly positive (score grade 3 or 4) in approx 24–27% of INR cases. No significant correlation was found between serum RAST or RAST score and INR. No significant differences in the RAST were found with respect to the individual allergens *(63,65,66,69,88,90,127).*

6. The serum concentration of the total IgG antibodies was increased in 19% of the INR cases, of the total IgM in 0%, and of the total IgA in 1%. The serum concentration of the individual IgG subclasses did not change during most INR cases.

7. The blood eosinophil count increased (>300 × 10^6/L) during 5% of the INR cases *(63,66,88,127).*

8. The blood leukocyte count increased (>10 × 10^9/L) during 4% of the INR cases *(63,66,88,127).*

9. No increased body temperature (>37°C = >98.6°F axillary) or general malaise complaints were recorded during the positive INRs *(63,66,88,127).*

10. No significant changes of the concentrations of histamine have been recorded in the serum during the INR to allergen challenge *(63,127,146).*

11. The increased nasal mucosa responsiveness to histamine (PD_{20}), countervalue of which is the decreased nasal histamine threshold, was recorded in 31–59% of patients developing the INRs. The nasal histamine threshold varied mostly between 0.5 and 4.0 mg/mL (1.5–12 mmol/mL). The normal value of the nasal mucosa threshold for histamine is >4.0 mg/mL (>12 mmol/mL) *(63,66,85,86,89,127).*

12. The increased nasal mucosa responsiveness to methacholine bromide and/or chloride (PD_{20}), the countervalue of which is the decreased nasal methacholine bromide and/or chloride threshold, has been recorded in 11/14% of patients developing the INRs. The nasal threshold of methacholine bromide and/or chloride varied mostly between 0.5 and 2.0, and 1.0 and 8.0 mg/mL, respectively *(63).* The normal value of the nasal mucosa threshold for methacholine bromide is >4.0 mg/mL and for methacholine chloride >8.0 mg/mL *(84,127).*

Table 3
The Association of the Various Types of Nasal Response with Other Diagnostic Parameters (%)

	Nasal mucosa response to allergen challenge			
	Immediate, n = 148	Late, n = 131	Delayed, n = 63	Negative, n = 205
Response-related parameters				
Positive skin response				
Immediate	70			31
Late		65		9
Delayed			67	3
Increased total IgE in the serum (PRIST)	17	6	5	9
Positive specific IgE in the serum (RAST)	27	9	2	11
Total IgG	19	51	1	3
IgG$_1$	0	2	0	1
IgG$_2$	0	0^a	0	4
IgG$_3$	2	19	0	1
IgG$_4$	0	16	1	2
Total IgM	0	8	0	0
Total IgA	1	1	0	1
Increase in blood leukocytes	4	20	11	3
Increase in blood eosinophils	5	43	0	1
Increase in body temperature (more than 37°C = 98.6°F)	0	25	2	0
General malaise complaints	0	6	12	2
Aspects of the nasal mucosa				
Hyperemia	34	10	0	18
Violaceous aspect	59	90	100	1
Nasal mucosa hemorrhages	0	24	43	0
Patient-related parameters				
Increased reactivity of the nasal mucosa to histamine	31	23	2	89

^{a}IgG$_2$ in the serum decreased in 16% of the LNR cases.
References: *63–67,83–86,89–92,96–116,127,153,160–165,171,224.*

ASSOCIATION OF INR WITH OTHER ORGANS' RESPONSES

The INR was accompanied by headache in 26%, conjunctival irritation (injection or chemosis) in 27%, palpebral edema in 12%, middle ear response (otalgia, decrease in hearing, changes in the middle ear pressure as recorded by tympanometry) in 30%, pressure in the maxillary and frontal sinuses in 37%, changes on the X-ray of maxillary sinuses (increase in mucosal thickness or appearance of acute edema of the sinus mucosa) in 3%, changes on the echogram of maxillary sinuses in 5%, bronchial complaints (secondary dyspnea as recorded by spirography, sometimes wheezing and/or cough) in 5%, and other complaints (e.g., itching in the mouth, nasopharyngeal irritation, deglutitory complaints to a slight degree in 3% of the cases) (Table 4) *(50,53–59,63,65,66,68,69,72,83,90,95, 97,100,127,130–134).*

NASAL SECRETIONS (NS)

Cellular Aspects. The positive INR was accompanied by significant changes ($p < 0.05$) in the count of eosinophils (increase followed by decrease) in 67%, neutrophils (decrease followed by increase) in 40%, goblet cells (increase followed by decrease) in 41%, and basophils (decrease) in 13%, in the NS. The changes in the count of other cell types recorded in the NS during the positive INR, e.g., of lymphocytes in 2%, as well as of epithelial cells, plasma cells, and monocytes in 0%, were not sig-

Table 4
Survey of the Nasal Complaints and Other Organs' Response Accompanying
the Particular Types of Nasal Response to Allergen Challenge (%)

	Nasal response to allergen challenge			
	Immediate, n = 148	Late, n = 131	Delayed, n = 63	Negative, n = 205
Nasal complaints				
Obstruction	100	100	100	0
Sneezing	69	16	9	8
Hypersecretion	93	18	0	10
Itching	52	3	0	0
Conjunctival injection/chemosis	27	46	5	1
Palpebral edema	12	13	3	0
Middle ear response (otalgia, decrease in hearing, changes in middle ear pressure)	30	23	6	7
Pressure in the sinuses (maxillary and frontal)	37	18	22	7
Acute edema of sinus mucosa (X-ray)	3	11	14	1
Cephalgia	26	47	11	2
Bronchial complaints (mostly secondary bronchoconstriction, sometimes also wheezing and/or cough)	5	4	6	2
General malaise complaints	3	1	0	0

References: 63–67,90–92,96–116,127,130,132–134,153,160–165,171,224.

Table 5
Presence of Individual Cell Types in the Nasal Secretions and Changes
in Their Count During the Particular Nasal Response (%)

	Presence of the cells			Change in the cells' count between, before, and after the challenge		
	INR, n = 117	NNR, n = 83	PBS,[a] n = 200	INR, n = 117	NNR, n = 83	PBS,[a] n = 200
Eosinophils	85	19	48	68[b]	5	3
Neutrophils	71	17	40	37[b]	3	0
Basophils	16	91	31	3[b]	0	0
Epith. cells	68	23	25	9	7	4
Goblet cells	57	13	11	16[b]	4	2
Lymphocytes	11	4	7	2	3	0
Mast cells	4	2	3	0	0	0
Plasma cells	7	2	3	0	0	0
Monocytes	1	0	0	0	0	0

INR, immediate nasal response; NNR, negative nasal response; PBS, phosphate-buffered saline.
[a]Control.
[b]Statistically significant ($p < 0.05$).
References: 66,97,99,102,105,107,110–113,153,160,161.

nificant (Table 5, Fig. 4) (63,65,66,72,83,96,97,99, 102,105,107,109–113,117,118,135–137).

Immunological Aspects. The immunological aspects of the NS concern the factors and chemical compounds that may appear in the NS, can be detected, and whose changes in concentration can be related to the clinical event, e.g., the particular types of the nasal response to allergen, the nasal response owing to the nonspecific hyperreactivity, and so on. The study of these factors in the NS may contribute not only to the clarification of the mechanisms involved in and underlying the certain clinical event, but such knowledge can also be used for practical purposes, e.g., confirmation, verification, and prediction of a certain clinical event and for differential diagnosis. These factors are immunoglobulins, mediators, chemotactic factors, and ultimately all chemical compounds participating in the allergy or nonspecific hyperreactivity processes in the nose or being consequences of these processes, e.g., being released or generated by them or during them (63,66,127).

Immunological Aspects: The Immunoglobulins (Antibodies). The immunoglobulins (antibodies) have been studied frequently in nasal secretions. The appearance of total IgE, specific IgE, and sometimes also IgG and IgA in the NS of patients with allergic rhinitis repeatedly has been reported. Evidence has also been provided for a local production of IgE, IgG, and IgA antibodies in the nasal mucosa. Some investigators have concluded that local immunoglobulin production is higher in subjects with allergic rhinitis than in healthy subjects (138–143).

Unfortunately, there are only very few studies concerning the repeated determination of immunoglobulins in the NS during the INR, meaning before and repeatedly after a nasal challenge with a certain allergen (65,143). The appearance and changes of the particular immunoglobulin classes in the nasal secretions accompanying the INR have also been investigated by us. The data of these preliminary studies are prepared for publication (127).

In a group of 168 patients with positive INRs, before the allergen challenge (baseline), the total IgE antibodies were detected in NS in 12 cases (7.1%), specific IgE antibodies to the allergen used for challenge in 19 cases (11.3%), total IgG antibodies in 9 cases (5.3%), and total IgA in 2 cases (1.2%). No changes in the concentration of the total IgE, total IgG, or total IgA antibodies were recorded in the NS of any patient during the INR (postchallenge), but the concentration of specific IgE antibodies demonstrated changes during the 15 INR cases (8.9%), a decrease in 14 cases, and an increase in 1 case. However, all these changes were nonsignificant (127).

In the group of 82 patients with a negative nasal response, before the allergen challenge, the total IgE antibodies were found in NS in 7 cases (8.5%), specific IgE antibodies in 11 cases (13.4%), total

IgG in 6 cases (7.3%), and total IgA in no case. The concentration of specific IgE antibodies in NS decreased slightly to a nonsignificant degree in 2 cases (2.4%) after the allergen challenge, whereas no postchallenge changes in the concentration of the immunoglobulins of any class were recorded. No significant changes in concentration of any of the earlier-mentioned antibodies were recorded in NS during all 250 PBS control challenges (127).

Immunological Aspects: The Mediators. The INR may be accompanied by an increase in concentration of histamine, PGD_2, TAME-esterases, and kinins in NS. Sometimes also bradykinin, lysylbradykinin, prostaglandins (PGE_1, $PGF_{2\alpha}$), leukotrienes (LTB_4, LTC_4, LTD_4, LTE_4), thromboxanes (TXB_2), high-mol-wt neutrophil factor of anaphylaxis (HMWNF) may be found in NS during the INR (66,94,117,118,136,144–146). However, our data have indicated that the INRs may be associated with detectable changes in the concentrations of histamine in the NS in 69% of cases (103,106,127).

Biochemical and Biophysical Aspects. The NS produced during the INR have an increased viscosity and contain an increased concentration of the total protein in both ipsilateral and contralateral portions, an increased albumin percentage on the ipsilateral side, and increased relative proportions of lactoferrin and lysozyme on the contralateral side (71,147,148).

BIOPSIES

The following histologic changes have been recorded in the nasal mucosa during the INR. Before the allergen challenge (baseline), the nasal mucosa was compact and did not demonstrate any histologic or functional changes. In the upper layer of lamina propria, intact eosinophils, tissue mast cells, neutrophils, and lymphocytes were found to a very slight degree. During the positive INR, the following changes have been recorded: increased amount of thin serous secretions on the epithelial surface; enlarged ducti of mucosal glands; enlarged intercellular spaces in the epithelium; eosinophil and tissue mast cell accumulation, but not infiltrate forming, in the upper layer of lamina propria (approx 30% of eosinophils and 80% of mast cells were degranulated); dilated but not disrupted capillaries and perivascular edema to a slight degree in the lamina propria (as far as this could be evaluated); and an intact (not affected) basement membrane. These changes were of a "functional"

Table 6
Protective Effects of Basic Drugs on the INR, LNR,
and DYNR to Allergen Challenge

	INR	LNR	DYNR
Antihistamines			
H_1-receptor antagonists	±	−	−
H_2-receptor antagonists	−	−	−
H_1 + H_2-receptor antagonists	−	−	−
Anticholinergics			
Systemic (oral)	−	−	−
Topical	−	−	−
Calcium channel blockers	0	0	0
Acetylsalicylic acid	0	0	0
cAMP modulators	0	0	0
α_2-sympathomimetics	−	−	−
Disodium cromoglycate (DSCG)	+++	++	−
Nedocromil sodium (NDS)	++	+++	±
Corticosteroids			
Systemic			
Oral	−	−	−
Injection (iv, im)	±	±	±
Topical	−	+++	+++
Immunotherapy	±	−	−

−, No effect; ±, slight or partial effects (without significance); +, positive effects
($p < 0.05$); ++, distinctly significant effects ($p < 0.01$); +++, highly significant effects
($p < 0.001$); 0, lack of data.

and transient character, in contrast to those recorded during the LNR or DYNR (107,115,149).

THE PHARMACOLOGIC MODULATION OF THE INR/ENR

The INR can be prevented highly significantly by intranasal (topical) disodium cromoglycate (DSCG) (Rynacrom®, Lomusol®, Intal®, Nasalcrom®), whereas topical corticosteroids, such as beclomethasone dipropionate (BDA) (Beconase®, Viarin®, Aldecin®, Vancenase®), budesonide (BSA/BUD) (Rhinocort®), fluticasone dipropionate (FLD), flunisolide (FLN), or tixocortol pivalate (TCP) are not capable of preventing or significantly affecting the INR, as has been demonstrated repeatedly in our (Table 6, Figs. 3, 5, and 6) as well as in other investigators' clinical studies (65,66,83,90,97,99,105,109,113,117,127, 132,144,150).

Recently, a new compound, nedocromil sodium (NDS) (disodium salt of a novel pyranoquinoline dicarboxylic acid), demonstrating a number of unique pharmacologic properties, including a variety of antiallergic and anti-inflammatory effects, has been shown to prevent significantly the

INR (recent, preliminary, and unpublished data) (63,151,152).

H_1-receptor antagonists, oral, such as promethazine hydrochloride (Phenergan®), dexchlorpheniramine (Polaramine®), chlorphenamine maleate (Methyrit®), chlorpheniramine maleate (Chlortrimeton®), clemastine (Tavegil®), mequitazine (Mircol®), mebhydroline napadisilate (Incidal®), alimenazine (Nedeltran®), cyproheptadine hydrochloride (Periactin®), dimethindene maleate (Fenistil®), ketotifen (Zaditen®), cinnarizine (Cinnipirine®), astemizole (Hismanal®), terfenadine (Triludan®, Seldane®), acrivastine (Semprex®), loratadine (Claritin®), azelastine (Astelin®), cetirizine (Reactine®, Zyrtec®), and hydroxyzine hydrochloride (Atarax®), as well as topical, such as levocabastine hydrochloride (Livocab®), can diminish, and sometimes also prevent, some of the nasal complaints accompanying the INR, such as hypersecretion, sneezing, and itching, but they are, despite some investigators' reports, not capable of preventing significantly the nasal obstruction owing to the swelling of the nasal mucosa, being the most prominent aspect of the INR. The H_2- and H_3-receptor antagonist do not affect or prevent the

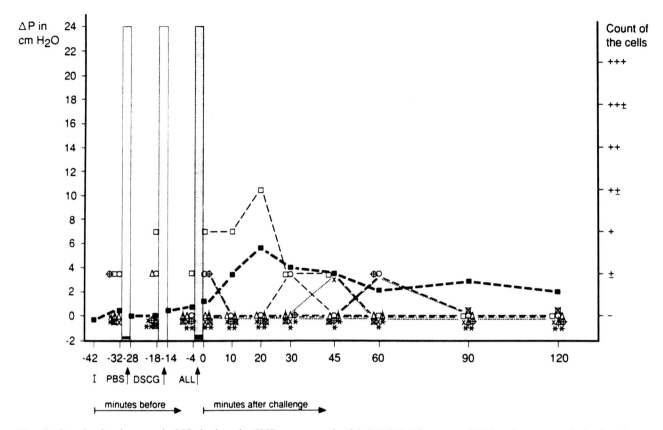

Fig. 5. Cytologic changes in NS during the INR pretreated with DSCG. The mean NPG values recorded after the allergen challenges pretreated with DSCG in 24 patients developing 24 INR. The mean changes in the counts of the particular cell types in the NS were calculated from 24 positive INR. I, Initial values; PBS, control challenge; ALL, allergen challenge. ■ – – – – ■, INR pretreated with DSCG (*n* = 24); □ – – – – □, eosinophils; △ _ _ _ △, basophils; ⟁ ._._._. ⟁, mast cells; ○ – – – ○, neutrophils; X · · · · · X, goblet cells; ⊠ · · · · · · · ⊠, lymphocytes; ⊕ · · · · · · · ⊕, epithelial cells; * · · · · · · · · · *, plasma cells; * · — · — · — · *, monocytes.

INR *(63,66,83,126,127,153–158).* However, the effects of particular H_1-receptor antagonists on the INR have not yet been studied sufficiently and only limited data concerning this topic are available in the literature *(158).* The effects of H_2- and H_3-receptor antagonists on the INR have not yet been documented *(127,158).* Anticholinergic drugs, such as oral thiazinamium hydrochloride or topical ipratropium bromide, as well as topical decongestants, such as xylomethazoline hydrochloride or oxymethazoline hydrochloride, did not demonstrate any significant protective effects on the INR *(127,153,156,159).* The possible protective effects of other drugs, such as calcium channel blockers, nonsteroidal anti-inflammatory agents, cAMP modulators, various antimediator agents, and inhibitors of 5-lipoxygenase pathways or thromboxane synthesis, on the INR have not yet been investigated sufficiently *(156).*

The immunotherapy may sometimes be effective in preventing nasal complaints accompanying the INR, especially INR owing to the particular pollen species, house dust mites, or animal danders, such as cat, dog, and horse.

MECHANISM(S) POSSIBLY INVOLVED IN THE INR

Regarding the earlier-presented data concerning various in vivo and in vitro parameters, accompanying the clinical INR as well as the pharmacologic modulation of INR and effects of various drugs on this type of nasal response, the immediate hypersensitivity (type I allergy) may be regarded as the most probable mechanism underlying the INR *(63,65,66,68,69,73,74,83,88,97,107,127).* The immediate hypersensitivity includes the tissue mast cells in the nasal mucosa as the basic immunocompetent cells and specific IgE antibodies being partly attached to the surface membrane of

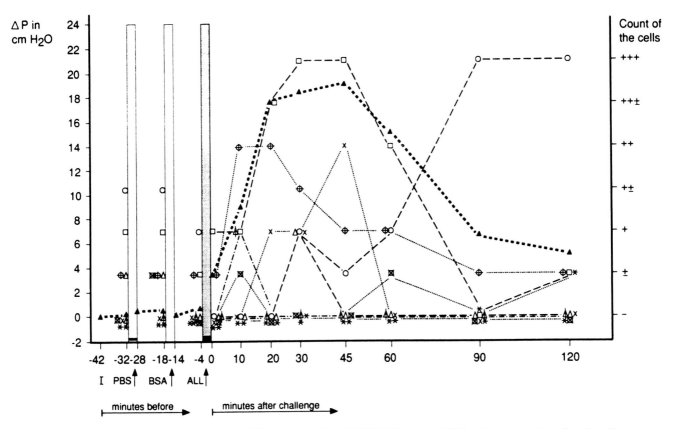

Fig. 6. Cytologic changes in NS during the INR pretreated with BUD. The mean NPG values recorded after the allergen challenges pretreated with BUD in 24 patients developing 24 INR. The mean changes in the counts of the particular cell types in the NS were calculated from 24 positive INR. I, Initial values; PBS, control challenge; ALL, allergen challenge. ▲____▲, INR pretreated with BUD (*n* = 24); □————□, eosinophils;⚠._._._.⚠, mast cells; ○———○, neutrophils; X······X, goblet cells;⊠·······⊠, lymphocytes; ⊕········⊕, epithelial cells; *········*, plasma cells; *·—·—·—·*, monocytes; △____△, basophils.

the mast cells and party free in the blood and tissue circulation *(63,65,72–74,83,97,107,117,118,127)*. The key role of the tissue mast cells in the INR has been supported by the finding of prostaglandin D_2 (PGD_2) in the nasal lavage fluid during the INR, a compound that is produced only by mast cell and not by basophil *(117,118,135,136)*. Moreover, (1) the significant protective effects of disodium cromoglycate on the INR, a compound protecting significantly both the mast cells and the basophils from their degranulation; (2) the lack of significant effects of H_1-receptor antagonists on the INR, compounds that antagonize predominantly the H_1-receptors, but do not affect or protect the mast cells or basophils; and, finally, (3) the absolute ineffectiveness of topical corticosteroids on the INR, receptors of which are not present both on the mast cells and on the basophils, may support strongly the presumed pivotal role of mast cells in

the immediate hypersensitivity mechanism leading to the INR *(65,66,72,83,90,102,103,105, 109,110,113,127,144,150–155,157,158)*.

Nevertheless, the participation of other cell types (such as eosinophils, neutrophils, platelets, epithelial cells, and endothelial cells—in various steps of immediate hypersensitivity, and in both simultaneous and sequential manners), is one of the necessary conditions for the development of the immediate hypersensitivity, a fact that has already been repeatedly confirmed by various research data from NS, nasal mucosa biopsies, and pharmacologic studies *(63,65, 66,83,96,97,102,107,110–112,115,117, 118,127,135–137,144–146,149,153,160,161)*.

The specific IgE antibodies, circulating and/or produced locally in the nasal mucosa, may undoubtedly play a key role in the immediate hypersensitivity mechanism leading to the INR *(63,65,69,74,83,138–141,143,153,160)*. However,

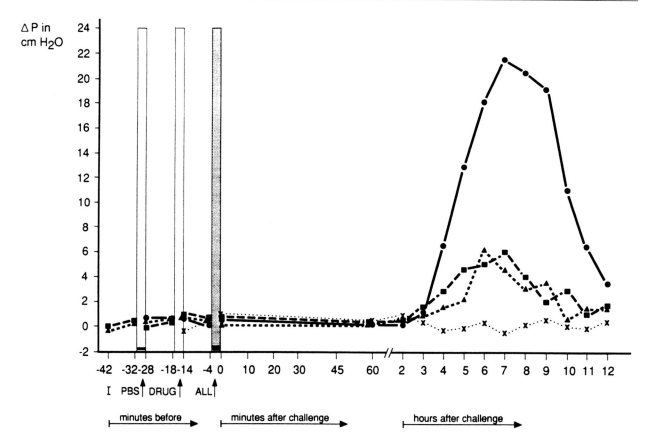

Fig. 7. The LNR to allergen challenge and protective effects of DSCG and BUD. The NPG values recorded after the nonpretreated and the pretreated allergen challenges and PBS control NPG values in 26 patients developing 26 positive LNR. I, Initial values; PBS, control challenge; ALL, allergen challenge. ● ———— ●, Nonpretreated LNR (n = 26); ■ – – – – ■, LNR pretreated with DSCG (n = 26); ▲ _ _ _ ▲, LNR pretreated with BUD (n = 26); X · · · · · · X, PBS control challenge (n = 26).

with respect to some recently gathered data demonstrating the lack of specific IgE antibodies both in the blood circulation and in the NS, on one hand, and the increased concentration of IgG and/or IgM antibodies in the NS during some cases of the INR, on the other hand, the possible participation of other antibody classes, different from IgE class, such as IgG and/or IgM, in the mechanism underlying the INR, cannot be more excluded *(63,69,83,140–142)*.

LNR

This type response regularly plays an important role in the nasal complaints of allergic rhinitis, is often overlooked in the practice, and may be responsible for the failure of the usual treatment in these patients.

OCCURRENCE, CLINICAL FEATURES, CHARACTERISTICS, AND FORMS

The LNR occurs in approx 41% of the patients with allergic rhinitis *(63–66)*. The clinical course

of the LNR, recorded by rhinomanometry, is as follows: onset within 4–6 h, maximum within 6–10 h, and resolving within 24 h (Table 1, Figs. 7 and 8) *(63–66)*. The LNR occurs either as an "isolated late response," or it can be preceded by an immediate response *(63–66)*. The LNR is usually accompanied by various acute nasal complaints appearing simultaneously with the course of the clinical response. However, the nasal obstruction owing to the distinct swelling of the nasal mucosa is the most prominent symptom, whereas the other nasal symptoms, such as hypersecretion, sneezing, and itching, are present to a lesser degree (Table 2) *(63–67,86,91,95,97,98,102,104,106,108,110,114, 115,117,118,127,135,136,144–146)*.

DETECTION OF LNR

The existence of LNR to a particular allergen in a certain patient can only be confirmed by the NPT (challenge) performed by means of rhinomano-

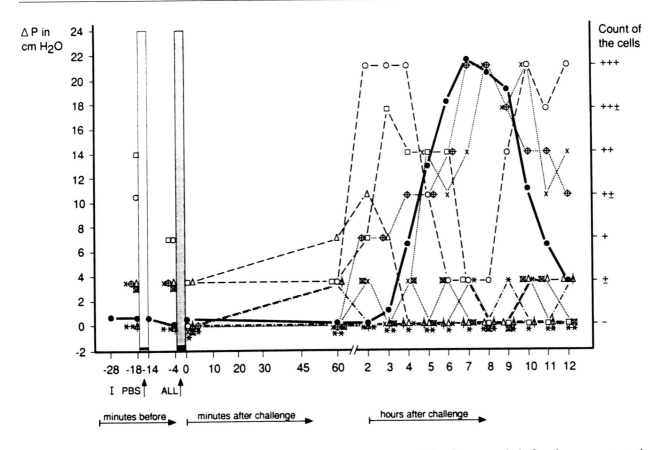

Fig. 8. Cytologic changes in NS during the nonpretreated LNR. The mean NPG values recorded after the nonpretreated allergen challenges in 26 patients developing 26 positive LNR. The mean changes in the counts of the particular cell types in the NS were calculated from the 26 positive INR. I, Initial values; PBS, control challenge; ALL, allergen challenge. ●————●, nonpretreated LNR (*n* = 26); □———□, eosinophils; △ _ _ _ △, basophils; △ . _ . _ . _ .△, mast cells; ○ – – – ○, neutrophils; X · · · · · · X, goblet cells; ⊠ · · · · · · · ·⊠, lymphocytes; ⊕ · · · · · · · ⊕, epithelial cells; * · · · · · · · · *, plasma cells; * · — · — · — · *, monocytes.

metry. The rhinomanometric parameters should be recorded before and after the allergen challenge, for a sufficiently long period of time, in the case of LNR, being at least 12 h.

Association of LNR
with Other Diagnostic Parameters

The LNR is associated with other diagnostic parameters in vivo and in vitro to different degrees, as summarized in Tables 3 and 4.

1. The positive disease history to the allergen causing the LNR was found in 40% of the LNR cases, in 27% of which the history was indicative of the late onset of nasal complaints *(63,66)*.

2. Anterior rhinoscopy and/or nasoscopy: During the LNR; the nasal mucosa in a majority of patients (±90%) was found to be violaceous and of a rather dry aspect owing to the diminished amount of secretions. Sometimes solitary small

mucosal hemorrhages may be observed on the middle and/or inferior turbinate. Sporadically also small lacunas of very viscous secretions can be found on the nasal mucosa *(63–66)*.

3. Skin tests: The late skin response (induration) was found in approx 65% of the LNR cases, and that of a small size (+) in 9%, a medium size (++) in 20%, a large size (+++) in 31%, and a very large size (++++) in 5% *(63–66)*.

4. The concentration of total IgE antibodies in the serum (PRIST) was found to be significantly increased (>500 IU/mL) in only 6% of LNR cases *(63–66)*.

5. The specific IgE antibodies in the serum (RAST, CAP) to the same allergen as that causing the LNR was significantly positive (score grade 3 or 4) in approx 9% of the LNR cases *(63–66)*.

6. The serum concentration of total IgG antibodies was increased in approx 51% of the LNR cases, of

total IgM antibodies in 8%, and that of total IgA antibodies in approx 1%. The serum concentration of the individual IgG subclasses during the LNR was recorded as follows: IgG_1 was elevated in 2%, IgG_3 in 19%, and IgG_4 in 16%, whereas IgG_2 was decreased in 11% *(63–66)*.

7. The increased blood eosinophil count (>300 × 10^6/L) has been recorded during 63% of the LNR cases *(63,66)*.
8. The increased blood leukocyte count (>10 × 10^9/L) has been recorded during 20% of the LNRs *(63,66)*.
9. The increased body temperature (>37°C = >98.6°F axillary) has been recorded during 2% of the LNRs *(63,66)*, whereas the general malaise complaints have been recorded in 6% of LNR cases *(63,66)*.
10. No significant changes in the concentrations of histamine have been recorded in the serum during the LNR to allergen challenge *(146)*.
11. The increased nasal mucosa responsiveness to histamine (PD_{20}) or its countervalue, the so-called decreased nasal histamine threshold, has been recorded by us in only 23% of the patients developing LNR, and that to a moderate degree (up to 4 mg/mL = 12 mmol/mL) *(66,85,86,89)*.
12. The increased nasal mucosa responsiveness to methacholine bromide has been found in 4% and that to methacholine chloride in 7% of patients developing the LNR. The nasal thresholds of both compounds varied between 4 and 8 mg/mL *(84,127)*.

ASSOCIATION OF LNR WITH OTHER ORGANS' RESPONSES

The LNR may be accompanied by headache in 47% of cases, conjunctival irritation (conjunctival injection or chemosis) in 46%, palpebral edema in 13%, middle ear response (otalgia, decrease in hearing, changes in the middle ear pressure as recorded by tympanometry) in 23%, pressure in the maxillary and frontal sinuses in 18%, changes on the sinus X-ray (increase in mucosal thickness or appearance of acute edema of the sinus mucosa) in 11 and 18%, respectively, and/or changes on the echogram of the sinuses in 16%, bronchial complaints (usually secondary dyspnea owing to the secondary induced bronchial constriction as recorded by spirography, sometimes also wheezing and/or cough) in 4% of the cases, and general malaise complaints in 6% of cases *(63–66,83,*

91,95,97,127,130,132–134). A review of other organs' responses is presented in Table 4.

NASAL SECRETIONS

Cellular Aspects. The positive LNR was accompanied by significant changes in the count of neutrophils in 84% of the cases (increase immediately before and decrease during the appearance of LNR, followed by increase again during the resolution of LNR), eosinophils in 58% (increase immediately before and decrease during appearance of LNR), epithelial cells in 73% (increase followed by decrease, running parallel with the clinical course of LNR), goblet cells in 63% of the cases (increase followed by decrease), basophils in 8%, and lymphocytes in 6% (both of them demonstrated a slight increase during the LNR) in the NS. No significant changes in the count of other types of cells in the NS (monocytes, plasma cells, mast cells) were recorded during most of the LNR cases (Table 7, Fig. 8) *(63,65–67,97,98,104,108,110,114,115,117, 118,135–137,153,160–163)*.

In most of the cells appearing in NS during the positive LNR, various intracellular and other changes, such as degranulation, disappearance of the cytoplasmic granules, vacuolization, diminished intake of stain, wrinkling of the cellular membrane, and sometimes cellular disruption, were recorded. The neutrophils were degranulated during 94% of the positive LNR cases, eosinophils in 49%, and basophils in 3%, whereas during the negative nasal response, the neutrophils were degranulated in 7% of the cases, eosinophils in 7%, and basophils in 0% *(63,102,108,110,163)*.

Immunologic Aspects: Immunoglobulins in NS During LNR. The LNR has been accompanied by an increased concentration of total IgE antibodies in 8.4%, specific IgE antibodies in 12.5%, total IgG antibodies in 46%, and IgA antibodies in 4.2% in the NS *(63,66,162,164)*.

Immunologic Aspects: Mediators and Other Factors in NS During LNR. The LNR has been accompanied by an increase in concentration of histamine, kinins, TAME-esterases, neutrophil chemotactic factor, major basic protein (MBP), and LTB_4, whereas bradykinin, lysylbradykinin, and PGF2α may also be detected in NS *(117,118, 136,144,145)*.

Biochemical and Biophysical Aspects. In general, there is a great dearth of data concerning this topic *(66)*. In some patients developing the LNR

Table 7
Presence of Particular Cell Types in the Nasal Secretions and Changes
in Their Count During the Appropriate Nasal Response (%)

	Presence of the cells			Change in the cells' count between, before, and after the challenge		
	LNR, n = 104	NNR, n = 83	PBS,[a] n = 187	LNR, n = 104	NNR, n = 83	PBS,[a] n = 187
Eosinophils	61	19	49	58[b]	5	1
Neutrophils	96	17	45	84[b]	3	2
Basophils	15	9	10	8[b]	0	0
Epith. cells	100	23	41	73[b]	4	1
Goblet cells	82	13	35	63[b]	3	0
Lymphocytes	18	4	9	6[b]	0	0
Mast cells	3	2	1	0	0	0
Plasma cells	4	2	1	0	0	0
Monocytes	1	0	0	0	0	0

LNR, late nasal response; NNR, negative nasal response; PBS, phosphate-buffered saline.
[a]Control.
[b]Statistically significant ($p < 0.05$).
References: 63,66,67,97,98,102,104,110,114,153,160,162,163.

($n = 12$) as well as the INR ($n = 14$), the author and colleagues have examined the biochemical and biophysical properties of NS. During the LNR, the viscosity of the NS increased approximately seven times with respect to that measured during the INR, the density increased approximately three times, pH showed a slight increase in acidity, albumin concentration increased about twice, and the total protein concentration did not demonstrate any significant changes (63,66).

BIOPSY

The following changes have been found in the biopsies of nasal mucosa during the LNR as compared with the "prechallenge" baseline: the epithelium was edematic and its compactness was damaged, intercellular spaces were enlarged, some breaches appearing in the epithelium were filled with fluid, some epithelial cells and some goblet cells were expelled, and the epithelial surface showed empty holes; the compactness of the basement membrane was irregular, with single breaches; the edematic subepithelial layer of the lamina propria contained mixed eosinophil-neutrophil infiltrates and single mast cells, basophils, monocytes, and lymphocytes; the lamina propria showed a perivascular edema, dilation of the terminal parts of the capillaries, and sometimes rupture of the small capillaries with erythrocyte excavation (63,65–67,115).

The changes recorded in the nasal mucosa during the LNR differed distinctly from those observed by us during both the INR and the DYNR. The changes in the nasal mucosa during the INR were pronounced to a slight degree only and were of a "functional" and transient character, whereas those found during LNR were largely pronounced and also slight tissue damage of the nasal mucosa with inflammatory components was recorded (63,66,67,115).

PHARMACOLOGIC MODULATION OF THE LNR

The LNR can be prevented very significantly both by the topical intranasal DSCG (Rynacrom, Lomusol, Intal, Nasalcrom) (63,65,66,91,104, 108,114), and by the topical intranasal corticosteroids, such as BDA (Beconase, Viarin, Vancenase), Budesomide [BSA/BUD] (Rhinocort) or FLD, as demonstrated in our previous clinical studies (Table 6, Figs. 7, 9, and 10) (63,65,66,91,104, 108,114,127,165) and later confirmed by results of other investigators (75,135,156,166). Interestingly, FLN did not demonstrate any significant protective effects on the LNR (63,83,153).

Some authors have also reported significant protective effects of oral corticosteroids (prednisone) on the LNR and the associated influx of the cells and mediators into NS or nasal lavage fluid (117,144,167), whereas other investigators have failed to demonstrate such effects (145). However,

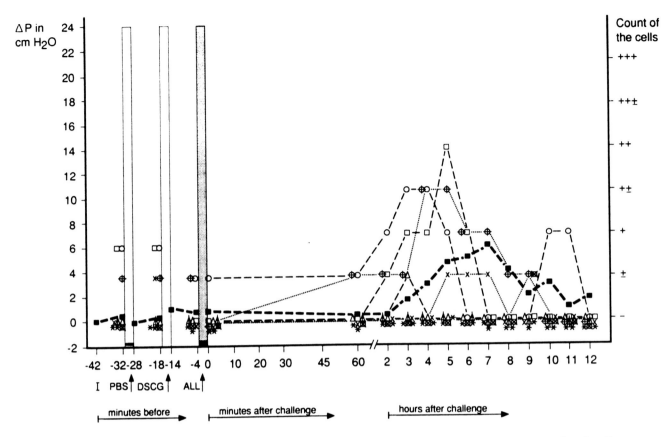

Fig. 9. Cytologic change in NS during the LNR pretreated with DSCG. The mean NPG values recorded after the allergen challenges pretreated with DSCG in 26 patients developing 26 LNR. The mean changes in the counts of the particular cell types in the NS were calculated from 26 positive LNR. I, Initial values; PBS, control challenge; ALL, allergen challenge. ■ --- ■, LNR pretreated with DSCG (n = 26); □ --- □, eosinophils; △ ___ △, basophils; ⚠ . _ . _ . _ . ⚠, mast cells; ○ --- ○, neutrophils; X · · · · · · X, goblet cells; ⊠ · · · · · · · ·⊠ , lymphocytes; ⊕ · · · · · · · ⊕, epithelial cells; * · · · · · · · · *, plasma cells; * · — · — · — · *, monocytes.

the systemic corticosteroids should be regarded as being to heavy treatment of LNR. Recently, a new compound, nedocromil sodium, has demonstrated highly significant protective effects on the LNR (data of our preliminary studies have not yet been published) (63,83,153).

The H_1-receptor antagonists, such as orally administered promethazine hydrochloride, clemastine, chlorphenamine maleate, cinnarizine, astemizole, terfenadine, loratadine, azelastine, hydroxyzine hydrochloride, mebhydroline napadisilate, alimenazine, and dimentidene maleate, or topically administered levocabastine hydrochloride did not demonstrate any significant protective effects on the LNR (Table 6) (63,66,83,153). Surprisingly, according to preliminary results, cetirizine seems to be capable of affecting both the LNR and the eosinophil count in the nasal secretions (126).

The effects of H_2- and H_3-receptor antagonists on the LNR have not yet been sufficiently studied. However, with respect to our knowledge of their mode of action and pharmacologic effects, these drugs would not be expected to affect the LNR.

The anticholinergic drugs, both those administered orally, such as thiazinamium hydrochloride, and those administered topically, such as ipratropium, do not affect the LNR (63,66,83,153,159). Also, the topical decongestants, such as xylomethazoline hydrochloride and oxymethazoline hydrochloride, have failed to demonstrate any effects on the LNR (63).

The possible protective effects of other drugs, such as β_2-sympathomimetics, calcium channel blockers (Nifedipine, Verapamil), nonsteroidal anti-inflammatory drugs (acetylsalicylic acid and its derivatives, indomethacin, ibuprofen),

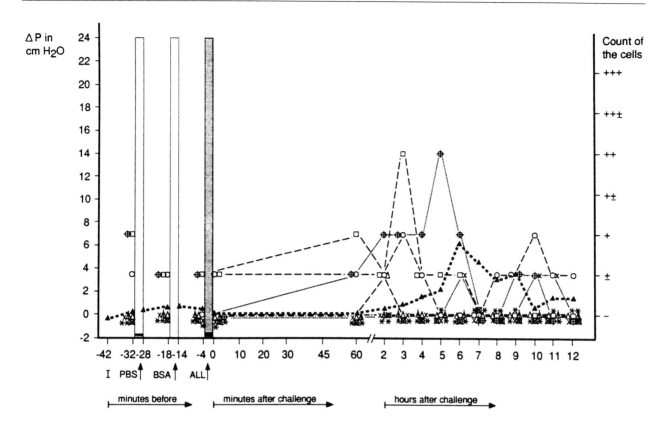

Fig. 10. Cytologic changes in the NS during the LNR pretreated with BUD. The mean NPG values recorded after the allergen challenges pretreated with BUD in 26 patients developing 26 LNR. The mean changes in the counts of the particular cell types in the NS were calculated from 26 positive LNR. I, Initial values; PBS, control challenge; ALL, allergen challenge. ▲ _ _ _ ▲, LNR pretreated with BUD (*n* = 26); □ – – – □, eosinophils; △ – – – △, basophils; ⬕._._._.⬕, mast cells; ○–––○, neutrophils; X · · · · · · X, goblet cells; ⊠· · · · · · · ⊠, lymphocytes; ⊕ · · · · · · · ⊕, epithelial cells; * · · · · · · · · · *, plasma cells; * · — · — · — · *, monocytes.

eicosapentaenoic acid (EPA), cAMP modulators, prostaglandin suppressing compounds, new experimentally synthetized mediator antagonists, inhibitors of the 5-lipoxygenase pathway products, or thromboxane-synthesis inhibitors, on the LNR and/or the underlying mechanisms have not yet been confirmed and/or sufficiently investigated *(66)*.

No convincing evidence has been provided for any effects of the immunotherapy on the clinical LNR and/or on the underlying mechanism, until now. The immunotherapy should therefore be considered as a nonestablished and unproven treatment for the LNR.

Possible Mechanism(s) Underlying the LNR

The views on the pathogenetic and immunologic mechanisms, presumably underlying the clinical LNR, vary *(64–66,73,75,83,91,97)*. The LNR should be regarded as a clinical phenomenon, defined by the appearance of nasal complaints, predominantly obstruction, accompanied by other symptoms and changes, within 4–12 h after the allergen exposure/antigen–antibody interaction, which may be induced by a complex mechanism(s) *(64–66,83,91,97)*.

Although the pathogenetic and immunologic mechanisms leading to the LNR can be different, the late-type hypersensitivity, including the IgG and/or IgM antibodies, particular IgG subclasses, some of the components or parts of the complement system (such as C_{12}, C3, C3a, C5, C5a), and the particular cell types (such as basophils, eosinophils, neutrophils, platelets, epithelial, and endothelial cells), should be regarded as one of the possible mechanisms involved in the clinical LNR, but far from being the only ones *(64–67,78,81,91,97,102,104, 110,114,153,160,164)*. Moreover, various primary, secondary, and tertiary mediators, such as prostaglandins, leukotrienes, thromboxanes, TAME-esterases, PAF, components of kallikrein system, clotting factors, major basic protein, eosinophil cationic protein, eosinophil-derived cationic protein, eosinophil proteases, cyclic nucleotides (cAMP, cGMP); chemotactic factors, such as eosinophil and neutrophil chemotactic factors; cytokines, including IL-1, IL-2, IL-3, IL-4, IL-5, IL-6, IL-8, GM-CSF, TGFα, TGFβ, INF-γ, PGF2α, LTC$_4$, LTB$_4$, LTD$_4$, and LTE$_4$; and, finally, adhesion glycoproteins, such as ICAM-1, ICAM-2, LFA-1, ELAM-1, VCAM-1, GMP-140, VLA-2,-5,-6, and PECAM-1, may also participate in the mechanism(s) underlying the clinical LNR *(64–66,83, 97,98,104,106,108,110,114,115,117,118, 127,135–137,144,145,160,164–167).*

With respect to the results concerning various in vivo as well as in vitro parameters generated from the nasal challenges, nasal secretions, nasal mucosa biopsies, and pharmacologic studies, the evidence for the involvement of the late hypersensitivity mechanism, or at least parts of it, in the clinical LNR, is growing *(64–67,83,91,104,108,110,114, 115,127,160,163).* From clinical, morphologic, immunologic, and pharmacologic points of view, the LNR shows various similarities to the late asthmatic response (LAR) *(168,169)* and differs distinctly from the INR, described earlier, which then shares some clinical features with the immediate asthmatic response (IAR) *(170).*

The data that may support the involvement of late hypersensitivity in the clinical LNR may include:

1. The differences in the clinical course, features, symptoms, complaints, and various in vivo and in vitro parameters accompanying the LNR, and the differences having been recorded during the other nasal response types (INR and DYNR);
2. The significant changes in the count of neutrophils, eosinophils, basophils, epithelial, and goblet cells during the LNR, the majority of these cell types also expressing intracellular changes;
3. The lack of significant changes of the specific IgE antibody concentration both in the blood and in the nasal secretions during the LNR, whereas some cases of the LNR have been accompanied by changes in the concentration of the IgG antibody in the blood and in nasal secretions;
4. The appearance of some mediators and other compounds in nasal secretions exclusively during the LNR, such as eosinophil-derived neurotoxin

(EDN), eosinophil cationic protein (ECP), prostaglandin F2α (PGF2α), and GM-CSF;
5. The typical histologic changes in the nasal biopsies accompanying the LNR, which represent slight and reversible tissue damage and differ distinctly from the histologic changes observed during other types of nasal response (INR, DYNR); and
6. The differences in the (protective) effects of various drugs on the LNR and the other nasal response types (INR, DYNR), as well as the pattern of their pharmacologic modulation *(64–67,83,91,97,102, 104,108,110,114,115,127,153,156,160,163,164).*

The possible involvement of the specific IgE antibodies and the IgE-mediated immediate hypersensitivity (type I allergy) in the mechanisms underlying the LNR, as has been suggested by some investigators, seems to us, regarding our data as well as the results of other investigators, to be unlikely and not convincingly documented *(64,66,83,91).*

DYNR

The DYNR to allergen challenge was first observed and described by the author and colleagues *(64).* This type of nasal response occurs less frequently than the INR or LNR in patients with allergic rhinitis. In earlier studies, the author and colleagues have observed the DYNR in 2% of patients *(64).* However, results of later studies have indicated that approx 14% of patients with allergic rhinitis may develop the DYNR *(66,92).* The DYNR may play an important role in the nasal complaints of some rhinitis patients and may also be responsible for the failure of the usual treatment in these patients *(92).* This type of response is also often overlooked in the practice, because the nasal challenges are not yet carried out as a part of routine diagnostic procedure of the nasal allergy in most of the particular clinics, departments, and allergy practices *(64,66,92).*

Clinical Features, Characteristics, and Forms

The DYNR, recorded by rhinomanometry, shows the following clinical course: it begins within 24–30 h, reaches its maximum within 30–40 h, and resolves within 60 h after the allergen challenge in most of the subjects (Table 1, Figs. 11,12) *(64,66, 83,92,101,115,116,171).* The DYNR occurs in two forms, either as an isolated delayed nasal response (IDYNR) in approx 6% of subjects, or as a dual delayed nasal response (DDYNR) in approx 8% of patients, where an immediate nasal response

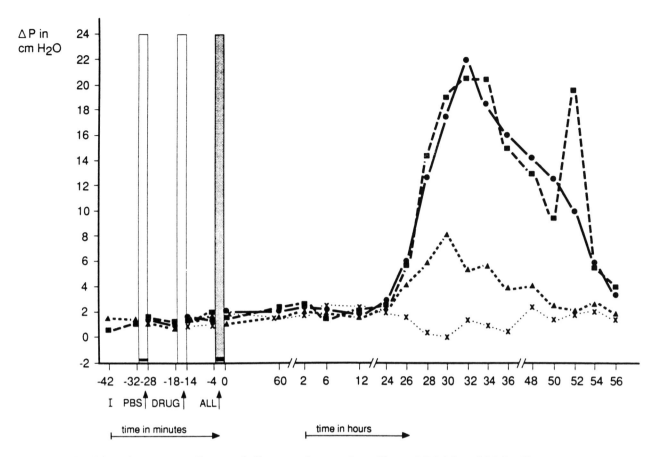

Fig. 11. The delayed DYNR to allergen challenge and protective effects of DSCG and BUD. The mean NPG values recorded after the nonpretreated and the pretreated allergen challenges and PBS control NPG values in 18 patients developing 18 positive DYNR. I, Initial values; PBS, control challenge; ALL, allergen challenge. ●———●, Nonpretreated DYNR (n = 18); ■————■, DYNR pretreated with DSCG (n = 18); △ _ _ _ △, DYNR pretreated with BUD (n = 18); X $\cdots\cdots$ X, PBS control challenge (n = 18).

(IDDYNR) appears within 2 h and then after a symptom-free interval of 22–28 h, the delayed nasal response (DDDYNR) occurs *(64,92,101,171)*.

Similar to the DLNR (*see* paragraph concerning the INR), the previously presumed existence of the DDYNR as a compact response of two phases may be doubted, regarding our recent data concerning the pharmacologic modulation of the dual asthmatic responses and our preliminary data concerning the nasal responses *(128,129)*. The recent data are indicative of an existence of two independent responses, INR and DYNR, owing to different mechanisms, being activated by an allergen at the same time. Although both the responses develop independently in the patient, their projection simulates a two-phase reaction.

The DYNR is accompanied by nasal complaints, predominantly by nasal obstruction and to a slight degree by hypersecretion, whereas sneezing and itching are absent (Table 2) *(64,66,92,101,116,171)*.

DETECTION OF DYNR

The existence of DYNR to a particular allergen in a certain patient can only be confirmed by the NPT (challenge) combined with rhinomanometry, by means of which the pre- and postchallenge parameters may be recorded for at least 36 h *(64,66,92)*.

THE ASSOCIATION OF DYNR WITH OTHER DIAGNOSTIC PARAMETERS

The DYNR may be associated with various in vivo and in vitro diagnostic parameters, to different degrees, as presented in Tables 3 and 4.

1. Positive disease history to the same allergen was found in 53% of the DYNR *(64–66,92,101)*.

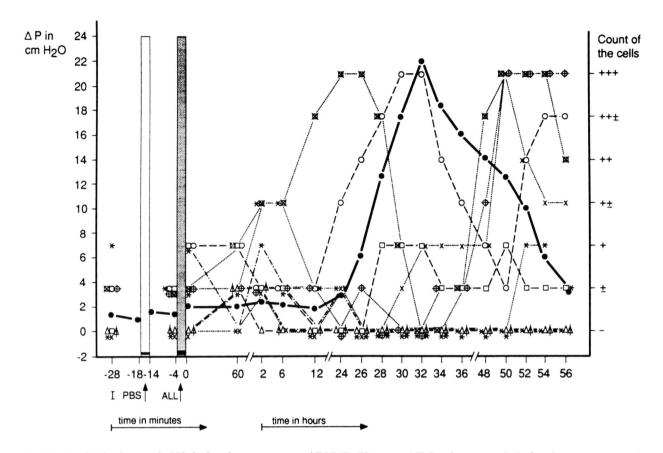

Fig. 12. Cytologic changes in NS during the nonpretreated DYNR. The mean NPG values recorded after the nonpretreated allergen challenges in 18 patients developing 18 positive DYNR. The mean changes in the counts of the particular cell types in the NS were calculated from 18 positive DYNR. I, Initial values; PBS, control challenge; ALL, allergen challenge. ● ——— ●, Nonpretreated DYNR (n = 18); □ – – – □, eosinophils; △ _ _ _ △, basophils;⚠ . _ . _ . _ . ⚠ , mast cells; ○ - - - ○, neutrophils; X · · · · · · X, goblet cells;⊠ · · · · · · ·⊠, lymphocytes; ⊕ · · · · · · · · ⊕, epithelial cells; * · · · · · · · · *, plasma cells; * · · - · · · · *, monocytes.

2. Anterior and posterior rhinoscopy and/or naso-scopy: In all cases of DYNR, a very pronounced violaceous aspect of the nasal mucosa was accompanied by a distinct mucosal edema or induration, very limited amount of NS (mucosal dryness), and in some cases, by small multiple mucosal hemorrhages localized on all three turbinates, and sometimes also on the nasal septum (Table 3) *(64–66,92,101,116,127)*.

3. Skin tests: The positive delayed skin response infiltration was found in approx 59% of the DYNR. The size of the delayed skin response may be divided into the following degrees: a slight grade (+) in 10%; medium grade (++) in 16%; a high grade (+++) in 27%; and a very high grade (++++) in 6% *(64–66,92,127)*.

4. The concentration of the total IgE antibodies in the serum (PRIST) was found to be significantly increased (>500 IU/mL) in only 5% of the DYNR cases *(64–66,127,164)*.

5. The specific IgE antibodies in the serum (RAST, CAP) to the same allergen as that causing the DYNR were found to be significantly positive (score grade 3 or 4) in 2% of the DYNR cases *(64–66,127,164)*.

6. Immunoglobulins of other classes: The increased concentrations of the total IgG, IgM, IgA, and the IgG subclasses in the serum during the DYNR were recorded only very sporadically *(63–66,127,164)*.

7. The blood eosinophil count did not increase (>300 × 10^6/L) in any of the DYNR cases *(64–66,127,164)*.

8. The blood leukocyte count increased (>10 × 10^9/L) during the 11% of the DYNR cases *(64–66, 127,164)*. The leucocyte differential count in

blood demonstrated a slight lymphocytosis during 23% of the DYNR cases (63–66,83,127).

9. Body temperature increased (>37°C = >98.6°F axillary) during 2% of the DYNR cases (Table 4, section INR) (63–66,127). General malaise complaints (tiredness, weakness, hyporeactivity, muscular pain) were recorded during 12% of the DYNR cases (64–66,127).

10 No significant changes of the histamine concentration have been recorded in the serum of the patients demonstrating the DYNR, either before or during the DYNR (127,146).

11. The increased nasal mucosa responsiveness to histamine (PD_{20}) or its reciprocal value, the decreased nasal histamine threshold (NHT), has been recorded only sporadically (<1%) in patients demonstrating the DYNR (115,127).

12. The increased nasal mucosa responsiveness to methacholine bromide or chloride, or its countervalue, the decreased nasal threshold for these compounds, has not been recorded in patients developing the DYNR (85,86,115,127).

ASSOCIATION OF DYNR
WITH OTHER ORGANS' RESPONSE

The DYNR was accompanied by pressure in the maxillary and frontal sinuses (22%), acute edema of mucosal membrane in maxillary sinuses (X-ray of sinuses or echography) (14%), general malaise complaints (tiredness, hyporeactivity, muscular pain, weakness, and so forth) (12%) (Tables 4 and 5, section LNR), headache (11%), bronchial complaints (dyspnea and bronchoconstriction recorded by spirography, wheezing, and sometimes coughing) (6%), middle ear response (otalgia, decrease in hearing, and changes in the middle ear pressure as recorded by tympanometry) (6%), conjunctival irritation (conjunctival injection or chemosis) (5%), and palpebral edema (3%) (Table 4) (64–66, 92,101,116,127,153,171).

NASAL SECRETIONS

Few data are available concerning the DYNR in general or illustrating the appearance of particular cell types and the changes in their count in NS during the DYNR in particular. Our studies of the DYNR are probably the only ones in the literature, since the first description of this type of nasal response was reported by us (101,116,171).

Cellular Aspects. The positive DYNR was accompanied by significant changes in the count (p < 0.05) of lymphocytes (77%) (gradual increase reaching its maximum immediately before the onset of DYNR, followed by a rapid decrease during the appearance of the response, and then by an increase during the resolving of DYNR), neutrophils (53%) (an increase immediately before the onset of DYNR, followed by a decrease, running parallel with the clinical course of DYNR, and then by an increase during the resolving of the clinical response), and epithelial cells (37%) (slight increase during the appearance of the DYNR, followed by distinct increase during the resolving of the clinical response) in the NS. The changes in the count of the other cell types, such as goblet cells (18%), eosinophils (12%), and monocytes (6%) were not significant, whereas the count of mast cells, basophils, and plasma cells was very low and did not change (Table 8, Fig. 12) (2,101,116,127, 153,171).

Immunological Aspects. The immunological aspects of the NS concern primarily the immunoglobulins and mediators. No significant appearance or changes in the concentration of immunoglobulins of any class or subclass have been recorded in NS during the DYNR (64,127,164). No significant concentration of histamine or changes in its concentration have been found in the NS before or during the DYNR (106,127). No other mediators and factors have been investigated in NS during this type of nasal response. Studies dealing with this type of nasal response are not numerous, and various aspects concerning the DYNR have not yet been investigated sufficiently.

Biochemical and Biophysical Aspects. These aspects and properties of NS and their changes during the DYNR have not yet been investigated.

BIOPSIES

There is also a dearth of information concerning the histologic changes in the nasal mucosal membrane during the DYNR. The following histologic changes in the nasal mucosa have been recorded during the DYNR: edematic epithelium showing decreased compactness, enlarged intercellular spaces, breaches and empty holes; expelled epithelial and goblet cells; hemorrhages (erythrocytes) in the epithelial layer; distinct edema of the subepithelial layer; several breaches in the basement membrane; perivascular edema and infiltrates in the upper layer of the lamina propria formed by polymorphonuclear leukocytes, predominantly small lymphocytes, neutrophils, and, sometimes, plasma

Table 8
Presence of Particular Cell Types in the Nasal Secretions and Changes
in Their Count During the Appropriate Nasal Response (%)

	Presence of the cells			Change in the cells' count between, before, and after the challenge		
	DYNR, n = 83	NNR, n = 71	PBS,[a] n = 83	DYNR, n = 83	NNR, n = 71	PBS,[a] n = 83
Eosinophils	26	10	12	12	3	1
Neutrophils	59	13	11	53[b]	7	2
Basophils	2	1	0	1	0	0
Epith. cells	73	14	10	37[b]	4	2
Goblet cells	60	11	7	18	0	0
Lymphocytes	86	13	14	77[b]	8	4
Mast cells	2	1	1	0	0	0
Plasma cells	10	4	2	0	0	0
Monocytes	16	3	1	6	1	0

DYNR, delayed nasal response; NNR, negative nasal response; PBS, phosphate-buffered saline.
[a]Control.
[b]Statistically significant ($p < 0.05$).
References: *101,116,153,171.*

cells; and disrupted wall of several capillaries accompanied sometimes by erythrocyte excavation. These changes may be qualified to be a distinct damage of the nasal mucosal membrane owing to a distinct inflammatory component *(115,127).*

PHARMACOLOGICAL MODULATION OF THE DYNR

The DYNR can be prevented significantly ($p < 0.01$) by intranasal topical corticosteroids, such as BUD (Rhinocort) or BDA (Beconase, Viarin, Aldecin, Vancenase) (Table 6, Figs. 11, 13, and 14) *(63–66,83,92,116).* Surprisingly, the systemic glucocorticosteroids, administered either orally (Prednisolone in a daily dose of 30 mg for 7 d) or by means of a single intramuscular injection (Methylprednisolone = Solu-Medrol 40 mg im) have been shown to be able to prevent the DYNR only partially ($p = 0.05$) (unpublished data). The intranasal DSCG (Lomusol, Rynacrom, Intal, Nasalcrom), did not demonstrate any significant protective effects on the DYNR ($p > 0.05$) *(63–66,83,92,116,153).* The oral anticholinergics (thiazinamium methyl-sulfate = THM), topical anticholinergics (ipratropium bromide), topical decongestants (xylomethazoline hydrochloride, oxymethazoline hydrochloride), H_1-, H_2-, and H_3-receptor antagonists did not affect the DYNR *(153).* The possible protective effects of intranasal nedocromil sodium (NDS) on DYNR have not yet been satisfactorily investigated (Table 6) *(153).*

POSSIBLE MECHANISM(S) UNDERLYING THE DYNR

Since the first report of the existence of the DYNR *(64),* we have regularly studied this type of nasal response from various points of view *(2,64,92,101,106,115,116,127,146,153,164,171).*

Fig. 13. *(opposite page)* Cytologic changes in the NS during the DYNR pretreated with DSCG. The mean NPG values recorded after the allergen challenges pretreated with DSCG in 18 patients developing 18 DYNR. The mean changes in the counts of the particular cell types in the NS were calculated from 18 positive DYNR. I, Initial values; PBS, control challenge; ALL, allergen challenge. ■ – – – – ■, DYNR pretreated with DSCG ($n = 18$); □ – – – □, eosinophils; △ _ _ _ △, basophils;△ . _ . _ . _ .△, mast cells; ○ – – – ○, neutrophils; X · · · · · · X, goblet cells;⊠· · · · · · · ⊠, lymphocytes; ⊕ · · · · · · · ⊕, epithelial cells; * · · · · · · · · *, plasma cells; * · – · – · – · *, monocytes.

Fig. 14. *(opposite page)* Cytologic changes in the NS during the DYNR pretreated with BUD. The mean NPG values recorded after the allergen challenges pretreated with BUD in 18 patients developing 18 DYNR. The mean changes in the counts of the particular cell types in the NS were calculated from 18 positive DYNR. I, Initial values; PBS, control challenge; ALL, allergen challenge. △ _ _ _ △, DYNR pretreated with BUD ($n = 18$); □ – – – □, eosinophils; △ – – – △, basophils;△ . _ . _ . _ .△, mast cells; ○ – – – ○, neutrophils; X · · · · · · X, goblet cells; ⊠ · · · · · · · ⊠, lymphocytes; ⊕ · · · · · · ⊕, epithelial cells; * · · · · · · · · *, plasma cells; * · – · – · – · *, monocytes.

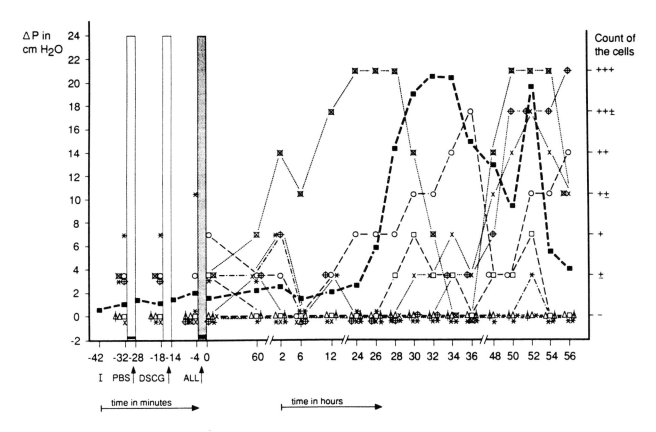

Fig. 13.

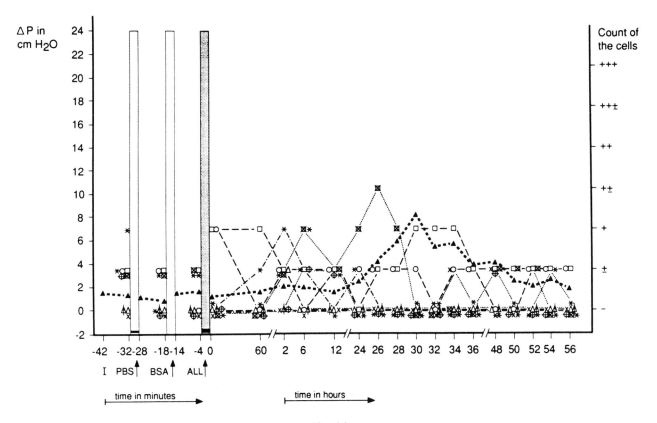

Fig. 14.

Despite some progress, the exact pathogenetic mechanism(s) underlying the DYNR is not yet fully understood. The DYNR shares some clinical, immunologic, and pharmacologic features with the delayed asthmatic response (DYAR), described recently by us *(172–174)*. Generally, there is a dearth of information concerning the role of delayed (cell-mediated) hypersensitivity mechanism(s) in the nasal mucosa and nasal allergy.

The DYNR differs principally in several aspects, such as clinical course and features, association with other in vivo and in vitro diagnostic parameters, morphologic and immunologic aspects of nasal secretions, histologic changes of the nasal mucosa, and pharmacologic modulation, both from the INR *(63,65,66,68,69,72,83,87,88,90,94–97, 99,102,103,105–107,109–113,115,117,118, 127,130,132–137,144–146,149,153–155,160, 161,164)* and from the LNR *(63–67,72,83,91,95, 97,98,102,104,106,108,110,114,115,117,118,127, 130,132–137,144–146,160–164,167)*. The DYNR begins approx 26 h after the allergen challenge, the time at which the LNR is usually resolved *(66)*.

A distinction should be made between the DYNR and the delayed-type hypersensitivity (DTH) (cell-mediated reactions, type IV allergy) *(66,73,76,77,82)*. The DYNR should be regarded as a clinical phenomenon, characterized by appearance of nasal symptoms, predominantly nasal obstruction, accompanied by other parameters within 26–56 h after the allergen exposure (challenge) *(64)*. The DYNR may be induced by complex mechanisms *(64)*. Although the pathogenetic and immunologic mechanisms leading to the development of the clinical DYNR have not yet been satisfactorily clarified, the cell-mediated (delayed type) hypersensitivity may be regarded as one of the possible mechanisms involved in this type of nasal response, but far from the only one *(64–66,92,101,115,116,127,153,171)*. This assumption can be supported by findings of other investigators from the animal asthma model *(175–179)*, in patients with allergic bronchial asthma *(175,180, 181)*, or in asthmatics after the bronchial challenge with allergen *(182)*, in patients with allergic rhinitis *(181,183)*, or after the nasal provocation with allergen *(184,185)*, and finally from various in vitro studies *(186,187)*.

In the cell-mediated immunity (CMI) or the DTH, the antigen, presented by an APC, enters into an interaction with the antigen-specific activated

(sensitized) T-lymphocytes (the lymphokines producing subset, usually the T helper subset [T_{h1}], and/or the cytotoxic subset including the NK subsuset) *(73,76,77,79,80,175,180–182,188)*. They release then a variety of factors, so-called lymphokines, a group consisting of interleukines (IL-2–IL-5, IL-9, IL-10) and M-CSF, GM-CSF, IFN-γ, TNF-β), and lymphotoxines, acting then through various pathways and cells on the other systems and effector organs, resulting in an immunological tissue injury and appearance of the clinical manifestation of the delayed hypersensitivity *(73,76,77,79–81,175,179,180,187–189)*. Regarding these facts, there is no doubt about the pivotal role of the activated T-lymphocyte in the cell-mediated ("delayed") hypersensitivity mechanism *(73,76,79,80,186,188,189)*.

Nevertheless, the evidence for the involvement of T-lymphocytes and other DTH mechanisms in allergic disorders of the respiratory tract, especially in allergic bronchial asthma and allergic rhinitis, is growing *(64,65,73,76,78,80,92,101,116,171– 177,183–186,188,190–195)*.

In most of the patients demonstrating DYNR, similar to those developing the DYAR *(172–174)*, the serum concentrations of particular immunoglobulin classes (total IgE, specific IgE, total IgG, IgA, and IgM), as well as of IgG subclasses, were not elevated and did not change during the DYNR in any patient *(64,65,92,101,116,127,164,171)*. These findings would not support a direct involvement or participation of these immunoglobulins in the mechanism(s) underlying the clinical DYNR *(64,65,92)*.

The other diagnostic parameters accompanying the clinical DYNR can be summarized as follows:

1. The increase in the leukocyte count and the appearance of a slight lymphocytosis in the peripheral blood during DYNR;
2. The nonincreased count of eosinophils in peripheral blood during all DYNR cases;
3. The appearance of lymphocytes, neutrophils, and epithelial cells in the nasal secretions, demonstrating significant changes in their count during the most cases of DYNR;
4. The histologic changes in the nasal mucosal membrane (biopsy) consisting of a distinct damage of the nasal epithelium, distinct edema of the subepithelial layer, and perivascular infiltrates in the upper layer of the lamina propria, formed pre-

dominantly by lymphocytes and neutrophils *(64,65,92,101,115,116,127,153,171)* may also be indicative of the possible role of the activated lymphocytes in the mechanisms involved in the DYNR *(64,65,92).*

The possible role of lymphocytes in the mechanisms leading to the development of the clinical DYNR may also be supported by results of pharmacologic modulation of the DYNR *(65,92,116, 153).* The antihistamines, anticholinergics, and even cromolyn (DSCG) did not demonstrate any significant protective effects on the DYNR ($p > 0.05$) *(65,92,116,153).* The effects of intranasal nedocromil sodium (NDS) on the DYNR have not yet been satisfactorily investigated *(153).* In contrast, the topical glucocorticosteroids (BUD and BDA) have prevented DYNR very significantly ($p < 0.01$) *(65,92,116,153).* These results may be considered very important additional data with respect to the known pharmacologic effects of these drugs. Cromolyn (Disodium cromoglycate, DSCG), through its stabilizing effects, prevents and inhibits the IgE-mediated degranulation of the mast cells and basophils. With subsequent mediator release, DSCG also seems to promote other pharmacologic effects, such as decreasing the neutrophil chemotactic activity and stimulation of factors that increase the exogenous cAMP and/or decrease the exogenous cGMP. There is also evidence for the possible increase of both the membrane-associated cAMP and the intracellular cAMP in some other cell types, such as neutrophils, eosinophils, platelets, cells in the lung, and nasal mucosal membrane, by DSCG *(196,197).*

NDS possesses a number of unique pharmacologic properties, including various anti-inflammatory effects, such as inhibition of histamine release from chopped human lung, and inhibition of activation of eosinophils, neutrophils, human alveolar macrophages, blood monocytes, and platelets *(197,198).*

There is no evidence for a pharmacologic modulation of activated lymphocytes either in vitro or in vivo by DSCG or NDS in animals or humans *(196–198).* A direct pharmacologic effect of either DSCG or NDS, an inhibition or suppression of the activated lymphocytes, especially of the T-lymphocytes, their particular subsets, and their products (lymphokines), has not yet been reported. From this point of view, the

lack of protective effects of the above-mentioned drugs on the DYNR is not surprising.

The antihistamines (H_1-receptor antagonists), as well as anticholinergics, would not be expected to demonstrate any direct effects on the activated lymphocytes. The effects of H_2-receptor antagonists (e.g., Cimetidine) on the activated lymphocytes unfortunately have not yet been investigated satisfactorily *(157,158,199).*

In contrast, the glucocorticosteroids (GCS) possess manifold anti-inflammatory, immunosuppressive, and immunoregulatory effects *(200–202).*

In addition to other effects that are discussed in detail henceforth, the GCS affect the lymphocytes, especially the T-cells and their products, by several ways and on different levels, mostly by antagonizing and suppressing their activation and proliferation *(200–202).*

The corticosteroids decrease the number of lymphocytes in asthmatics, not only in the peripheral blood, through their redistribution, but also in the airway tissue. They inhibit macrophage functions, inhibit the production of IL-1 and expression of Ia antigens by macrophages (products stimulating the $CD4^+$ cells), inhibit the secretion of Il-2 (which induces proliferation of T-lymphocytes), diminish the number of circulating helper/inducer ($CD4^+$) T-cells, and probably inhibit (indirectly) the NK activity *(200–202).*

The corticosteroids have also demonstrated manifold effects on various cytokines, their production or elaboration, and their effects. They reduce elevated serum cytokine level, mostly of GM-CSF; inhibit lymphocyte growth and activating factors (including IL-1, IL-2, and INF-γ), IL-3, synthesis of RNA, which is necessary for production of some cytokines, especially for IL-2 and INF-γ; and probably antagonize the effects of IL-5 *(200–202).* They also inhibit expression of low-affinity IL-2 receptors and rapidly induced IL-2 expression on cultured T-lymphocytes in vitro. They are also able to inhibit the macrophage-derived TNF *(202).* The results of these pharmacologic studies, the results of the inability of DSCG to influence the DYNR, and the capacity of the GCS to affect significantly this type of nasal response, taken together with the known effects of GCS on the activated T-lymphocytes and their products, could be suggestive for the possible participation of T-lymphocytes in the DYNR mechanism(s) *(65,92).*

Our presumption of a possible involvement of activated T-lymphocytes in the development of the DYNR may also be supported by other investigators' findings, providing evidence for an important, if not pivotal, role of the activated T-cells and cytokines in the skin test model in patients with various allergic disorders *(181,195,203)*, in patients with allergic bronchial asthma *(175,180–182, 188,192–195,204)*, and, finally, in patients with allergic rhinitis *(181,183–185,190)*.

THE BASIC TYPES OF NASAL RESPONSE TO FOODS

The role of food allergy and of foods in general in subjects with various allergic disorders, especially in those suffering from rhinitis *(66,100,205, 206)*, otitis media *(100,207)*, sinusitis *(59)*, bronchial asthma *(208–211)*, atopic eczema *(208,212, 213)*, urticaria *(214)*, entero-colitis *(208)*, and general malaise complaints *(100,205,209,215)*, is still underestimated. The reasons for this underestimation may include:

1. The classical hypothesis that the majority of allergic disorders may be attributed to the immediate hypersensitivity (Type I allergy) mechanisms and that the allergens suspected have been inhalant allergens;
2. There may be various mechanisms by means of which the foods can cause the clinical disorders in patients, and the hypersensitivity mechanisms are only one group of them;
3. The diagnosis of food allergy and its confirmation in the symptomatology of patients are not so easy and require both the clinical experience and a sufficiently equipped diagnostic system and procedure of a high quality *(100)*.

Definition

Food allergy or hypersensitivity may be defined as the clinical manifestation of an immunologic process in which foods or their parts are able to act as an antigen or hapten to stimulate the production of antibodies or to sensitize the particular T-cells, and then they are capable of interacting with these antibodies or cells, a process resulting in an allergic (hypersensitivity) reaction. By this way, the foods may be responsible for the immunologic injury by any of the classical types of hypersensitivity reaction *(66,100,205,209)*.

A distinction must be made between the genuine food allergy, being the result of an immunologic mechanism, and other disorders that can also be caused by foods, their parts, or factors related to them that can produce even similar symptoms, but are, however, owing to completely different mechanisms (Table 9) *(66,100,205,209)*.

There are two basic forms of food allergy: the primary and the secondary forms *(100)*. (1) The primary form, in which the food alone causes the defined complex of symptoms through an immunologic (hypersensitivity) mechanism—in such a case, the food is the primary and sole cause of the hypersensitivity mechanism and the resulting symptoms; and (2) the secondary form, in which one or more foods potentiate the already existing hypersensitivity mechanism(s) caused by different antigens, e.g., inhalant allergens. The foods may act through different pathways in potentiating the particular responses. In such a case, the food allergy is only a complementary event to another hypersensitivity state, which is the primary and basic event. The secondary form of food allergy occurs more frequently than the primary form and it is regularly overlooked in the practice *(100)*.

Immunological Features of the Food Allergy

1. The foods usually enter into the body via the digestive tract, which means by ingestion. However, the foods can also cause the hypersensitivity reactions by contact with the skin, gingiva, lips, or tongue, or by inhalation on and in the nasal or bronchial mucosa *(100)*.
2. The antibodies involved in the food allergy have classically been understood to be of the IgE class. However, later evidence has been provided for a possible participation, not only of antibodies of other classes, such as IgG, IgM, or IgA, but also immune complexes and T-lymphocytes in the hypersensitivity mechanism(s) owing to the foods *(66,100,205,209)*.
3. All four basic types of hypersensitivity (Type I, II, III, IV) may be involved in the food allergy and can lead to the clinical symptoms. However, the immediate (Type I) and the late (Type III) reactions have mostly been investigated and documented. Recently, the delayed type of hypersensitivity has also been shown to be a presumable mechanism that may cause the delayed type of response in subjects with rhinitis, bronchial

Table 9
Survey of the Disorders Caused by Foods, Their Ingredients, or Factors Relating
to Them that Can Lead to Symptoms Similar to Those Resulting from the Food Allergy Mechanism

Idiosyncrasy
Intolerance (e.g., enzymatic)
Nonspecific hyperreactivity (e.g., histamine or other mediator liberators, food additives)
Toxicity
    By noncontrolled chemical compounds (e.g., insecticides, contaminants)
    By microorganisms
    By products of microorganisms
        Bacterial toxins
        Mycotoxins
    By controlled chemical compounds exceeding their permitted threshold or individual subjects having increased
        susceptibility to these compounds (e.g., disinfectants) caused by other metabolic disorders
Adverse nonimmunological reaction to additives (controlled chemical compounds)
    Preservation and conservation compounds
    Coloring compounds
    Flavoring compounds
    Consistency correcting compounds, emulsifiers, and stabilizers
    Antioxidants
    Adjuvants
Psychological disorders

References: *66,100,205–207,209–211.*

asthma, atopic eczema, urticaria, migraine, and other disorders *(66,100,205,209).*

The terms "food allergy" or hypersensitivity imply already an immunologic mechanism, but in many instances, the exact immunopathologic mechanisms by which the foods produce the symptoms and complaints in the particular subjects remain unknown. It would therefore be more appropriate to use the term "adverse reactions to foods" where the genuine food hypersensitivity would represent one of the suspected mechanisms *(66,100).*

The food allergy may also be differentiated from the nonspecific hyperreactivity reactions to foods and from the reactions to chemical additives, both groups being nonimmunologic mechanisms *(66,100).*

The chemical additives present in foods form a special problem, not only with respect to their frequent occurrence in the manufactured foods and their heterogeneity, but also because of the lack of understanding concerning their mode of action as well as the mode of production of clinical symptoms (Table 10). There is clear evidence that the additives may cause symptoms in various organs, as has already been demonstrated by clinical oral challenge studies. Although the clinical manifestations are significantly related to the ingestion of

additives, the antibodies of the IgE or other classes or sensitized T-lymphocytes have not yet been unequivocally found in the clinically affected patients *(100).* Moreover, the disodium cromoglycate, administered orally, has been shown to prevent significantly various symptoms owing to the food allergy, whereas this drug has been found to be completely ineffective on the symptoms following oral challenge with additives *(66,100, 206,210,211,213,214).* This suggests that additives may produce the symptoms through nonimmunologic mechanisms, such as nonspecific hyperreactivity, direct mediator release without preceding antigen–antibody interaction, direct effects on the effector organs, or through a direct pharmacologic action, e.g., subtoxic effects *(100).*

Nasal Response to the Foods

Three basic types of the nasal response, following the food ingestion challenge, have been recorded and already reported by us:

1. INR, occurring within 70 min, reaching the maximum within 105 min, and resolving within 180 min;
2. LNR, starting within 6 h, reaching its maximum within 10 h, and resolving within 24 h; and
3. DYNR, beginning within 24–28 h, with a peak within 32–36 h, and resolving within 48–52 h

Table 10
Review of the Most Frequently Appearing Additives in Foods

Coloring agents	Flavoring agents	Preservatives	Stabilizers/emulsifiers/others
Tartrazine	trans-Anethole	Benzoic acid	Calcium salts
Coccine	Malic acid	EDTA derivatives	Agar-agar
Amaranth	Acetic acid	O-Phenylphenol	Carbonates
Sunset Yellow	Benzaldehyde	Formic acid	Diacetyl tartaric acid
Pyrazole	Benzyl compounds	Nitrate compounds	Phosphate compounds
Hydrozy aromatic acids	Cyclamate	Propionic acid	Glycerol derivatives
Annatto	Ethylmaltol	Sulfites	Lecithin
Anthocyanins	Ethylvanillin	4-Hydroxybenzoic acid	
Azorubine	Fumaric acid	Benzene sulfuric acid	*Consistency corrigents*
Brilliant Blue FCF	*l*-Glutamates	Sodium sulfuric acid	Carrageenan
Brilliant Black PN	Maltol	Sodium benzoate	Aluminum compounds
Brilliant Black	Amylbutyrate		Cellulose compounds
Food Green S	Benzyl acetate		
Allura Red AC	D-Camphor		*Antioxidants*
Chlorophyll	Citronellol		Butylated hydroxyanisole
Citral	Ethyl acetoacetate		Acetone peroxide
Ponceau 4R	Ethyl proprionate		Citric acid
Food Green 3	α Ionone		Gallates
Food Red 14	γ Undecanone		
Indigotin	2,4-Undecadienal		*Others*
Carminic acid	Δ Nonalactone		Bacitracin
Patent Blue	Propyl propionate		
Indigo Carmine	Methyl thiopropionate		
Wool Green B	2-Pentenol		
	n-Heptenal		

Reference: *100.*

Table 11
The Time-Course of the Individual Clinical Types
of Nasal Response to the Food Ingestion Challenge[a]

	Onset	Maximum	Resolving
Immediate	10–20 min	30–45 min	90–120 min
Late	4–6 h	6–10 h	12–24 h
Delayed	24–28 h	32–36 h	48–52 h

[a]The time is expressed in minutes or hours after a 60-min waiting interval following the ingestion challenge.
References: *100,125,205,206,208.*

after the food ingested (Table 11, Figs. 15–17) *(66,100,205,208).*

The INR occurs in approx 35%, the LNR in 55%, and the DYNR in 10% of the patients with allergic rhinitis, in whom the foods participate in the nasal complaints *(66,100,205,208).*

The particular types of nasal response to food have been associated with other in vivo and in vitro diagnostic parameters to various degrees, as reviewed in Table 12 *(66,100,205).*

With respect to the high variation and mostly insufficient correlation of various diagnostic parameters with the particular types of nasal response to foods, it should be emphasized that the definitive diagnostic confirmation of the role of a certain food in the complaints of the patient, such as nasal, bronchial, and other symptoms, should be provided by the ingestion challenge with the particular foods *(66,100,205,209).* The food ingestion challenge should not only be regarded as (1) an exclusive method for demonstrating the existence

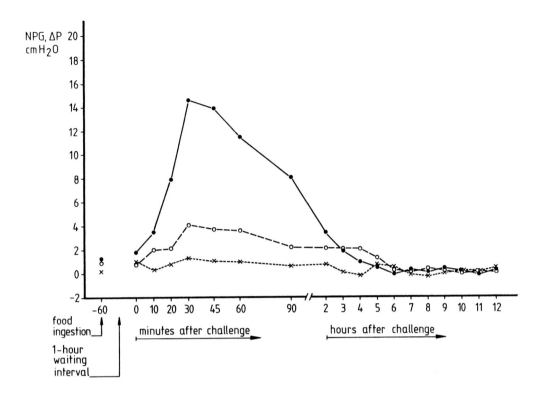

Fig. 15. The INR to food ingestion challenge and protective effects of oral DSCG. The mean NPG values recorded during the nonpretreated and pretreated INR owing to the foods ingested and PBS control NPG values in 28 patients developing 28 INR. ●————●, Nonpretreated INR to foods ingested ($n = 28$); ○ — — — ○, INR pretreated with oral DSCG ($n = 28$); X · · · · · · X, PBS control challenge ($n = 28$).

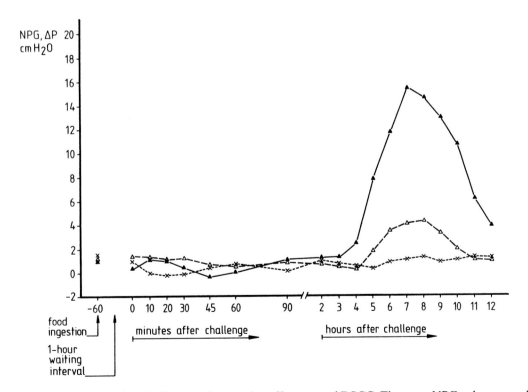

Fig. 16. The LNR to food ingestion challenge and protective effects or oral DSCG. The mean NPG values recorded during the nonpretreated and pretreated LNR owing to the foods ingested and PBS control NPG values in 25 patients developing 25 NR. ▲————▲, Nonpretreated LNR to foods ingested ($n = 25$); △ — — — △, LNR pretreated with oral DSCG ($n = 25$); X · · · · · · X, PBS control challenge ($n = 25$).

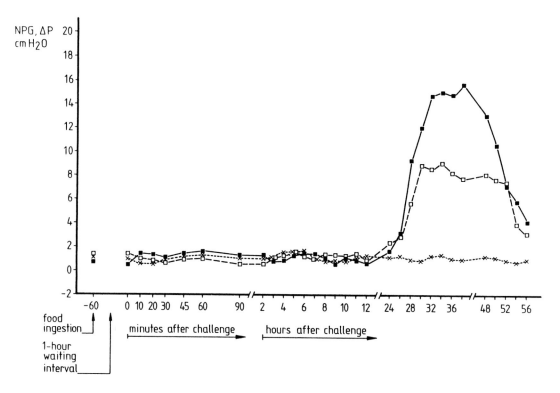

Fig. 17. The DNR to food ingestion challenge and protective effects of oral DSCG. The mean NPG values recorded during the nonpretreated and pretreated DYNR owing to the foods ingested and PBS control NPG values in 16 patients developing 16 DYNR. ■———■, Nonpretreated DYNR to foods ingested ($n = 16$); □–––□, DYNR pretreated with oral DSCG ($n = 16$); X······X, PBS control challenge ($n = 25$).

Table 12
The Association of the Particular Types of Nasal Response to Food Ingestion Challenge
with Other In Vivo and In Vitro Diagnostic Parameters

	Nasal mucosa response to food ingestion			
	Immediate, n = 267	*Late,* n = 203	*Delayed,* n = 164	*Negative,* n = 309
Positive skin response	146			48
		98		11
			69	3
Increase in total serum IgE (PRIST)	11	1	0	3
Increase in specific serum IgE (RAST)	38	3	1	4
Increase in blood eosinophils	14	17	2	2
Increase in blood leukocytes	10	18	11	3
Aspects of the nasal mucosa				
Hyperemia	97	47	1	5
Violaceous aspect	168	55	163	0
Nasal mucosa hemorrhages	0	42	2	0
Nasal secretions changes in count of				
Eosinophils	201	128	53	21
Mast cells/basophils	53	30	6	0
Neutrophils	208	182	41	15
Goblet cells	113	49	14	2
Lymphocytes	9	5	46	0

References: *66,100,125,205,206,208,209.*

Table 13
The Nasal Complaints and the Other Organs' Responses Accompanying the Particular Types
of the Nasal Response to Food Ingestion Challenge

	Nasal mucosa response to food ingested			
	Immediate, n = 267	Late, n = 203	Delayed, n = 164	Negative, n = 309
Nasal complaints				
Obstruction	267	203	164	0
Sneezing	19	1	0	1
Hypersecretion	193	166	39	16
Itching	181	75	145	13
General malaise complaints	22	54	49	1
Conjunctival irritation	35	18	6	0
Middle ear response (otalgia, decrease of hearing, change of middle ear pressure)	31	19	13	10
Pressure in the sinuses (maxillary and frontal, acute edema of sinus mucosa)	45	32	33	7
Cephalgia	56	91	125	42
Urticaria	4	7	8	5
Angio-edema (labial, palpebral or elsewhere)	9	6	3	3
Increase in body temperature	4	21	1	0
Bronchial complaints	13	15	12	8
Other complaints	2	1	2	0

References: *66,100,125,205,206,208.*

of the particular types of the organ response, e.g., nasal response owing to the food, but in combination with other parameters, such as X-ray of sinuses *(59)*, echography *(59)*, tympanography *(207)*, lung functions *(209,215)*, and so forth, but, (2) it should also be considered as the sole method for the confirmation of the causal role of the nasal mucosa and nasal response in other organs and their response to foods, such as middle ear, paranasal sinuses, bronchial tree, and eyes *(59,66,100,205, 208,214,215)*.

The nasal response to foods may also be regularly accompanied by other organs' symptoms, such as conjunctival injection or chymosis, palpebral edema, otalgia, pressure in the sinuses, cephalgia, gastrointestinal symptoms (nausea, vomiting, diarrhea), and sometimes also bronchial obstruction, migraine, general malaise complaints, or other symptoms, as presented in Table 13 *(66,100,205,209)*.

The pharmacologic modulation of the particular types of nasal response to food ingested has also been intensively studied by us. DSCG (Nalcrom®),

in a daily dose of 4 × 200 mg, has protected very significantly both the INR and the LNR, whereas it has protected the DYNR to a slight degree only (Figs. 15–17) *(66,100,206)*. The H_1- and H_2-receptor antagonists as well as topical GCS have not been able to prevent significantly any of the particular types of nasal response to foods. Furthermore, the oral corticosteroids have prevented the food-related LNR and DYNR, but not the INR, whereas iv administered corticosteroids have prevented significantly both the LNR and the DYNR, and have also partly influenced the food-related INR (our unpublished data) *(59,100,224)*.

SINUS RESPONSE OWING TO THE HYPERSENSITIVITY (ALLERGY) MECHANISM(S)

As has been already mentioned, the sinus disease in which the hypersensitivity mechanisms play the main causal role may include two forms. The primary form of the sinus disease, where the whole immunologic event, beginning with the antigen–

antibody (or sensitized T-lymphocyte) and resulting in the clinical response of the particular sinuses, is located in the mucosal membrane of the involved sinuses, whereas the secondary form of the sinus disease is induced by the immunologic event that takes place primarily in the nasal mucosa *(53–57)*.

Occurrence

According to the author's data, consistent with the other investigators' results, the acute sinusitis, being mostly the result of the viral or bacterial infections, occurs both in children and in adults, without any significant differences between both groups *(1–8,30,216–222)*. However, some investigators have reported a higher frequency of acute sinusitis in children (4–13%) than in adults *(216–218)*, with respect to higher frequency of the upper airway infections in children *(7,45)*. In most cases of the acute sinusitis, both in children and in adults, the rhinitis owing to the same bacterial or viral infection may also be observed, either as an accompanying or a preceding disorder *(7,30,45,216–218)*. In the latter case, the acute sinusitis, being in fact a secondary form, may usually be considered a complication of the acute rhinitis *(30,33,45,219)*. An acute sinusitis without any accompanying nasal infection, being in fact a primary form, can be seen very rarely *(1–6)*. The acute bacterial or viral sinusitis is diagnosed most frequently in the maxillary sinuses and to a lesser degree in the frontal sinuses *(2,3,6,8,45,220–222)*. The origin of the infection in the maxillary sinuses is nasal (90%), dental (4%), traumatic (4%), or systemic (2%) *(2,42,43)*. The acute frontal sinusitis is often associated with homolateral anterior ethmoidal cells and maxillary sinus infections *(2)*. Infections of the ethmoid sinuses seldom occur as a separate clinical entity in adults, but they are relatively common in children *(2,3)*. In adults, the ethmoid sinuses are often involved when the other sinus types are infected *(2,28,33)*. It can be concluded that most cases of acute sinusitis owing to the bacterial or viral infections occur in the sinuses that open into the middle meatus *(2,6,33,46,60)*, the area between the lower and the middle turbinate. The sequence of the frequency of the particular sinus types is the following: the maxillary, the anterior and middle ethmoid, and finally the frontal sinuses *(2,45,46,60,220–222)*. The middle meatus is the site of the major

passage of the inspiratory nasal air flow and, therefore, it is also one of the most exposed areas in the nose *(32,33,60)*.

It has also been postulated that the infection of the maxillary and frontal sinuses may frequently be either accompanied or probably even preceded by disease of the ipsilateral anterior and middle ethmoid sinuses, including bulla ethmoidalis, suggesting a rhinogenic origin *(23–25,33,46,60)*.

In contrast to the acute infectious sinusitis, the acute sinus disease in which the hypersensitivity mechanism(s) may play the major causal role, occurs very rarely *(222)*. The immunologically mediated acute sinus disease is usually of the secondary form, which has been induced by the primary nasal response to the inhalant allergen, such as pollen species, house dust mites, or particular kinds of animal dander *(53–58)*. This type of sinus disease, concerning almost exclusively the maxillary sinuses, occurs usually in children and young adults, mostly after a sudden and mass exposure to one of the inhalant allergen *(40,42,43)*.

The chronic sinus disease differs from the acute sinus disease from various points of view, such as etiology, causal agents and processes, features, clinical picture, and accompanying in vivo, as well as in vitro, clinical parameters.

The incidence of the chronic sinus disease owing to the bacterial infections (the chronic viral infection does not exist) is distinctly lower than that of acute chronic disease *(43,218,219,223,224)*. In contrast, the chronic sinus disease, in which the hypersensitivity mechanisms may play the major causal role, is observed much more frequently than the immunologically induced acute form *(43,224)*. Our not yet published data may indicate that the incidence of the bacteriologically induced chronic sinus disease would not exceed 15%, whereas the immunologically induced chronic form may be observed in approx 80% of cases *(224)*. The chronic sinus disease owing to the hypersensitivity mechanisms is a very common disorder in adults *(43)*. However, this form may also be observed in children, with an incidence of 10–15%, especially in those suffering from allergic rhinitis, bronchial asthma, or serious otitis media *(1,2,6–12,43)*.

The immunologically mediated chronic sinus disease may also be observed in two forms: a primary form without any preceding or accompanying nasal allergic response, and in a secondary form that may be induced by the hypersensitivity mecha-

Table 14
Nasal and Sinus Responses After the Nasal Challenge with Allergen

Patients, n = 78, and nasal challenges, n = 193	Sinus response			
	Maxillary	Frontal	Maxillary + frontal	Negative
69 Patients				
149 Positive NR	121	3	14	11
15 Negative NR	4[a]	1[a]	1[a]	9
9 Patients				
29 Negative NR	6[a]	0	2[a]	21
78 PBS	0	0	0	78

NR, nasal response.

[a]Primary or "nonassociated" form of the sinus response (SR); the remaining responses are secondary or "associated" forms of the sinus response. The agreement between positive NS and SR as well as negative NS and SR was statistically distinctly significant ($p < 0.01$).

References: 56,127,224.

nism taking place primarily in the nasal mucosa (Table 14) (33,56,219,224).

The secondary or "associated" form of the immunologically induced chronic sinus disease occurs in approx 95%, whereas the primary or "nonassociated" form appears in approx 5% of subjects suffering from this disorder (53–58). Although the incidence of the primary form of the chronic sinus disease owing to the hypersensitivity mechanism does not exceed 5%, it is distinctly more frequent than the immunologically mediated primary form of the acute sinus disease (33,53,56, 58,219,224).

No differences in the incidence of the particular forms of the immunologically induced chronic sinus disease have been observed between children and adults (53–58,224).

The chronic sinus disease resulting from the hypersensitivity mechanisms (allergic reactions) has been observed by us most frequently in the maxillary sinuses only (in approx 85% of which 65% is a bilateral form and 20% a monolateral form), sometimes in both maxillary and frontal sinuses (approx in 14%, almost always as a bilateral form), and sporadically in the frontal sinuses only (approx in 1%, always as a bilateral form), without any significant differences between adults and children (Table 14) (55,224).

No sufficient data are available in the literature concerning the ethmoid as well as the sphenoid sinus disease, either acute or chronic, owing to the immunologic mechanisms. The dearth of such information may probably be caused by a variety of factors, such as a difficult accessibility of these sinuses with respect to their topographic location, incomplete knowledge of their physiologic, as well as pathologic, functions, and a lack of reliable diagnostic parameters to confirm such disorder (224).

Basic Types of the Paranasal Sinus Response

The sinus disease in which the hypersensitivity mechanisms play the causal role belongs almost exclusively to the chronic sinus disease (2,6,30, 43,53–58,63,223). Patients with the chronic sinus disease when challenged intranasally by allergens or exceptionally by nonspecific hyperreactivity agents, may develop different types of the paranasal sinus responses (53–58,224).

THE PRIMARY OR SO-CALLED "NONASSOCIATED" FORM OF THE PARANASAL SINUS RESPONSE TO THE INTRANASAL ALLERGEN CHALLENGE

This, without any preceding or accompanying nasal response, occurs in <5% of all positive paranasal sinus responses, and may be observed only in maxillary sinuses (53–58,224). We have never observed the primary form of response in the frontal sinuses (224). The primary form can be induced only by intranasal challenge with an allergen, but not with a nonspecific hyperreactivity agent (224).

Two types of the primary form of maxillary sinus response may be observed, an early response in approx 4% and a late response in approx 1% of the cases (53–58,224).

***The Early Response of Maxillary Sinuses
(ER-MS).*** The clinical course of the ER-MS,
recorded by echography in combination with radiography, is as follows: onset within 60 min, maximum within 1–2 h, and resolution within 8–10 h
after the allergen challenge *(53–58,224).* The
ER-MS has been accompanied by changes in the
following in vivo and in vitro diagnostic parameters and symptoms *(53–58,224):*

1. Echography: a decreased passage of the sound
   through the sinus cavity indicating an increase in
   the thickening of the anterior part of the maxillary
   sinus mucosa;
2. Radiographs: an increase in the thickening of the
   sinus mucosal membrane indicating mucosal
   edema and/or infiltration, whereas the other
   changes, such as decreased aeration or increase in
   opacification, are not usually observed in this type
   of sinus response;
3. Suspect disease history for the maxillary sinus
   response to the particular allergen(s) has been
   found in 70% of these cases;
4. Subjective complaints: usually a sharp pain to a
   slight degree, without pressure, located in the
   maxillary sinuses; the pain may progress sporadically into the skin of the face, inferior palpebrae,
   or gingival area;
5. Rhinoscopy, anterior as well as posterior, has not
   revealed any significant changes in the aspect of
   the nasal mucosa or maxillary ostium;
6. Except for a slight hypersecretion, no other nasal,
   other organs', or general symptoms have been
   observed;
7. No significant changes in the NS cytology of any
   cell types have been observed;
8. The transparent NS contained very few cells
   and a low concentration of albumin, however,
   no immunoglobulins or histamine have been
   found; and
9. Other diagnostic parameters, such as intradermal
   tests, eosinophil, and leukocyte counts in the NS
   and in the blood, serum concentrations of the
   particular immunoglobulin classes, IgG subclasses and specific IgE, and the changes in the
   blood concentration of histamine, did not demonstrate any significant changes or any significant
   correlation with the ER-MS.

***The Late Response of Maxillary Sinuses
(LR-MS).*** The clinical course of the LR-MS
recorded by echography in combination with X-ray is

as follows: onset within 6–10 h, maximum within
8–12 h, and resolution within 24 h after the allergen
challenge *(53–58,224).* The LR-MS has been associated with the following in vivo and in vitro diagnostic parameters, symptoms, and complaints
(53–58,224):

1. Echography: an increase in the thickening of the
   mucosal membrane in the maxillary sinuses;
2. Radiographs: an increase in the thickening of the
   mucosal membrane and sometimes a slightly
   decreased aeration and/or increased opacification;
3. The disease history suspect for maxillary sinus
   response to a certain allergen has been found in
   65–70% of these cases, with only a few patients
   indicating the late onset of complaints;
4. Subjective complaints accompanying this type
   of maxillary sinus response: usually a sharp
   pain to a moderate degree, without pressure,
   and sometimes a slight pulsation, located in
   the maxillary sinuses; the pain may progress
   sporadically into the skin of the face, inferior
   palpebrum, external ear, and gingival area;
5. Rhinoscopy, anterior as well as posterior, did not
   demonstrate any significant changes in the aspect
   of nasal mucosa or maxillary ostium;
6. No nasal, other organs', or general symptoms
   have been recorded during the LR-MS;
7. Small amounts of watery nasal secretions may be
   observed sometimes;
8. No immunoglobulins of any class or subclass
   or histamine have been detected in the NS or
   nasal washing fluid during this type of sinus
   response;
9. The NS contained a very few cells, mostly
   sporadical eosinophil, neutrophil, or epithelial
   cell, without any significant changes in their
   counts; and
10. The intradermal tests, the eosinophil, and leu-
    kocyte counts in the NS and in the blood, the
    serum concentrations of the immunoglobulins
    and histamine did not demonstrate any signifi-
    cant changes or any significant correlation with
    the LR-MS.

The Secondary or So-Called "Associated" Form of the Paranasal Sinus Response

This is induced by the hypersensitivity mecha-
nism(s) appearing primarily in the nasal mucosa, in
response to the intranasal allergen exposure (challenge), and leading to the development of one of the
basic types of nasal response *(33,53–58,219,224).*

Table 15
Particular Types of the Nasal and Sinus Responses and Their Relationships (*see also* Table 14)

Nasal response	Sinus response					
	Maxillary, n = 135[a]			Frontal, n = 17[b]		
	ESR	LSR	DYSR	ESR	LSR	DYSR
149 Positive NR						
51 Immediate/early	44	3	1	3	3	0
15 Immediate + late	6	4	0	1	2	0
67 Late	0	61	3	0	5	0
7 Immediate + delayed	1	0	4	1	0	1
9 Delayed	0	0	8	0	0	1
	Maxillary, n = 13[c]			Frontal, n = 4[d]		
44 Negative NR	5[e]	7[e]	1[e]	3[e]	1[e]	0

NR, nasal response; ESR, early sinus response; LSR, late sinus response; DYSR, delayed sinus response.
[a] 135 = 121 + 14.
[b] 17 = 3 + 14.
[c] 13 = 4 + 6 + 1 + 2.
[d] 4 = 1 + 1 + 2.
[e] Primary or "nonassociated" form of sinus response; the remaining responses are of the secondary or "associated" form.
References: *56,127,224.*

In such case, the nasal response owing to the hypersensitivity mechanism acts not only as a preceding, but also as an accompanying causal factor that then induces the secondary sinus response *(53–58,224)*. The secondary form of paranasal sinus response is a very common disorder in both adults and children, and may be observed in 95% of subjects suffering from immunologically mediated chronic sinus disorders *(33,53–58,219,224)*. The secondary form of the paranasal sinus response, in contrast the primary form, is not limited to the maxillary sinuses only, but may also sometimes include the frontal sinuses *(33,53–58,224)*. The secondary form of paranasal sinus response, both in the maxillary and in the frontal sinuses, induced by the primary nasal response, occurs in the majority of cases (70%) bilaterally and in a minority of cases (30%) monolaterally *(224)*.

Three types of the secondary form of sinus have been recorded: an early, a late, and a delayed type *(53–58,224)*. All three types are associated with the preceding and inducing nasal response of the appropriate type (Table 15) *(53–58,224)*. However, the clinical course of the particular sinus response, especially its onset, is usually shifted in time, and the sinus response appears 10–30 min later than the corresponding nasal response type *(53,58,224)*.

In most subjects suffering from immunologically mediated chronic sinus disease, an allergic rhinitis and, in some cases, other additional disorders (on participation of hypersensitivity mechanism[s]) may also be observed. These additional disorders may include bronchial asthma in approx 12%, allergic conjunctivitis in 7%, and serous otitis media in 6% *(53–58,224)* (Table 16). However, some of the in vivo and in vitro diagnostic parameters, symptoms, and other organs' symptoms are related both to the initial nasal mucosa response and to the secondary induced sinus response, whereas some of the parameters and symptoms are related to only one *(53–58,224)*.

The Early Sinus Response (ESR). The ESR, induced by and associated with the INR/ENR, may be recorded either in the maxillary sinuses only (88%) (ESR-MS), both in the maxillary and the frontal sinuses (10%) (ESR-MFS), or finally in the frontal sinuses only (2%) (ESR-FS) *(53–58,224)*.

The clinical course of the ESR, recorded by the echography and supplemented by the radiography is as follows *(53–58,224)*: onset within 30–60 min, maximum within 2 h, and resolution within 8–10 h, sporadically within 24 h, after the intranasal allergen challenge (Figs. 18A–C and 19A–D). The ESR

Table 16
Other Organs' and General Symptoms Accompanying the Particular Types of Sinus Response (%)

	Sinus response to nasal challenge with allergen					
	Maxillary sinuses			Frontal sinuses		
	ESR, n = 56	LSR, n = 75	DYSR, n = 17	ESR, n = 8	LSR, n = 11	DYSR, n = 2
Nasal obstruction	92	91	94	62	91	100
Conjunctival injection or chemosis	7	13	12	0	9	0
Palpebral edema	2	5	6	12	9	50
Middle ear response (otalgia, hypacusia, changes in middle ear pressure)	13	15	12	0	9	0
Pressure in the sinuses	91	100	100	75	100	100
Bronchial complaints (mostly secondary bronchoconstriction, sometimes also wheezing and/or cough)	9	11	6	0	0	0
Headache	2	12	12	75	91	100
Pharyngeal irritation	0	3	6	0	0	0
General malaise complaints	0	13	12	0	9	0

ESR, early sinus response; LSR, late sinus response; DYSR, delayed sinus response.
References: *55,56,58,127,224.*

has been associated with the changes of the following in vivo and in vitro parameters (53–58,224):

1. Echography: a distinct increase in the thickening of the mucosal membrane in the particular sinus types (Fig. 19A–D);
2. Radiographs: a distinct increase in the thickening of the sinus mucosal membranes indicating a mucosal edema and/or infiltration and, in the majority of cases, a slightly decreased aeration of the particular sinuses (Fig. 18A–C);
3. The disease history suspect for sinus response may be found in approx 55% of the cases, whereas that suspect for the early nasal response may be found in 80% of the cases;
4. The following subjective complaints may be observed during the ESR: a blunt pain to a slight degree and/or slight pressure in the particular sinuses, sometimes with propagation into the corresponding skin area, inferior palpebrum, and/or gingival area, accompanied by a slightly painful palpation and percussion of the particular sinuses, and sometimes also a hypophonia to a slight degree;
5. Anterior and posterior rhinoscopy may reveal a characteristic picture of the nasal mucosa, a distinct hyperemia of the nasal mucosal membrane, especially on the turbinates, which may be covered by an abundant transparent NS and edematic ostia of the particular sinuses;

6. Nasal complaints: nasal obstruction to a moderate degree, distinct hypersecretion of the watery transparent secretions, distinct sneezing, and sporadic nasal itching;
7. Other organs' and general symptoms are listed in Table 16;
8. The transparent NS contained low concentration of albumin, and sometimes also histamine and specific IgE antibodies;
9. The cytology of the nasal secretions may reveal changes in the count of the particular cell types as already described in the INR section;
10. The positive intradermal tests (immediate skin response) with the allergen causing the INR and secondary induced ESR have been found in 69% of cases, the increased concentration of total IgE antibody in the serum in 23%, the positive specific IgE antibody in 41%, the increased count of eosinophils in the peripheral blood in 58%, and leukocytes in 3%, with no changes in the serum concentration of immunoglobulins of other classes or histamine having been recorded during the positive ESR associated with positive INR; and
11. The concentrations of other mediators, cytokines, neuropeptides, or other factors, either in the serum, in the NS, or in the lavage fluid from the sinuses and their possible changes during this type of the sinus response have not yet been investigated sufficiently.

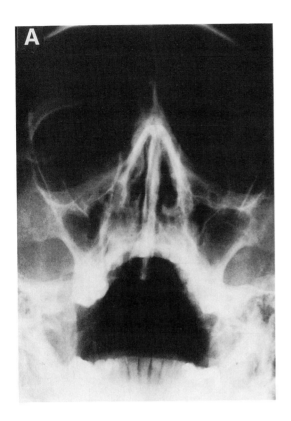

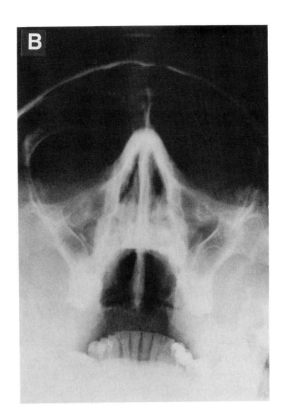

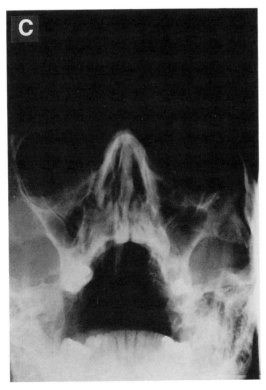

Fig. 18. Radiographs of maxillary sinuses of a patient (C. J.) developing the secondary or associated form of the ESR-MS, induced by the primary INR to the nasal challenge with grass pollen in a concentration of 1000 BU/mL. **(A)** Before the allergen challenge; **(B)** 1 h after the allergen; **(C)** 2 h after the allergen.

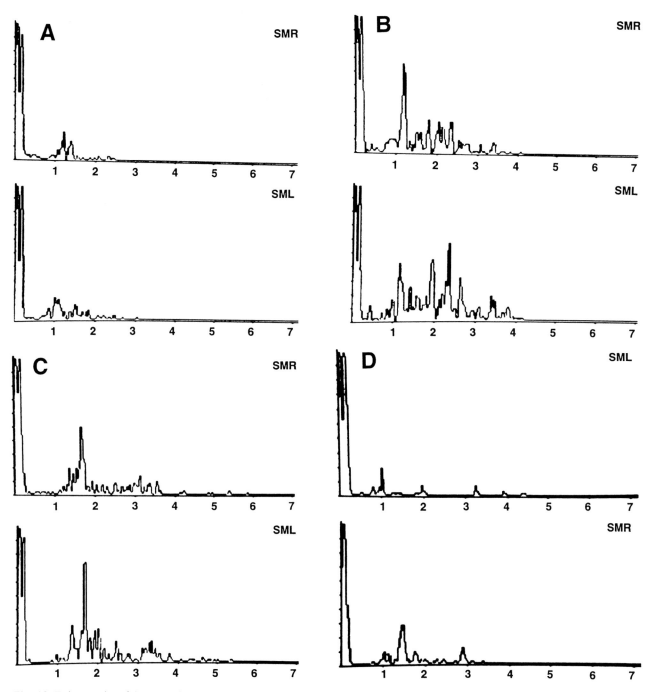

Fig. 19. Echographs of the maxillary sinuses in the same patient (C. J.) developing the associated form of the ESR-MS, induced by the primary INR to the grass pollen (1000 BU/mL). **(A)** Before the allergen challenge; **(B)** 1 h after the allergen challenge; **(C)** 2 h after the allergen; **(D)** 6 h after the allergen.

The Late Sinus Response (LSR). The LSR, induced by and associated with the LNR, may be recorded in a majority of cases in the maxillary sinuses (83%) (LSR-MS), sometimes both in the maxillary and the frontal sinuses, as a combined clinical event (14%) (LSR-MFS), or sporadically in the frontal sinus only (3%) (LSR-FS) *(53–58,224)*.

The clinical course of LSR, recorded by the echography and supplemented by the radiography, can be characterized as follows: onset within 5–8 h, maximum within 8–12 h, and resolution within 24 h, sometimes within 48 h, after the intranasal allergen challenge (Figs. 20A–D and 21A–D) *(53–58,224)*.

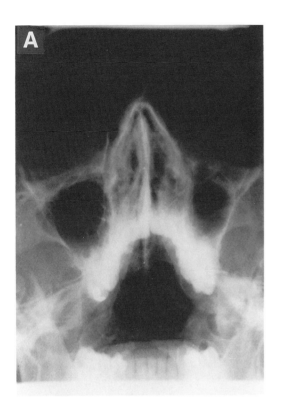
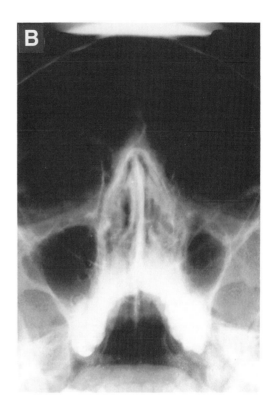
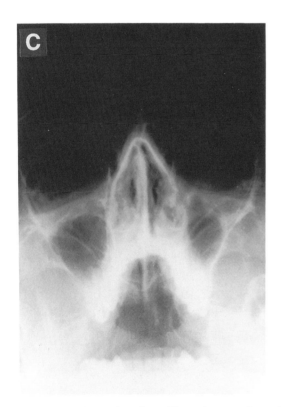
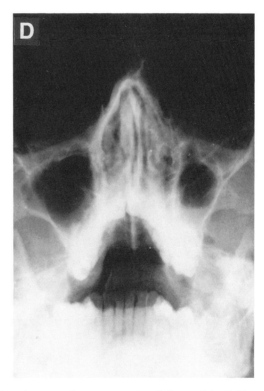

Fig. 20. Radiographs of maxillary sinuses of a patient (A. V.) developing the secondary or associated form of the LSR-MS, induced by the primary LNR to the nasal challenge with cat danders in a concentration of 0.5 mg/mL. **(A)** Before the allergen challenge; **(B)** 1 h after the allergen; **(C)** 6 h after the allergen; **(D)** 24 h after the allergen.

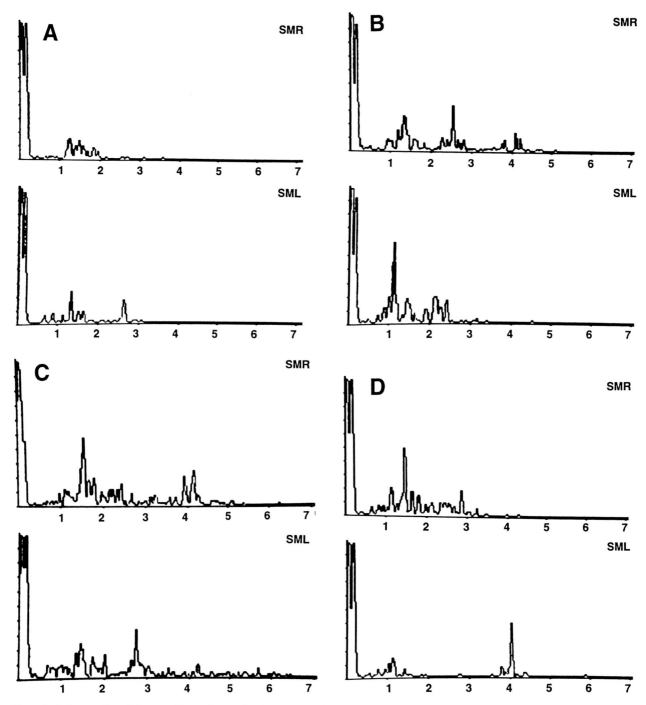

Fig. 21. Echographs of the maxillary sinuses in the same patient (A. V.) developing the associated form of the LSR-MS, induced by the primary LNR to the cat danders (0.5 mg/mL). **(A)** Before the allergen challenge; **(B)** 1 h after the allergen; **(C)** 6 h after the allergen; **(D)** 24 h after the allergen.

The LSR has been accompanied by the following changes of the in vivo and in vitro diagnostic parameters, symptoms and complaints *(53–58,224)*:

1. Echography: a distinct increase in the thickening of the mucosal membrane in the particular sinuses,

accompanied sometimes by a transient accumulation of the secretions on the bottom of the maxillary sinuses, which can even imitate the air–fluid level, and can be recorded in sporadical cases (Fig. 21A–D);
2. Radiographs: a distinct increase in the thickening of the sinus mucosal membrane, a distinctly

decreased aeration, and a slightly increased opacification (Fig. 20A–D);

3. The disease history suspect for the sinus disease found in approx 40% of the cases, whereas that suspect for the LNR may be found in 65% of the cases;

4. The LSR is usually associated with the following complaints: a moderate pressure in the particular sinus, sometimes pulsating and increasing intensity in some body positions, such as horizontal lying or forward bend, and associated with a painful palpation and percussion of the appropriate sinus; sometimes also hypophonia may be observed;

5. Rhinoscopy reveals a violaceous and edematic aspect of the nasal mucosa, especially that on the middle turbinates, edematic ostia which are usually oppressed by the swollen margins, and a small amount of the tough secretions dispersed on the nasal mucosa surface;

6. Nasal complaints accompanying the LNR are mostly a distinct nasal obstruction (blockage) and a limited hypersecretion, without sneezing and nasal itching;

7. Other organs' and general symptoms are summarized in Table 16;

8. Nasal secretions are usually of a higher viscosity grade and sometimes contain IgG antibodies, but no specific IgE antibodies;

9. The changes in the count of particular cell types in the nasal secretions are identical with those having been described in the LNR section;

10. The positive intradermal tests (late skin response) with the allergen causing the LNR and secondary induced LSR have been found in 65% of the cases, the increased concentration of total IgE antibody in the serum in 6%, the positive specific IgE antibody in the serum in 9%, the increasing concentration of total IgG in the serum in 51%, IgG_3 in 19% and IgG_4 in 16% of the cases, the increased count of eosinophils in the peripheral blood in 43% and leukocytes in 20%, and changes in the histamine concentration in the serum in 2% of the cases; and

11. The concentrations of other mediators, cytokines, neuropeptides, or other factors in the blood, NS, or in the lavage fluid both from the nose and from the sinuses, and their changes during the LSR and accompanying LNR, have not yet been studied.

The Delayed Sinus Response (DYSR). The DYSR, induced by and associated with the DYNR, has been recorded predominantly in the maxillary sinuses (88%) (DYSR-MS) and sometimes simultaneously in the maxillary and frontal sinuses (12%) (DYSR-MFS), but not solely in the frontal sinuses *(58,224)*.

The clinical course of the DYSR, recorded by the echography and supplemented by the radiography, is as follows: onset within 26–30 h, maximum within 36–48 h, and resolution usually within 60–72 h (Figs. 22A–D and 23A–D) *(58, 224)*. The DYSR has been associated with the changes of the following in vivo and in vitro parameters *(58,224)*:

1. Echography: a very pronounced increase in the thickening of the mucosal membrane in the appropriate sinuses and sometimes the opposite mucosal parts contact each other, and sporadically a small amount of the fluid in the maxillary sinus (monolateral) may be detected (Fig. 23A–D);

2. Radiographs: a very pronounced increase in the thickening of the mucosal membrane in the particular sinus, reducing distinctly the air content of the sinus, which indicates a large infiltration of the mucosal membrane in the particular sinus and a distinct decrease in aeration, and a pronounced opacification is observed; occasionally a small amount of fluid on the elevated bottom of the maxillary sinus is recorded as a transient finding (Fig. 22A–D);

3. The disease history suspect for sinus response may be found in approx 45% of the cases, whereas that for the DYNR may be found in 30% of the cases;

4. The DYSR usually may be accompanied by a pronounced pressure localized in the sinus, however with propagation into the nasal cavity, gingival area, and buccal area of the skin, and sometimes also into the middle ear (secondary otalgia) and orbita; the palpation and/or percussion of the appropriate sinuses usually is painful, the pressure intensity increasing in a horizontal lying or forward bend position; the nasal blowing can be difficult and painful; and only a small amount of secretions usually may be produced;

5. The aspect of the nasal mucosa, as evaluated by rhinoscopy, is distinctly violaceous and

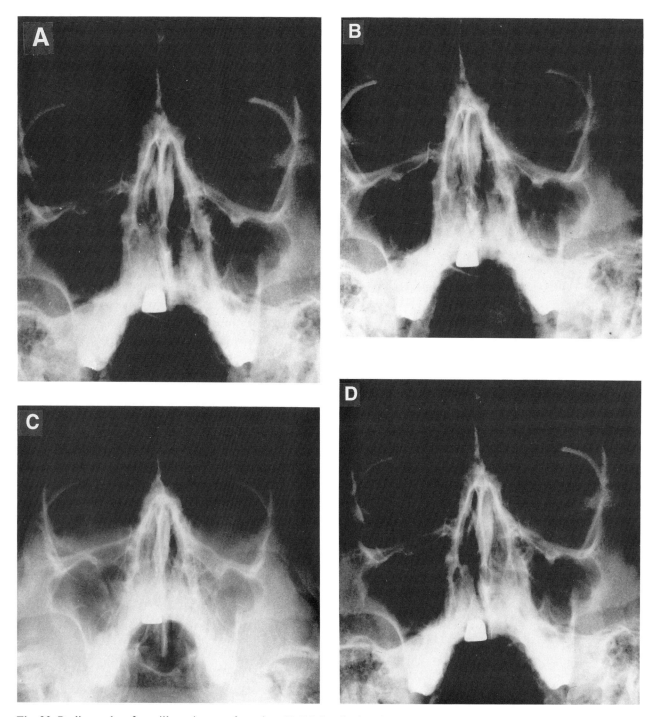

Fig. 22. Radiographs of maxillary sinuses of a patient (P. B.) developing the secondary or associated form of the DYSR-MS, induced by the primary DYNR to the nasal challenge with mites *(Dermatophagoides pteronyssinus)* in a concentration of 100 NU/mL. **(A)** Before the allergen challenge; **(B)** 24 h after the allergen; **(C)** 36 h after the allergen; **(D)** 56 h after the allergen.

edematic, and small mucosal hemorrhages are found regularly, predominantly on the inferior and middle turbinate; the maxillary ostia are almost fully closed by the swollen margins; and

almost no secretions may be seen on the surface of the nasal mucosa;

6. Nasal complaints accompanying the DYNR are represented almost solely by a very severe

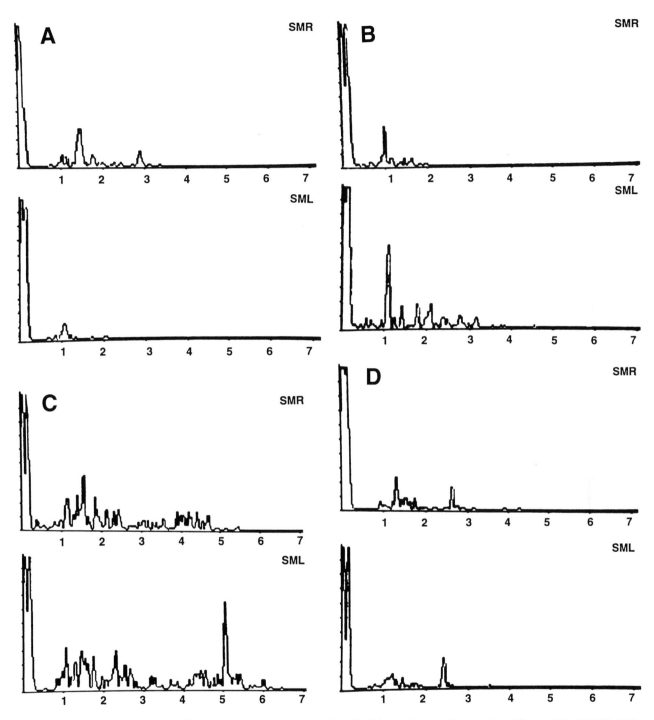

Fig. 23. Echographs of the maxillary sinuses in the same patient (P. B.) developing the associated form of the DYSR-MS, induced by the primary DYNR to the *Dermatophagoides pteronyssinus* (100 NU/mL). **(A)** Before the allergen challenge; **(B)** 24 h after the allergen; **(C)** 36 h after the allergen; **(D)** 56 h after the allergen.

obstruction (blockage) on full absence of other nasal complaints;

7. Other organs' and general symptoms are presented in Table 16;

8. A very small amount of highly viscous and opaque NS have been detected during the DYNR. No antibody of any class have been detected in the NS obtained during the DYNR;

9. The cytologic changes recorded in the nasal secretions are identical with those having been reported in the DYNR section;

10. The positive intradermal tests (delayed skin response) with the allergen causing the DYNR and secondary induced DYSR have been found in 67% of the cases, the increased serum concentration of total IgE antibody in 5%, positive specific IgE antibody in the serum in 2%, increased serum concentrations of total IgG in 1%, particular IgG subclasses in <1%, an increased count of eosinophils in the peripheral blood in 0%, and leukocytes in 11%, mostly with a distinct lymphocytosis, with no changes in the blood concentrations of histamine having been recorded; and

11. The changes in the concentrations of other mediators, chemotactic factors, cytokines, neuropeptides, or other factors in the blood, nasal secretions, nasal, or sinus lavage fluid, during the DYSR and DYNR, have not yet been investigated.

DIAGNOSTIC PROCEDURE

The reliable diagnostic procedure should meet some necessary conditions, such as:

1. It should be as complex as possible to cover most of the important aspects of that disorder;

2. The in vivo diagnostic parameters should be considered to be the basic data, being supported by in vitro data;

3. The relative values are of higher diagnostic importance than the absolute values, especially when they are related to a certain, well-defined event or factor, such as allergen challenge; this may be called a comparison principle;

4. The diagnostic parameters recorded repeatedly in time, the so-called "dynamic parameters" and forming the time–response curves, are distinctly superior and much more important than the single-recorded so-called "static or single-phase parameters."

5. The diagnostic confirmation of a certain pathologic process may be considered to be of an equal value to the diagnostic exclusion of the same pathologic process; this may be called the reciprocal diagnostic values *(63,66,100,220–232)*.

General Examination

DISEASE HISTORY

The disease history may not only be focused on the paranasal sinuses, but also on other organs and states, and it may include certainly the following parts: family history; past medical history; personal and social state; profession history and circumstances; house and all internal as well as external factors related, such as construction, location, neighborhood, furnishing, pets, and so on; habits; present disease history and condition of all organs; use of drugs; nutrition and use of basic and supplementary foods; hobbies; and use of personal and care means, such as washing powders, soaps, shampoos, after shave, bath foams, shaving foams, cosmetics, deodorants, perfumes, make-up preparations, creams, and toothpaste *(4,6,30,37,45,47,56,63,66,100,220, 224,232)*.

GENERAL, ALL-ROUND EXAMINATION *(4,6,30,37,45,47,56,66)*

The general examination should include the all-round physical examination, basic laboratory, X-ray, and supplementary examinations, such as lung and sinus radiogram, electrocardiogram, basic pulmonary functions, bacteriological examination of the sputum, nasal secretions, and pharyngeal smear *(4,6,14,25–27,31,33,47,53–58,64–66,98,220,224)*.

Allergologic and Immunologic Examination

BASIC OR SCREENING STEPS

In vivo part, consisting of:

1. Skin tests: prick tests or cutaneous (scratch) test followed by the intradermal tests, if the scratch tests have been negative, with basic inhalant allergen extracts and if indicated with basic food extracts *(45,53–58,64,66,95,98,99,165)*. If indicated, skin tests with other allergen extracts can also be carried out, such as unusual allergens (patient's own house dust or pet danders, and so on), less common allergens (exotic animals), individual pollen kinds, particular mould kinds, and others *(53–58,66)*.

2. Anterior and/or posterior rhinoscopy *(30,45,47, 54,56,57,220,231)*.

3. Endoscopic examination of the sinuses on indication, which can be combined with the lavage of the sinus for histologic, cytologic, immunologic, and bacteriologic purposes *(3,5,32,37,47,220,225, 229,231)*.

In vitro part, consisting of:

1. Determination of immunoglobulins (so-called basic immunoglobulin profile) of various classes and types, such as total IgE; allergen-specific IgE,

IgG, IgM, IgA, and IgD, IgG subclasses; precipitating antibodies (mostly IgG, but sometimes also IgM); in various media, such as blood serum, nasal secretions, nasal lavage fluid, and sinus lavage fluid; and by means of a variety of established techniques, including radioimmunoassay (PRIST, RAST) immunoenzymatically (ELISA, CAP), double immunodiffusion (Ouchterlony technique), radial immunodiffusion (Mancini technique), and some other new techniques, being recently investigated (HPLC, flow cytometry, and so forth). The accuracy of the immunoglobulin determination, qualitative, semiquantitative, and quantitative, depends both on the technique selected and on method of processing of the particular medium *(45,56,66,138,143,164,230,232).*

2. Cytologic examination of the nasal secretions, performed repeatedly *(6,30,45,46,56,66,97–99,101,111,135,137,171,230).*

3. Repeated eosinophil, leukocyte, and leukocyte differentiation count in the blood *(53–58,66).*

PRINCIPAL STEPS OR DEFINITE CONFIRMATION

In vivo part, consisting of:

1. NPT with a representative of the nonspecific hyperreactivity, such as histamine, methacholin, or cold air, which may definitely confirm the participation of the nonspecific hyperreactivity component in the nasal symptoms, and in some exceptional cases, also indirectly in the sinus response *(84–88,127).*

2. NPT with various inhalant allergens, such as house dust, mites *(Dermatophagoides pteronyssinus, Dermatophagoides farinae)*, various pollen species, various kinds of animal danders, particular kinds of moulds, and so on, performed in combination with the registration of various parameters indicating the changes in the nasal functions, for various time intervals, as has already been discussed. The nasal challenges with allergen should be considered to be a definite confirmation of the causal role of a certain allergen in the particular type of nasal response owing to the hypersensitivity mechanisms, and being represented by a certain complex of nasal symptoms in the particular patient.

3. The NPT, especially those with inhalant allergens, can be supplemented by a simultaneous recording of other diagnostic parameters by means of which the response of other organs can be detected and monitored. In this way, the pos-

sible causal role of the nasal mucosa and/or the hypersensitivity reaction, taking place primarily in the nasal mucosa, in the secondarily induced response of the other organ can be demonstrated and confirmed *(47,53–56,63,64,69,87,116,130–133).*

4. The NPT can be combined with recording of a variety of other diagnostic parameters, such as radiography, echography, and other sinus imaging techniques to monitor a possible secondarily induced response of the sinuses; tympanometry to record the secondarily induced response of the middle ear; or spirography to follow the secondarily induced bronchospasm. The nasal challenges can also be supplemented routinely by recording of general diagnostic parameters, such as body temperature, eosinophil and leukocyte count in the circulating blood, and leukocyte differentiation count in the blood, as well as by recording of parameters related exclusively to the primary hypersensitivity reaction in the nasal mucosa, such as cytologic changes in the NS, histologic changes in the nasal mucosa (biopsies), and, finally, determination of various compounds, such as particular mediators and the changes of their concentrations, in the NS, accompanying the particular types of the nasal response *(53–58,66,130–133).*

5. Ingestion challenges with foods (FICH) suspected to participate in the hypersensitivity mechanism(s) leading either to primary response of the individual organs, such as nasal mucosa, sinus mucosa, middle ear, conjunctivae, or to a primary response of the nasal mucosa, which then may induce the secondary response of another organ, such as sinus mucosa, middle ear response, or conjunctival response. The food ingestion challenge (FICH), may, of course, be performed on an indication or serious suspicion *(59,100,125,134,205–215).*

In vitro part consisting of:

1. Cytologic examination of NS, nasal lavage fluid, and/or sinus lavage fluid to record the influx of various cell types and the dynamic changes in their counts *(30,46,56,60,63,66,67,96–118).*

2. Immunologic examination of NS, nasal lavage fluid, and/or sinus lavage fluid to record the appearance of the basic mediators and the changes in their concentrations *(13,15,24,60,63,66,67,94,100,103,117).*

COMPLEMENTARY STEPS

These include a variety of heterogeneous techniques and tests, which may contribute, if necessary, to the confirmation, explanation, or interpretation of the primary sinus response owing to the hypersensitivity mechanisms and/or the secondary sinus response induced by the primary nasal mucosa response owing to the hypersensitivity event. These techniques and tests may include the recording of a number of compounds, such as cytokines, chemotactic factors; constituents released by the particular cells involved in the particular types of hypersensitivity; lymphocyte typing; examination of the activation degree of the particular cell types; biochemical and biophysical examination of the NS and/or secretions obtained from the particular sinuses and their composition; investigation of various receptors, molecules, and other structures on the membrane surface of particular relevant cells; determination of adhesive molecules; intravital microscopy of the nasal and/or sinus mucosa; measurement of intramucosal temperature, measurement of the blood circulation and microcirculation in the mucosal membrane of the nose and/or sinuses; and others (13,15,46,47,66,67,72,106,107, 144–146,149,164,166,167,183–185,190, 191,230,232).

Monitoring of the Paranasal Sinus Response

The response of the paranasal sinuses can be followed and recorded by means of the so-called imaging techniques. There are several techniques for imaging of the sinuses, diagnostic values of which, however, differ and depend not only on the purposes for which they should be used, but also on the investigator's experience, department facilities, and financial (budget) aspects. The basic rule of the use of these techniques for the investigation of the role of an allergy reaction (hypersensitivity mechanism[s]) in sinus disease concerns their repeated application before and after a principal event, which is the allergen exposure or challenge (56). With respect to our data, the combination of one of the sinus imaging techniques with the monitored nasal provocation tests seems to be a very interesting diagnostic approach revealing very useful and sometimes surprising information on the role of allergy, either directly or indirectly through the nasal mucosa, in the sinus disease (Table 17) (53–59). The hypersensitivity mechanism, including

Table 17
Survey of Radiographic and Echographic Changes in the Maxillary Sinuses (Increase in the Thickening of the Mucosal Membrane)[a]

	Changes	
	Radiographic	Echographic
21 Patients		
29 Positive NR	26	22
4 Negative NR	2	1
3 Patients		
5 Negative NR	1	0

NR, nasal response.
[a]The agreement between the radiographs and the echographs was statistically significant (p < 0.05).
References: 55,58.

various consequent steps, is a very dynamic process necessitating a dynamic approach, which means repeated recording of the particular parameters before and after a certain event or agent, in time (66). In contrast, a single application of the sinus imaging techniques delivers information on the temporary state of the particular sinus and its mucosal membrane only, thus being a static parameter that is, however, fully insufficient and unable to be used as a criterion of a dynamic process like allergy (66).

The diagnostic imaging of paranasal sinuses may include the following techniques:

1. Transillumination (4,6,45);
2. Radiography (conventional X-ray or so-called plain film) (4,6,14,25–27,31,33,47,53–59,220, 224,225,227);
3. Plain tomography (31,33);
4. Computed tomography (CT) (14,31,33,37, 227,231);
5. Ultrasonography or so-called echography (6,14, 20–22,29,30,45,55,57,58,220,225);
6. Magnetic resonance imaging (MRI) (31,33,47, 227,228); and
7. Single photon emission computerized tomography (SPECT) (40,41).

The particular imaging techniques and their practical performance and application are described in detail in another chapter of this book. The brief description of the techniques in this chapter will therefore be limited to their capability and their usefulness for the registration of the changes in the sinuses owing to the hypersensitivity reactions.

Transillumination may be considered to be a satisfactory inexpensive screening technique for the general state of maxillary and frontal sinuses, especially to discriminate between an absence and a presence of a suspect pathologic process *(4)*. However, this technique cannot generate more detailed data concerning the fine changes in the thickening of the sinus mucosa, opacification, and aeration of the sinuses, and the state of the bones building the particular sinuses *(2)*. Moreover, this technique cannot be used for examination of other sinus types than maxillary and frontal sinuses. This technique should therefore be considered an incompetent method for the earlier-mentioned purpose *(4,6,45)*.

Radiography—conventional X-ray or plain film— is the most common technique for imaging of almost all sinus types *(4,6,14,25–27,31,45,47,220, 224,225,227)*. This technique is not expensive, can be repeated up to a certain number, the modern equipment produces a very limited radiation (especially when the nonrelevant parts of the head are shielded), the basic radiologic equipment is present in practically all hospitals and clinics, and the detailed results obtained by this technique are reliable and reproducible. This technique may be considered to be suitable for the recording and consideration of the changes both of the mucosal membrane and of the whole sinuses owing to the hypersensitivity (allergy) reactions. Our experience with conventional X-ray of maxillary and frontal sinuses would not confirm the disadvantages of this technique reported by some investigators. The most commonly used projections for these purposes are the Water's projection (postero-anterior or so-called occipito-mental), followed by the Caldwell's projection (angled postero-anterior), and sporadically the Towne's (occipito-frontal) or lateral projections *(31,220)*. Nevertheless, the radiation, even limited up to the minimal degree, remains to be the disadvantage of this technique.

Plain tomography *(31,33)* and more accurate CT, or so-called "computed tomography" scan including its modification "screening computed tomography" *(14,31,33,37,47,227,231)*, characterized by a limited number of slices and a low-dose technique, may be considered to be the standard imaging technique for the paranasal sinus disease. The costs and the radiation doses of the CT do not differ substantially from those of the plain tomography, but the CT has much greater accuracy. The coronal thin sections usually demonstrate excellent delineation of lesions in the ostiomeatal complex, which is considered to be a very important site in the pathophysiology of the recurrent and chronic disease of paranasal sinuses *(31)*. The axial sections are important for the evaluation of the periorbital and infraorbital complications of the sinus disease *(31)*. The most common and important indication of the tomography and even of the CT is the preoperative assessment *(32,33)*. Despite the ability of CT to measure precisely the thickening of the mucosal membrane in the sinuses, this technique cannot be considered to be a suitable routine parameter for the diagnostic evaluation of the changes of the mucosal membrane in the sinuses owing to the hypersensitivity mechanism(s), with respect to the costs, radiation doses, and therefore its inability to be performed repeatedly within a short period of time.

Ultrasonography (ultrasound imaging, echography) may be considered to be a satisfactory noninvasive, inexpensive, time- and labor-saving technique, without using any ionizing radiation and guaranteeing optimal convenience for the patient *(55,58,59)*. There are two basic types of ultrasound techniques: A-scan and B-scan. The A-scan is a one-dimensional method, modulating the amplitude, whereas the B-scan modulates the brightness in a two-dimensional manner *(225)*. The author and colleagues, like many other investigators, are using the A-scan with respect to its reliable evaluation of the mucosal thickening and presence of fluid in the sinuses, and its simple operation. This technique is utilizable for the evaluation of the mucosal thickening and air–fluid level in the maxillary sinuses, as well as of the mucosal thickening in the frontal sinuses, but not applicable for other sinus types. One of the most important advantages of this technique, especially for its use in the case of the sinus disease owing to the hypersensitivity mechanism(s) (allergy reaction), is its unlimited use both in the time and number.

This technique seems to be clearly suitable for the repeated evaluation of the changes of and in the mucosal membrane of the maxillary and frontal sinuses *(55,58)*. Our previous data (Table 17) *(55,58)*, as well as recently gathered data (Table 18) *(224)*, demonstrating a correlation of 76 and 92% between the echographic and radiographic findings, respectively, in the maxillary sinuses, are in agreement with some investigators' results *(20–*

Table 18
Radiographic and Echographic Changes Recorded During Particular Types
of Sinus Response (Increase in the Thickening of the Mucosal Membrane)[a]

	Changes		
	Radiographic only	Echographic only	Radiographic + echographic
Maxillary sinus			
Early SR, $n = 56$	3	1	52
Late SR, $n = 75$	4	2	69
Delayed SR, $n = 17$	1	0	16
Frontal sinus			
Early SR, $n = 8$	2	0	6
Late SR, $n = 11$	0	1	10
Delayed SR, $n = 2$	0	0	2
Total $n = 169$ (100%)	10 (6%)	4 (2%)	155 (92%)

SR, sinus response.
[a]The agreement between the radiographs and the echographs was highly significant both for the total comparison ($p < 0.01$) and for the particular types of SR ($p < 0.02$).
Reference: 224.

22), whereas they disagree with other data reported (28). The possible reasons for the unsatisfactory correlation of the echography and radiography reported by some authors may be the insufficient diagnostic procedure and definition of their patients; only a single and not repeated recordings being carried out; the target of their studies being different from ours; and, finally, no supplementary diagnostic parameters, such as nasal secretion cytology, being used as the third and control tool (6,14,20–22,28–30,45,55–58,220,225).

MRI may be considered a sophisticated and advantageous technique without the use of ionizing radiation. Although the MRI supersedes the CT in resolving the soft tissue structures, it is superior in differentiation between the bacterial and fungal sinus disease, and offers the best contrast in the case of neoplasms and inflammation. This technique also has several limitations, such as high cost, long imaging times, the inability to display directly the bony landmarks, and, finally, it is not suitable for the repeated use within a short period of time. This technique, being the only practical cross-sectional method for generating the directly obtainable sagittal scans, is, however, not suitable for the evaluation of the primary or secondary sinus response owing to the hypersensitivity mechanism(s) (31,33,47,227,228).

SPECT, having been introduced by Slavin and coworkers, is a new technique for the imaging of

the paranasal sinuses by means of the isotope (40,41). This promising technique is still in the research stage (40,41). However, with respect to the data received thus far, this technique might be an interesting supplement to the already existing diagnostic possibilities of the evaluation of the role of allergy in the sinus disease (40,41).

Invasive techniques of sinus imaging include various modifications of endoscopy, which can be combined with other techniques and performed either for diagnostic or for therapeutic purposes. The diagnostic endoscopy may be used not only for the direct examination and evaluation of the sinus content and mucosal membrane, but, in combination with the rinsing of the sinus by saline, also for the collection of the sinus lavage fluid for various cytologic and/or immunologic tests and studies (23–25,32,47,225,229). The endoscopy can also be used for therapeutic purposes, such as mechanical enlargement of the ostia, resulting in an improved gas and fluid drainage from the particular sinuses, or it can be combined with the therapeutic irrigation of the particular sinuses by, e.g., saline and instillation (administration) of certain drugs or therapeutic agents (32,219,220,233). The further description of these techniques and their clinical applications will exceed the scope of this chapter. These techniques are discussed in detail in other chapters of this book.

THERAPEUTIC APPROACH AND NONSURGICAL TREATMENT OF SINUS DISEASE RESULTING FROM ALLERGY

The therapeutic control in general and the treatment of the individual cases of sinus disease owing to the hypersensitivity mechanism(s) represent a complex and multiple affair, being characterized not only by a variety of aspects, but also by a variety of solutions depending on the points of view from which this target would be approached (224).

This section will therefore be restricted to the basic and auxiliary antiallergic treatment of the primary or "nonassociated," and secondary or "associated" forms of the sinus disease owing to the hypersensitivity mechanisms, including the treatment of the primary allergic disorders of the nasal mucosa, which may induced secondarily the associated form of the sinus disease.

Generally, there is a great dearth of data concerning the pharmacologic control and treatment of sinus disease owing to the hypersensitivity mechanisms. The lack of such data has probably been caused by the poor understanding of the role of allergy, and the allergic reactions in the nasal mucosa, in the sinus disease in the past (56). The recognition and recent confirmation of such roles have allowed us to exploit this relationship for the diagnostic, as well as therapeutic, approaches to the immunologically mediated sinus disease in the practice (53–59). Therefore, the therapeutic measures recommended in this section are based predominantly on our clinical experience and results, which have not yet been published in full extension (57,58,153,224). Unfortunately, therapeutic data comparable with our results have not yet been found by us in the literature (224).

The treatment of sinus disease owing to allergy should be considered to be a logical consequence of the reliable diagnostic conclusions resulting from the reliable diagnostic procedure (58,66,83,100,224). This treatment should be as complex as possible to include aspects and features of the basic disorder, as well as disorders playing the causal role in the basic disorder, associated disorders, and finally the disorders being secondary induced by the basic disorder (58,66,83,100,219,224).

The choice of the particular drugs, their combinations, and supplementary therapeutic measures, in the case of sinus disease owing to the hypersensitivity mechanism(s), depends on a variety of factors, the most important of them being the outcomes of the reliably performed diagnostic procedure (224).

The Therapeutic Arsenal Available for this Target

GENERAL MEASURES

These are rinsing of the nose with the buffered physiologic solution (saline) to improve directly the nasal and indirectly also the sinus mucociliary clearance and the general function of the nasal mucosa (37,45,46,63,219,220,235).

ANTIALLERGIC MEASURES

The confirmed and/or highly suspected allergens should be eliminated as far as possible, and their exposure should be avoided by the subject (63,66, 234–236).

Pharmacologic Agents (Drugs). (See Tables 19–22).

Pharmacologic Agents (Drugs): Histamine-Receptor (H) and Mediator Antagonists (Tables 19 and 21).

1. The H_1-receptor antagonists (generally called antihistamines) can be divided into "three generations" (45,46,66,126,153–158,235). The "first generation" includes such drugs as promethazine hydrochloride, chlorphenamine maleate, clemastine, ketotifen, cinnarizine, triprolidine, chlorpheniramine, oxatomide, buclizine, meclizine, azatadine, and mebhydroline. The "second generation" consists of terfenadine, astemizole, acrivastine, and azelastine. The "third generation" includes cetirizine, loratadine, and levocabastine.
2. The H_2-receptor antagonists are represented by such drugs as cimetidine and ranitidine (46,153, 156–158,235).
3. The anticholinergic drugs include thiazinamium hydrochloride, oxyphenonium bromide, and ipratropium bromide (46,66,153,156,159,199, 219,236,241).

Pharmacologic Agents (Drugs): Disodium Cromoglycate (DSCG, Cromolyn). For topical and oral cromolyn, see Tables 19 and 22 (46,66, 90,92,100,104,105,108,109,113,114,125,153, 156,196,197,235,236).

Pharmacologic Agents (Drugs): Nedocromil Sodium (NDS). See Tables 20 and 22 (151–153, 156,197,198,235,237).

Table 19
Daily Doses of Some Antiallergic and Supplementary Drugs Recommended for Adults

Drug			
H$_1$-receptor antagonist			
First generation			
Promethazine	OR	1–3 × 12.5	mg or 1 × 25 mg
Chlorphenamine	OR	1–2 × 12	mg
Clemastine	OR	1–2 × 1	mg
Ketotifen	OR	1–2 × 1	mg
Cinnarizine	OR	1–2 × 25	mg
Triprolidine	OR	1 × 10	mg
Chlorpheniramine	OR	1–2 × 6	mg
Oxatomide	OR	1–2 × 30	mg
Azatidine	OR	1–2 × 1	mg
Mebhydroline	OR	2–4 × 50	mg
Hydroxyzine	OR	2 × 25	mg
Brompheniramine	OR	3 × 4	mg
Dexchlorpheniramine	OR	3–4 × 1–2	mg
Dimethindene	OR	3 × 1–2	mg
Second generation			
Astemizole	OR	1 × 10	mg
Terfenadine	OR	1–2 × 60	mg
Azelastine	OR	2 × 2	mg
Acrivastine	OR	3 × 8	mg
Third generation			
Cetirizine	OR	1 × 10	mg
Loratadine	OR	1 × 10	mg
Levocabastine	OR	2 Puffs (0.5 mg/mL) each nostril; 2× daily	
Ebastine	OR	1 × 5	mg
H$_2$-receptor antagonists			
Cimetidine	OR	1–3 × 300	mg
Ranitidine	OR	2 × 150	mg
Anticholinergic agents			
Thiazinamium	OR	1–3 × 100–200 mg	
Oxyphenonium	OR	2–4× daily × 5–10 mg	
Ipratropium	TOP[a]	4 × 40–80	mcg
Disodium cromoglycate			
Nasal drops 2%			
(20 mg/mL)	TOP	2 Drops—each nostril; 4–6× daily	
Nasal spray 2%			
(20 mg/mL)	TOP	2 Sprays—each nostril; 6× daily	
Nasal spray 4%			
(40 mg/mL)	TOP	1–2 Sprays—each nostril; 4–5× daily	
Powder (1 caps = 10 mg)	TOP	1 Capsule divided between both nostrils; 4× daily	
Oral formulation (powder			
in capsules or solution)		4 × 100–200 mg	

Administration: OR, oral; TOP, topical (intranasal).
[a]Commercial formulation is not yet available.

Pharmacologic Agents (Drugs): Glucocorticosteroids (GCS) (Tables 20 and 22). These are: (1) Systemic: (a) oral, such as prednisone, prednisolone, cortisone acetate, betamethasone, dexamethasone, triamcinolone, hydrocortisone; (b) parenteral, such as cortisone acetate, triamcinolone acetonide, betamethasone acetate, dexamethasone sodium-phosphate, paramethasone

Table 20
Daily Doses of Some Antiallergic and Supplementary Drugs Recommended for Adults

Drug		
Nedocromil sodium	TOP[a]	2 Sprays of 1%—each nostril—4× daily[a]
Glucocorticosteroids		
Systemic		
Prednisone	OR	0.5–1 mg/kg daily divided into 2–4 doses
Prednisolone	OR	0.5–0.8 mg/kg daily divided into 2–4 doses
Dexamethasone	OR	0.5–9 mg daily (up to 2 × 16 mg) divided in 2 doses
Topical		
Beclomethasone dipr	TOP	2 × 50 mcg—each nostril 2–3× daily
Budesonide	TOP	2 × 50 mcg—each nostril 2–3× daily
Flunisolide	TOP	2 × 25 mcg—each nostril 2–3× daily
Fluticasone	TOP	1 × 50 mcg—each nostril 2× daily
Triamcinolone	TOP	1–2 × 25 mcg—each nostril 4× daily
Decongestants		
Xylometazoline	TOP	1–2 Drops of 0.1%—each nostril 2–3× daily
Oxymetazoline	TOP	1–3 Drops of 0.05%—each nostril 1–3× daily
Naphazoline	TOP	1–2 Sprays—each nostril 2–3× daily
Tetrahydrozoline	TOP	1–2 Sprays—each nostril 2–3× daily
Phenylephrine	TOP	1–2 Sprays—each nostril 4× daily
Varia		
Acetylsalicyl acid	OR	1–3 × 500 mg
Indomethacine	OR	1 mg/kg/24 h divided into 2–3 doses
Ibuprofen	OR	2–6 × 200 mg

Administration: OR, oral; TOP, topical (intranasal).
[a]Commercial formulation is not yet available.

acetate, methylprednisolone acetate, prednisolone sodium-succinate, hydrocortisone sodium-succinate, triamcinolone acetonide, triamcinolone-diacetate, and methylprednisolone sodium-succinate (45,46, 144,145,167,200–202,238,239); and (2) Topical corticosteroids, such as beclomethasone dipropionate, budesonide, flumisolide, fluticasone propionate, and triamcinolone acetonide (46,66, 90–92,104,105,108,109,113,114,153,156,165, 219,236,238,239).

SUPPLEMENTARY PHARMACOLOGIC MEASURES AND AGENTS (TABLES 20 AND 22)

1. Decongestants (usually α-sympathomimetics) with α2 activity: xylometazoline, oxymetazoline, naphazoline, or tetrahydrozoline, or α1 activity: phenylephrine (37,45,46,156,219,235,236,240);
2. Some of the mucokinetic, mucolytic and mucoregulatory agents, such as cysteine derivatives and bromhexine (156,219);* and

*However, the therapeutic rationale and clinical effects of these compounds on the sinus mucosa or nasal mucosa response owing to the hypersensitivity mechanisms have not yet been confirmed and established (66,156,219).

3. Nonsteroidal anti-inflammatory drugs (acetylsalicylic acid and its derivatives, indomethacin, flurbiprofen, ibuprofen, prostaglandin-suppressing compounds), cAMP modulators, calcium channel blockers (nifedipine, verapamil), β-2-sympathomimetics, neuropeptide antagonists, thromboxanesynthesis inhibitors, inhibitors of 5-lipoxygenase pathway products, and other mediator antagonists (anti-PAF, antileukotrienes, antiserotonin, antikinins, and so on) (66,156,219).*

The Therapeutic Approach to the Particular Forms of the Sinus Disease Resulting from Hypersensitivity Mechanism(s)

The primary or "nonassociated" form of the sinus response can be divided into the responses caused by inhalant allergens and responses resulting from the adverse reactions to foods. The therapeutic possibilities in the case of inhalant allergens are rather limited and may include the avoidance of the suspected allergen(s), irrigation of the nose with saline (2–3 times daily),

Table 21
Daily Doses of Some Antiallergic and Supplementary Drugs Recommended for Children

Drug		<12 yr	12–16 yr
H_1-receptor antagonists			
First generation			
Promethazine	OR	1–3 yr = 2–4 × 1–2 mg; 3–12 yr = 2–4 × 2–4 mg	2–4 × 4 mg
Chlorphenamine	OR	X	1 × 12 mg
Clemastine	OR	1–3 yr = 1–2 × 0.25 mg; 3–12 yr = 1–2 × 0.5 mg	1–2 × 1 mg
Ketotifen	OR	>3 yr; 0.025 mg/kg/–24 h	1–2 × 1 mg
Cinnarizine	OR	>3 yr = 1 × 12.5 mg	1–2 × 12.5 mg
Triprolidine	OR	X	1 × 10 mg
Chlorpheniramine	OR	1–2 × 2.5 mg or 0.35 mg/kg/24 h	1 × 6 mg
Oxatomide	OR	1 mg/kg/24 h divided into 2 doses	1–2 × 15–30 mg
Azatidine	OR	1–2 × 0.5 mg	1–2 × 1 mg
Mebhydroline	OR	1–2 × 50 mg	2–3 × 50 mg
Hydroxyzine	OR	>2 yr = 1–2 × 25 mg; 2–6 yr = 2 mg/kg/24 h— divided into 2 doses	2 mg/kg 24 h divided into 2 doses
Brompheniramine	OR	X/NE	X/NE
Dexchlorpheniramine	OR	2–12 yr 2 × 1 mg repetabs	2–3 × 1 mg
Dimethindene	OR	1–3 yr = 3 × 0.5 mg; 3–12 yr = 3 × 0.75 mg	3 × 1 mg
Second generation		<6 yr = 0.2 mg/kg/24 h	
Astemizole	OR	2–6 yr = 0.2 mg/kg/24 h; 6–12 yr = 1 × 5 mg divided into 2 doses	1 × 10 mg
Terfenadine	OR	3–6 yr = 2 × 15 mg; 6–12 yr = 1–2 × 30 mg	1–2 × 30 mg
Azelastine	OR	X/NE	1 × 2 mg
Acrivastine	OR	X/NE	1–3 × 8 mg
Third generation			
Cetirizine	OR	X/NE	1–2 × 5 mg
Loratadine	OR	<30 kg = 1 × 5 mg; >30 kg = 1–2 × 5 mg	1–2 × 5 mg
Levocabastine	TOP	>3 yr = 1 puff (0.5 mg/mL) each nostril 2× daily	2 Puffs (0.5 mg/mL) each nostril 2× daily
Ebastine	OR	X/NE	1 × 5 mg
H_2-receptor antagonists			
Cimetidine	OR	X/NE	2–3 × 100 mg or 20 mg/kg/24 h divided in 3 doses
Ranitidine		UK[a]	UK[a]
Anticholinergic agents			
Thiazinamium	OR	6–12 yr = 2 × 100 mg	2–3 × 100 mg
Oxyphenonium	OR	6–12 yr = 2 × 2.5 mg	2–3 × 2.5 mg
Ipratropium	TOP	UK[a]	UK[a]

Administration: OR, oral; TOP, topical (intranasal); X, not used; UK, unknown; NE, the dose has not yet been clinically established.

[a]Not yet commercially available.

Table 22
Daily Doses of Some Antiallergic and Supplementary Drugs Recommended for Children

Drug		<12 yr	12–16 yr
Disodium cromoglycate			
Nasal drops 2% (20 mg/mL)	TOP	2 Drops—each nostril 4× daily	2 Drops—each nostril 4–6× daily
Nasal spray 2% (20 mg/mL)	TOP	2 Sprays—each nostril 4× daily	2 Sprays—each nostril 6× daily
Nasal spray 4% (40 mg/mL)	TOP	1 Spray—each nostril 4× daily	1–2 Sprays—each nostril 4× daily
Powder (1 cap = 10 mg)	TOP	>3 yr = 1 capsule divided between both nostrils— 4× daily	1 Capsule—divided between both nostrils—4× daily
Oral formulation	OR	4 × 50–100 mg	4 × 100–200 mg
Nedocromil sodium	TOP	NE[a]	NE[a]
Glucocorticosteroids			
Systemic			
Prednisone	OR	0.1–0.2 mg/kg/24 h	0.5 mg/kg/24 h divided into 2 doses
Prednisolone	OR	0.1–0.2 mg/kg/24 h divided in 2 doses	0.5 mg/kg/24 h divided into 2 doses
Dexamethasone	OR	2–4 yr = 4 × 1 mg; 5–7 yr = 4 × 1.6 mg; 8–11 yr = 4 × 2.5 mg daily divided into 2 doses	4 × 3 mg daily divided into 2 doses
Topical			
Beclomethasone dipr	TOP	2 × 50 mcg—each nostril 2× daily	2 × 50 mcg—each nostril 2× daily
Budesonide	TOP	2 × 50 mcg—each nostril 2× daily	2 × 50 mcg—each nostril 2× daily
Flunisolide	TOP	6–12 yr = 1 × 25 mcg—each nostril 2× daily	2 × 25 mcg—each nostril 2× daily
Fluticasone	TOP	X/NE	1 × 100 mcg—each nostril 1× daily
Triamcinolone	TOP	X/NE	X/NE
Decongestants			
Xylometazoline	TOP	>2 yr 1–2 drops of 0.05%—each nostril 1–3× daily	1–2 Drops of 0.1%—each nostril 2–3× daily
Oxymetazoline	TOP	>2 yr 1 drop of 0.025%—each nostril 2–3× daily	1–3 Drops of 0.05%—each nostril 1–3× daily 1–2 Sprays—each nostril 1–3× daily
Naphazoline	TOP	X/NE	1–2 Sprays—each nostril 1–3× daily
Tetrahydrozoline	TOP	UK/X/NE	X/NE
Phenylephrine	TOP	UK/X/NE	X/NE
Varia			
Acetylsalicyl acid	OR	>3 yr 1–3 × 50 mg daily	1–3 × 200 mg daily
Indomethacine	OR	>3 yr 1 mg/kg/24 h divided into 2 doses	1 mg/kg/24 h divided into 2 doses
Ibuprofen	OR	X/NE	1–3 × 200 mg

Administration: OR, oral; TOP, topical (intranasal); X, not used; UK, unknown; NE, the dose has not yet been clinically established.

[a]Not yet commercially available.

155

topical decongestants, oral antihistamines, and, in the extreme situation or acute exacerbation, a short-term treatment with oral corticosteroids (for 6–10 d) *(45,46,55,219,224,238)*.

However, even in the case in which the sinus response is not preceded or accompanied by a nasal response, but some indicators for the activation of the nasal mucosa, such as an aspect of the nasal mucosa, disturbed sinus drainage, and/or edematic ostia, are observed, the nasal mucosa might be taken into therapeutic account. In such a condition, it is imaginable that the initial antigen–antibody interaction takes place in the nasal mucosa or simultaneously in the nasal and sinus mucosal membrane, and is followed by sequential steps of the hypersensitivity mechanisms occurring already exclusively in the sinus mucosa, where they result in the sinus response, without any clinical nasal manifestation or a nasal response. In such, fortunately sporadical, cases of the nonassociated sinus response, a therapeutic attempt should be made to treat, at least experimentally, the nasal mucosa, for example, with a combination of topical cromolyn and topical GCS in the form of nasal sprays, in addition to the already earlier-mentioned measures *(55,224)*. According to our practical experience, this drug combination has been found to be very effective in this form of sinus response *(224)*.

The therapeutic possibilities for controlling adverse reactions to foods are somewhat more favorable than in the case of inhalant allergens, and they may include, in addition to the avoidance of the suspected food(s), irrigation of the nose with the saline and oral antihistamines, the administration of oral DSCG (Nalcrom) in a daily dose of 4 × 200 mg, either 4 × 2 capsules containing 100 mg DSCG powder, or 4 × 1 ampules containing 200 mg dissolved DSCG, or 4 × 2 ampules containing 100 mg dissolved DSCG *(66,100,206,224)*.*

The secondary or "associated" form of the sinus response induced by the primary response in the nasal mucosa has a different background than the previous forms and can also be divided into the responses caused by the inhalant allergens and those owing to the adverse reactions to foods. In this form, the therapeutic regimen is focused pre-

dominantly on the nasal mucosa and the hypersensitivity reactions occurring there *(224)*.

In the case of the inhalant allergens, the important criterion determining the choice of the basic antiallergic and anti-inflammatory drugs is the type of the primary nasal and the induced sinus mucosa response to allergen challenge in the individual patient, meaning INR, LNR, or DYNR. (1) The general therapeutic measures common for patients demonstrating these forms of sinus response may consist of: the avoidance of the suspected allergen(s) *(45,46,66,219)*, irrigation of the nasal cavities with the saline (2–3× daily) *(45,46,219)*, oral antihistamines, or, in some cases in which the oral antihistamines produce some of the side effects or are not well tolerated, the topical antihistamines, and sporadically also decongestants *(45,46,63,126, 157,158,219,224,235)*. (2) The specific antiallergic treatment depends on the type of the primary nasal mucosa and the induced sinus mucosa response: INR and ISR responses may excellently be controlled by the intranasal DSCG (Lomusol, Nasalcrom), either in the powder form stored in capsules (1 capsule = 10 mg DSCG) and delivered into the nose by means of special insufflator (in a daily dose of 4 × 1 capsule divided between both the nasal cavities), or in the aerosol form (nasal spray), existing as a 2% (Lomusol) or 4% (Lomusol forte®, Nasalcrom) formulation. The 2% cromolyn should be administered in a daily dose of 6 × 2 nasal sprays in each of the nasal cavities, whereas the 4% cromolyn should be administered in a daily dose of 4 × 2 nasal sprays *(63,66,105,109,113,153,224,242)*.

LNR and LSR responses can be effectively controlled both by the intranasal DSCG (Lomusol, Nasalcrom) in the above recommended daily doses, and by the intranasal topical corticosteroids, such as Beclomethasone dipropionate (BDA) (Beconase, Viarin, Aldecin, Vancenase) in a daily dose of 2–3 × 2 nasal sprays in each of the nasal cavities (1 spray = 42 or 50 mcg), Budesonide (Rhinocort) aerosol or vapor in a daily dose of 2–3 × 2 nasal sprays (1 spray = 50 mcg) in each of the nostrils, Triamcinolone acetamide (Nasacort®) in a daily dose of 4 × 1 nasal sprays (1 spray = 55 mcg), or Fluticasone propionate (Flunase®, Flixonase®) in a daily dose of 2 × 2 nasal sprays (1 spray = 50 mcg) *(45,63,66,91,104,108, 114,153,165,219,224,238,239)*.

DYNR and DYSR can only be controlled by the intranasal topical GCS in the earlier-recommended daily doses, which could, if necessary, be increased

*The oral cromolyn formulation is not yet available in the US, whereas it is available in almost all European countries as well as former members of the British Commonwealth.

by one supplementary dose daily. In some highly resistant cases of the DYNR and DYSR, a short-time treatment with oral corticosteroids is, however, inevitable to support and accelerate the effects of the topical GCS. The intranasal cromolyn usually does not have sufficient protective or therapeutic effects on this type of nasal and/or sinus response (66,92,116,153,224).

According to our practical experience, the therapeutic approach in the patients demonstrating this form of nasal and sinus response can be summarized as follows:

1. In patients demonstrating only the immediate or immediate and late responses, cromolyn is used as the first-choice drug and topical corticosteroids are usually added only temporarily during some special periods, such as exposure to a high concentration of the allergen(s), acute exacerbation of the disease, appearance of other related allergic disorder, such as secretory otitis media or allergic conjunctivitis, or increase in the edema of the nasal and/or sinus mucosa despite cromolyn administration (224);
2. The patients demonstrating the late responses only are initially treated with a combination of cromolyn and topical GCS, for at least 3–4 mo, then GCS are gradually reduced until withdrawal, and cromolyn administration only is continued. Also in these patients, the GCS are temporarily added for some weeks during some special periods, as listed above (224); and
3. In patients showing only the delayed type of responses, the topical corticosteroids are administered permanently. The patients demonstrating the immediate and delayed responses are usually treated with a permanent combination of topical GCS and cromolyn (63,66,153,224).

In the case of the food allergens, the foods, their parts, or their ingredients may cause the primary nasal response, which then induces the secondary sinus and/or sinus mucosa response. In these patients, in addition to the general measures described, the oral DSCG (Cromolyn, Nalcrom), either in capsules or in solution, has been shown to be very effective in the primary nasal and the secondary induced sinus response, especially those of the immediate and the late type (66,100, 125,206,224).

Recently, a new compound, NDS (disodium salt of a novel pyranoquinoline dicarboxylic acid), has been found by some investigators and also by the author's group to be a very promising drug in the treatment of the nasal allergy (151,152), especially that being represented by the LNR (127). This drug has demonstrated a number of unique pharmacologic properties, including a variety of the anti-allergic and anti-inflammatory effects. In two preliminary studies, the data of which have not yet been finally published, we have investigated the possible protective effects of NDS in the nasal spray on the LNR ($n = 14$) and the INR ($n = 18$), as well as on the cellular changes in the NS accompanying both nasal response types, after a 2-wk pretreatment in a daily dose of 16 mg, divided equally between both the nasal cavities (4×1 puff containing 2 mg of NDS in each nostril daily = 4×2 mg $\times$ 2 = 16 mg). The NDS has prevented significantly the INR ($p < 0.05$) and highly significantly the LNR ($p < 0.001$) (127,224). Moreover, NDS has significantly reduced the influx of eosinophils, neutrophils, mast cells, and basophils into the NS during the INR, whereas it has almost completely prevented the influx of neutrophils, eosinophils, and basophils, and decreased significantly the count of epithelial and goblet cells in NS, during the LNR (127,224,235).

Immunotherapy

This one of the oldest antiallergic treatment remains, however, still a controversial issue. Moreover, the exact mechanism through which the immunotherapy should affect the immunologic system is not yet fully clarified, and views on this matter vary greatly (239).

In the literature, there is a dearth of data concerning the possible effects of immunotherapy on the sinus disease owing to the allergy mechanisms.

Finally, the so-called oral immunotherapy, a technique by means of which allergenic extracts are administered orally, or the sublingual immunotherapy, should be considered the nonestablished and nonproven method, which includes some uncontrolled risks for the patient, and should therefore be rejected (224,243).

Nonspecific Hyperreactivity

This mechanism plays a causal role in sinus disease very rarely. In some sporadic cases, in which this mechanism participates in the pathophysiologic processes underlying the sinus mucosa response, this participation is not of a direct character, but is almost exclusively through the nasal mucosa. The treatment of such cases may include the irrigation of the nasal cavities with saline (2–3 times daily) *(46,47,219)*, decongestants, such as xylomethazoline hydrochloride in 0.1% dilution for adults or 0.05% for children (2–3 × 1 nasal spray or drop daily) *(46,47,127,219,224)*, or anticholinergic drugs administered either orally, such as thiazinamium hydrochloride (2–3 × 100 mg) or oxyphenonium bromide (2–3 × 5 mg), or topically, such as ipratropium bromide (2–4 × 80 mcg daily, divided between both the nasal cavities) *(46,47, 127,159,219,224,241)*. Sometimes, antihistamines (H_1-receptor antagonists) administered either orally or topically, such as levocabastine hydrochloride (2 × 2 nasal sprays daily), may also be effective in controlling this condition *(83,127,153,219,224)*.

REFERENCES

1. Slavin RG. Sinusitis in adults. J Allergy Clin Immunol 1988;81:1028–1032.
2. English GM. Nasal polyps and sinusitis. In: Middleton E Jr, Reed CE, Ellis EF, eds., Allergy, Principles and Practice, 2nd ed. St. Louis, MO: CV Mosby, 1983; pp. 1215–1248.
3. Wald ER. Microbiology of acute and chronic sinusitis. Immunol Allergy Clin N Am 1994;14(No 1):31–45.
4. Ballenger JJ, Harding HB. Paranasal sinus infection. In: Ballenger JJ, ed., Diseases of the Nose, Throat and Ear, 12th ed. Philadelphia: Lea & Febiger, 1977; pp. 155–167.
5. White JA. Paranasal sinus infections. In: Ballenger JJ, ed. Diseases of the Nose, Throat, Ear, Head and Neck, 14th ed. Philadelphia: Lea & Febiger, 1991; pp. 184–202.
6. Slavin RG. Nasal polyps and sinusitis. In: Middleton E, Reed ChE, Ellis EF, Adkinson EF, Yunginger JW, Busse WW, eds., Allergy, Principles and Practice, 4th ed. St. Louis, MO: Mosby-Year Book, 1993; pp. 1455–1470.
7. Fireman P. Diagnosis of sinusitis in children: emphasis on the history and physical examination. J Allergy Clin Immunol 1992;90(No 3, Part 2):433–436.
8. Shapiro GG. Sinusitis in children. J Allergy Clin Immunol 1988;81:1025–1027.
9. Rachelefsky GS, Siegel SC, Katz RM, Spector MD, Rohr AS. Chronic sinusitis in children (abstract). J Allergy Clin Immunol 1991;87:219.
10. Middleton E Jr. Chronic rhinitis in adults. J Allergy Clin Immunol 1988;81:971–975.
11. Rachelefsky GS, Katz RM, Siegel SC. Chronic sinusitis in children with respiratory allergy: the role of antimicrobials. J Allergy Clin Immunol 1982;69:382–387.
12. Pearlman DS. Chronic rhinitis in children. J Allergy Clin Immunol 1988;81:962–966.
13. Harlin SL, Ansel DG, Lane SR, Myers J, Kephart GM, Gleich GJ. A clinical and pathologic study of chronic sinusitis: the role of the eosinophil. J Allergy Clin Immunol 1988;81:867–875.
14. Kuhn JP. Imaging of the paranasal sinuses: current status. J Allergy Clin Immunol 1986;77:6–8.
15. Lober P. Histology and pathology of the nose and sinuses. In: Paparella MM, Shumrick DA, eds. Otolaryngology, vol 1. Philadelphia: WB Saunders 1973;551–562.
16. Aust R. Oxygen exchange through the maxillary ostium in man. Rhinology 1974;12:25–37.
17. Aust R. Measurements of the ostial size and O_2 tension in the maxillary sinuses. Rhinology 1976;14:43,44.
18. Rohr AS, Spector SL. Paranasal sinus anatomy and pathophysiology. Clin Rev Allergy 1984;2:387–395.
19. Graney DO. Anatomy of the paranasal sinuses. Immunol Allergy Clin N Am 1994;14(No 1):1–15.
20. Mann W, Beck C, Apostolidis T. Liability of ultrasound in maxillary sinus disease. Arch Otorhinolaryngol 1972;215:67–74.
21. Revonta M. Ultrasound in the diagnosis of maxillary and frontal sinusitis. Acta Otolaryngol 1980;370 (suppl):1–54.
22. Jannert M, Andreasson L, Holmer N-G. Ultrasonic examination of the paranasal sinuses. Acta Otolaryngol 1982;389(suppl):1–51.
23. Kennedy DW, Zinreich SJ, Rosenbaum AE, Johns ME. Functional endoscopic sinus surgery. Arch Otolaryngol 1985;111:576–582.
24. Stammberger H. Endoscopic endonasal surgery—concepts in treatment of recurring rhinosinusitis. Part 1. Anatomic and pathophysiologic considerations. Otolaryngol Head Neck Surg 1986;94:143–147.
25. Bolger WE, Butzin CA, Parsons DS. Paranasal sinus bony anatomic variations and mucosal abnormalities: CT analysis for endoscopic sinus surgery. Laryngoscope 1991;101:56–64.
26. Laszlo I. Radiology of the paranasal sinuses. In: Ballenger JJ, ed. Diseases of the Nose, Throat and Ear, 12th ed. Philadelphia: Lea & Febiger 1977; pp. 155–167.
27. Zizmor J, Noyek AM. Radiology of the nose and paranasal sinuses. In: Paparella MM, Shumrick DA, eds. Otolaryngology, vol 1. Philadelphia: WB Saunders, 1983; pp. 1043–1095.
28. Shapiro GG, Furukawa CT, Pierson WE, Gilbertson E, Bierman CW. Blinded comparison of maxillary sinus radiography and ultrasound for diagnosis of sinusitis. J Allergy Clin Immunol 1986;77:59–64.
29. Landman MD. Ultrasound screening for sinus diseases. Otolaryngol Head Neck Surg 1986;94:157–164.
30. Druce HM. Diagnosis of sinusitis in adults: History, physical examination, nasal cytology, echo, and rhinoscope. J Allergy Clin Immunol 1992;90(No 3, Part 2):436–441.
31. Diament MJ. The diagnosis of sinusitis in infants and children: X-ray, computed tomography, and magnetic resonance imaging. J Allergy Clin Immunol 1992;90 (No 3, Part 2):442–444.
32. Lusk RP. Endoscopic approach to sinus disease. J Allergy Clin Immunol 1992;90(No 3, Part 2):496–505.
33. Zinreich J. Imaging of inflammatory sinus disease. Immunol Allergy Clin N Am 1994;14(No 1):17–29.
34. Friedman WH, Slavin RG. Diagnosis and medical and surgical treatment of sinusitis in adults. Clin Rev Allergy 1984;2:409–428.

35. Williams HL. Infections and granulomas of the nasal airways and paranasal sinuses. In: Paparella MM, Shumrick DA, eds. Otolaryngology, vol 3, Philadelphia: WB Saunders, 1973; pp. 27–38.

36. Steiner D, Feehs K, Georgitis JW. Immunodeficiency in children with recurrent sinusitis and otitis (abstract). J Allergy Clin Immunol 1989;83:276.

37. Goodman GM, Slavin RG. Medical management in adults. Immunol Allergy Clin N Am 1994;14(No 1):69–87.

38. Williams HL. Nasal physiology. In: Paparella MM, Shumrick DA, eds. Otolaryngology, vol 1. Philadelphia: WB Saunders, 1973; pp. 329–346.

39. Slavin RG. Clinical disorders of the nose and their relationship to allergy. Ann Allergy 1982;49:123–126.

40. Slavin RG, Zilliox AP, Samuels LD. Allergic sinusitis: does it exist? (abstract) N Engl Reg Allergy Proc 1988;9:253.

41. Slavin RG, Zilliox AP, Samuels LD. Is there such an entity as allergic sinusitis? J Allergy Clin Immunol 1988;81:284(abstract No 466).

42. Furukawa CT. The role of allergy in sinus in children. J Allergy Clin Immunol 1992;90(No 3, Part 2):515–517.

43. Spector SL. The role of allergy in sinus in adults. J Allergy Clin Immunol 1992;90(No 3, Part 2):518–520.

44. Holmström M, Lund VJ, Scadding G. Nasal ciliary beat frequency after nasal allergen challenge. Am J Rhinol 1992;6:101–105.

45. Schapiro GG, Virant FS. Medical management in children. Immunol Allergy Clin N Am 1994;14(No 1):47–68.

46. Minotti DA. Allergic rhinitis and sinusitis. Immunol Allergy Clin N Am 1994;14(No 1):113–127.

47. Pinczower EF, Weymuller EA. Nasal obstruction. Immunol Allergy Clin N Am 1994;14(No 1):129–142.

48. Shapiro GG. Role of allergy in sinusitis. Pediatr Infect Dis 1985;4:55–58.

49. Fusijawa T, Kephart GM, Gray BH, Gleich GJ. The neutrophil and chronic allergic inflammation. Immunochemical localization of neutrophil elastase. Am Rev Respir Dis 1990;141:689–697.

50. Savolainen S. Allergy in patients with acute maxillary sinusitis. Allergy 1989;44:116–122.

51. Jeney GR, Meredith S, Baraniuk J, Kaliner M. Nasal secretions in recurrent sinusitis (abstract). J Allergy Clin Immunol 1989;83:214.

52. Sacha RF, Trembray NF, Jacobs RL. Chronic cough, sinusitis, and hyperreactive airways in children: an overlooked association. Ann Allergy 1985;54:195–198.

53. Pelikan Z. Nasal challenge with allergen (NPT) in patients with chronic sinusitis maxillaris (abstract 018). N Engl Reg Allergy Proc 1988;9:253.

54. Pelikan Z. Role of nasal allergy in chronic sinusitis maxillaris (CSM)—diagnostic value of nasal challenge with allergen (NPT). J Allergy Clin Immunol 1989;83 (No 1):214(abstract 171).

55. Pelikan Z. Chronic sinusitis maxillaris (CSM) and nasal allergy—comparison of the echography and radiographs during the nasal challenge with allergen (NPT). Proceedings of the 13th Congress of European Rhinologic Society, incl. the IXth ISIAN & combined with BSACI & EAFS, London, June 24–29, 1990;225.

56. Pelikan Z, Pelikan-Filipek M. Role of nasal allergy in chronic maxillary sinusitis—diagnostic value of nasal challenge with allergen. J Allergy Clin Immunol 1990;86:484–991.

57. Pelikan Z, Pelikan-Filipek M. The role of nasal allergy in chronic sinusitis maxillaris (CSM)—X-ray and echography during the nasal response to allergen challenge. Allergy Clin Immunol News 1991(suppl 1); 334(abstract 933).

58. Pelikan Z, Pelikan-Filipek M, Ossekoppele R. Chronic sinusitis maxillaris (CSM)—the role of nasal allergy and the diagnostic value of echography and radiographs. Allergy Clin Immunol News 1994(suppl 2);415(abstract 1500).

59. Pelikan Z, Pelikan-Filipek M, van Stigt HJ. The maxillary sinus (MS) response due to the food allergy. J Allergy Clin Immunol 1995;95(No 1, Part 2):328 (abstract 750).

60. Wagenmann M, Naclerio RM. Anatomic and physiologic considerations in sinusitis. J Allergy Clin Immunol 1992;90(No 3, Part 2):419–423.

61. Rachelefsky GS, Golbert M, Katz RM, Boris G, Gyepes MT, Shapiro MJ, Mickey MR, Finegold SM, Siegel SC. Sinus disease in children with respiratory allergy. J Allergy Clin Immunol 1978;61:310–314.

62. Melen I, Ivarsson A, Schrewelins C. Ostial function in allergic rhinitis. Acta Otolaryngol (Stockh) 1992;492 (suppl):82–85.

63. Pelikan Z. Late nasal response to allergen challenge (LNR)—clinical features and pharmacologic modulation. Proceedings of the 13th Congress of European Rhinologic Society, incl. the IXth ISIAN & combined with BSACI & EAFS, London, June 24–29, 1990;226.

64. Pelikan Z. Late and delayed responses of the nasal mucosa to allergen challenge. Ann Allergy 1978;41:37–47.

65. Pelikan Z. The role of immediate, late and delayed reactions in allergic nasal diseases. In: Pepys J, Edwards AM, eds. The Mast Cell, Its Role in Health and Disease. Tunbridge Wells: Pitman Medical Publ, 1979; pp. 772–777.

66. Pelikan Z. Late nasal response—its clinical characteristics, features, and possible mechanisms. In: Dorsch W, ed. Late Phase Allergic Reactions. Boca Raton, FL; CRC, 1990; pp. 111–155.

67. Pelikan Z, Pelikan-Filipek M. Late nasal response to allergen challenge (LNR)—cytologic changes in the nasal secretions (NS) and histologic changes in the nasal mucosa. Proceedings of the 7th International Congress of mucosal Immunology, Prague, Czechoslovakia, August 16–20, 1992;185.

68. Pelikan Z. Feenstra L, Barree GOF. Response of the nasal mucosa to allergen challenge measured by two different methods of rhinomanometry. Ann Allergy 1977;38:263–267.

69. Pelikan Z, Pelikan-Filipek M. The diagnostic approach to the immediate hypersensitivity in patients with allergic rhinitis: a comparison of nasal challenges and serum RAST. Ann Allergy 1983;50:395–400.

70. Davies J. Embryology and anatomy of the face, palate, nose and paranasal sinuses. In: Paparella MM, Shumrick DA, eds. Otolaryngology, vol 1, Philadelphia: WB Saunders 1973; pp. 150–178.

71. Kaliner MA. Human nasal host defence and sinusitis. J Allergy Clin Immunol 1992;90(No 3, Part 2):424–430.

72. Despot JE, Lemanske RF. Inflammatory mediators in allergic rhinitis. Immunol Allergy Clin N Am 1987; 7:37–55.

73. Shearer WT, Huston DP. The immune system. In: Middleton E, Reed ChE, Ellis EF, Adkinson NF, Yunginger JW, Busse WW, eds. Allergy, Principles and Practice, 4th ed. St Louis, MO: Mosby-Year Book, 1993; pp. 3–21.

74. Siraganian RP. Mechanism of IgE-mediated hypersensitivity. In: Middleton E, Reed ChE, Ellis EF, Adkinson NF, Yunginger JW, Busse WW, eds. Allergy, Principles and Practice, 4th ed. St. Louis, MO: Mosby-Year Book, 1993; pp. 105–134.

75. Lemanske RF, Kaliner MA. Late phase allergic reactions. In: Middleton E, Reed ChE, Ellis EF, Adkinson NF, Yunginger JW, Busse WW, eds. Allergy, Principles and Practice, 4th ed. St. Louis, MO: Mosby-Year Book 1993; pp. 320–361.

76. Askenase PW. Effector and regulatory mechanisms in delayed type hypersensitivity. In: Middleton E, Reed ChE, Ellis EF, Adkinson NF, Yunginger JW, Busse WW, eds. Allergy, Principles and Practice, 4th ed. St. Louis, MO: Mosby-Year Book 1993; pp. 362–389.

77. Zweiman B, Levinson AI. Cell-mediated immunity in health and disease. In: Middleton E, Reed ChE, Ellis EF, Adkinson NF, Yunginger JW, Busse WW, eds. Allergy, Principles and Practice, 4th ed. St Louis, MO: Mosby-Year Book, 1993; pp. 963–989.

78. Lawley TJ, Frank MM. Immune complexes and allergic disease. In: Middleton E, Reed ChE, Ellis EF, Adkinson NF, Yunginger JW, Busse WW, eds. Allergy, Principles and Practice, 4th ed. St Louis, MO: Mosby-Year Book, 1993; pp. 990–1006.

79. Goodman JW. The immune response. In: Stites DP, Terr AI, eds. Basic and Clinical Immunology, 7th ed. Norwalk, CT: Appleton & Lange, 1991; pp. 34–44.

80. Oppenheim JJ, Ruscetti FW, Faltynek C. Cytokines. In: Stites DP, Terr AI, eds. Basic and Clinical Immunology, 7th ed. Norwalk, CT: Appleton & Lange, 1991; pp. 78–100.

81. Terr AI. Mechanisms of inflammation. In: Stites DP, Terr AI, eds. Basic and Clinical Immunology, 7th ed. Norwalk, CT: Appleton & Lange, 1991; pp. 131–140.

82. Coombs RRA, Gell PGH. Classification of allergic reactions responsible for clinical hypersensitivity and disease. In: Gell PGH, Coombs RRA, Lachmann PJ, eds. Clinical Aspects of Immunology, 3rd ed. Oxford: Blackwell Scientific Publications, 1975; pp. 761–781.

83. Pelikan Z. Differential diagnosis of nasal hyperreactivity and allergy, in allergic rhinitis. Proceedings of the Symposium "Facts about the nose," Brugge, Nov 18, 1989, Huizing EH, ed. Astra, The Netherlands, 1991;45–53.

84. Pelikan Z. Non-specific hyperreactivity of the nasal mucosa (N-SH)-comparison of histamine and metacholine challenges in rhinitis patients. Allergy Clin Immunol News 1991;(suppl 1):335(abstract 934).

85. Pelikan Z. Allergic and non-specific hyperreactivity (N-SH) component in patients with chronic rhinitis. Allergy Clin Immunol News 1991;(suppl 1):335 (abstract 935).

86. Pelikan Z, Pelikan-Filipek M. Non-specific hyperreactivity (N-SH) and basic types of nasal response to allergen challenge in rhinitis patients. J Allergy Clin Immunol 1992;89(No 1, Part 2):179(abstract 140).

87. Pelikan Z. Provocation tests—a definitive confirmation of the role and involvement of a certain allergen or a non-specific hyperreactivity agent in the complaints of patients with an allergy disorder. Abstracts of the International Seminar on the Immunological System as a Target for Toxic Damage. (An International Seminar organized by the Commission of the European Communities, WHO and the United States Environmental Protection Agency), Luxembourg, November 6–9, 1984;122–126.

88. Pelikan Z. Immediate hypersensitivity and non-specific hyperreactivity in the nose and bronchial tree,—a possible double role of the mast cells and basophils,—the place and role of the chemicals. Abstracts of the International Seminar on the Immunological System as a Target for Toxic Damage. (An International Seminar organized by the Commission of the European Communities, WHO and the United States Environmental Protection Agency), Luxembourg, November 6–9, 1984;127–130.

89. Pelikan Z. Participation of allergy (ALL) and non specific hyperreactivity [N-SH] components in rhinitis. Allergy Clin Immunol News 1994;(suppl 2):415 (abstract 1499).

90. Pelikan Z, Pelikan-Filipek M. The effects of disodium cromoglycate and beclomethasone dipropionate on the immediate response of the nasal mucosa to allergen challenge. Ann Allergy 1982;49:283–292.

91. Pelikan Z, Pelikan-Filipek M. The effects of disodium cromoglycate and beclomethasone dipropionate on the late response of the nasal mucosa to allergen challenge. Ann Allergy 1982;49:200–212.

92. Pelikan Z. The effects of disodium cromoglycate (DSCG) and beclomethasone dipropionate (BDA) on the delayed nasal mucosa response to allergen challenge. Ann Allergy 1984;52:111–124.

93. Solomon W, McLean JA. Nasal provocative testing. In: Spector SL, ed. Provocative Challenge Procedures: Background and Methodology. Mount Kisco, NY: Futura Publ, 1989; pp. 569–625.

94. Pelikan Z, Bruijnzeel PLB, Verhagen J. Leukotrienes (LTC_4/LTD_4, LTB_4) in the nasal secretions. Ann Allergy 1985;55:336(abstract 443).

95. Pelikan Z, Pelikan-Filipek M. A new disease—a nasal form of pigeon breeder's disease. Allergy 1983;38: 309–318.

96. Pelikan Z. The changes in the nasal secretions' eosinophils during the immediate nasal response to allergen challenge. J Allergy Clin Immunol 1983;72:657–662.

97. Pelikan Z, Pelikan-Filipek M. Cytologic changes in the nasal secretions (NS) during the immediate (INR) and the late nasal response (LNR) to allergen challenge. In: Nijkamp FP, Engels F, Hendrickx PAV, Oosterhout AJM, eds. Mediators in Airway Hyperreactivity. Basel, Switzerland: Birkhäuser Verlag 1990; pp. 55–62.

98. Pelikan Z, Pelikan-Filipek M. Cytologic changes in the nasal secretions during the late nasal response. J Allergy Clin Immunol 1989;83:1068–1079.

99. Pelikan Z, Pelikan-Filipek M. Cytological changes in the nasal secretions during the immediate nasal response. J Allergy Clin Immunol 1988;82:1103–1112.

100. Pelikan Z. Rhinitis and secretory otitis media: a possible role of food allergy. In: Brostoff J, Challacombe SJ, eds. Food Allergy and Intolerance. London: Baillière Tindall, Sanders, 1987; pp. 467–485.

101. Pelikan Z, Pelikan-Filipek M. Nasal secretions (NS) cytology during the delayed nasal response to allergen challenge (DNR). Allergy Clin Immunol News 1991; (suppl 1):334(abstract 930).

102. Pelikan Z, Pelikan-Filipek M. Intracellular changes in some cell types in nasal secretions (NS) during the immediate (INR) and late (LNR) nasal response to allergen challenge. Allergy Clin Immunol News 1991;(suppl 1):273(abstract 689).

103. Pelikan-Filipek M, Pelikan Z. Histamine in nasal secretions (NS) during the immediate nasal response to allergen challenge (INR). J Allergy Clin Immunol 1992; 89(No 1, Part 2):333(abstract 754).

104. Pelikan Z, Johansson S-A. Effects of Disodium cromoglycate (DSCG) and Budesonide (BSA) on the late nasal response (LNR) and nasal secretions cytology (NS). Allergy 1992;47(No 12, suppl):3(abstract).

105. Pelikan Z, Pelikan-Filipek M. The effects of disodium cromoglycate (DSCG) and Budesonide (BSA) on the immediate nasal response (INR) and nasal secretions cytology (NS). Allergy 1992;47(No 12, suppl):284 (abstract).

106. Pelikan Z. Histamine (NS) in nasal secretions (NS) and its changes during the basis types of nasal response (NR) to allergen challenge. Allergy 1992;47(No 12, suppl):304(abstract).

107. Pelikan Z, Pelikan-Filipek M. Immediate nasal response to allergen challenge (INR)—cytologic changes in the nasal secretions (NS) and histologic changes in the nasal mucosa. Proceedings of the 17th International Congress of Mucosal Immunology, Prague, Czechoslovakia, August 16–20, 1992;184.

108. Johansson SA, Pelikan Z. The effects of Cromolyn (DSCG) and Budesonide (BSA) on the late nasal response (LNR), changes in the cell count in the late nasal response (LNR), changes in the cell count in the nasal secretions (NS) and their intracellular changes. J Allergy Clin Immunol 1993;91(No 1, Part 2):259 (abstract 475).

109. Pelikan-Filipek M, Pelikan Z. The effects of Cromolyn (DSCG) and Budesonide (BSA) on the immediate nasal response (INR), the appearance of cell-types in nasal secretions (NS) and their intracellular changes. J Allergy Clin Immunol 1993;91(No 1, Part 2):300 (abstract 636).

110. Pelikan Z, Pelikan-Filipek M. Intracellular changes of eosinophils (EO), neutrophils (NE) and basophils (BS) in nasal secretions (NS) during the early (ENR) and late (LNR) nasal response. Allergy Clin Immunol News 1994;(suppl 2);336(abstract 1205).

111. Pelikan-Filipek M, Pelikan Z. Intracellular changes in some cell types in nasal secretions (NS) accompanying the immediate nasal response (INR). J Allergy Clin Immunol 1990;85(No 1, Part 2):300(abstract 626).

112. Pelikan Z. Intracellular changes of eosinophils, neutrophils and basophils in nasal secretions during the immediate nasal response to allergen challenge. N Engl Reg Allergy Proc 1988;9(No 4):442.

113. Pelikan-Filipek M, Pelikan Z. Nasal secretions cytology (NS) during the immediate nasal response (INR), pretreated with Disodium cromoglycate (DSCG) and Budesonide (BSA). J Allergy Clin Immunol 1991;87 (No 1, Part 2):144(abstract 24).

114. Pelikan Z, Pelikan-Filipek M. Cytologic changes in nasal secretions (NS) during the late nasal response (LNR) pretreated with disodium cromoglycate (DSCG) and beclomethasone dipropionate (BDA) or budesonide (BSA). J Allergy Clin Immunol 1991;87(No 1, Part 2):281(abstract 566).

115. Pelikan Z. Histologic changes in the nasal mucosa during the immediate (INR), late (LAR) and delayed (DNR) nasal response to allergen challenge. Allergy Clin Immunol News 1991;(suppl 1);132(abstract 158).

116. Pelikan Z, Pelikan-Filipek M. Cytologic changes in nasal secretions (NS) during the delayed nasal response (DNR) pretreated with disodium cromoglycate (DSCG) and beclomethasone dipropionate (BDA) or budesonide (BSA). Allergy Clin Immunol News 1991;(suppl 1): 334(abstract 932).

117. Walden SM, Proud D, Bascom R, Lichtenstein LM, Kagey-Sobotka A, Adkinson NF, Naclerio RM. Experimentally induced nasal allergic responses. J Allergy Clin Immunol 1988;81:940–949.

118. Togias A, Naclerio RM, Proud D, Pipkorn U, Bascom R, Illiopoulos O, Kagey-Sobotka A, Norman PS, Lichtenstein LM. Studies on the allergic and non-allergic nasal inflammation. J Allergy Clin Immunol 1988; 81:782–790.

119. Cole P, Havas T. Nasal resistance to respiratory airflow: a plethysmographic alternative to the face mask. Rhinology 1987;25:159–166.

120. Eccles R. Rhinomanometry and nasal challenge. In: Mackay I, ed. Rhinitis: Mechanisms and Management. London: Royal Society of Medical Services Ltd 1989; pp. 53–67.

121. Schumacher MJ. Advances in tests for evaluation of rhinitis. Immunol Allergy Clinics N Am 1987; 7: 15–35.

122. Olsson P, Bende M, Ohlin P. The laser Doppler flowmeter for measuring microcirculation in human nasal mucosa. Acta Otolaryngol (Stockh) 1985;99:133–139.

123. Hilberg O, Jackson AC, Swift DL, Pederson OF. Acoustic rhinomanometry: evaluation of nasal cavity geometry by acoustic reflexion. J Appl Physiol 1989;66: 295–303.

124. Lenders H, Pirsig W. Diagnostic value of acoustic rhinometry: patients with allergic and vasomotor rhinitis compared with normal controls. Rhinology 1990;28: 5–16.

125. Pelikan Z, Pelikan-Filipek M, Venmans BJW. Nasal response due to the food ingestion challenge and protective effects of oral disodium cromoglycate (DSCG). Ann Allergy 1988;60:149(abstract 25).

126. Pelikan Z. Effects of Cetirizine (CZ) on the immediate (INR) and late nasal response (LNR) and on the eosinophils in the nasal secretions (NS). J Allergy Clin Immunol 1993;91(No 1, Part 2):193(abstract 210).

127. Pelikan Z. The immediate/early, late and delayed nasal response to allergen challenge, their occurrence and association with various "in vivo" and "in vitro" diagnostic parameters, other organs' responses, and non-specific hyperreactivity, and pharmacologic control. In preparation as a monograph.

128. Pelikan Z, Johansson S-A. The effects of budesonide (BSA) on the late asthmatic response (LAR), administered before and at various points in time after allergen challenge (abstract). Allergy Clin Immunol News 1991;(suppl 1):180.

129. Pelikan Z, Knottnerus I. Inhibition of the late asthmatic response by nedocromil sodium administered more than two hours after allergen challenge. J Allergy Clin Immunol 1993;92:19–28.

130. Pelikan Z. Allergic conjunctivitis-relationship to allergic rhinitis and the effect of disodium cromoglycate (DSCG). Abstracts of the XIth International Congress of Allergology and Clinical Immunology. London and Basingstoke: The Macmillan Press Ltd, 1982; Abstract 392P.

131. Fireman P. Allergic rhinitis. In: Bluestone CD, Stool SE, eds. Pediatric Otolaryngology, 2nd ed. Philadelphia: WB Saunders, 1990; pp. 793–804.

132. Pelikan M, Pelikan Z. The role of the nasal mucosa in some cases of allergic conjunctivitis and the effects of disodium cromoglycate (DSCG). J Allergy Clin Immunol 1985;75(No 1, Part 2):186(abstract).

133. Pelikan Z. Changes in middle ear pressure (MEP) due to the nasal allergen challenge in patients with secretory otitis media (SOM) and otalgia. J Allergy Clin Immunol 1987;79:258(abstract).

134. Pelikan Z, Pelikan-Filipek M. Middle ear response due to the food ingestion challenge. J Allergy Clin Immunol 1989;83:239(abstract).

135. Bascom R, Wachs M, Naclerio RM, Pipkorn U, Galli SJ, Lichtenstein LM. Basophil influx occurs after nasal antigen challenge. Effects of topical corticosteroid pretreatment. J Allergy Clin Immunol 1988;81:580–589.

136. Iliopoulos O, Proud D, Adkinson NF, Norman PS, Kagey-Sobotka A, Lichtenstein LM, Naclerio RM. Relationship between the early, late and rechallenge reaction to nasal challenge with antigen: observation on the role of inflammatory mediators and cells. J Allergy Clin Immunol 1990;86:851–861.

137. Meltzer EO, Orgel AH, Jalowayski A. Cytology. In: Mygind N, Naclerio RM, eds. Allergic and Non-allergic Rhinitis—Clinical Aspects. Copenhagen: Munksgaard, 1993; pp. 66–81.

138. Mygind N, Weeke B, Ullman S. Quantitative determination of immunoglobulins in nasal secretion. Int Arch Allergy 1975;49:99–107.

139. Mygind N. Nasal Allergy, 2nd ed. Oxford: Blackwell Sci, 1979.

140. Platts-Mills TAE, Mur RK von, Ishizaka K, Norman PS, Lichtenstein LM. IgA and IgG anti-ragweed antibodies in nasal secretions. J Clin Invest 1976;57:1041–1050.

141. Deutschl H, Johansson SGO. Specific IgE antibodies in nasal secretion from patients with allergic rhinitis and with negative or weakly positive RAST in the serum. Clin Allergy 1977;7:195–202.

142. Platts-Mills TAE. Local production of IgG, IgA and IgE antibodies in grasspollen hay fever. J Immunol 1979;122:2218–2225.

143. Houri M, Msyer ALR, Houghton LE, Jacobs D. Correlation of skin, nasal and inhalation tests with IgE in the serum, nasal fluid and sputum. Clin Allergy 1972;2:285–298.

144. Bascom R, Pipkorn U, Proud D, Dunnette S, Gleich GJ, Lichtenstein LM, Naclerio RM. Major basic protein and eosinophil-derived neurotoxin concentrations in nasal-lavage fluid after antigen challenge: effects of systemic corticosteroids and relationship to eosinophil influx. J Allergy Clin Immunol 1989;84:338–346.

145. Freeland HS, Pipkorn U, Schleimer RP, Bascom R, Lichtenstein LM, Naclerio RM, Peters SP. Leukotriene B_4 as a mediator of early and late reactions to antigen in humans: the effect of systemic glucocorticoid treatment in vivo. J Allergy Clin Immunol 1989;83:634–642.

146. Pelikan Z, Pelikan-Filipek M. Histamine in the serum and the changes in its concentration accompanying the basic types of the nasal mucosa response to allergen challenge. Prepared for the presentation.

147. Brofelt S, Mygind N. Viscosity and spinability of nasal secretions induced by different provocation tests. Am Rev Respir Dis 1987;136:353–356.

148. Raphael GD, Igarashi Y, White MV, Kaliner MA. The pathophysiology of rhinitis. V. Source of protein in allergen-induced nasal secretions. J Allergy Clin Immunol 1991;88:33–42.

149. Lozewicz S, Gomez E, Chalstrey S, Gathland D, Davies RJ. Time course of cellular infiltration in the nasal mucosa during the immediate allergic reaction. Int Arch Allergy Appl Immunol 1991;95:273–277.

150. Small P, Barrett D. Effects of high doses of topical steroids on both ragweed and histamine-induced nasal provocation. Ann Allergy 1991;67:520–524.

151. Ruhno J, Denborg J, Dolovich J. Intranasal nedocromil sodium in the treatment of ragweed-allergic rhinitis. J Allergy Clin Immunol 1988;81:570–574.

152. Kaulbach HC, Igarashi Y, Mullol J, White MV, Kaliner MA. Effects of nedocromil sodium on allergen-induced rhinitis in humans. J Allergy Clin Immunol 1992;89:599–610.

153. Pelikan Z, Pelikan-Filipek M. Cytologic changes in the nasal secretions (NS) during the immediate (INR), late (LNR) and delayed nasal response (DYNR) to allergen challenge and their pharmacologic modulation by various drugs. In preparation for publication.

154. Majchel AM, Proud D, Kagey-Sobotka A, Lichtenstein LM, Naclerio RM. Ketotifen reduces sneezing but not histamine release following nasal challenge with antigen. Clin Exp Allergy 1990;20:701–705.

155. Naclerio RM, Proud D, Kagey-Sabotka A, Freidhoff L, Norman PS, Lichtenstein LM. The effect of cetirizine on early allergic response. Laryngoscope 1989;99:956–599.

156. Meltzer EO, Schatz M. Pharmacotherapy of rhinitis—1987 and beyond. Immunol Allergy Clin N Am 1987;7:57–91.

157. Simons FER, Simons KJ. H_1-receptor antagonist treatment of chronic rhinitis. J Allergy Clin Immunol 1988;81:975–980.

158. Simons FER, Simons KJ. Antihistamines. In: Middleton E, Reed ChE, Ellis EF, Adkinson NF, Yunginger JW, Busse WW, eds. Allergy, Principles and Practice, 4th ed. St. Louis, MO: Mosby-Year Book, 1993; pp. 856–892.

159. Borts MR, Druce HM. The use of intranasal anticholinergic agents in the treatment of non-allergic perennial rhinitis. J Allergy Clin Immunol 1992;90:1065–1070.

160. Pelikan Z, Pelikan-Filipek M. Cytologic changes in the nasal secretions (NS) during the immediate (INR) and the late (LNR) nasal response. Proceedings of the 13th Congress of European Rhinologic Society, incl. the IXth ISIAN & combined with BSACI & EAFS, London, June 24–29, 1990;227.

161. Pelikan Z. Nasal secretions cytology during the immediate and late nasal response to allergen challenge. J Allergy Clin Immunol 1989;83(No 1):243(abstract 287).

162. Pelikan Z, Pelikan-Filipek M. Cytological changes in the nasal secretions during the late nasal response. J Allergy Clin Immunol 1986;77(No 1, Part 2):245 (abstract 497).

163. Pelikan Z, Pelikan-Filipek M. Intracellular changes in some cell types in nasal secretions (NS) during the late nasal response (LNR) to allergen challenge (NPT). Clin Exp Allergy 1990;20(suppl 1):60(abstract P 131).

164. Pelikan Z, Pelikan-Filipek M. The antigen-specific IgE antibodies and antibodies of other classes in the nasal secretions (NS) and in the serum, and the changes in their concentrations during the particular types of nasal response (INR, LNR, DYNR) to allergen challenge. In preparation for publication.

165. Pelikan Z, Boorsma M. Effects of intranasal budesonide (BUD) on the early (ENR) and late nasal response (LNR) to challenge (NPT) with bird faeces extracts. J Allergy Clin Immunol 1994;93(No 1, Part 2):165(abstract 14).

166. Bisgaard H, Gronberg H, Mygind N, Dahl R, Lindquist N, Venge P. Allergen-induced increase of eosinophil cationic protein in nasal lavage fluid: effect of the glucocorticoid budesonide. J Allergy Clin Immunol 1990;85:891–895.

167. Bascom R, Pipkorn U, Lichtenstein LM, Naclerio RM. The influx of inflammatory cells into nasal washings during the late response to antigen challenge. Effect of systemic steroid pretreatment. Am Rev Respir Dis 1988;138:406–412.

168. Pelikan Z, Pelikan-Filipek M. The late asthmatic response to allergen challenge—part I. Ann Allergy 1986;56:414–420.

169. Pelikan Z, Pelikan-Filipek M. The late asthmatic response to allergen challenge—part II. Ann Allergy 1986;56:421–435.

170. Pelikan Z, Pelikan M, Kruis M, Berger MPF. The immediate asthmatic response to allergen challenge. Ann Allergy 1986;56:252–260.

171. Pelikan Z, Pelikan-Filipek M. Cytologic changes in the nasal secretions (NS) during the delayed nasal response to allergen challenge (DNR). Clin Exp Allergy 1990; 20(suppl 1):27(abstract P52).

172. Pelikan Z. Delayed asthmatic response and its pharmacologic modulation. J Allergy Clin Immunol 1989;83 (No 1):224(abstract 290).

173. Pelikan Z. Delayed asthmatic response (DAR) and its pharmacologic modulation. In: Nijkamp FP, Engels F, Hendricks PAV, Oosterhout AJM, eds. Mediators in Airway Hyperreactivity (suppl 31 to Agents and Actions). Basel, Switzerland: Birkhäuser Verlag 1990; pp. 49–54.

174. Pelikan Z, Pelikan-Filipek M. A new clinical phenomenon—a delayed type of asthmatic response to allergen challenge (DAR) and its pharmacologic modulation. J Allergy Clin Immunol 1991;87(No 1, Part 2):249(abstract 437).

175. Holt PG, McMenamin C, Schon-Hegrad MA, Strickland D, Nelson D, Wilkes L, Bilyk N, Oliver J, Holt BJ, McMenamin PG. Immunoregulation of asthma: control of T-lymphocyte activation in the respiratory tract. Eur Respir J 1991;4(suppl 13):65–159.

176. Enander I, Nygren H, Ahlstedt S. Immunological suppression of delayed hypersensitivity responses in mouse lungs as reflected by numbers of mononuclear cells, mast cells and mucus-producing cells. Int Arch Allergy Appl Immunol 1988;85:99–103.

177. Enander E, Nefgren A, Nygren H, Larsson P, Holmdahl R, Klareskog L, Ahlstedt S. Regulation by T cells delayed hypersensitivity reaction in mouse lung as reflected by mononuclear cells, mast cells and mucus-producing cells. Int Arch Allergy Appl Immunol 1988;85:374–380.

178. Loveren van H, Garssen J, Nijkamp FP. T-cell-mediated airway hyperreactivity in mice. Eur Respir J 1991;4(suppl 13):169–265.

179. Hutson PA, Church MK, Clay TP, Miller P, Holgate ST. Early and late-phase bronchoconstriction after allergen challenge of non-anaesthetized guinea pigs. I. The association of disordered airway physiology to leukocyte infiltration. Am Rev Respir Dis 1988;137:548–557.

180. Corrigan CJ, Kay AB. T-lymphocyte activation in acute severe asthma is accompanied by elevated serum concentrations of Gamma-interferon and Interleukin-2 receptor. Clin Exptl Allergy 1990;20(suppl 1):117 (abstract S 12/8).

181. Sustiel A, Rocklin RE. T cell responses in allergic rhinitis, asthma and atopic dermatitis. Clin Exp Allergy 1989;19:11–18.

182. Frew AJ, Corrigan CJ, Maestrelli P, Tsai J-J, Kurihara K, O'Hehir RE, Hartnell A, Cromwell O, Kay AB. T-lymphocytes in allergen-induced late-phase reactions and asthma. Int Arch Allergy Appl Immunol 1989; 88:63–67.

183. Holm AF, Fokkens WJ, Rijntjes E, Vrom ThM. Activated T-cells in allergic rhinitis. Abstracts of the 13th Congress European Rhinology Society, including the IXth ISIAN & combined with British Society of Allergology and Clinical Immunology & European Association of Facial Surgery, London, June 24–29, 1990;94.

184. Bentley AM, Cumberworth V, Varney VA, Jacobson MR, Sudderick RM, Kay AB, Durham SR. Studies during the pollen season in understanding allergic rhinitis. In: Gordard Ph, Bousquet J, Michel FB, eds. Advances in Allergology and Clinical Immunology. Carnforth, Lancaster, UK: Parthenon 1992; pp. 457–464.

185. Varney VA, Jacobson MR, Sudderick RM, Robinson DS, Irain AM, Schwartz LB, Mackay IS, Kay AB, Durham SR. Immunohistology of the nasal mucosa following allergen-induced rhinitis. Am Rev Respir Dis 1992;146:170–176.

186. Kapsenberg ML, Jansen HM, Bos JD, Wierenga EA. Role of type 1 and type 2 T-helper cells in allergic diseases. Curr Opinion Immunol 1992;4:788–793.

187. Benner R, Savelkoul HFJ. Regulation of IgE production in mice. Eur Respir J 1991;4(suppl 13):973–1043.

188. Kay AB, Corrigan CJ, Frew AJ. Immunoregulation of asthma: control of T-lymphocyte activation in the respiratory tract. Eur Respir J 1991;4(suppl 13):1053–1123.

189. Corrigan CJ, Kay AB. Lymphocytes. In: Middleton E Jr, Reed ChE, Ellis EF, Adkinson NF, Yunginger JW, Busse WW, eds. Allergy, Principles and Practice, 4th ed. St. Louis, MO: Mosby-Year Book, 1993; pp. 206–211.

190. Hellquist HB, Karlsson MG, Rudblad S, Ekedahl C, Davisson A. Activated T-cells in the nasal mucosa of patients with grass-pollen allergy. A pilot study. Rhinology 1992;30:57–63.

191. Kemeny DM, Diaz-Sanchez D, Holmes BJ. CD8[+] T cells in allergy. Allergy 1992;47:12–21.

192. Crump JW, Pueringer RJ, Hunninghake GW. Broncho-alveolar lavage and lymphocytes in asthma. Eur Respir J 1991;4(suppl 13):39s–46s.

193. Frew AJ, O'Hehir RE. What can we learn from studies of lymphocytes present in allergic-reaction sites? J Allergy Clin Immunol 1992;89:783–788.

194. Gerblich AA, Salik H, Schnyer MR. Dynamic T-cell changes in peripheral blood and bronchoalveolar lavage after antigen bronchoprovocation in asthmatics. Am Rev Respir Dis 1990;141:970–977.

195. Frew AJ, Kay AB. Eosinophils and T-lymphocytes in late-phase allergic reactions. J Allergy Clin Immunol 1990;85:533–539.

196. Brogden RN, Speight TM, Avery GS. Sodium cromoglycate (Cromolyn Sodium): a review of its mode of action, pharmacology, therapeutic efficacy and use. Drugs 1974;7:188–282.

197. Foreman JC, Pearce FL. Cromolyn and Nedocromil. In: Middleton E Jr, Reed ChE, Ellis EF, Adkinson NF, Yunginger JW, Busse WW, eds. Allergy, Principles and Practice, 4th ed. St. Louis, MO: Mosby-Year Book, 1993; pp. 926–940.

198. Auty RM. The clinical development of a new agent for the treatment of airway inflammation, nedocromil sodium (Tilade®). Eur Respir J 1986;69(suppl No 147):120–131.

199. Gross NJ, Boushey HA, Gold WM. Anticholinergic drugs. In: Middleton E Jr, Reed ChE, Ellis EF, Adkinson NF, Yunginger JW, Busse WW, eds. Allergy, Principles and Practice, 4th ed. St Louis, MO: Mosby-Year Book, 1993; pp. 941–962.

200. Schleimer RP, Claman HN, Oronsky A. Anti-inflammatory Steroid Action, Basic and General Aspects. San Diego: Academic, 1989.

201. Goldstein RA, Bowen DL, Fauci AS. Adrenal corticosteroids. In: Gallin JI, Goldstein IM, Snyderman R, eds. Inflammation: Basic Principles and Clinical Correlates, 2nd ed. New York; Raven, 1992; pp. 1061–1081.

202. Schleimer RP. Glucocorticosteroids, their mechanisms of action and use in allergic diseases. In: Middleton E Jr, Reed ChE, Ellis EF, Adkinson NF, Yunginger JW, Busse WW, eds. Allergy, Principles and Practice, 4th ed. St Louis, MO: Mosby-Year Book, 1993; pp. 893–925.

203. Gaga M, Frew AJ, Varney VA, Kay AB. Eosinophil activation and T lymphocyte infiltration in allergen-induced late phase skin reactions and classical delayed-type hypersensitivity. J Immunol 1991;147:816–822.

204. Gonzalez MC, Diaz P, Gallequillos FR, Ancic P, Cromwell O, Kay AB. Allergen-induced recruitment of bronchoalveolor helper (okt 4) and suppressor (okt 8) T-cells in asthma. Am Rev Respir Dis 1987;136:600–604.

205. Pelikan Z. Nasal response to food ingestion challenge. Arch Otolaryngol Head & Neck Surg 1988;114:525–530.

206. Pelikan Z, Pelikan-Filipek M. Effects of oral cromolyn on the nasal response due to foods. Arch Otolaryngol Head & Neck Surg 1989;115:1238–1243.

207. Pelikan Z, Pelikan-Filipek M. Middle ear response due to the food ingestion challenge. J Allergy Clin Immunol 1989;83(No 1):239(abstract 269).

208. Pelikan-Filipek M, Pelikan Z. A comparison of double-blind and open techniques of food ingestion challenge upon recording of objective and subjective parameters. J Allergy Clin Immunol 1994;93(No 1, Part 2):303 (abstract 844).

209. Pelikan Z, Pelikan-Filipek M. Bronchial response to the food ingestion challenge. Ann Allergy 1987;58:164–172.

210. Pelikan Z, Pelikan-Filipek M, Knottnerus I. Asthmatic response to food ingestion challenge (FICH) and protective effects of oral cromolyn. Allergy Clin Immunol News 1991;(suppl 1):108(abstract 71).

211. Pelikan-Filipek M, Pelikan Z. Protective effects of oral cromolyn on the immediate and late asthmatic response due to the food ingestion challenge. Allergy 1993;48:113(abstract 2071).

212. Pelikan Z, Pelikan-Filipek M. The involvement of foods in atopic eczema. N Engl Reg Allergy Proc 1988;9(No 4):327.

213. Pelikan Z, Pelikan-Filipek M. Protective effects of oral disodium cromoglycate (DSCG) in atopic eczema due to food ingested. N Engl Reg Allergy Proc 1988;9(No 4):327.

214. Pelikan Z, Pelikan-Filipek M. Urticaria (NT) due to the food allergy and effects of oral cromolyn (DSCG, Nalcrom®). Allergy 1992;47(No 12, suppl):50.

215. Pelikan Z, Knottnerus I. Protective effects of oral cromolyn (DSCG) on migraine due to the adverse reactions to foods. J Allergy Clin Immunol 1993;91:(No 1, Part 2):150(abstract 38).

216. Wald ER, Guevra N, Byers C. Upper respiratory tract infections in young children: duration of and frequency of complications. Pediatrics 1991;87:129–133.

217. Friday G, Fireman P, Sukanich A, Steinberg M. Sinusitis. In: Naspitz CK, Tinkelman DG, eds. Childhood Rhinitis and Sinusitis. New York: Marcel Dekker, 1990;199–215.

218. Gwaltney JM, Scheld WM, Sande MA, Sydnor A. The microbial etiology and antimicrobial therapy of adults with acute community-acquired sinusitis: A fifteen year experience at the university of Virginia and review of other selected studies. J Allergy Clin Immunol 1992;90:457–462.

219. Zeiger RS. Prospects for ancillary treatment of sinusitis in the 1990s. J Allergy Clin Immunol 1992;90:478–495.

220. Lund VJ. Sinusitis: diagnosis and treatment. In: Mackay I, ed. Rhinitis; Mechanisms and management. London: Royal Society of Medicine Services Ltd. 1989; pp. 153–167.

221. Katz RM, Patnaik M, Siegel S, Rachelefsky G, Corren J, Schanker H, Spector S. The treatment of acute sinusitis in adults. Allergy Clin Immunol News 1994;(suppl No 2):515(abstract 1892).

222. Suonpää J, Suonpää S. The role of nasal allergy in acute frontal sinusitis. N Engl Reg Allergy Proc 1988;9: 253(abstract 17).

223. Goldenhersch MJ, Rachelefsky G, Dudley J, Brill J, Katz R, Rohr A, Spector S, Siegel S, Feingold S. Bacteriology of chronic maxillary sinusitis in children with respiratory allergy. J Allergy Clin Immunol 1989;83: 214(abstract 170).

224. Pelikan Z, Pelikan-Filipek M. The basic types of the paranasal sinus response to nasal challenge with allergens and non-specific agents, their occurrence, association with various "in vivo" and "in vitro" diagnostic parameters, diagnostic procedure and treatment. In preparation for publication.

225. Draf W, Strasding G. Radiology, ultrasound and endoscopy in the diagnosis of diseases of the nose and paranasal sinuses. In: Mackay I, eds. Rhinitis: Mechanisms and Management, London: Royal Society of Medicine Services Ltd. 1989; pp. 81–96.

226. Druce HM. Diagnosis and management of chronic sinusitis and its complications. Immunol Allergy Clinics N Am 1987;7(No 1):117–132.

227. Clement P, Van der Veken P, Iwens P, Buisseret Th. X-ray, CT-scan, MR-imaging. In: Mygind N, Naclerio RM, eds. Allergic and Non-allergic Rhinitis, Clinical Aspects. Copenhagen: Munksgaard, 1993; pp. 58–65.

228. Katz R, Fridman S, Diament M, Rohr A, Siegel S, Rachelefsky G, Spector S. A comparison of sinus imagery in chronic sinusitis. J Allergy Clin Immunol 1989; 83:213(abstract 168).

229. Wald ER. Microbiology of acute and chronic sinusitis in children. J Allergy Clin Immunol 1992;90:452–460.

230. Slavin RG. Asthma and sinusitis. J Allergy Clin Immunol 1992;90(No 3, Part 2):518–520.

231. Vinning EM, Kennedy DW. Surgical management in adults. Immunol Allergy Clin N Am 1994;14(No 1): 97–111.

232. Reid TE, Shearer WT. Recurrent sinusitis and immunodeficiency. Immunol Allergy Clin N Am 1994;14 (No 1):143–170.

233. Richardson MA. Surgical management in children. Immunol Allergy Clin N Am 1994;(No 1):89–95.

234. Evans R. Environmental control and immunotherapy for allergic disease. J Allergy Clin Immunol 1992;90: 462–468.

235. Wong DA, Dolovich J. Topical medical management of allergic conditions of the nose. Part 1: Topical medical treatment (excluding intranasal steroids). In: Mackay I, ed. Rhinitis: Mechanisms and Management. London: Royal Society of Medicine Services Ltd. 1989; pp. 169–182.

236. Warner JO. Nasal allergy in children. In: Mackay I, ed. Rhinitis: Mechanisms and Management. London: Royal Society of Medicine Services Ltd. 1989; pp. 215–224.

237. Donnelly AL, Casale TB, Bernstein DI, Goldstein S, Grossman J, Schwartz HJ. Nedocromil sodium 1% nasal solution reduces symptoms of ragweed seasonal allergic rhinitis within 24 hours. J Allergy Clin Immunol 1994;93(No 1, Part 2):272(abstract 659).

238. Cauwenberge van P. The use of systemic corticosteroids in the treatment of rhinitis. In: Mackay I, ed. Rhinitis: Mechanisms and Management. London: Royal Society of Medicine Services Ltd. 1989; pp. 199–213.

239. Mackay IS: Topical medical management of allergic conditions of the nose. Part 2: Intranasal steroids. In: Mackay I, ed. Rhinitis: Mechanisms and Management. London: Royal Society of Medicine Services Ltd. 1989; pp. 183–204.

240. Malm L, Änggard A. Vasoconstrictors. In: Mygind N, Naclerio RM, eds. Allergic and Non-Allergic Rhinitis-Clinical Aspects. Copenhagen: Munksgaard, 1993; pp. 95–100.

241. Dolovich J, Mygind N. Anticholinergic medication. In: Mygind N, Naclerio RM, eds. Allergic and Non-Allergic Rhinitis—Clinical Aspects. Copenhagen: Munksgaard, 1993; pp. 105–110.

242. Pelikan Z, Pelikan-Filipek M. Disodium cromoglycate (DSCG)-comparison of 2% and 4% formulations in seasonal allergic rhinitis. Clin Exp Allergy 1990;20(suppl 1):100(abstract P243).

243. Grieco MH. Diagnosis of upper respiratory tract allergy: classical versus controversial. Immunol Allergy Clin N Am 1987;7:1–13.

7

Diagnosis and Treatment of Acute and Subacute Sinusitis in Children and Adults

Gary A. Incaudo, MD
and L. Gretchen Wooding, MD

CONTENTS

INTRODUCTION

Sinusitis is one of the most common health complaints in the United States *(1)*. Primary care physicians represent that part of the medical community most frequently called on to diagnose and treat sinus disease (87% of cases) *(2)*. In fact, 33–50% of all visits to primary care physicians are for problems or complaints related to the head and neck region, particularly the upper respiratory tract *(3)*. Primary care physicians are ill-prepared for this duty for two major reasons. Medical schools pay little attention to diseases of the upper airway except when presented in more fulminant forms.

From: *Diseases of the Sinuses* (M. E. Gershwin and G. A. Incaudo, eds.), ©1996 Humana Press Inc., Totowa, NJ.

This is particularly true among internists, whose training is mostly in-patient in character. Second, experts in the area of sinus disease have failed to present a uniform voice on how to diagnose and treat sinusitis most effectively in the primary care setting. Problems arise especially from the realization that imaging studies, antral puncture with fluid analysis, or endoscopy is commonly necessary to establish the diagnosis of sinusitis with certainty, procedures that require increased costs and/or specialized skills.

The lack of extensive epidemiologic data describing the natural history of sinus disease in both adults and children adds to the problem of developing proven sinusitis treatment techniques and algorithms of care. For example, bacterial invasion of the paranasal sinuses is commonly present in individuals with purulent rhinorrhea persisting for more than 3–7 d following the onset of a common cold. Yet, 40–45% of proven acute sinusitis cases in children and adults may spontaneously resolve *(4,5)*. Under such circumstances, how does the physician choose which patient to treat and from which to withhold antibiotic therapy?

In pediatrics, the problem of who to treat is compounded by the practical and ethical issues surrounding the endoscopic and radiographic imaging procedures commonly needed to diagnose sinus disease accurately. Furthermore, there is a paucity of natural history data concerning sinus disease available for this age group. It is clear that the incidence of sinusitis in children <5 yr of age is significantly greater than children >12 yr of age. Such data create a tendency among pediatricians to shy away from aggressive forms of sinusitis intervention during prepubertal years.

Further problems in choosing the "best" therapeutic approach in acute and subacute sinusitis arise from the fact that a prescription for antibiotics alone may be insufficient therapy for what is presumed to be a bacterial infection within a closed space. Even in an acute care setting, the examining physician must continually keep in mind the potential diversity of origins of sinus-related disease to optimize the long-term therapeutic outcome. A question to ask when caring for a patient with historically responsive, but recurrent sinus disease is: When does acute sinusitis demand a more detailed examination? We hope this chapter will clarify these issues, and allow the creation of a reasonable protocol for the first-line medical management of acute and subacute sinusitis in both children and adults.

DEFINITION

Paranasal sinusitis is an inflammatory reaction of the mucosal lining of the paranasal sinuses. Such reactions can be infectious or noninfectious. Infectious sinusitis may be suppurative or nonsuppurative, and temporally separated into acute, subacute, and chronic (Table 1). An acute infection in adults is generally present for <2–4 wk, a subacute infection can last up to 2–3 mo, and a chronic infection is reserved for infections >3 mo in duration. These definitions are generally based on historical data. An additional reference may be made to the sinus involved when known (e.g., frontal, ethmoid, maxillary, sphenoid, or "pan-sinusitis"). Finally, recurrent sinusitis is used to describe an acute infection frequency of >2–4 episodes/yr in adults and 4–6 episodes/yr in children.

Controversy still exists concerning a standardized definition of chronic sinusitis in children. A consensus report of Otolaryngologists and Allergists from the United States and European Nations presented to the 15th European Rhinologic Congress in 1994 defined chronic childhood sinusitis as: (1) 2 mo of chronic purulent rhinorrhea unresponsive to a minimum of 3 wk of antibiotic treatment or (2) six acute episodes of clinically diagnosed sinusitis in a 12-mo period with at least one episode documented with a sinus computed tomography (CT) scan.

When faced with a case of bacterial sinusitis, it is helpful to consider that the disease process may arise as a primary or secondary event. Primary events, such as bacterial seeding during or following a viral upper respiratory infection (URI) or as a consequence of a dental infection, are common examples. Secondary sinus infection arises as a complication of another nasal or systemic disease process that interrupts the normal mucociliary cleansing mechanisms (Table 2). These clinical problems include eosinophilic rhinitis (allergic, nonallergic with or without ASA sensitivity, allergic fungal sinusitis), immunoglobulin deficiency states (most commonly selective IgG subclass deficiency, selective IgA deficiency, common variable immunodeficiency), complement deficiencies, leukocyte abnormalities, ciliary defects, nasosinus structural defects (cleft palate, septal

Table 1
Temporal Definition of Sinusitis

Acute	<2–4 wk
Subacute	1–3 mo
Chronic	>3 mo

Table 2
Diagnostic Considerations in Sinus Disease

Structural evaluation
Allergy evaluation
Immunologic evaluation
Ancillary disease entity

deviation, conchae bullosae, paradoxically curved middle turbinate, von Haller cell formation), cystic fibrosis, AIDS, and foreign bodies or nasal polyps. Whatever the cause, the primary pathophysiology appears to be an interruption in normal nasosinus hygiene giving rise to overgrowth of one or more of the normal bacterial inhabitants of the nasal passage.

Carefully formulated definitions are useful standardizations when drafting a treatment plan. For example, many investigators feel that chronic purulent sinusitis in adults is likely to require surgical intervention to achieve adequate long-term clinical control. Similarly, recurrent sinusitis, whether suppurative or nonsuppurative, suggests a need for further diagnostic investigation for inflammatory and noninflammatory causes. However, difficulties arise when clinicians begin to accept the labeling of all patients with head congestion, rhinorrhea, and/or postnasal drainage as having "sinus problems." As the use of this term becomes more common among the public, it is imperative that the physician ultimately confirm that the patient's signs and symptoms are consistent with true sinus disease. Only then can a meaningful management plan be formulated to treat the pathophysiology in question appropriately. Without such diagnostic care, the prescription of antibiotics with or without antihistamine/decongestants may be inappropriate therapy, and lead to wasteful medical costs and/or increased risks of complications or surgical requirements in the future.

INCIDENCE

Acute sinusitis presents most commonly as a bacterial infection of the paranasal sinuses follow-

ing a viral upper respiratory tract infection. On this basis, it seems reasonable to assume that the incidence of acute sinusitis is higher in children than adults, since children experience viral infections more frequently, especially in the first 5 yr of life. The precise incidence of sinusitis in children remains elusive because of the ethical conflicts in using routine radiographic imaging for surveying pediatric populations. Based on the assumption that prolonged upper respiratory tract symptoms following a viral illness might equate with sinusitis, it has been suggested that 6–13% of children experience sinusitis in the first 3 yr of life and that .5–5% of all URIs in children are complicated by acute sinus disease (6).

The estimation of the frequency of bacterial sinusitis as a complication of the common cold has been hampered by the inability to perform direct, noninvasive, precise measurements of infection of the paranasal sinuses in children. Wald et al. have suggested that a useful clinical marker of acute sinusitis in children 2–16 yr of age is a history of respiratory symptoms that have not improved over 10 d or persisted beyond 15 d (7). Children in a daycare or preschool environment are particularly prone to frequent and protracted respiratory symptoms. Van Cauwenberge noted that, in a random sampling of preschool children, 22% will have mucopurulent secretions on inspection, and most of those will have a positive CT scan (8). The clinical relevance of a positive CT scan of the sinuses at any one point in time will be discussed in a later section entitled Diagnostic Aides.

The incidence of sinus disease in adults is no less elusive. The National Center for Health Statistics estimates that approx 31.2 million people in the United States are afflicted with sinus disease accounting for 16 million office visits in 1989 (1). During the same year, Americans spent approx $150 million on "cold" products their physicians prescribed or recommended for the treatment of sinus disease (2). Almost $100 million were spent on products containing antihistamines, despite the fact that histamine levels do not increase during common viral respiratory tract infections. The accuracy of this data is clouded by the lack of rigid criteria used in defining "sinus" disease. It is clear that "sinus problems" are a very common and varied malady as viewed by the public and primary care physicians, and represent a significant expenditure of the health care budget in the United States.

PATHOPHYSIOLOGY

The sinus openings, or ostia, are the focal point for sinus disease. Pronounced obstruction of sinus ostia is seen in approx 50% of patients with uncomplicated acute rhinitis, more often in acute and subacute sinusitis, and almost always in chronic sinusitis *(9)*. The size and number of the ostia for a particular sinus may also vary congenitally and influence the efficiency with which adequate sinus cleansing can occur. Aust and Drettner showed that the time required for spontaneous elimination of contrast media in a maxillary sinus is shorter in those with large ostia compared to those with smaller ostia *(10)*. Since relative sterility of the paranasal sinuses is maintained by mucociliary flow out of these ostia, anything that disrupts that flow will promote mucous stasis. The nasal cavity is an excellent reservoir for bacteria. The theoretical conclusion is that sinusitis is typically a secondary seeding of bacteria from the nasal cavity that are capable of thriving in a hypoxic, hypercarbic, and mildly acidic pH created when the sinus ostia are obstructed.

The precise mechanism on which bacterial seeding develops is not fully understood. Viral infections and allergic disease, the two most common sources of acute sinusitis, can promote prolonged ostial obstruction through mucosal edema. Negative pressure may ultimately develop within the closed sinus space, and hypoxia can develop. During sniffing or nose blowing, if the ostia are opened transiently during the period of increased intranasal pressure, bacterially laden nasal secretions could gain entrance to the respective sinus cavity. Impaired mucociliary flow and altered mucosal immunity induced by viral or allergic inflammation may represent an additional mechanism for promoting intrasinus bacterial overgrowth *(11)*. It appears that most bacteria recovered from infected sinuses thrive in low-oxygen environments. Hypoxia, hyperbaria, and a mildly acidic pH have been shown to be a suitable biochemical environment for the growth of *Streptococcus pneumoniae* and *Haemophilus influenzae*, two of the most common bacterial isolates in maxillary sinusitis *(12)*. Furthermore, bacteriological studies have revealed that the more chronic the sinus disease, the more polymicrobial and anaerobic the organisms found within the involved sinus tend to be *(13)*.

Table 3
Causes of Acute Community-Acquired Sinusitis as Determined by Maxillary Antral Puncture

Organism	Percentage of cases	
	Adults	Children
S. pneumoniae	20–41%	36%
H. influenzae	6–50%	23%
H. influenzae and *S. pneumoniae*	1–9%	
Anaerobic bacteria	0–10%	
M. catarrhalis	2–4%	19%
Streptococcus pyogenes	1–8%	2%
Other *Streptococcal* sp.	2%	
S. aureus	0–8%	
Gram-negative bacteria	0–24%	2%
Rhinovirus, influenzae virus, parainfluenzae virus, adenovirus	0–10%	0–7%

MICROBIOLOGY

The majority of microbiology data concerning acute and subacute sinusitis are based on examination of maxillary sinus aspirates (Table 3). Current thought suggests that maxillary sinus data can be assumed to be representative of the other paranasal sinuses as well. Studies suggest that children who present with either persistent or severe respiratory symptoms and demonstrate significantly abnormal sinus radiographs (e.g., sinus opacification or air–fluid levels on plain sinus films) will yield a high density of bacteria recoverable in up to 70% of the aspirates *(14)*. Figures <60% are commonly quoted for culture positive aspirates in adults under similar circumstances *(15)*. Additional data derived from studies using maxillary antral aspirates further demonstrate the difference between purulent and nonpurulent secretions obtained. Bacterial growth can be achieved in nearly all purulent aspirates in a clinical setting consistent with sinusitis, whereas up to 25% of nonpurulent aspirates will fail to yield bacterial growth on culture. If nonpurulent aspirates are examined by gram stain, however, 75% will still reveal demonstrable bacteria making this distinction less clinically useful.

The organisms recovered tend to be nosocomial inhabitants of the nasal airway who prefer low-oxygen climates, such as *S. pneumoniae, Moraxella catarrhalis, H. influenzae,* and *Streptococcal* species in children, and *S. pneumoniae, H. influenzae,* anaerobes, and *Streptococcal* species in adults. The

Table 4
Clinical Diagnosis of Sinusitis

Signs and symptoms	Diagnostic tests
Major criteria	Major criteria
Purulent nasal discharge	Water's radiograph with
Purulent pharyngeal drainage	opacification, air–fluid level,
Cough	or thickened mucosa filling
Minor criteria	≥50% of antrum
Periorbital edema[a]	Coronal CT scan with
Headache[b]	thickening or mucosa or
Facial pain[b]	opacification of sinus
Tooth pain[b]	Minor criteria
Earache	Nasal cytologic study
Sore throat	(smear) with neutrophils
Foul breath	and bacteria
Increased wheeze	Ultrasound studies
Fever	
Probable sinusitis	Probable sinusitis
Signs and symptoms: 2 major	Diagnostic tests: 1 major =
criteria or 1 major and ≥2	confirmatory, 1 minor =
minor criteria	supportive

CT, computed tomography.
[a]More common in children.
[b]More common in adults.
Reproduced with permission from ref. 20.

H. influenzae found in sinus aspirates tend to be nontypable organisms, further suggesting that their probable source is the nasopharynx. Both *H. influenza* and *M. catarrhalis* may be β-lactamase-producing organisms making them penicillin and amoxacillin resistant. *Staphylococcus aureus* is rarely if ever encountered in acute or subacute sinusitis in children, and infrequently seen (0–8%) in adults *(16)*. The culturing of anaerobic organisms generally suggests coexisting chronic disease when encountered in the acute setting.

Viral illness may represent the most common triggering mechanism of acute and subacute sinus disease. The sinus tends to be involved in at least one-quarter of the natural rhinovirus infections (colds) that persist symptomatically into the second week. Several families of viruses have been directly implicated in the pathogenesis of acute sinusitis by virtue of being recovered from sinus aspirates in patients with acute, community acquired, sinus disease. In experimental rhinovirus infections, Turner et al. demonstrated mucosal thickening or fluid accumulation in the sinuses by MRI scanning in one-third of volunteers *(17)*. Influenzae virus is the next most common isolate in acute sinus disease, followed by parainfluenzae and, rarely,

adenovirus *(18,19)*. The resultant sinus inflammation may be exclusively the result of direct viral invasion of the sinus mucosa or involve additionally a secondary bacterial invasion of nasopharyngeal organisms.

DIAGNOSIS

The clinical diagnosis of acute sinusitis has been defined by certain major and minor criteria for symptoms that exist for longer than 7 d as shown in Table 4 *(20)*. Five to 7 d represent the typical uncomplicated time-course for a viral-induced upper respiratory tract infection. The presence of two major criteria or one major and two or more minor criteria is highly suggestive of acute or subacute sinus disease. It is important to note the differences in criteria between children and adults as shown in Table 4.

The Clinical Presentation of Acute and Subacute Sinusitis in Children

The "classic" clinical presentation of sinusitis in children differs considerably from that of adults. This difference is best described as the lack of pain and the prominence of a cough. Rhinorrhea and cough represent the most common clinical presentation of sinus disease in children *(21)*. It is the cough that follows 5–7 d of an upper respiratory tract infection that commonly prompts the parent to seek medical attention. The cough may be wet or dry, occur day or night, although it is typically worse at night when the child first goes to bed. Once asleep, the child will usually sleep through the night unless "bronchitis" or bronchospasm is a coexisting feature of the disease process. The rhinorrhea is typically purulent, but may be clear and, in cases of severe congestion, minimal or even absent. Other less frequent complaints are fever, periorbital edema, fetid oralis, irritability, pallor, and wheezing. In children old enough to localize discomfort, complaints of headache, sore throat, or earache may be elicited. In common clinical practice, the complaints of fever, headache, and facial pain are infrequently encountered as primary complaints in pediatric sinus disease, especially under the age of 8 yr *(21,22)*. When present, the physician should be alerted to look for possible sinusitis complications.

In children with pre-existing atopic disease, the presentation of acute or subacute sinus disease may be more confusing. Rachelefsky et al. showed that over 50% of allergic children will have some abnormality of the sinuses by plain radiography with 21% having complete opacification of one or more of the sinus cavities *(23)*. Because most of these children have chronic respiratory complaints, the clinician should consider sinus disease when the patient with allergic rhinitis or asthma does not clear with the usual historically effective treatment methods, or when clearing with allergy or asthma medications is followed by a rapid return of symptomatology. Directing treatment to the infected sinuses will often return the child to his or her former state of medication responsiveness.

Physical Findings in Acute and Subacute Sinusitis in Children

The physician treating a child with an upper respiratory tract infection that appears to be more severe than normal or the mildly ill child with persistent rhinorrhea and/or cough for more than 10–15 d can typically find direction for treatment through available physical findings. A careful examination of the head and neck region may reveal turbinate erythema accompanied by purulent pooling of secretions in the floor of the nasal passage

and/or in the posterior nasopharynx. In the clinical setting of a child who has been symptomatic for more than 10 d, this would be unusual for nonbacterial sources of infection. A similar statement can be made for the observation of thick purulent discharge and erythema of the posterior oropharynx.

Even though purulence in the nasal passage in the appropriate clinical setting is presumptive evidence of sinusitis, direct visualization of mucopus emanating from the middle meatus is more confirmatory. This is rarely achieved in clinical pediatric practice because:

1. Physicians are typically poorly trained in the physical exam of the nose and understand little of its anatomy;
2. Children under the age of 6–8 yr commonly resist examination of their nose with a nasal or ear speculum (other than with their finger);
3. Direct visualization of the middle meatus, especially in the congested nose, usually requires decongesting and examination with a fiberoptic rhinoscope.

Because fiberoptic rhinoscopy requires complete patient cooperation, it is even more difficult to perform in the preadolescent child.

Facial pallor with dark periorbital circles and edema have been described in association with sinus disease. However, such "soft" physical findings can be the consequence of any source of upper airway congestion engorging the normal venous and lymphatic drainage. For example, "allergic shiners," "adenoidal facies," and periorbital edema of sinusitis have very similar clinical features, yet represent diverse sources of disease.

The middle ear space should be given careful attention in the child with suspected sinus disease. The middle ear space may be viewed as another sinus cavity with a translucent window for viewing. Even before the advent of CAT scanning, otolaryngologists have noted the strong association of disease of the middle ear and disease of the sinus in children *(24)*.

The Clinical Presentation of Acute Sinusitis in Adults

As the patient population with sinusitis progresses into adolescence and adulthood, the clinical signs and symptoms of sinus disease become more focalized to the structures involved. Nasal congestion, mucous purulence, and sinus pain and/or tenderness become prominent complaints. Severe infections may present themselves with headache, high temperature, restlessness, and delirium. More commonly, the presenting syndrome is more subtle congestion with nasal mucous purulence and facial pain. The pain of acute sinusitis is typically stabbing or aching, and is commonly located over the infected sinus, although radiation to other areas of the head and neck is common. The intensity of the pain may increase with straining, bending, or coughing, and is most prominent in the late morning and afternoon hours.

Pain location may provide a valuable clue as to which of the sinuses are involved. Typical maxillary sinus pain extends from the inner canthus of the eye to the molars or even the ear. Ethmoid sinus disease localizes pain over the bridge of the nose and behind the eyes, and may increase with eye movement. Frontal sinus pain typically radiates from the forehead to the temple and occasionally to the occiput. Isolated sphenoid sinusitis is rare. Sphenoid involvement leads to pain in many diverse areas from the head to the shoulder and may present as simply an ill-defined chronic headache or as meningitis.

It should be remembered that pain from sinusitis, much like otitis media, is especially prominent when the sinus is under pressure from a suppurative infection with a closed ostium. Purulent sinusitis with a patent ostium, in contrast, may have minimal associated pain and discomfort. Under these circumstances, the signs and symptoms of sinusitis are the consequence of purulent drainage, and take the form of nasal congestion, fetor oris, sore throat, cough, and occasional nausea. Merely prolonging the coryzal symptoms in conjunction with nasal obstruction following a typical viral upper respiratory tract infection should suggest paranasal sinus edema, but not necessarily irreversible purulent sinus disease. The probability of bacterial sinusitis being present would be enhanced if the congestive symptoms occurred after flying, diving, swimming, nasal packing, nasal intubation, or an upper molar dental procedure.

Physical Findings in Acute and Subacute Sinusitis in Adults

Examination of the mucosal lining of the nose in acute and subacute sinus disease typically reveals an irregular bright red appearance. Adult patients with acute sinusitis will commonly have mucopus in the nares or the nasopharynx, unless drainage is impeded or intermittent owing to swelling of the turbinates. Dehydration of nasal secretions after airway heating and cooling, often enhanced by the inhibition of ciliary clearing by inflammatory mediators, may lead to purulent-appearing crusts throughout the nasal vestibule. Such a finding in conjunction with generalized nasal erythema may serve as the only physical suggestion of purulent sinus disease.

Under the best of circumstances, only a small portion of the nasal surface area can be seen through a nasal speculum. Even the anterior tip of the middle turbinate, displaced posteriorly, may be obscured by the swollen inferior turbinate. Decongesting with a topical α-adrenergic agonist spray, such as oxymetazoline, is helpful in visualizing the anterior tip of the middle turbinate and the middle meatus. The positioning of the nasal septum relative to the middle turbinate and the patency of the meatal drainage tract can be better appreciated in the decongested nose. Furthermore, decongesting may help visualize pus emanating directly from the middle meatus.

Direct visualization of the middle turbinate and middle meatus, enhanced by decongesting, can also help in identifying potential structural causes of sinus disease. For example, a nasal polyp may extrude anteriorly from the middle meatus and be readily visible. However, differentiating a nasal polyp from a turbinate can be a source of confusion when examining the nose with an otoscope. Probing the structure in question with a blunt instrument, the examining physician will find that a polyp is soft, pliable, and without sensation in contrast to a turbinate, which has a firm cartilaginous undersurface and is sensitive to touch. More skilled observers may appreciate potential sources of sinus disease arising from the configuration of the middle turbinate. For example, a large concha bullosae may be visible as a bulbous anterior tip of the middle turbinate. A septal deviation may compress the middle turbinate and lateralize its position, resulting in a compromise in middle meatal drainage. The hyperplastic appearance of the middle turbinate in chronic allergic disease may be a distinguishing insight into the allergic pathophysiology of a particular sinusitis problem.

Palpation of the affected sinus in search of tenderness is a poor indicator of underlying sinus infection. If the inflammation extends beyond the confines of the sinus, there may be pain and swelling of the adjacent tissues. The so-called "Pott's Puffy Tumor" of acute frontal sinusitis, as well as periorbital cellulitis or proptosis from ethmoid disease are examples of such disease extension. In maxillary sinusitis, examination and palpation of the upper molars may be important, since infection may spread from an infected tooth directly into the maxillary antrum and vice versa.

There is a growing base of information linking sinus disease with asthma instability. The group of patients who appear to be at greatest risk for asthma instability as a result of sinusitis are steroid-dependent asthmatics, asthma patients with aspirin sensitivity, and individuals with known nasal polyposis. The mechanism by which sinusitis activates asthma is not clear (25). It is speculated that bacteria from the sinuses can seed the lungs to cause an increase in asthma severity. Reflex bronchospasm might also be a mechanism through the parasympathetic nervous system via common pathways of enervation of the sinuses and lower airways. Some researchers have suggested that infection of the sinuses may reduce β-adrenergic function leading to increased airway obstruction. Using rabbits as an animal model, the most likely explanation is the passage of mediators elaborated from activated inflammatory cells in the upper airway into the lower airway tree (26). Whatever the mechanism in humans, auscultation of the chest should be undertaken in all cases of suspected sinusitis, particularly if there are accompanied pulmonary symptoms or if the patient falls into one of the three classifications noted earlier. Findings may vary from totally normal breath sounds, to coarse rhonchi suggestive of "bronchitis," to frank wheezing suggestive of bronchospasm.

Diagnostic Aides

Nasal Cytology

Microscopic examination of nasal secretions can provide a useful clue to the cause of respiratory complaints in both adults and children. In bacterial sinusitis, nasal cytology shows a predominance of neutrophils with intracellular bacteria suggestive of active phagocytosis. Studies by Wilson et al. in 55 patients (35 children and 20 adults) comparing nasal cytology with sinus X-rays revealed a 79% correlation when there was more than 1 neutrophil/high power field on smear. The correlation improved to 90% if the nasal cytology revealed >6 neutrophils/high power field and bacteria were present (27). Specificity and sensitivity were 0.79 in this investigation. The sampling of the nasal mucosa was from the inferior turbinate with a Rhinoprobe® and stained with modified Wright-Giemsa. Gill and Neiburger, using nasal secretions discharged into wax paper, examined 300 children and adults correlating the results with sinus radiographs and number of neutrophils per high power field. These authors demonstrated an 86% sensitivity and 40% specificity when >5 neutrophils/high power field were used as the distinguishing criteria for a positive sinus radiograph (28).

Neutrophilia without intracellular bacteria can be seen in viral respiratory infection or after exposure to mucosal irritants at home or in the work place. The presence of small amounts of bacteria and neutrophils may be normal in nasal secretions from infancy through adulthood. The major pitfall in the procedure is failure to sample sufficiently posterior on the inferior turbinate and/or sampling secretions only. The primary disadvantage of exclusively using nasal cytology to diagnose sinusitis is the 11–14% false-negative readings obtained using plain sinus radiographs as the standard, which, in itself, has limitations. Most authors still conclude that large numbers of neutrophils and bacteria when viewed on a Wright-Giemsa stain of nasal secretions, especially if obtained by scraping the medial portion of the inferior turbinate, most likely represent the presence of true purulent sinus disease (29). More definitive studies using maxillary antral puncture and CAT scanning are needed to clarify the place of nasal cytology in the diagnosis of sinusitis in children and adults.

Both Wilson et al. and Gill and Neiburger noted that positive sinus X-rays were commonly associated with an eosinopenic appearance to the nasal smear. The presence of eosinophils alone, or >10% of the white blood cells counted on a nasal smear correlates well with the presence of atopy in children. Eosinophilia in nasal secretions is less specific in adults where secretory eosinophilia may be found in patients with nasal polyposis, nonallergic rhinitis with eosinophilia (NARES), or chronic "intrinsic" asthma with no evidence of significant IgE-mediated involvement. As a corollary, the absence of nasal eosinophilia does not exclude the diagnosis of underlying allergic disease.

Transillumination

Transillumination of the paranasal sinuses is not a reliable indicator of sinus disease. Unilateral opacification of the maxillary antrum may be the one exception, provided agenesis of the maxillary sinus in question is not present (30). However, in a study by McNeill comparing transillumination, sinus X-ray, and antral lavage findings, transillumination was found to be an unacceptable diagnostic tool (31). Since one cannot transilluminate the ethmoids or sphenoid sinuses, and asymmetry or absence of the frontal sinus is common, there is little, if any, use for transillumination in the diagnosis of acute or subacute sinus disease in children or adults.

Ultrasonography

The use of A-mode ultrasonography has been studied in detail over the past 15 yr, but has yet to find a place in the diagnosis and management of sinus disease. In 1980, Revonta from Finland reported a statistically significant correlation between the presence of mucosal thickening on plain sinus radiographs and on ultrasonic imaging (32). The presence of fluid within the maxillary antrum proven by antral puncture correlated very well with ultrasound echo findings in this study. Jannert et al. from Sweden, using antral puncture data, demonstrated equally encouraging ultrasound correlations (33). However, this was not reproduced in another Swedish study by Berg and Carenfelt (34) or in an English study by Pfleidrer et al. (35).

Experience in the United States with A-mode ultrasonography and maxillary antral disease was also encouraging at first (36,37). Subsequent studies soon dampened enthusiasm. Rohr et al. (38) and Druce and Rutledge (39) studying adults with maxillary sinus disease found the specificity of A mode ultrasonography to range from 93 to 61%, respectively. However, the diagnostic sensitivity in both of these studies was unacceptably low, varying from 61 down to 29% in the first investigation depending on which commercial instrument was used and 34% in the second study cited. Shapiro et al., studying mostly pediatric patients with allergic rhinitis who had signs and symptoms suggestive of sinus disease, found equally discouraging data (40). Correlating A-mode ultrasonography with a Water's view of the paranasal sinus, these authors found the technique to be lacking in sensitivity and

specificity. Wald et al. (21) and Berger and Weiss (41) came to similar conclusions that A-mode ultrasound is typically diagnostic when complete opacification of the maxillary antrum is present and not particularly useful for the more common mucoperiosteal swelling seen in sinus disease.

A-mode ultrasonography may still have a place in evaluation of the obstetric patient with rhinitis. Pregnancy is complicated by a sixfold increase in the incidence of sinusitis (42). Rhinitis of pregnancy and rhinosinusitis during pregnancy may be difficult to differentiate, a problem enhanced by a justifiable reluctance to use ionizing radiation in pregnancy for diagnostic purposes. Since ultrasonography is typically a part of routine obstetric practices, the use of A-mode ultrasound may represent a cost-effective (and safe) approach to the diagnosis and monitoring of sinus disease in the pregnant population as long as the limitations inherent with this technique are recognized.

Radiography

The diagnosis of sinusitis from infancy through adulthood by X-ray, computed tomography, and magnetic resonance imaging is discussed elsewhere in this text in detail. However, the timing and type of study chosen and its interpretation deserve comment.

Doubt has been cast on the utility of conventional sinus radiographs for defining the presence or absence of sinusitis both in terms of overestimating and underestimating disease. In a study by McAlister et al., comparing simultaneously obtained plain sinus radiographs and CT scans in children during a posttreatment period for recurrent chronic sinus disease, the authors found that 75% of the patients had findings on plain radiographs that did not correlate with those on CT scans (43). Approximately 45% of the patients had normal findings on conventional radiographs of at least one sinus with the corresponding sinus being abnormal on the CT scan. Conversely, approx 35% of the patients had an abnormality on plain radiographs that proved normal on simultaneous CT scanning. More recently, Garcia et al. found in 70 children with chronic sinusitis that, compared with CT scan findings, plain sinus radiographs detected diseases in 1 of 5 (20%) frontal and 0 of 12 sphenoidal sinuses (44). For ethmoiditis, radiographs were positive in 17 of 31 (54%) cases with 7 false-positive and 14 false-negative results. Using criteria of a minimum of 40–50% of sinus volume taken up by mucosal edema or sinus opacification, plain sinus radiographs detected maxillary disease in 37 of 49 (75%) cases with 3 false-positive and 12 false-negative results.

The interpretation of plain sinus radiographs pose many problems to the examining physician. The sloping contours of the maxillary sinus may appear on the Water's view as mucosal thickening. A hypoplastic maxillary sinus will appear as opacification by plain radiography. The appearance on the Caldwell view of partial ethmoidal clouding or opacification can be caused by superimposed ethmoidal air cells, slight rotation, nasal secretions, and mild mucous membrane thickening. A small sphenoid sinus may appear partially opacified on lateral sinus radiographs. The maxillary sinus appears to be the "best" sinus studied by conventional radiography. Still, in comparison to CT scanning, small amounts of mucosal thickening can be missed even in this area. Furthermore, if the theory that the ethmoid sinuses are the focal point of chronic or recurrent sinus disease proves correct, the use of plain radiography in the clinical evaluation of the extent and site of sinusitis is open to question (45). Nevertheless, as a screening exam for a pediatric population with chronic respiratory complaints, especially when considering cost and radiation exposure, a Water's view remains an acceptable diagnostic procedure. Since the maxillary sinus is the second most common site involved (the ethmoid sinus is first) in sinusitis, Garcia et al. showed that a Water's view would miss only 24% of cases of significant sinus disease (44).

The CT scan has emerged as the "gold standard" for imaging of sinus disease, although even this technique can underestimate (46) or overestimate disease (47) (Table 5). Diament et al. prospectively evaluated the CT scans of 137 consecutive asymptomatic pediatric patients. In the 1–2-yr-old age group, 69% had abnormal scans compared to 14% of adolescent patients (age 13–17 yr). Thirty-seven to 49% of the in-between age groups revealed at least one opacified sinus with an overall incidence of sinus abnormalities compatible with "sinusitis" in 45% of the children studied (48). Glasier et al. in a similar study found a 31% incidence of sinus abnormalities in asymptomatic pediatric patients, 22% if children <1 yr were excluded (49). Glasier et al. looked at infants <1 yr. Excluding by history and physical examination all

Table 5
Comparison of CT Studies of Paranasal Sinus Disease

	Ages studied	Abnormal
Symptomatic patients		
McAlister et al. (43)	4 mo to 19 yr	81%
Lazar et al. (54)	14 mo to 6 yr	75%
van der Veken et al. (53)	3–14 yr	64%
Calhoun et al. (47)	18–72 yr	62%
Garcia et al. (44)	2–17 yr	63%
Asymptomatic patients		
Glasier et al. (50)	<1 yr	68%
Glasier et al. (49)	1 d to 16 yr	31%
Diament et al. (48)	<18 yr	45%
Lesserson et al. (52)	<18 yr	41%
Calhoun et al. (47)	18–72 yr	16%
Havas et al. (57)	>18 yr	43%

evidence of intercurrent URI, these authors still found 59% of maxillary and 39% of ethmoid sinuses opacified (50). Such findings may still represent asymptomatic temporary changes following a URI (51). Recently, Lesserson et al. studied 142 pediatric patients symptomatically free of sinus disease, but with a history of recurrent sinusitis and, in contrast to the earlier studies, did not find a statistically significant difference across age groups (52). These authors found an overall incidence of 41% of scans with some mucosal thickening or opacification of at least one sinus. If more strict criteria were used, such as requiring at least one-third of the volume of an affected sinus be opacified before a diagnosis of sinusitis can be made, only 20% of their patients would have been included in the abnormal group. Nevertheless, these authors concluded that radiographic abnormalities of the sinuses in all asymptomatic children are incidental and, without clinical correlation, are not predictive of clinically significant sinus disease.

Children with symptomatic sinus disease show a better correlation with the findings on their paranasal sinus CT scans. McAlister et al. prospectively studied 70 children with recurrent sinusitis during a posttreatment period and found 81% had abnormal coronal CT scans (43). Van der Veken et al. reviewed children (age 3–14 yr) with clinically suspected rhinosinusitis and found 64% with at least one sinus abnormality (53). In a similar group of pediatric patients age 14 mo to 6 yr whose CT scans were retrospectively reviewed, Lazar et al. found 93% contained evidence of sinus disease (54).

Asymptomatic mucosal cysts, polyps, air–fluid levels, and mucoperiosteal thickening >3 mm in depth may be seen in 10–20% of adults referred for an MRI scan of the brain *(55,56)*. Looking exclusively at adult patients, free of respiratory symptoms, undergoing axial CT with contrast for neurological complaints, Havas et al. found 43% with some paranasal sinus abnormality *(57)*. Calhoun et al. compared symptomatic and asymptomatic adult patients studied by coronal CT scan and found 62% of the "sinusitis patients" had some sinus abnormality, whereas 16% of the asymptomatic group revealed a positive finding *(47)*. It is important to remember that imaging as described above represents a point in time whose significance must be interpreted in the face of the clinical history. Like the pediatric patient group, paranasal sinus CT findings in adults must be still interpreted in light of the clinical history.

The clinical usefulness of obtaining a sinus CT scan in the acute sinusitis setting in children and adults appears to be restricted. In those cases where a complication of sinusitis extension beyond its bony confines is suspected, a CT scan is clearly indicated. A CT scan is also useful in the face of recurrent acute disease when documentation is needed for surgical considerations. The timing of the CT scan under this circumstance can be during the acute illness for documentation if the diagnosis is open to question and to identify the probable sinuses involved for future surgical direction. Alternatively, some physicians prefer to time the imaging study in their patients with a history of recurrent or chronic sinus disease after intensive medical treatment has been completed in an attempt to document the presence or absence of true persistent inflammation, as well as to scan simultaneously for fixed anatomical abnormalities.

Basic X-ray examination of the paranasal sinuses may still have a place in pediatric practice. This study included three films: the Water's (occipitomental) for maxillary and frontal sinus viewing, the Caldwell (angled posteroanterior) for ethmoid imaging, and the Lateral to evaluate adenoidal size relative to the nasopharyngeal space (adenopharyngeal ratio). Because CT scanning in infants and children is limited by the need for sedation, plain sinus radiographs remain useful for the pediatric patient with uncomplicated recurrent or chronic upper respiratory symptoms being evaluated in an ambulatory care setting. However, the limitations of this technique both in overestimating or underestimating sinus disease, particularly with reference to evaluating the ethmoid sinuses, must be constantly kept in mind. McAlister et al. showed that 23% of pediatric patients with normal maxillary sinuses on Water's view still had ethmoidal disease on CT scanning *(43)*. Conventional radiography of the sinuses are generally poor for evaluating the ethmoid sinuses in all age groups, but especially in the pediatric population *(58)*.

There is probably no role for basic sinus radiography in the diagnosis and treatment of acute sinus disease for any age group if CT scanning is available. The superiority of CT scanning compared to the clinically useful information derived by plain sinus radiography has induced some institutions, such as ours, to provide screening axial CT examinations of the sinuses for the patient with suspected recurrent or chronic sinus disease. Such screening CT scans are offered at a cost and radiation exposure competitive with plain film studies, while providing the accuracy in description of the sinuses inherent with this technique.

ENDOSCOPY

The value of flexible and rigid fiberoptic endoscopy in the diagnosis and treatment of sinus disease is discussed elsewhere in this text. This technique clearly represents an advancement by enabling the physician to perform a more complete examination of the nasopharynx and, as a result, limiting the need for more costly and sometimes more difficult diagnostic and/or imaging procedures *(59)*. Furthermore, Vining et al. found abnormal endoscopic findings indicative of sinus disease in 9% of 100 consecutive patients in the context of a negative CT examination, underscoring the value of this procedure as a diagnostic tool *(60)*. Findings such as a septal spur obstructing the middle meatus, nasal polyps, narrow middle meatus with mucosal contact between the middle turbinate and the uncinate process, hypertrophied inferior turbinate significantly narrowing the nasal cavity, and adenoidal hypertrophy obstructing the choanae may all be appreciated on nasal endoscopy, but missed on inspection of the CT scan. Considering the incidence of abnormal sinus CT findings in asymptomatic patients and normal CT exams encountered in some symptomatic patients, the endoscopic exam of the nasopharynx has become an indispensable tool for the diagnosis and treatment of sinus disease.

Table 6
Organisms Most Likely to Be Found in Sinusitis

Acute	Subacute	Acute recurrence of chronic dx	Nosocomial
S. pneumoniae			⟶
H. influenzae			⟶
M. catarrhalis			⟶
S. pyogenes			⟶
	S. aureus		⟶
	Anaerobes[a]		⟶
		Other gram-negative organisms	⟶
			Fungal

[a]Less likely to be seen in childhood disease.

TREATMENT

The mainstay of treatment for presumed bacterial sinusitis is antimicrobial possibly combined with adjunctive therapy. A culture and sensitivity of infected material from the sinus involved would normally direct antibiotic selection, but random nasal swabs have shown unreliable correlation with cultures obtained by direct sinus puncture (61). Since sinus aspiration is not usually indicated as first-step therapy, empiric antibiotic selection is indicated. A detailed review of the history, physical examination, and severity can direct initial antibiotic selection. The microbiology of sinusitis can be suggested by the:

1. Duration of illness (Table 4);
2. Type of acquisition (nosocomial or community—Table 6);
3. Particular sinus involvement;
4. Age of patient (Table 6);
5. Dental history; and
6. Immunocompetence.

Numerous new antibiotics have flooded our formularies making empiric antibiotic selection confusing and their injudicious use of clinical concern for potential development of increasing bacterial resistance. Individual protocols directing therapy can be derived by a review of current antibiotics and their efficacy studies in sinusitis and otitis media, providing a rational approach to sinusitis treatment.

The microbiology of acute and subacute sinusitis has been well defined (Tables 3 and 6), and the importance of certain bacterial species has not changed appreciably during the past several decades. However, when choosing an antibiotic for treatment, certain points demand review. Some bacterial species have changed their susceptibility to antimicrobial agents, and some newer organisms, such as chlamydia, have been occasionally isolated. S. pneumoniae (30–40% of isolates), H. influenzae (about 20%), and M. catarrhalis (about 20%), however, remain the most common pathogens in acute and subacute community-acquired sinusitis in children and adults as previously discussed, although a variety of additional bacterial and viral isolates have been observed (group A streptococci, group C streptococci, streptococci viridins, peptostreptococci, Moraxella species, and Eikenella corrodens) in isolated studies (62). Mixed anaerobic infections have been seen in adults, possibly of dental origin. Furthermore, children in the acute setting tend to have a higher frequency of M. catarrhalis. Even S. aureus, rarely implicated in acute community-acquired maxillary sinusitis, can be seen in up to 29% of cultures from sphenoid sinusitis (63). Finally, Chlamydia pneumoniae (strain TWAR) has been recognized recently as an important respiratory pathogen. Clinical sinusitis has been seen in 16% of 19 older children and adults with C. pneumoniae infection, but is still considered an uncommon sinus pathogen under age 5 (64).

Clinical situations where sinus infection occurs in the intubated hospitalized patient and the immunocompromised host require special consideration. Acute nosocomial sinusitis seen in association with nasotracheal and nasogastric tubes yields a higher than expected incidence of gram-negative organisms (Pseudomonas, Enterobacter, Klebsiella, and Bacteroides species) as well as Staphlococcus epidermidis and Staphlococcus aureus (65,66).

Fungal sinus infections are seen more frequently in diabetes mellitus. A variety of gram-negative bacteria and fungal agents have caused recalcitrant sinusitis in AIDS patients along with such unusual organisms as *Legionella* and *Acanthamoeba* *(67,68)*. *H. influenzae* and *S. pneumoniae*, however, remain the common bacterial isolates in acute sinusitis even among these unique clinical settings.

Knowledge of antibiotic resistance patterns within each community are important in antibiotic selection. *H. influenzae* organisms have been found to produce β-lactamase in 5–30% of isolates, resulting in resistance to the penicillins and some cephalosporins. Seventy-five percent of *Moraxella branhemella* isolates, particularly common among preschool children, produce β-lactamase. Penicillin resistance even among pneumococci has alarmingly increased from a 4–5% incidence in 1988 to a 20% incidence in 1992 secondary to their production of altered penicillin-binding proteins. These penicillin-resistant strains may also be resistant to cephalosporins with the level of resistance varying according to the drug as indicated by their respective minimum inhibitory concentrations (MICs) *(69)*.

With a knowledge of the pathogens most likely to cause acute and subacute sinusitis, one must ask which antibiotics would be logical choices based on the likely flora as well as resistance patterns within each individual community. With the variety of new antibiotics available, a review of their pharmacodynamic properties, antimicrobial spectra, and toxicities is presented (Table 7). This information will allow a sensible and cost-effective approach for the treatment of acute, subacute, and nosocomial sinusitis to be formulated.

AMINO-PENICILLINS

Standard initial therapy for acute sinusitis has been ampicillin or amoxicillin because their spectrum of activity covers the major organisms responsible for acute sinusitis in most clinical settings. Gastric acid destroys ampicillin, but not amoxicillin, which, with its tid dosage schedule, improves compliance and makes this the more ideal agent to achieve adequate blood levels of drug.

Mode of Action

Amino-penicillins affect cell-wall synthesis by binding to penicillin-binding proteins, and each has a common β-lactam ring. As such, the most common form of resistance is through exposure to the enzyme, β-lactamase.

Spectrum of Activity

The amino-penicillins are active against *streptococci*, pneumococci, and most strains of *H. influenzae* (β-lactamase-negative). These drugs are not effective against most staphylococcal infections, *M. catarrhalis*, and some *H. influenzae* species seen in sinus disease because of the high frequency of β-lactamase production among these organisms.

Sinus Penetration

Ampicillin has been shown, in limited studies, to penetrate into maxillary antral secretions in sufficient amounts to eradicate sensitive bacterial agents responsible for acute sinus disease *(70)*.

Efficacy Studies

Amoxicillin has become the standard against which most drugs are compared in the treatment of acute sinusitis. Studies in adults and children with 10 d of amoxicillin reveals favorable bacteriologic "cure" in 60–100% of cases *(19,71)*. Comparative studies of amino-penicillins with antimicrobial agents effective against β-lactamase-producing organisms commonly fail to demonstrate superiority in the treatment of acute sinusitis in children and adults. Wald felt that this discrepancy arises from the 40–50% spontaneous cure rate in acute sinus disease, inducing a significant resolution of sinusitis in even those patients harboring β-lactamase-producing organisms *(62)*. On this basis, studies with larger populations of subjects should reveal the expected improvement in efficacy of the broader spectrum antimicrobials.

AUGMENTED PENICILLINS

Spectrum of Activity

The addition of the β-lactamase inhibitor, clavulanate potassium, to amoxicillin (Augmentin) extends the spectrum of antimicrobial activity to include more species, such as *H. influenzae* (β-lactamase-resistant), *M. catarrhalis*, *E. coli*, *Klebsiella*, *Bacteroides fragilis*, and other anaerobes. It is also active against *staphylococci* that produce β-lactamase, but are not methicillin-resistant.

Sinus Penetration

Amoxicillin-clavulanate has been shown to penetrate into sinus tissue *(72)*.

Table 7
Oral Antibiotic Agents Used in Treatment of Acute Sinusitis

Drug	Deficiency in antimicrobial spectrum	Significant precaution, drug interactions, and side effects	Dose
Amino-penicillins			
Ampicillin	All β-lactamase-producing H. influenzae, M. catarrhalis, and S. aureus	Destroyed by gastric acid; Diarrhea (10–15%), skin rash; Contraindicated in penicillin allergy	Adults: 500 mg tid; Children: 40 mg/kg/d in divided doses q 6 h
Amoxicillin	All β-lactamase-producing H. influenzae, M. catarrhalis, and S. aureus	Diarrhea (10–15%); Skin rash; Contraindicated in penicillin allergy	Adults: 500 mg tid; Children: 40 mg/kg/d in divided doses q 8 h
Augmented penicillins			
Amoxicillin-clavulate (Augmentin)	Rare H. influenzae	Diarrhea (10–15%)—50% incidence diarrhea if wrong dose or closed too close; Skin rash; Contraindicated in penicillin allergy	Adults: 500 mg (based on amoxicillin component) q 8 h; Children: 40 mg/kg/d (based on amoxicillin component) in divided doses q 8 h with meals
Cephalosporins **First generation**			
Cephalexin (Keflex)	H. influenzae	GI—2%; Eosinophilia 9%; Contraindicated in those with immediate-type penicillin allergy	Adult: 500 mg q 6 h; Children: 25–50 mg/kg/d q 6 h
Cefadroxil (Duricef)	H. influenzae	Same as cephalexin	Adults: 500 mg bid; Children: 30 mg/kg/d q 12 h
Second generation			
Cefaclor (Ceclor)	Some β-lactamase-producing H. influenzae	Serum sickness-like reaction (<1:100) (children > adults); GI—2%; Contraindicated in those with immediate-type penicillin allergy	Adults: 500 mg tid; Children: 40 mg/kg/d in 3 divided doses
Cefprozil (Cefzil)	Some β-lactamase-producing H. influenzae	GI—2%; Pt. with increased creatinine, further increase in 5%; Rest same as cefaclor	Adults: 250–500 mg bid; Children: 30 mg/kg/d in 2 divided doses
Cefuroxime (Ceftin)	Rare H. influenzae	GI—10%; skin rash; unpleasant taste crushed tab; Contraindicated in those with immediate-type penicillin allergy	125 mg bid if age < 5 yr; 250 mg bid if age 5–10 yr; 250–500 mg bid if age >10 yr
Loracarbef (Lorabid)	Rare H. influenzae	GI—10–15%; skin rash; Contraindicated in those with immediate-type penicillin allergy	Adults: 200–400 mg bid; Children: 15–30 mg/kg/d 2 divided doses
Third generation			
Cefixime (Suprax)	S. aureus and some S. pneumoniae	GI—(5–15%); skin rash; Contraindicated in those with immediate-type penicillin allergy	Adults: 400 mg qd; Children: 8 mg/kg/d in one dose or divided bid

Drug	Activity	Side Effects/Interactions	Dosage
Cefpodoxime (Vantin)	Pseudomonas	GI—(~8%); increase creatine (3.6%) Contraindicated in those with immediate-type penicillin allergy	Adults: 200 mg bid Children: 10 mg/kg/d in 2 divided doses
Macrolides/Azalides			
Erythromycin	*H. influenzae* and some *M. catarrhalis*	Frequent GI side effects; drug interactions with astemizole (Hismanel), terfenadine (Seldane), digoxin, and theophylline Cholestatic jaundice esp. with erythro estolate	Adults: 250–500 mg qid (or 400 mg ethyl succinate) Children: 40 mg/kg/d in 4 divided doses
Azithromycin (Zithromax)	Some *H. influenzae*, limited data	Fewer GI side effects than erythromycin, overall 12% May have drug interactions same as erythromycin Do not give with food	Adults: 500 mg on day 1, then 250 mg/d on days 2–5 Children: only if age >15 yr then adult dose
Clarithromycin (Biaxin)	Some *H. influenzae*, less active than azithromycin against *H. influenzae*, limited data	GI—(13%) Drug interactions same as erythromycin Headache (2%)	Adults: 500 mg bid Children: 15 mg/kg/d divided bid
Fluroquinolones			
Ciprofloxicin (Cipro)	Streptococci in general, including *S. pneumoniae*, and *S. viridans*, anerobes	GI—(1.5%); drug interactions with cimetidine, caffeine, theophylline Decreased levels if given with antacids, sucrafate, Ca^{2+}, Fe^{2+}	Adults: 500–750 mg bid Children: not approved for age <18 yr 20–30 mg/kg/d in 2 divided doses
Ofloxacin (Floxin)	Same as Cipro except possibly better against streptococci, less active pseudomonas	Similar to Ciprofloxacin Take with no food	Adults: 200–400 mg bid Children: not approved
Lomefloxacin (Maxaquin)	Same as Ciprofloxacin, less active against pseudomonas, limited data	Similar to Ciprofloxacin except no interaction with theophylline, caffeine	Adults: 400 mg q d Children: not approved
Sulfonamide combinations			
TMP/SMX (Septra)	Some resistant *S. pneumoniae* and *H. influenzae*, limited anaerobic coverage	Skin rash, leukopenia Cannot use G6PD deficiency Interactions with phenytoin sodium, warfarin Contraindicated in sulfa allergy	Adults: 1 DS tab bid Children: 8–12 mg TMP/40–60 mg SMX/kg/d in 2 divided doses
Erythromycinethyl-succinate/sulfisoxa-zole acetyl (Pediazole)	Same as erythromycin and TMP/SMX	Same as erythromycin and TMP/SMX	Children: 40 mg/kg/d of erythromycin component
Others			
Clindamycin	*H. influenzae* and other gram-negative rods	GI—(diarrhea 7%, pseudomembranous colitis with toxic megacolon rare), rash	Adults: 150–450 mg q 6 h Children: 20–30 mg/kg/d q 6 h
Tetracyclines (e.g., doxycycline)	Some resistant *S. pneumoniae*, *H. influenzae*, and *S. aureus*	GI—skin rash, phototoxicity, but less than TCN, deposition in teeth, contraindicated in pregnancy-hepatotoxicity, gastric binding with antacids	Adults: 100 mg bid Children: Pts >8 yr 2–4 mg/kg/d q 12 h on 1st day, then 1/2 dose q 24 h

qd, once daily; bid, twice daily; tid, three times daily; qid, four times daily.

Efficacy Studies

Clinical efficacy studies in children have shown the drug to be equally effective as amoxicillin *(4)*, and cefaclor (Ceclor) in the treatment of acute maxillary sinusitis *(73)*. In adults with acute maxillary sinusitis, bacteriologic cure rates of 87 and 84% have been demonstrated for amoxicillin-clavulanate (Augmentin) and cefuroxime (Ceftin), respectively *(74)*.

General Precautions

These agents are usually well tolerated, but can cause antibiotic-associated diarrhea, hypersensitivity reactions (rash—3%), and rare anaphylactic reactions. Diarrhea can be helped by taking the amoxicillin-clavulanic acid in combination with food *(75)*.

CEPHALOSPORINS/CARBACEPHEMS

Mode of Action

Cephalosporins and other β-lactams (carbacephems, i.e., loracarcef) have the same mechanism of action as penicillin (inhibition of cell-wall synthesis).

Spectrum of Activity

The oral cephalosporins can be divided into generations according to their spectrum of biological activity. Generally speaking, first-generation cephalosporins are most active against gram-positive bacteria, and third-generation compounds have better gram-negative coverage.

First-Generation Agents (Cefadroxil, Cephalexin)

SPECTRUM OF ACTIVITY

The first-generation agents are the most active of the cephalosporins against *S. aureus* (nonmethicillin-resistant strains). Their spectrum includes *S. pneumoniae, K. pneumoniae, E. coli,* and *Proteus mirabilis*. They are active against some anaerobes (i.e., *peptostreptococcus*), but not including the *B. fragilis* group. They have no activity against *M. catarrhalis, P. aeruginosa,* methicillin-resistant *staphylococci,* and very poor activity against *H. influenzae.*

SINUS PENETRATION

There is little comparative information on the tissue penetration of these agents. Studies have shown measurable levels of cephalexin in purulent sinus secretions *(76)*.

EFFICACY STUDIES

Cephalexin (Keflex) has been used in acute and acute-chronic sinusitis with an 83% clinical response rate shown in one study *(77)*. However, the predominant organisms recovered from patients in this study were *streptococcus* and *staphylococcus* species with very few isolates of *H. influenzae,* clouding the interpretation of these figures. This spectrum of pathogens differs from most other bacteriological studies in which *Staphylococcus* species were found to be unusual in acute and subacute sinusitis.

Cefadroxil (Duricef) is considered a first-generation agent. One clinical trial produced a 90% cure rate in patients with acute and acute-chronic sinusitis (30 patients included) *(78)*. However, the validity of this study is open to question, since the culture data revealed no *H. influenzae* and six patients with *M. catarrhalis,* presumably resistant to cefadroxil, still improved. It can be dosed twice daily, but is more expensive than other first generation cephalosporins.

Second-Generation Agents (Cefaclor, Cefprozil, Cefuroxime, Lorcarbef)

SPECTRUM OF ACTIVITY

The second-generation agents extend the gram-negative spectrum of the first-generation compounds, particularly in their activity against *H. influenzae* and *M. catarrhalis*. Cefaclor (Ceclor), one of the earliest second-generation cephalosporins, has activity against both β-lactamase-positive and β-lactamase-negative strains of *H. influenzae*. However, sporadic resistance has been noted. Cefaclor has been demonstrated to be less active against *H. influenzae* than amoxicillin-clavulanic acid and trimethoprim/sulfamethoxazole in susceptibility studies *(79)*. In contrast, cefuroxime axetil (Ceftin) and cefprozil (Cefzil) exhibit excellent activity against the organisms most frequently responsible for acute and subacute sinusitis, including *H. influenzae* and *M. catarrhalis*. Loracarbef (Lorabid), a β-lactam compound with a carbacephem nucleus that improves chemical stability, is equivalent to other second-generation cephalosporins in its bacteriologic spectrum.

SINUS PENETRATION

As with the first-generation compounds, limited data are available regarding sinus penetration levels, but all drugs appear in the sinus mucosa on administration. However, sinus tissue penetration studies have shown wide ranges of antibiotic concentrations. Sudderick et al. *(80)* showed that the median sinus mucosal cefuroxime concentration exceeded the desired MIC of 90 mg/L for *S. pneumoniae* and *H. influenzae*, but not for *M. catarrhalis*. This discrepancy with clinical cure rates may be explained by bioavailability (when taken after food, bioavailability is 50–60% and is reduced to 30–40% when taken with food), delayed gastric emptying, and higher blood levels compared to tissue levels (β-lactams act primarily extracellularly since the bacteria are also primarily extracellular). The penetration of cefprozil into tissue fluid (skin blister fluid) exceeds the MICs for susceptible pathogens *(81)*, but studies are not available for sinus tissue.

The chemical alteration in loracarbef results in significantly greater chemical stability. High serum and tissue levels are obtainable (including sinus tissue) with the drug delivered twice daily *(82)*.

EFFICACY STUDIES

Bacteriologic efficacy studies have shown cefaclor to be inferior to cefuroxime axetil in the treatment of acute bacterial maxillary sinusitis *(83)*, but equal to amoxicillin-clavulanate *(84)*. Cefuroxime has been shown to be equally effective to amoxicillin-clavulanate in the treatment of adults with acute maxillary sinusitis with bacterial eradication rates of 84 and 87% *(85)*. A noncomparative study utilizing two dose levels of cefprozil showed a satisfactory clinical response in 87% of the low-dose group compared to 100% in the high-dose group *(86)*. Loracarbef appears to have comparable efficacy to amoxicillin-clavulanate in the treatment of acute bacterial maxillary sinusitis *(87)*.

Third-Generation Agents (Cefixime, Cefpodoxime)

SPECTRUM OF ACTIVITY

Both of the agents, cefixime and cefpodoxime proxetil, are considered third-generation cephalosporins. They surpass the second-generation cephalosporins in some of their gram-negative coverage and include activity not only against *Haemophilus* species and *Moraxella* species (high stability in presence of beta lactamase) but some enterobacteriaeceae, *E. coli*, *Proteus mirabalis*, and *Klebsiella* species. Cefixime (Suprax), like most

third-generation cephalosporins, has poor activity against gram-positive organisms, such that this drug is not active against *S. aureus* and it is less active against *S. pneumoniae* than first- and second-generation cephalosporins and penicillins. Cefpodoxime (Vantin) has a broad range of activity against both gram-positive and gram-negative bacteria. Unlike cefixime (Suprax), cefpodoxime proxetil (Vantin) has greater activity against *streptococci* (4- to 16-fold greater in in vitro studies) and has been shown to have fourfold greater activity against methicillin-sensitive *staphylococci (88)*.

SINUS PENETRATION

Sinus penetration studies of cefixime have not been performed, but percentage penetration was high (132.6%) into inflammatory fluid utilizing a blister-fluid model *(89)*. This percentage is comparable to the oral quinolones, which are generally regarded as having good tissue-penetrating ability including the paranasal sinuses. Low protein binding of cefpodoxime allows the drug to obtain good tissue penetration. The concentration of cefpodoxime in maxillary sinus tissue has been shown to be greater than the MIC 90 (the minimum inhibitory concentration against 90% of tested strains) for *S. pneumoniae*, *S. pyogenes*, *H. influenzae*, *M. catarrhalis*, and other gram-negative rods *(90)*.

EFFICACY STUDIES

Clinical trials have not been done utilizing cefixime in the treatment of sinusitis. However, in acute otitis media, a parallel microbial situation, cefixime was about as effective as amoxicillin in eradicating *M. catarrhalis* and β-lactamase-negative *H. influenzae* and more effective against β-lactamase-positive *H. influenzae*. It had poor activity against *S. pneumoniae*; 7 (37%) of 19 patients with pneumococcal infection had positive cultures during treatment with cefixime, compared to 1 (6%) of 18 with amoxicillin. Disturbingly, nine patients grew *S. aureus* from on-therapy cultures and, in seven of these patients, *S. aureus* was not present on the pretreatment culture. This did not happen in the amoxicillin group *(91)*. In a multicenter, randomized, double-blind European study of 250 adult outpatients with acute sinusitis, cefpodoxime was compared with cefaclor. Cefpodoxime-treated patients had a higher clinical cure rate (84 vs 68%). However, the bacteriologic cure rates were equivalent—95% for cefpodoxime and 91% for cefaclor *(92)*.

GENERAL PRECAUTIONS

The cephalosporins in general should never be used in individuals with a history of anaphylaxis to penicillin or in those whom positive skin testing to penicillin determinants have been documented. Diarrhea and nausea are frequent side effect complaints (5–10% of patients) for all generations of cephalosporins.

MACROLIDES

This group of antibiotics includes erythromycin, clarithromycin (Biaxin), and azithromycin (Zithromax—also referred to as azalide).

Mode of Action

As a class, the macrolide antibiotics exert their antimicrobial activity by binding to the 50S subunit of the 70S ribosome, which interferes with protein synthesis of susceptible organisms.

Spectrum of Activity

Erythromycin is widely utilized to treat upper and lower respiratory infections. It has a broad spectrum of antimicrobial activity, including *S. pneumoniae*, *M. catarrhalis*, *Mycoplasma pneumoniae*, *Chlamydia species*, and some *S. aureus* and anaerobes. Unfortunately, erythromycin exhibits variable activity against *H. influenzae*, is inactive against some *M. catarrhalis*, and *S. pneumoniae* and *staphylococci* are rapidly developing resistance to its activity. Azithromycin and clarithromycin expand the spectrum of erythromycin, and have better gastrointestinal tolerance. Clarithromycin is active against *S. pneumoniae*, *M. pneumoniae*, and methicillin-sensitive *S. aureus*. It has in vitro activity against *M. catarrhalis, Legionella* species, and *Chlamydia pneumoniae*. It is more effective against *H. influenzae* than erythromycin. The spectrum of activity of azithromycin exceeds that of clarithromycin. Not only does it cover typical sinusitis pathogens such as *S. pneumoniae, H. influenzae* (four- to eightfold more active than clarithromycin against *H. influenzae*) and *M. catarrhalis*, but it also has activity against Mycoplasma species, Legionella species, and enhanced activity against Chlamydia *(93)*. Its in vitro activity also includes anaerobes, such as *peptostreptococci, Clostridium perfringes, C. difficile*, and some members of the *B. fragilis* group. Unfortunately, as with erythromycin, heavy clinical use

has resulted in rapid emergence of resistance and many of the erythromycin-resistant organisms are becoming crossresistant to clarithromycin and azithromycin *(94)*.

Sinus Penetration

There is limited information suggesting that the penetration of erythromycin into the sinus mucosa and sinus secretions is adequate, but somewhat less than the concentration of ampicillin *(95)*. Clarithromycin has been shown to penetrate very well into sinus mucosa and, with its range of activity, it is theoretically an effective agent in the treatment of sinusitis *(96)*. Azithromycin also penetrates well into tissues and is concentrated in phagocytes, which may transport the drug directly to the site of infection *(97)*. Because the drug is highly concentrated in tissue and slowly released, it has a long biologic half-life and low serum levels. These properties result in an antibiotic that appears to be active against a variety of organisms, despite low serum levels.

Efficacy Studies

Clarithromycin has been shown by Karma et al. to be as equally effective as amoxicillin in the treatment of acute maxillary sinusitis with bacteriological cure rates of 88 and 91% of evaluatable patients with clarithromycin and amoxicillin, respectively *(98)*. However, patients from whom β-lactamase-producing strains were isolated were excluded from the study. Another study, presented in abstract form only, showed clarithromycin to be as effective as amoxicillin and amoxicillin-clavulanate in patients with maxillary sinusitis *(99)*.

Dubois et al. also compared a 2-wk regimen of clarithromycin (500 mg bid) with amoxicillin-clavulanate (500 mg tid) in a single-blind, randomized, multicenter study of 497 adults with acute maxillary sinusitis *(100)*. Sinusitis had to be documented by a combination of clinical history as well as a positive sinus radiograph, and a positive culture of sinus fluid obtained endoscopically or by antral puncture. Clinical success was noted in 97% of the clarithromycin group and 93% of the amoxicillin-clavulanate recipients with respective pathogen eradication rates of 87 and 90%. Gastrointestinal upset was seen less frequently in the clarithromycin recipients.

Another study using limited antral puncture specimens showed azithromycin (5 doses/5-d regimen) to be as effective clinically and bacteriologically in the treatment of sinusitis and other infections of the upper respiratory tract, as a 30 dose/10-d treatment with amoxicillin or a 40 dose/10-d treatment with erythromycin *(101)*. There was no lower incidence of adverse effects in the azithromycin treatment group in this comparative study with gastrointestinal side effects being the most common complaint among all patients.

General Precautions

Drug interactions are common with the macrolide group of antibiotics because they utilize the cytochrome P-450 oxidase mechanism of liver metabolisms. Increased drug concentrations result when multiple drugs are administered that use this same pathway of elimination. Clarithromycin, like erythromycin, may elevate theophylline and digoxin levels when used concomitantly. The effect of azithromycin on the plasma levels of theophylline (when steady-state levels are achieved) are incompletely studied. Prudent medical practice indicates that levels of these compounds be followed closely at all times when administered with the macroloide group of antibiotics. Administration of clarithromycin or azithromycin with either terfenadine (Seldane) or astemizole (Hismanal) is not recommended because of the potential of these antihistamines to cause cardiac arrhythmias at high plasma levels.

Adverse events are as common with the macrolide group of antibiotics as amoxicillin-clavulanate in the treatment of sinus disease. However, gastrointestinal side effects generally appear less frequently with the macrolides when amoxicillin-clavulanate is compared with clarithromycin and azithromycin.

FLUOROQUINOLONES

Ciprofloxacin (Cipro) and ofloxacin (Floxin) are the two most useful agents in upper respiratory infections, and lomefloxacin (Maxaquin) has recently appeared on the US market.

Mode of Action

The fluroquinolones inhibit the bacteria's DNA replication process and are bactericidal.

Spectrum of Activity

Ciprofloxacin is active in vitro against a wide range of clinically relevant bacteria, particularly aerobic gram-negative organisms. *H. influenzae*, *K. pneumoniae*, *Neisseria* species, *Moraxella* species, and *Pseudomonos aeruginosa* are highly susceptible to the drug. Gram-positive cocci are generally less susceptible to ciprofloxacin than are gram-negative species. Nevertheless, the drug has shown good activity against methicillin-sensitive *S. aureus* and coagulase-negative *staphylococci*. Its initial promise, however, with infection caused by methicillin-resistant *S. aureus* and *P. aeruginosa* has been tempered by the development of resistance of these organisms. Against anaerobic bacteria, the fluroquinolones have little or no activity, and they are not highly active against *streptococci*, which are common pathogens in sinus infections. Treatment of *S. pneumoniae* infections with a fluroquinolone has resulted in clinical failures. Therefore, they are not recommended for empiric treatment of community-acquired pneumonia or acute sinusitis *(102)*. Ofloxacin's spectrum of activity is similar to ciprofloxacin, except it has less activity against *P. aeruginosa*. It is also thought to be more effective against *S. pneumoniae* and *Chlamydia pneumoniae*, although it is still not recommended in the therapy of pneumococcal pulmonary disease. Lomefloxacin (Maxaquin) has even less activity against pseudomonas than ciprofloxacin or ofloxacin, and *S. pneumoniae* exhibits in vitro resistance to lomefloxacin as do most Group A, B, D, and G *streptococci*. Clinical resistance to the quinolones has become increasingly common in infections caused by *S. aureus*, *P. aeruginosa*, and *Serratia marcesiens*. The prevalence of fluoroquinolone-resistant *S. aureus* increased from 0 to 35% and even up to 79% in some American hospitals within a few years after the initial use of such drugs *(103)*. This rapidly developing rate of resistance may be secondary to person-to-person transmission of resistant strains of *S. aureus* rather than acquisition of resistance during treatment (mutation type) *(104)*. Hence, these drugs are considered inappropriate initial therapy for common outpatient infections (i.e., otitis media, sinusitis, and pharyngitis) that can be treated with ordinary antimicrobials. They should be reserved for their unique role against pseudomonas, susceptible strains of methicillin-resistant *S. aureus*, and upper respiratory infection in patients with severe β-lactamase allergy. Focused therapy may reduce the rising resistance rate and salvage the usefulness of this family of drugs.

Sinus Penetration

Ciprofloxacin has been shown to achieve excellent penetration into paranasal sinus mucosa. Maxillary sinus mucosal levels were nearly twice as high as corresponding blood levels in a study by Dan et al. *(105)*. Ofloxacin and lomefloxacin concentration in sinus mucosa have been investigated in only a limited number of patients, and these studies, published in Japanese, show similar results to that of ciprofloxacin *(106,107)*.

Efficacy Studies

Unfortunately, no clinical studies have been done comparing the efficacy of fluroquinolones in acute and subacute sinusitis with known therapeutic agents. A recent abstract presented at the 15th European Rhinologic Congress has shown that ciprofloxacin was as effective as amoxicillin-clavulanate in the treatment of acute exacerbations of chronic sinusitis with overall cure rates of 64.7% for ciprofloxacin and 51.2% for amoxicillin-clavulanate, and clinical success rates of 67.6 and 56.1%, respectively *(108)*.

General Precautions

The interactions between other drugs and the fluoroquinolones should be taken into account. Ciprofloxacin, ofloxacin, and lomefloxacin all interact with cimetidine, cyclosporine, and warfarin. Their absorption is impaired by antacids, sucrafate, Fe^{2+}, and Ca^{2+}. Theophylline levels need to be followed with ciprofloxacin, less likely with ofloxacin, and not with lomefloxacin.

SULFONAMIDE COMBINATIONS

Mode of Action

The combination of trimethoprim and sulfamethoxazole (TMP/SMX) acts by interfering with folate metabolism and nucleic acid synthesis of susceptible microorganisms. TMP/SMX may be bactericidal for some organisms, whereas either drug alone may be bacteriostatic; this synergistic effect may be observed even when organisms are resistant to one agent or the other. Erythromycin is the other drug commonly combined with a sulfonamide.

Spectrum of Activity

The spectrum of in vitro activity of sulfonamide combinations tends to be broad and includes the commonly isolated pathogens of sinusitis: *S. pneumoniae*, *H. influenzae* (including β-lactamase producing), and *M. catarrhalis*. TMP/SMX also is active against *S. aureus*, gram-negative bacilli, especially the *Enterobacteriaceae* (*E. coli*, *Klebsiella*, and *Proteus*), *Neisseria meningitidis*, and some anaerobes, although clinical efficacy is not established. *P. aeruginosa* is resistant. The newly emerging penicillin-resistant pneumococci are often equally resistant to non-β-lactam antibiotics, such as TMP/SMX and erythromycin with incidences as high as 20 and 50%, respectively, in children with otitis media *(79,109)*.

Sinus Penetration

Tissue penetration studies of TMP/SMX into sinus mucosa are not available, but the compounds are distributed throughout the body and enter the cerebrospinal, synovial, pleural, and peritoneal fluids in concentrations that approximate 80% of serum levels. The penetration capacity of the macrolide group of antibiotics has been discussed.

Efficacy Studies

Clinical efficacy studies comparing TMP/SMX to amoxicillin and ampicillin in the treatment of acute maxillary sinusitis in adults have shown good clinical and bacteriologic responses to all three regimens *(110)*. TMP/SMX has also been shown to be an adequate alternative to amoxicillin in the treatment of chronic sinusitis in children with respiratory allergy *(111)*.

The fixed combination of erythromycin and sulfonamide has been successfully and conveniently used in children in the treatment of acute otitis media and sinusitis. Erythromycin penetrates well into most tissues, and concentrations achieved in sinus secretions and middle ear exudates are adequate to treat susceptible *S. pneumoniae*, but not to eradicate *H. influenzae*. Combinations of erythromycin and sulfonamides have been shown to be comparable to ampicillin and amoxicillin in the treatment of acute otitis media, regardless of the causative organism *(112)*. The combination has also been shown to be more effective than cefaclor for β-lactamase-positive *H. influenzae* and *M. catarrhalis*, and penicillin-sensitive *S. pneumoniae* isolates from middle-ear effusions in children with acute otitis media *(113)*.

General Precautions

Serious adverse reactions associated with the use of TMP/SMX in patients without AIDS are rare; they include anaphylaxis, severe cutaneous eruptions, and hematologic effects, such as thrombocytopenia, leukopenia, and hemolytic anemia. The drug should not be given to patients with glucose-6-phosphate dehydrogenase deficiency. Erythromycin is one of the safest antimicrobial agents in use. Dose-related gastrointestinal distress occurs most commonly.

CLINDAMYCIN

Mode of Action

Clindamycin binds to bacterial ribosomes and suppresses protein synthesis.

Spectrum of Activity

Clindamycin is effective against many strains of *S. aureus* and has excellent activity against most anaerobic species. It also inhibits chlamydiae growth, but is poorly effective against strains of *H. influenzae.*

Sinus Penetration

No data concerning sinus penetration are available.

Efficacy Studies

Clinical efficacy studies are not currently available. The use of clindamycin to treat sinus infections empirically is not recommended because of *H. influenzae* resistance to this agent. Clindamycin appears to be an alternative if macrolide resistance is present, and the patient cannot be treated with β-lactam antibiotics. It has been used favorably in some children with otitis media who have not responded to several courses of antibiotics *(114)*.

General Precautions

Although the major adverse reaction of clindamycin is the potential for severe pseudomembranous colitis, this effect can be encountered with other potent antimicrobials used for sinusitis and is not unique to clindamycin.

TETRACYCLINES

Mode of Action

Tetracyclines are bacteriostatic agents that inhibit protein synthesis by binding to bacterial ribosomes. Resistance to the tetracyclines is mediated by plasmids and appears slowly. Microorganisms that acquire resistance to one tetracycline are usually resistant to the other tetracyclines as well.

Spectrum of Activity

Tetracyclines are effective in vitro against a great variety of bacteria, including gram-positive, gram-negative, aerobic bacteria, anaerobic bacteria, mycoplasma, chlamydia, legionella, and some protozoa. Doxycycline and minocycline (second-generation agents) are more active, in general, than the parent compound against a variety of organisms. Doxycycline has some activity against *B. fragilis*, whereas minocycline has improved activity against *S. aureus*. In general, however, the tetracyclines are not recommended for treatment of streptococcal or staphylococcal infections because of an observed increasing rate of resistance. Up to 15% of strains of *S. pneumoniae* and 10% of Group A *streptococci* are not sensitive to tetracycline *(115,116)*.

Sinus Penetration

The long-acting tetracyclines (doxycycline and minocycline) penetrate tissues well because of their lipid solubility. Doxycycline penetrates sinus mucosa and secretions adequately in the setting of acute maxillary sinusitis *(117)*.

Efficacy Studies

Doxycycline is commonly prescribed in Europe for sinusitis where bacteria, presumably, are still somewhat sensitive. The Scandinavian Study Group evaluated doxycycline vs loracarbef in the treatment of acute bacterial maxillary sinusitis. The clinical response rate (cure or improvement) was 98.2% for patients receiving loracarbef and 92.2% for those who received doxycycline *(118)*.

General Precautions

The tetracyclines should not be given to pregnant women, and their use is contraindicated in children <8 yr of age because of mottling of the permanent teeth.

ACUTE SINUSITIS

Controversies concerning the treatment of acute sinusitis include antimicrobial therapy, timing of intervention, and ancillary methods of control.

Observations supporting the use of antimicrobials in acute sinusitis appear conclusive, and include a substantial decrease in orbital and intracranial complications from sinusitis since the onset of the antimicrobial era, an increase in the clinical improvement rate when comparing treatment with amoxicillin or amoxicillin-clavulanate to placebo, and the possible prevention of the evolution toward more chronic sinus disease. The timing of antimicrobial intervention, however, is more open to question and cannot always be subjected to an algorithmic approach. Wald has suggested that upper respiratory symptoms in children that have not improved over a 10-d period is highly suggestive of sinusitis. One might make a similar judgment for adults by 7 d according to Table 3. Ancillary therapeutic approaches as discussed in another chapter of this text are sometimes combined with antibiotic therapy, but there remains no confirmed evidence that these additions make a major impact on the clinical outcome.

Concerns over the frequency of β-lactamase producing *H. influenzae* and *M. catarrhalis* and the emergence of antibiotic-resistant organisms in all clinical forms of sinusitis have prompted many physicians to use liberally the broadest-spectrum antibiotic available. However, it can be argued that since the overall rate of spontaneous clinical recovery from acute sinusitis is high (40–45%) and not all organisms found in acute sinusitis are β-lactamase producers, there is no reason to deviate from the usual initial empirical treatment with amoxicillin (or erythromycin plus a sulfonamide in true penicillin allergic patients) for community-acquired disease. Erythromycin and the tetracyclines, if used alone, miss a large percentage of *H. influenzae*, and TMP/SMX should not be used alone if infection with Group A *streptococcus* is suspected or proven. In fact, a study comparing amoxicillin with amoxicillin-clavulanate (Augmentin) failed to show any increase in efficacy by providing a β-lactamase inhibitor. Furthermore, there is a growing concern that the liberal use of the broadest-spectrum antibiotics available induces the emergence of resistant organisms with increasingly greater frequency.

Guidelines for selecting an alternative to amoxicillin or the other drugs listed above as first-line therapy would include:

1. No clinical response within 48–72 h of initiating antibiotic treatment;

2. A clinical history of early recurrences or treatment failures of acute sinusitis following amoxicillin therapy;

3. A patient with a history of frequent courses of multiple antibiotics; and

4. A high incidence of β-lactamase-producing organisms in the community.

Under these circumstances, an alternative, broader-spectrum antibiotic should be chosen (*see* Fig. 1).

Amoxicillin-clavulanate is a logical choice as an alternative broad-spectrum antibiotic because of its effectiveness against potential β-lactamase pathogens. TMP/SMX can be used as an alternative second-line drug provided that prior treatment included coverage for Group A *streptococcus*.

Alternative and often more costly second-line regimens, some with broader antimicrobial coverage, include the cephalosporins, newer macrolide agents, and possibly the fluroquinolones. Clinical efficacy studies have been performed utilizing these drugs and have shown them to be clinically effective. However, many of these studies suffer from small numbers of patients and commonly revealed these drugs to be no more effective when compared with the response to amoxicillin or amoxicillin-clavulanate.

A number of cephalosporins are currently available for use in sinusitis. Utilizing clinical studies of sinusitis and in vitro sensitivity data, cefuroxime would be the first-line choice among the cephalosporin family of drugs. Cefaclor has been shown to have a significantly lower bacteriologic cure rate than cefuroxime in acute maxillary sinusitis, and resistance to cefaclor by *H. influenzae* has been on the rise. Faden et al. showed a 17% incidence of cefaclor-resistant *H. influenzae* in children not previously exposed to antibiotic treatment *(79)*. Cefaclor has the added disadvantage of causing a serum sickness-like illness in children for up to 6 wk after therapy is completed. Cefprozil (Cefzil) has been shown to be as effective as amoxicillin-clavulanate in otitis media in a single study. However, other authors have observed a higher failure rate with this agent when compared with amoxicillin-clavulanate, and there are insufficient studies utilizing cefprozil in sinusitis *(119)*. Loracarbef (Lorabid) has comparable efficacy to amoxicillin-clavulanate, but demonstrates less activity against penicillin-resistant *S. pneumoniae* than cefuroxime or cefprozil. Cefixime (Suprax) could be used as a

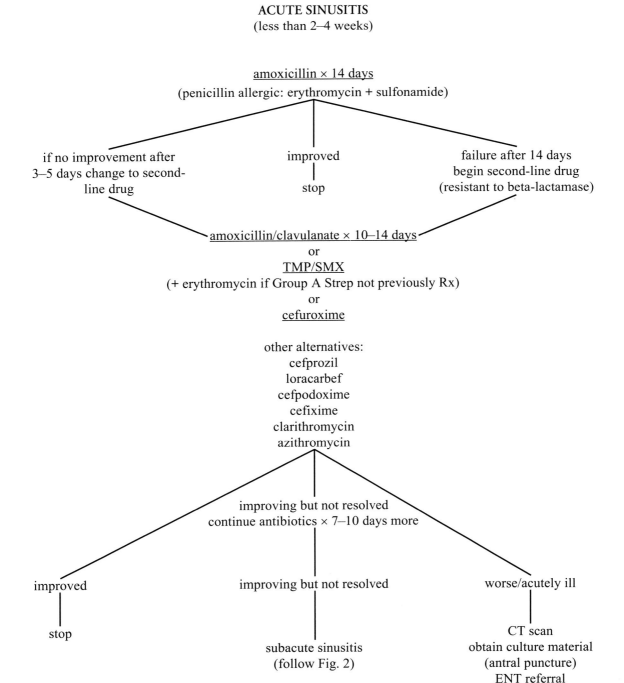

ACUTE SINUSITIS
(less than 2–4 weeks)

amoxicillin × 14 days
(penicillin allergic: erythromycin + sulfonamide)

if no improvement after   improved   failure after 14 days
3–5 days change to second-   begin second-line drug
line drug   stop   (resistant to beta-lactamase)

amoxicillin/clavulanate × 10–14 days
or
TMP/SMX
(+ erythromycin if Group A Strep not previously Rx)
or
cefuroxime

other alternatives:
cefprozil
loracarbef
cefpodoxime
cefixime
clarithromycin
azithromycin

improving but not resolved
continue antibiotics × 7–10 days more

improved   improving but not resolved   worse/acutely ill

stop   CT scan
                  subacute sinusitis   obtain culture material
                  (follow Fig. 2)   (antral puncture)
                                                       ENT referral

Fig. 1. Algorithm of care for acute sinusitis.

second-line agent after initial treatment with an agent that covers *S. pneumoniae* and *S. aureus* for which it lacks sufficient activity. Cefpodoxime (Vantin) retains activity against *streptococci* and methicillin-sensitive *staphylococci* and, like cefixime, surpasses second-generation cephalosporins in gram-negative coverage making this drug a more viable alternative. It should be cautioned that oral cephalosporins are demonstrating increasing inactivity against penicillin-resistant *S. pneumoniae*, but the extent of resistance varies from one cephalosporin to another. Cefprozil (Cefzil) and cefuroxime axetil (Ceftin) demonstrate lower MICs against penicillin-resistant *S. pneumoniae* than cefaclor (Ceclor) and loracarbef (Lorabid). Cefixime (Suprax), of all the cephalosporins, is the least active against *S. pneumoniae*.

The new macrolides, clarithromycin and azithromycin, offer microbiologic advantages over erythromycin, but presently they are not approved in the United States for sinusitis. Clinical data are insufficient to establish these drugs as alternatives to such agents as TMP/SMX, amoxicillin-clavulanate, or the cephalosporins in the treatment of sinusitis. However, in vitro sensitivity studies, ease of administration, and the need for alternatives in penicillin-allergic patients makes these newer macrolides attractive alternatives. Azithromycin, with its greater activity against *H. influenzae* and easier dosing regimen, might be utilized initially. Drug interactions, however, need to be addressed with these agents as previously discussed. The judicious use of these broader-spectrum and clinically unproven agents is crucial because of the cost and potential for developing future bacterial resistance.

The role of the fluroquinolones in the treatment of acute sinusitis should be reserved for those patients who are allergic or historically unresponsive to the β-lactam agents, sulfonamides, tetracyclines, and macrolides. Ciprofloxacin has been shown to be efficacious for acute exacerbations of chronic sinusitis, although it was not superior when compared with amoxicillin-clavulanate therapy in limited studies *(120)*. If ciprofloxacin or ofloxacin is utilized, its lack of activity against anaerobes and *streptococci* should be kept in mind.

The duration of antibiotic treatment for acute sinusitis has not been clearly established, but recommendations vary from treating for 7–10 d beyond clinical improvement to simply treating for a total of 2–4 wk (your choice). Usually as one progresses along the temporal framework of sinusitis, the recommended duration of treatment increases. Antral puncture studies have shown that maxillary sinuses can be sterilized in 7–10 d with antibiotic treatment in acute disease, although some patients require longer therapy. Similar data are not available for the ethmoid, sphenoid, or frontal sinuses. As a general rule, it is the consensus of most authors to prolong therapy beyond the 7–10 d typically recommended for respiratory infections to a minimum of 2 wk of antibiotic treatment in true purulent sinus disease.

ACUTE NOSOCOMIAL SINUSITIS

Acute sinusitis is generally thought of as an outpatient infection. However, up to 5.5% of critically ill patients housed in an ICU for only 48 h develop sinusitis *(121)*. Clinical presentation includes fever, leukocytosis, and presence or absence of purulent rhinorrhea. The major predisposing factor appears to be the presence of nasoenteric tubes. However, one study noted an equal occurrence rate with oropharyngeal tubes in patients undergoing prolonged mechanical ventilation *(122)*. Infection rates reported are 18.6/1000 patient days for patients with tubes compared with only 1/1000 patient days for those without nasoenteric tubes *(121)*. Diagnosis can be confirmed by standard radiographic imaging usually as the maxillary sinus is typically involved. CT scanning is helpful in assessing ethmoid or sphenoid involvement. Most commonly the microbiology reveals a polymicrobial infection with mixed enteric gram-negative bacilli, *S. aureus*, *P. aeruginosa*, and *Bacteroides* species being isolated. Younger patients undergoing emergency blind nasotracheal intubation had a higher incidence of *staphylococci* infection. Gram-negative organisms predominated in electively intubated older patients whose procedure was performed under operating room or ICU conditions *(123)*.

Treatment is often empiric, but the infecting pathogens should be identified by sinus aspiration. Frequently, patients are already receiving antibiotic therapy at the time of diagnosis, making antral puncture even more important for organism identification and susceptibility. Antral irrigation can be performed at the time of sampling allowing drainage and cleansing of the diseased sinus. In addition to antibiotic therapy and therapeutic lavage, treatment includes removal of the offending tubes. Some authors have also suggested the concomitant use of topical and systemic decongestants.

ACUTE SINUSITIS IN AIDS

Sinusitis in immunodeficient HIV-infected patients is an increasingly well-recognized entity. Although *H. influenzae* and *S. pneumoniae* are still the most commonly isolated organisms, community-acquired *P. aeruginosa* is being reported *(124)*. These patients usually present acutely ill with fever and severe headache. All the patients reported had been on powerful antibiotics for other

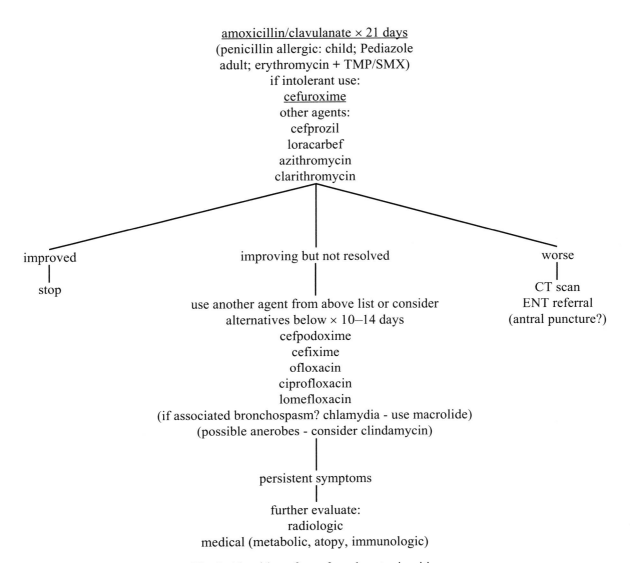

SUBACUTE SINUSITIS
(30–120 days duration)

amoxicillin/clavulanate × 21 days
(penicillin allergic: child; Pediazole
adult; erythromycin + TMP/SMX)
if intolerant use:
cefuroxime
other agents:
cefprozil
loracarbef
azithromycin
clarithromycin

improved   improving but not resolved   worse

stop   CT scan
                                                                            ENT referral
                    use another agent from above list or consider   (antral puncture?)
                    alternatives below × 10–14 days
                    cefpodoxime
                    cefixime
                    ofloxacin
                    ciprofloxacin
                    lomefloxacin
                    (if associated bronchospasm? chlamydia - use macrolide)
                    (possible anerobes - consider clindamycin)

                    persistent symptoms

                    further evaluate:
                    radiologic
                    medical (metabolic, atopy, immunologic)

Fig. 2. Algorithm of care for subacute sinusitis.

purposes and presumably no longer had "community" flora in their nasopharynx. Culture obtained by antral puncture should be performed readily and empiric treatment to cover the usual organisms, anaerobes, and *P. aeruginosa* instituted. Fungal disease and other "opportunistic organisms" should be sought.

SUBACUTE SINUSITIS

When sinusitis becomes subacute (30–120 d duration), the microbial etiology remains similar to that of an acute infection, but with a shift in predominance to gram-negative pathogens, particularly *H. influenzae* and *M. catarrhalis*, and, rarely, to *S. aureus*. Anaerobes may be seen occasionally in adult populations. A history of prolonged disease and previous antibiotic therapy raises the spectra of antibiotic resistance. In this clinical setting, the alternative, broader-spectrum second-line drug regimens discussed under the treatment of acute sinusitis should be considered for initial therapy (*see* Fig. 2).

If sinusitis symptoms persist despite adequate coverage for the usual bacterial organisms, difficult to grow organisms, such as anaerobes, or newly recognized agents, such as *C. pneumoniae* (strain TWAR) and penicillin-resistant *S. pneumoniae*, should be considered. When an anaerobic infection is unresponsive or untreatable with amoxicillin-clavulanate, clindamycin would be the drug of choice. Clindamycin would also be recommended for penicillin-resistant *S. pneumoniae* that is resistant to cephalosporins. *C. pneumoniae* should be entertained particularly in an older child or adult with prolonged cough and bronchospasm. Erythromycin is the drug of choice in this clinical setting, but azithromycin, clarithromycin, and possibly the fluoroquinolones can also be considered.

Most clinicians agree that the duration of treatment of subacute sinusitis should be 3–4 wk rather than the usual 10–14 d commonly recommended for acute sinus disease. If the patient again develops recurrent symptoms, he or she should be carefully scrutinized for possible anatomical abnormalities and contributing medical disorders, such as allergic rhinitis, thyroid dysfunction, and immunodeficiency. Referral to an allergist and/or otolaryngologist is indicated at this juncture.

ANCILLARY MEDICAL PROBLEMS

Treatment of underlying allergic rhinitis needs to be addressed prior to sending a patient for surgical intervention for recurrent disease. The strong association between sinusitis and atopy has already been reviewed in another chapter of this text. In the atopic individual who fails environmental control and pharmacotherapy, an immunotherapy program may be indicated. However, there remain no controlled studies demonstrating the efficacy of allergen immunotherapy in the prevention or treatment of sinusitis. Nevertheless, aggressive allergy treatment should not be withheld from the atopic patient who is experiencing recurrent or chronic sinus disease.

A careful screening for immunodeficiency diseases should also be undertaken concurrent with any surgical referral. Various forms of immunologic aides are available to the practicing physician. Parenteral immunoglobulin availability and efficacy have been expanded with the advent of intravenous γ-globulin. However, this expensive form of immunosupplementation should be reserved only for patients with bona fide IgG

deficiency. Since many children with selective immunoglobulin deficiency (e.g., IgG subgroup deficiency) have transient disease, prophylactic antibiotics may be adequate for this group. Prophylactic antibiotics may also be appropriate in children who develop recurrent sinusitis with every upper respiratory infection, since growth seems to have a beneficial effect on sinusitis frequency in childhood. No studies focusing on this approach have been done, but conclusions drawn from antibiotic prophylaxis in acute otitis media might suggest similar success rates in sinusitis. Amoxicillin, 10–20 mg/kg up to 500 mg, or TMP/SMX at bedtime have been suggested. Prophylaxis with low-dose continuous antibiotics, such as amoxicillin, TMP-SMX, or tetracyline, is appropriate for fixed immunodeficiency disorders in adults where purulent complications of the upper respiratory tract are observed.

Immunoprophylaxis should also be considered, particularly in light of the increasing antimicrobial resistance to commonly used antibiotics. Pneumococcal vaccine may be an appropriate immunologic aide in children <2 yr of age and adults. However, studies proving its effectiveness in sinus disease have yet to be undertaken. The use of other forms of immunostimulants in recurrent or chronic respiratory disease awaits further research developments.

CONCLUSION

The criteria available to accurately diagnose sinusitis has been reasonably established. However, no single test should be considered conclusive unless the clinical history fits the diagnosis of sinusitis. As with all other disciplines of medicine, there remains an "art" to the timing and choice of the appropriate test and formulating an interpretation before a final diagnosis can be secured. If the criteria set forth in this chapter are followed, we believe that considerable benefit will follow in terms of cost savings from limiting the number of inaccuracies in diagnosis and, therefore, needless and sometimes harmful treatment schemes. The haphazard manner in which potent, broad-spectrum antibiotic preparations are prescribed in some medical communities is likely the reason for the observed emergence of more and more resistant organisms in the ambulatory care setting.

Once a diagnosis of acute sinusitis has been made, it is important to remember that 40–45% of patients will spontaneously recover with no treatment other than time. It is this fact that allows us to establish the conservative, cost-effective algorithm of care described in this chapter. We believe that the additional patient contact required for some patients when following this treatment scheme is justified based on two factors. First, there will be considerable cost savings from utilizing less expensive antibiotics. Second, there will likely be a reduction in the extent and frequency of drug-resistant organisms.

The temporal definition of sinusitis serves as an important focus from which a decision can be made justifying further investigation into causative factors. This may simply take the form of a more detailed clinical history (e.g., child suddenly in a day-care setting, diving, flying, occupational hazards), or a more detailed laboratory investigation (e.g., a CAT scan, immunological studies, or an allergy investigation). We believe that every patient with recurrent or chronic sinusitis should ultimately undergo a coronal CAT scan, endoscopic examination, and limited or extensive immunological testing (depending on the clinical and family history). The frequency with which atopy and sinusitis coexist suggest that allergic disease be regularly considered even if other causes of sinusitis are suspected in children and adults. The same statement cannot be made concerning other immunological studies at the present time. However, if there are suggestions from the clinical or family history of immunodeficiency (such as frequent ancillary infections or unusual infective organisms), then limited immunological studies, such as quantitative immunoglobulins, IgG subgroups, AIDS screening, and white blood cell count and differential, can be requested.

REFERENCES

1. Moss AJ, Parsons VL. Current estimates from the National Health Interview Survey, Unites States—1985. Hyattsville, MD: National Center for Health Statistics, 1986:66,67; DHHS publication no. (PHS) 86-1588 (Vital and Health Statistics; series 10; no. 160).
2. National Disease and Therapeutic index. Plymouth Meeting, PA: IMS, 1988–1989; pp. 487,488.
3. Wald ER. Epidemiology, pathophysiology and etiology of sinusitis. Pediatr Infect Dis 1985;4:551–554.
4. Wald ER, Chiponis D, Ledesma-Medina J. Comparative effectiveness of amoxicillin and amoxicillin-clavulanate potassium in acute paranasal sinus infections in children: a double-blind, placebo-controlled trial. Pediatrics 1986;77:795–800.
5. Sykes DA, Wilson R, Chan KL, Mackay IS, Cole PJ. Relative importance of antibiotic and improved clearance in topical treatment of chronic mucopurulent rhinosinusitis. A controlled study. Lancet 1986;2:359,360.
6. Wald ER. Acute sinusitis in children. Adv Otolaryngol Head Neck Surg 1988;2:165–188.
7. Wald ER, Guerra N, Byrs C. Upper respiratory tract infections in young children: duration of and frequency of complications. Pediatrics 1991;87:129–133.
8. van Cauwenberge P. Prevalence and etiology in pediatric sinusitis (abstract). XV Congress of European Rhinological Society and XIII International Symposium on Infection and Allergy of the Nose 1994;254.
9. Dretner B. Pathophysiology of paranasal sinuses with clinical implications. Clin Otolaryngol 1980;5:277–284.
10. Aust R, Drettner B. Elimination of contrast medium from the maxillary sinus. Acta Otolaryngol 1975;81:468–475.
11. Holstrom M, Lund VJ, Scadding G. Nasal ciliary beat frequency after nasal allergen challenge. Am J Rhinol 1992;6:101–105.
12. Carrenfelt C, Lundberg C. Purulent and non-purulent maxillary sinus secretions with respect to PO_2, PCO_2, and ph. Acta Otolaryngol 1977;84:138–144.
13. Kennedy DW. First-line management of sinusitis: a national problem? Otolaryngol Head Neck Surg 1990;103,5 part 2:849.
14. Wald ER, Reilly JS, Casselbrant M, et al. Treatment of acute maxillary sinusitis in childhood: a comparative study of amoxicillin and cefaclor. J Pediatr 1983;104:297–302.
15. Evans FO, Sydnor B, Moore WEC, et al. Sinusitis of the maxillary antrum. N Engl J Med 1975;293:735–739.
16. Gwaltney JM. Microbiology of sinusitis. In: Sinusitis—Pathophysiology and Treatment, Druce HM, ed. Clinical Allergy and Immunology of series, New York: Marcel Dekker, 1993; p. 46.
17. Turner BW, Cail WS, Hendley JO, Hayden FG, Doyle WJ, et al. Physiologic abnormalities in the paranasal sinuses during experimental rhinovirus colds. J Allergy Clin Immunol 1992;90:474–478.
18. Hamory BH, Sande MA, Syndor A Jr, et al. Etiology and antimicrobial therapy of acute maxillary sinusitis. J Infect Dis 1979;139:197–202.
19. Wald ER, et al. J Pediatrics 1984;104:297–302.
20. Shapiro GG, Rachelefsky GS. Introduction and definition. J Allergy Clin Immunol 1992;90:417,418.
21. Wald ER, Milmoe GJ, Bower A, et al. Acute maxillary sinusitis in children. N Engl J Med 1981;304:749–754.
22. Kogutt MS, Swischuk LE. Diagnosis of sinusitis in infants and children. Pediatrics 1973;52:121–124.
23. Rachelefsky GS, Goldberg M, Katz RM. Sinusitis disease in children with respiratory allergy. J Allergy Clin Immunol 1978;61:310–314.
24. Horshaw TC, Nickman NJ. Sinusitis and otitis in children. Arch Otolaryngol 1974;100:194,195.
25. Slavin RG. Sinusitis in adults and its relation to allergic rhinitis, asthma and nasal polyps. J Allergy Clin Immunol 1988;82:950–956.
26. Irvin CG. Sinusitis and asthma: an animal model. J Allergy Clin Immunol 1992;90:521–533.

27. Wilson NW, Jalowayski AA, Hamburger RN. A comparison of nasal cytology with sinus X-rays for the diagnosis of sinusitis. Am J Rhinol 1988;2:55–59.

28. Gill FF, Neiburger JB. The role of nasal cytology in the diagnosis of chronic sinusitis. Am J Rhinol 1989;3:13–15.

29. Meltzer EO, Jalowayski AA. Nasal cytology in clinical practice. Am J Rhinol 1988;2:47–54.

30. Evans FO, Syndor B, Moore WEC. Sinusitis of the maxillary antrum. J Laryngol Otol 1963;77:1009–1013.

31. McNeill RA. Comparison of the findings on transillumination, X-ray and lavage of the maxillary sinus. J Laryngol Otol 1963;77:1009–1013.

32. Revonta M. Ultrasound in the diagnosis of macillary and frontal sinusitis. Acta Otolaryngol 1980;370 (suppl):1–54.

33. Jannert M, Andreasson L, Holmer N-G, et al. Ultrasonic examination of the paranasal sinuses. Acta Otolaryngol 1982;389(suppl):1–51.

34. Berg O, Carenfelt C. Etiological diagnosis in sinusitis: ultrasonography as clinical component. Laryngoscope 1985;95:851–853.

35. Pfleidrer AG, Drake-Lee AB, Lowe D. Ultrasound of the sinuses: a worthwhile procedure? A comparison of ultrasound and radiography in predicting the findings of proof puncture on the maxillary sinuses. Clin Otolaryngol 1984;9:335–339.

36. Isaacson S, Edell SL. A-mode ultrasound evaluation of maxillary sinusitis. ORL 1978;86:231–235.

37. Landman MD. Ultrasound screening for sinus disease. Otolaryngol Head Neck Surg 1986;94:157–164.

38. Rohr AS, Spector SL, Siegel SC, et al. Correlation between A-mode ultrasound and radiography in the diagnosis of maxillary sinusitis. J Allergy Clin Immunol 1986;78:58–61.

39. Druce HM, Rutledge J. Chronic sinusitis and rhinitis. Am J Rhinol 1989;3:163–166.

40. Shapiro GG, Furukawa CT, Pierson WE, et al. Blinded comparison of maxillary sinus radiography and ultrasound for diagnosis of sinusitis. J Allergy Clin Immunol 1986;77:59–64.

41. Berger W, Weiss J. A comparison of A-mode ultrasound and X-ray for screening of maxillary sinus disease (abstract). J Allergy Clin Immunol 1985;75:187.

42. Incaudo GA. The diagnosis and treatment of rhinosinusitis during pregnancy and lactation. In: Schatz M and Zeiger RS, eds., Asthma and Allergy in Pregnancy and Early Infancy. New York: Marcel Dekker, 1993; pp. 287–306.

43. McAlister WH, Lusk R, Muntz HR. Comparison of plain radiographs and coronal CT scans in infants and children with recurrent sinusitis. Am J Roentgenol 1989; 153:1259–1264.

44. Garcia DP, Corbett ML, Eberly SM, Joyce MR. Radiographic imaging studies in pediatric chronic sinusitis. J Allergy Clin Immunol 1994;94:523–530.

45. Andrew WK, Swart JG. Fallibility of sinus radiographs in demonstrating ethmoid sinusitis. S Afr Med J 1987; 72:158.

46. Mann WJ, Amedee RG, Jemma M. An assessment of radiologic discrepancies in patients with paranasal sinus disease. Am J Rhinol 1992;6:211–213.

47. Calhoun KH, Waggenspack GA, Simpson CB, Hokanson JA, Bailey BJ. CT evaluation of the paranasal sinuses in symptomatic and asymptomatic populations. Otolaryngol Head Neck Surg 1991;104:480–483.

48. Diament MJ, Senac JR, Gilsanz V, Baker S, Gillespie T, Larsson S. Prevalence of incidental paranasal sinus opacification in pediatric patients: a CT study. J Comp Asst Tomogr 1987;11:426–431.

49. Glasier CM, Archer DP, Williams KD. Incidental paranasal sinus abnormalities on CT of children: clinical correlation. Am J Neuroradiol 1986;7:861–864.

50. Glasier CM, Mallory GB, Steele RW. Significance of opacification of the maxillary and ethmoid sinuses in infants. J Pediatr 1989;114:45–50.

51. Kovatch AL, Wald ER, Ledesma-Medina J, Chiponis DM, Bedlingfield DM. Maxillary sinus radiographs in children with nonrespiratory complaints. Pediatrics 1984; 73:306–308.

52. Lesserson JA, Kieserman SP, Finn DG. The radiographic incidence of chronic sinus disease in the pediatric population. Laryngoscope 1994;104:159–166.

53. Van der Veken PJV, Clement PAR, Buisseret T, et al. CT scan study of the incidence of sinus involvement and nasal anatomic variations in 196 children. Rhinology 1990;28:177–184.

54. Lazar RH, Younis RT, Parvey LS. Comparison of plain radiographs, coronal CT, and intraoperative findings in children with chronic sinusitis. Otolaryngol Head Neck Surg 1992;107:29–34.

55. Rak KM, Newell JD, Yakes WF, Damiano MA, Luethke JM. Paranasal sinuses on MR images of the brain: significance of mucosal thickening. Am J Roentgenol 1991;156:381–384.

56. Cook LD, Hadley DM. MRI of the paranasal sinuses: incidental abnormalities and their relationship to symptoms. J Laryngol Otol 1991;105:278–281.

57. Havas TE, Motbey JA, Gullane PJ. Prevalence of incidental abnormalities on computed tomographic scans of the paranasal sinuses. Arch Otolaryngol Head Neck Surg 1988;114:856–859.

58. Som PM, Lawson W, Biller HF, Lanzieri CF. Ethmoid sinus disease: CT evaluation in 400 cases. Part I. Nonsurgical patients. Radiology 1986;159:591–597.

59. Imbeau SA, Lucas JL, Meyer S. Nasal endoscopy: an advancement in diagnosis and treatment of sinusitis. J S Carolina Med Assoc 1991;87:257–261.

60. Vining EM, Yanagisawa K, Yanagisawa E. The importance of preoperative nasal endoscopy in patients with sinonasal disease. Laryngoscope 1993;103:512–519.

61. Gwaltney JM, Sydnor A, Sande MA, et al. Etiology and antimicrobial treatment of acute sinusitis. Ann Otol Rhinol Laryngol 1981;90(suppl 84):68.

62. Wald ER. Sinusitis. Pediatr Rev 1993;14:345–351.

63. Lew D, Southwick FS, Montgomery WW, Weber AL, Baker AS. Sphenoid sinusitis. N Engl J Med 1983;309:1149–1154.

64. Hahn DL, Dodge RW, Golubjaatnikov R. Association of *Chlamydia pneumoniae* (strain TWAR) infection with wheezing, asthmatic bronchitis and adult-onset asthma. JAMA 1991;266:225–230.

65. Caplan ES and Hoyt NJ. Nosocomial sinusitis. JAMA 1982;247:639–641.

66. Linden BE, Aguilar EA, Allen SJ. Sinusitis in the nasotracheally intubated patient. Arch Otolaryngol Head Neck Surg 1988;114:860,861.

67. Schlanger G, Lutwick LI, Kurzman M, et al. Sinusitis caused by *Legionella pneumophilia* in a patient with the acquired immunodeficiency syndrome. Am J Med 1984; 77:952.

68. Gonzalez MM, Gould E, Dickinson G, et al. Acquired immunodeficiency syndrome associated with acanthamoeba infection and other opportunistic organisms. Arch Pathol Lab Med 1986;110:749.

69. Thornsberry C, Brown SD, Yee C, Bouchillon SK, Marler JK, Rich T. Increasing penicillin resistance in *streptococcus pneumoniae* in the US. Infec Med (suppl): 15–24.

70. Axelsson A, Brorson JE. The concentration of antibiotics in sinus secretions. Ann Otolaryngol 1974;83:323–330.

71. Scheld WM, Sydnor A, Farr B, Gratz JC, Gwaltney JM. Comparison of cyclacillin and amoxicillin for therapy of acute maxillary sinusitis. Antimicrob Agents Chemother 1986;30:350–353.

72. Iwasawa T. Fundamental and clinical studies with BRL25000 (Clavulanic acid-amoxicillin) in the otorhinologic field. Chemotherapy (Tokyo) 1982;30:612–625.

73. Wald ER, et al. Postgrad Med 1984;September–October:133–136.

74. Camacho AE, et al. Am J Med 1992;93:271–276.

75. Staniforth DH, Lillystone RJ, Jackson D. Effect of food on the bioavailability and tolerance of clavulanic acid/ amoxycillin combination. J Antimicrob Chemother 1982;10,131–139.

76. Kohonen A, Paavolainen M, Renkonen OV. Concentration of cephalexin in maxillary sinus mucosa and secretion. Ann Clin Res 1975;7:50–53.

77. Schaefer SD and Ronis ML. Cephalexin in the treatment of acute and chronic maxillary sinusitis. Southern Med J 1985;78:45–48.

78. Kaminszczik, I. Treatment of acute and chronic sinusitis with cefadroxil. Drugs 1986;32(Suppl. 3):33–38.

79. Faden H, Doern G, Wolf J, Blocker M. Antimicrobial susceptibility of nasopharyngeal isolates of potential pathogens recovered from infants before antibiotic therapy: implications for the management of otitis media. Pediatr Infect Dis J 1994;13:609–612.

80. Sudderick RM, Lund, VJ, et al. An evaluation of the penetration of cefuroxime axetil into human paranasal sinus tissue. Rhinology 1992;30:11–16.

81. Barriere et al. Pharmacology and pharmacokinetics of cefprozil. CID 1992;14(suppl 2):S18–S187.

82. Stenquist M, Lindahl D, Drikkson T, et al. Penetration of loracarbef into maxillary sinus fluid and tonsillary tissue after single dose administration. Abstract of the 17th International Congress of Chemotherapy, 1991.

83. Sydnor A, Gwaltney JM, Cocchetto DM, Scheld M. Comparative evaluation of cefuroxime axetil and cefaclor for treatment of acute bacterial maxillary sinusitis. Arch Otolaryngol Head Neck Surg 1989;115: 1430–1433.

84. Wald ER, Reilly JS, Casselbrant MC, Chiponis DM. Treatment of acute sinusitis in children: Augmentin vs cefaclor. Postgrad Med 1984;(Augmentin Sym suppl Sept–Oct):133–136.

85. Camacho AE, Cobo, R, Otte J, Spector SL, et al. Clinical comparison of cefuroxime axetil and amoxicillin/ clavulanate in the treatment of patients with acute bacterial maxillary sinusitis. Am J Med 1992;93:271–276.

86. Wijngaart W, Verbrugh H, Theopold HM, Bauernfeing A, et al. A noncomparative study of cefprozil at two dose levels in the treatment of acute uncomplicated bacterial sinusitis. Clin Ther 1992;14:306–312.

87. Sydnor TA, Scheld WM, Gwaltney J, Nielsen, Huck W, Therasse DG. Loracarbef (LY163892) vs amoxicillin/ clavulanate in bacterial maxillary sinusitis. Ear Nose Throat J 1992;71:225–232.

88. Sader HS, Jones RN, Washington JA, Murray PR, et al. In vitro activity of cefpodoxime compared with other oral cephalosporins tested against 5556 recent clinical isolates from five medical centers. Diagn Microbiol Infect Dis 1993;17:143–150.

89. Stone JW, Linong G, Andrews JM, Wise R. Cefixime, in-vitro activity, pharmacokinetics and tissue penetration. J Antimicrob Chemother 1989;23:221–228.

90. Del Beccarol MA. Cefpodoxime proxetil. Pediatr Ann 1993;22:187–196.

91. Howie VM, Owen MJ. Bacteriologic and clinical efficacy of cefixime compared with amoxicillin in acute otitis media. Pediatr Infect Dis J 1987;6:989–991.

92. Gehanno P, Depondt J, Barry B, Simonet M, Dewer H. Comparison of cefpodoxime proxetil with cefaclor in the treatment of sinusitis. J Antimicrob Chemother 1990;26(suppl E):87–91.

93. Hardy DJ, Hensey DM, Beyer JM, Vojtko C, McDonald EJ, Fernander PB. Comparative in vitro activities of new 14-, 15- and 16-membered macrolides. Antimicrob Agents Chemother 1988;32:1710–1719.

94. Moellering RC. Introduction: revolutionary changes in the macrolide and azalide antibiotics. Am J Med 1991;91(suppl 3A):3A-1S–3A-4S.

95. Axelsson A, Brorson JE. The concentration of antibiotics in sinus secretions; ampicillin, cephradine and erythromycinestolate. Ann Otolaryngol 1974;83:323–330.

96. Fraschini F, Scaglione F, Pintucci G, Maccarinelli G, Dugnani S, Demartini G. The diffusion of clarithromycin and roxithromycin into nasal mucosa, tonsil and lung in humans. J Antimicrob Chemother 1991;27 (suppl A):61–65.

97. Schentag JJ, Ballow CH. Tissue-directed pharmacokinetics. Am J Med 1991;91(suppl 3A):3A-5S-11S.

98. Karma P, Pukander J, Pentila M, Ylikoski J, et al. The comparative efficacy and safety of clarithromycin and amoxycillin in the treatment of outpatients with acute maxillary sinusitis. J Antimicrob Chemother 1991;27 (suppl A):83–90.

99. Dubois J, Saint-Pierre C, Devcich K. Clarithromycin in the treatment of acute maxillary sinusitis. Abstract presented Second International Conference on the Macrolides, Azalides and Streptogramins—Venice, Italy, January 1994.

100. Dubois J, Saint-Pierre C, Tremblay C. Efficacy of clarithromycin vs. amoxicillin/clavulanate in the treatment of acute maxillary sinusitis. ENT J 1993;72:1–5.

101. Felstead SJ, Daniel R, European Azithromycin Study Group. Short-course treatment of sinusitis and other upper respiratory tract infections with azithromycin: a

comparison with erythromycin and amoxycillin. J Int Med Res 1991;19:363–372.

102. Cooper B, Lawlor M. Pneumococcal bacteremia during ciprofloxacin therapy for pneumococcal pneumonia. Am J Med 1989;87:475.

103. Blumberg HM, Rimland D, Carroll DJ, Terry P, Wachsmith IK. Rapid development of ciprofloxacin resistance in methicillin-susceptible and -resistant *Staphylococcus aureus*. J Infect Dis 163;1991:1279–1285.

104. Shalit I, Berger SA, Gorea A, Frimerman H. Widespread quinoline resistance among methicillin-resistant S. aureus isolates in a general hospital. Antimicrob Agents Chemother 1989;33:593,594.

105. Dan M, Englander M, Gorea A, Harel M, Berger SA. Concentrations of ciprofloxacin in external ear granulation tissue and maxillary sinus mucosa. Rev Infect Dis 1989;2(suppl 5):S1080.

106. Sanbe B, Yoshihama H, Ueda R, Kobayashi K, Ito Y, Lkada J, Inafuku M. Experimental and clinical studies on DL-8280 in the field of otorhinolaryngology. Chemotherapy (Tokyo) 1984;32(suppl 1):1019–1029.

107. Futalo T, et al. Fundamental and clinical studies on NY-198 in the field of otorhinolaryngology. Chemotherapy 1988;36(suppl 2):1280–1288.

108. Klossek JM. The use of oral ciprofloxacin (CIP) for the treatment of chronic ENT infections. An overview of French data. Presented at the 15th European Rhinologic Congress Copenhagen, June 19–23, 1994.

109. Nelson CT, Mason EO, Kaplan SL. Activity of oral antibiotics in middle ear and sinus infections caused by penicillin-resistant *Streptococcus pneumoniae*: implications for treatment. Pediatr Infect Dis J 1994;13: 585–589.

110. Hammory BH, Sande MA, Sydnor A, Seale DL, Gwaltney JM. Etiology and antimicrobial therapy of acute maxillary sinusitis. J Infec Dis 1979;139:197–202.

111. Rachelefsky GS, Katz RM, Siegel SC. Chronic sinusitis in children with respiratory allergy: the role of antimicrobials. J Allergy Clin Immunol 1982;69:382–387.

112. Howie VM, Ploussard JH. Efficacy of fixed combination antibiotics versus separate components in otitis media. Clin Pediatr 1975;11:205.

113. Lambert-Zechovsky N, Mariani-Kurkdjian P, Doit C, Bourgeois F, Bingen E. J Hosp Pract 1992;22:89–97.

114. Shapiro GG. Sinusitis in children. J Allergy Clin Immunol 1988;81,5:1025–1027.

115. Daley CL, Sande M. The runny nose. Infection of the paranasal sinuses. Infect Dis Clin North Am 1988;2: 131–147.

116. Coonan KM, Kaplan EL. In vitro susceptibility of recent North American Group A streptococcal isolates to eleven oral antibiotics. Pediatr Infect Dis J 1994;13: 630–635.

117. Lundberg C, Gullers K, Malmborg AS. Antibiotics in sinus secretions. Lancet 1968;2:107,108.

118. Scandinavian Study Group. J Antimicrob Chemother 1993;31:949–961.

119. van den Wijngaart W, Verbrugh H, et al. A noncomparative study of cefprozil at two dose levels in the treatment of acute uncomplicated bacterial sinusitis. Clin Ther 1992;14:306–312.

120. Klossek JM. The use of oral ciprofloxacin (CIP) for the treatment of chromic ENT infections. An overview of French data. Presented at the 15th European Rhinological Congress. Copenhagen, June 19–23, 1994.

121. George DL, Falk PS, Nunally K, et al. Nosocomial sinusitis in medical intensive care unit (MICU) patients: a prospective epidemiologic study (abstract 13). Presented at the Second Annual Meeting of the Society of Hospital Epidemiologists of America. Baltimore MD, 1992.

122. Holzapfel L, Chevret S, Madinier G, Ohen F, Demingeon G, Coupry A, Chaudet M. Influence of long-term oro- or nasotracheal intubation on nosocomial maxillary sinusitis and pneumonia: results of a prospective, randomized, clinical trial. Crit Care Med 1993;21:1132–1338.

123. Deutschman CS, Wilton P, Sinow J, Dibbell D, Konstantinides FN, Cerra FB. Crit Care Med 1986;14: 111–114.

124. O'Donnell JG, Sorbello AF, Condoluci DV, Barnish MJ. Sinusitis due to Pseudomonas aeruginosa in patients with human immunodeficiency virus infection. Clin Infect Dis 1993;16:404–406.

8   Diagnosis and Medical Management of Recurrent and Chronic Sinusitis in Children

Sheldon C. Siegel, MD

CONTENTS

INTRODUCTION

Although the precise incidence of acute, recurrent, or chronic sinusitis in children has not been established, it is a very common problem in children because of their increased susceptibility to upper respiratory infections (URIs), which are frequently complicated by bacterial infections. Allergic rhinitis is another common disorder in children, and has also been implicated as a frequent predisposing factor for the development of recurrent or persistent sinusitis. Furthermore, because the symptoms of allergic disorders and sinus disease are similar, the diagnosis of one or the other will often be overlooked or misdiagnosed.

From: *Diseases of the Sinuses* (M. E. Gershwin and G. A. Incaudo, eds.), ©1996 Humana Press Inc., Totowa, NJ.

In an attempt to define better the prevalence of sinus disease, my associates and I prospectively evaluated 70 children, 3–16 yr of age, referred for an allergic evaluation *(1)*. In addition to a complete history and physical examination, laboratory tests, and skin tests, all patients had Water's (upright) and Caldwell (posteroanterior) sinus X-rays taken. A high prevalence of abnormal sinus X-rays was found; 37 subjects (53%) demonstrated some abnormality, with 15 (21%) having complete opacification of one or more maxillary sinus cavities. In a later study of 91 children referred for symptoms of persistent cough, chronic rhinorrhea, fatigue, and irritability, Shapiro *(2)* reported similar findings in that 64 (70%) were diagnosed as having sinusitis, which resolved when treated with antibiotics.

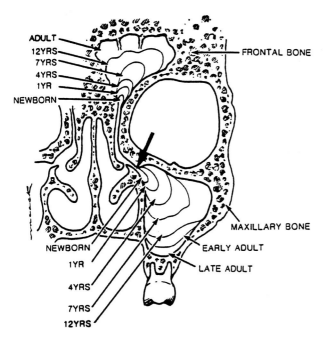

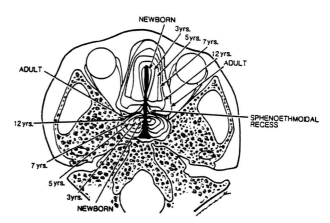

Fig. 1. Composite drawing in coronal projection shows temporal and morphologic changes that occur from birth to maturity during development of maxillary and frontal sinuses. Wide arrow shows ethmoidal infundibulum from which the maxillary sinus develops in an inferolateral direction. Reproduced by permission from Scuderi et al. *(3).*

Fig. 2. Composite drawing in axial projection shows temporal and morphologic changes from birth to maturity that occur during development of ethmoidal and sphenoidal sinuses. Reproduced by permission from Scuderi et al. *(3).*

PARANASAL SINUS DEVELOPMENT AND PHYSIOLOGY

The paranasal sinuses develop as outpouchings from the lateral walls of the nasal cavity and are lined with mucous membranes that are continuous with the lining of the nasal cavity. The maxillary and ethmoid sinuses form during the third and fourth month of gestation. During fetal life, they gradually enlarge and are readily visible radiographically at the time of birth. Although the frontal and sphenoidal sinuses also develop during gestation, they remain rudimentary for several years. The sphenoid sinuses begin to pneumatize about 3 yr of age. The frontal sinuses pneumatize later around 5–8 yr of age, but may remain hypoplastic until adulthood. However, the sphenoid sinuses are often not radiographically visible until the ninth year of life and the frontal sinuses before the fifth to seventh year of life. In Figs. 1 and 2, composite drawings of the growth of the sinuses from birth to maturity are shown. It is important to be aware that there is a great deal of variation in the shape and size of the sinuses at all ages. Rarely, development of the maxillary sinus, the most fre-

quently infected sinus in children, suddenly stops, producing a small sinus lumen (which is normally round and approx 4 mm at the sinus and 1 cm in length). Agenesis of the sinus may occur; its opaque appearance radiographically makes it difficult to differentiate from inflammatory sinus disease.

The ostia of the paranasal sinuses are always located at the sties of the embryonic evaginations from the nasal chamber. The drainage ostium for the maxillary, frontal, and anterior ethmoid sinuses is a tortuous channel about 6 mm long coursing from the maxillary sinuses through the anterior ethmoid sinuses to the middle meatus. This channel has been called the osteomeatal complex. In several parts of the osteomeatal complex, two mucosal layers come into close contact with one another, thus making it especially prone to obstruction (*see* Fig. 3). Secretions are retained leading to an increased risk of infection. The maxillary sinus is particularly prone to infection. Because the ostium of the maxillary sinus is located high up on the superior portion of the sinus, the cilia must beat and carry secretions against gravity into the nose. In contrast, the ostia of the ethmoidal, frontal, and sphenoid sinuses are located inferiorly, so drainage is aided by gravity.

PREDISPOSING FACTORS

Proper functioning of the sinuses depends on three key factors:

1. The patency of the ostia;
2. Normal ciliary function; and
3. The quality and quantity of secretions *(5).*

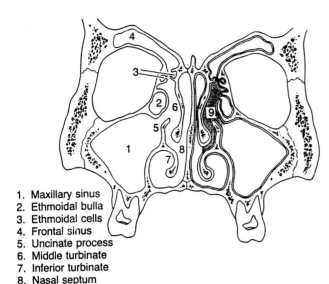

1. Maxillary sinus
2. Ethmoidal bulla
3. Ethmoidal cells
4. Frontal sinus
5. Uncinate process
6. Middle turbinate
7. Inferior turbinate
8. Nasal septum
9. Osteomeatal complex

Fig. 3. Coronal section of the nose and sinuses showing the nose and paranasal sinuses. Shaded area depicts the osteomeatal complex. Reproduced by permission from Wald *(4)*.

A number of medical and environmental conditions associated with impaired sinus function or immunity may also predispose to sinusitis. These factors, along with those causing obstruction of the ostia, are shown in Table 1. Although many conditions lead to obstruction of the ostia in children, URIs and allergic inflammation are the two most frequent causes.

Persistent obstruction of the sinus ostium ultimately leads to a negative intranasal pressure and congestion *(7)*. The negative pressure relative to atmospheric pressure may allow the introduction of bacteria into the sinus cavity. In addition, the altered intranasal pressure from sniffing, sneezing, and nose blowing increases the likelihood that pathogens can be introduced from the nasal cavity into the sinus cavity. Because of nasal congestion and obstruction of the sinus ostia, the sinus cavity becomes a relatively anaerobic site, which favors the growth of bacterial pathogens.

Disorders of mucociliary function are another important factor in causing sinus disease. The epithelium of the posterior two-thirds of the nasal cavity and sinuses are lined by ciliated columnar cells coated by a mucous layer. The normal motility of the cilia and adhesive properties of the mucous layer usually protect the sinuses from bacterial infection. Rare congenital defects of the cilial struc-

| Table 1 |
| Conditions Predisposing or Associated with Sinusitis |

Systemic diseases
  Viral URIs
  Allergic rhinitis and asthma
  Cystic fibrosis
  Aspirin and nonsteroidal anti-inflammatory drug
  Intolerance
  Immune disorders
    IgA deficiency
    Hypogammaglobulinemia
    Ataxia telangiectasia
    Human immunodeficiency virus infection
    Other
  Immotile cilia syndrome
  Down's syndrome
Local factors
  Mechanical obstruction
    Nasal polyps
    Choanal atresia
    Septal deviations
    Foreign bodies
    Tumors
      Benign
      Malignant
    Ethmoid bullae
    Hypertrophied adenoids
  Dental infection
  Trauma
    Facial fractures
    Oroantral fistula
    Barotrauma
  Swimming, diving
  Rhinitis medicamentosa
  Cold, dry air

[a]Modified from ref. *6*.

ture, such as occur with the immotile cilial syndrome, cause ciliary dysfunction with impaired secretion clearance. More often, the abnormal mucociliary transport is impaired by viral infections, cold or dry air, persistent use of topical decongestants, or by thick, tenacious purulent material from actively infected sinuses.

Abnormalities in both the quantity and quality of the mucous layer also affect sinus function. Kaliner *(8)* has recently summarized important roles and functions of human nasal secretions. He divided these functions in three categories: first, the mucus by coating the extracelluary surfaces protects the mucous membranes via humidification of inspired air, lubrication of the surface, waterproofing by trapping the aqueous layer beneath it, insulation, antioxidant (uric acid) activity, and by providing a proper medium for ciliary action. Second, the secretions provide barrier functions by acting as a macromolecular sieve, entrapping microorganisms and particulates, and transporting them for elimination. Finally, the secretions have important host-defense functions. The nasal secretions provide antimicrobial functions through the immunoglobulins (mainly IgA and IgG), other antimicrobial proteins, such as lysozyme and lactoferrin, secreted by the serous cells of the submucosal glands, and other antimicrobial plasma proteins that are deployed when processes, such as infection, lead to increase microvascular permeability.

UPPER RESPIRATORY INFECTIONS

There are several conditions that especially predispose children to chronic and recurrent sinusitis. Foremost among these factors are recurrent URIs, which occur more frequently in children under 5 yr of age (usually on the average of 6–8/yr) than in adults. It has been estimated that 5–10% of these infections are complicated by acute or chronic sinusitis and/or otitis media *(4)*. Young children who are cared for at day-care centers have an even greater incidence of URIs than children taken care of at home *(9,10)*. Although Wald et al. *(9)* did not investigate the incidence of sinusitis in their prospective study of the frequency and severity of infections in day care vs home care, it is of interest that 21% of children in day care required myringotomy and tube placement for recurrent acute middle ear disease and persistent effusion, whereas only 3% of the children in home care had to undergo this procedure. In a later study, Wald et al. *(11)*, using the clinical marker of acute sinusitis as "a history of respiratory symptoms lasting more than 10 days and not improving," which they had previously shown was associated with significant abnormal sinus radiographs in 88% of 2–6-yr-old children, found that nearly twice as many children had sinusitis in a day-care compared to a home-care setting. In investigating the cause of recurrent or chronic sinusitis in children, one must inquire whether the child attends day care, since this may be a major reason for recurrent respiratory infections and complicating sinusitis and/or otitis.

The mechanisms whereby the URIs frequently result in sinusitis relate to the edematous obstruc-tion of the sinus ostia and a decrease in the paranasal sinus ciliary action. As a consequence, there is an accumulation of mucus in the sinuses followed by secondary bacterial infection and conversion of mucus to mucopus. Mucopus further impairs ciliary function and increases the swelling around the ostia. Persistence of symptoms of URI for more than a week or two should alert one to suspect there is a bacterial infection of the paranasal sinuses.

ALLERGIC INFLAMMATION

Another common cause of chronic or recurrent sinusitis in both children and adults is an underlying allergic rhinitis. As with viral URIs, the IgE-mediated hypersensitivity involvement of the nasal mucous membranes produces inflammation, edema, and increases seromucous secretions that obstruct the sinus ostia and in turn lead to a secondary bacterial sinusitis. In our own study of 70 children referred for allergic rhinitis and/or asthma, 53% of the children had abnormal radiographs and 27% had opacification of one or both maxillary sinuses *(1)*. Certainly when any child has recurrent or chronic sinusitis, one should consider that the child may have an allergic rhinitis contributing to the chronicity of the problem.

IMMUNODEFICIENCY

Although less commonly encountered as a cause of recurrent or chronic sinus infections, the possibility that the sinusitis may be associated with an immunodeficiency is frequently overlooked. Deficiency in humoral or cell-mediated immunity, phagocyte disorders, or complement deficiencies, or a combination of these immunologic defects may predispose to sinus infections *(12)*. Signs and symptoms vary in these children. They may be similar to those encountered in the immunocompetent patient, but more often they are more severe and persistent. The immunodeficiencies most commonly associated with chronic sinusitis are the antibody deficiency states—Brutons X-linked congenital aggammaglobulinemia, common variable immunodeficiency, IgG subclass deficiency, and selective IgA deficiency. These patients are more likely to have infections with pyogenic bacteria with polysaccharide capsules, such as *Streptococcus pneumoniae, Haemophilus influenzae, Pseudomonas,* or *Neisseria meningitidis.*

Patients with primary abnormal cell-mediated immunodeficiencies, or secondary immunodeficiencies from corticosteroids, immunosuppressive, and cytotoxic drugs, or malignancies, are more susceptible to fungal, viral, and parasitic pathogens, such as *Pneumocystis carinii*. Pediatric HIV infections are increasing in frequency and are recognized as another cause of recurrent bacterial infections, including chronic sinusitis *(13)*. Unusual pathogens, such as *Pseudomonas* species, *Klebsiella* species, fungus, and protozoa, in addition to usual pathogens found in the immune competent patient, are commonly isolated in these patients.

CYSTIC FIBROSIS

Cystic fibrosis is a common cause of chronic pansinusitis and nasal polyps in children. Nasal polyps are rarely found in children, but occur in up to 12% of children with cystic fibrosis *(14)*. Whenever observed in a child, a sweat chloride should be performed to rule out this disease. Persistent opacification of sinuses in children also warrants a sweat test. Ledesma-Medina et al. *(15)* in a review of 187 cystic fibrosis patients found that 185 patients consistently had homogeneously opaque maxillary and ethmoid sinuses. Frequently, patients initially become infected with *Staphylococcus aureus* and *H. influenzae*. Subsequently, infectious organisms include *Escherichia coli, Klebsiella pneumoniae,* and almost always with progression of the disease, *Pseudomonas aeruginosa* and *Ps. cepaccia* pathogens predominate *(16)*.

DIAGNOSIS

The diagnosis of acute or chronic sinusitis in the pediatric age group, especially in infants and young children, may be difficult. In contrast to adults and adolescents, the commonly recognized symptoms of facial pain, headache, and fever are often absent. In the younger age groups, these complaints and findings are more subtle and nonspecific. In infants, irritability may be the only symptom.

In a study of 30 children who had upper respiratory tract symptoms, abnormal maxillary radiographic, and positive bacteriologic findings, Wald et al. found that cough, nasal discharge, and fetid breath were the most common signs, but fever was present inconsistently and low grade *(17)*. Facial pain or swelling and headache were the only prominent symptoms in older children.

Table 2
Clinical Diagnosis of Sinusitis[a]

Signs and symptoms
Major criteria
Purulent drainage
Purulent pharyngeal drainage
Cough
Minor criteria
Periorbital edema[b]
Headache[c]
Facial pain[c]
Tooth pain[c]
Earache
Sore throat
Foul breath
Increased wheeze
Fever
Diagnostic tests
Major criteria
Water's radiograph with opacification, air–fluid level, or thickened mucosa filling ≥50% of antrum
Coronal CT scan with thickening of mucosa or opacification of sinus
Minor criteria
Nasal cytologic study (smear) with neurophils and bacteremia
Ultrasound studies
Probable sinusitis
Signs and symptoms: 2 major criteria or 1 major and ≥2 minor criteria
Diagnostic tests: 1 major = confirmatory, 1 minor = supportive

CT, Computed tomography.
[a]Reproduced with permission from ref. *18*.
[b]More common in children.
[c]More common in adults.

Persistence of viral URI beyond the usual course of 5–7 d should suggest that a child has acute sinusitis. Nasal discharge can vary from grossly purulent to clear and thin. A dry or productive cough is often present during the day, but is usually worse at night. Postnasal drainage associated with frequent throat clearing or sore throat is also commonly observed.

Recently, Shapiro and Rachelefsky *(18)* proposed a schema for making the diagnosis of sinusitis based on major and minor signs and symptoms and diagnostic tests *(see* Table 2). They proposed that the presence of two major criteria (rhinorrhea, postnasal drip, and cough), or one major and two or more minor criteria (positive nasal cytology, ultrasound) for more than 7 d is highly likely to signify acute sinus disease, which is usually bacterial. If the signs and symptoms fulfill these criteria, the presence of one positive major diagnostic test is confirmatory, whereas the minor tests may be considered supportive.

ACUTE VS CHRONIC SINUSITIS

Depending on the duration of symptoms and signs, sinusitis has been arbitrarily divided into three categories; acute, subacute, and chronic *(19)*. In acute sinusitis, symptoms are present for < 3–4 wk and the patients usually have fever, purulent rhinorrhea, and other symptoms that are more severe than those observed with subacute or chronic sinusitis. Subacute sinusitis has been defined as disease with symptoms and signs lasting 4 wk to 3 mo. It is generally agreed that chronic sinusitis refers to disease lasting more than 3 mo.

In evaluating the patient with sinus disease, it is important to keep these different categories in mind, since the presenting symptoms and signs as well as the etiologic pathogens vary with the duration of the sinus disease and the age of the patient. Obviously, there is a continuum of symptoms and signs that makes the differentiation between acute and chronic somewhat arbitrary. Cough and rhinorrhea are almost always present in both acute and chronic disease, but are more likely to be present with more severe disease as determined by computed tomography (CT) scan *(20)*. On the other hand, fever, periorbital or facial swelling with or without sinus tenderness, or malodorous breath are less likely to be present in chronic than in acute sinusitis.

PHYSICAL FINDINGS

Unfortunately, the physical examination does not help very much in evaluating the extent of the inflammation of the sinuses in children. The mucosa is usually erythematous and boggy, and the throat may also be inflamed. Mucopurulent secretions along the nasal floor and/or crusting of the nasal passages may be observed. It is often helpful, after removing mucopurulent secretions for the nose, to apply a topical vasoconstrictor to the nasal mucosal for better visualization of the middle turbinate. The presence of purulent material in the middle meatus strongly suggests that diagnosis of sinusitis. Examination of the oropharynx may reveal purulent drainage and enlarged and inflamed tonsils. Usually cervical lymph nodes are not significantly enlarged or tender. Occasionally, in older children, facial tenderness can be detected when palpating or percussing over the paranasal sinuses. With chronic sinusitis, dark periorbital shiners and edema may be evident as a consequence of upper airway congestion impinging on normal venous and lymphatic drainage. This appearance can be intensified with lack of sleep from nighttime paroxysmal coughing. Because up to 50% of children with sinusitis have associated eustachian tube dysfunction complicated by middle ear effusions or acute otitis media, the middle ear should be carefully examined *(21–24)*.

DIAGNOSTIC PROCEDURES

When signs and symptoms suggest a diagnosis of acute, subacute, or chronic sinusitis, the following procedures may be helpful in confirming the diagnosis.

Imaging

Despite abnormal sinus radiographs being the most reliable method for confirming the diagnosis of sinusitis in children with respiratory symptoms, there remains much controversy as to the reliability of radiographic sinus abnormalities being diagnostic for sinus disease. Even in Caffey's latest ninth edition of *Pediatric X-ray Diagnosis (25)*, the author states that most pediatric radiologists are wary of making the diagnosis in children under 5 yr of age. On the other hand, pediatricians, otolaryngologists, and allergists place considerable significance on the radiographic findings when signs of URI or reactive airway disease are present.

The reasons for these differences of opinion relate to the frequent finding of similar abnormal radiographic findings occurring in apparently healthy children. For example, Diament et al. *(26)*, in reviewing CT cranial scans undertaken for complaints that would not warrant sinus films, found high rates of maxillary opacification. In another study by Kuhn *(27)*, almost 50% of children whose skulls were examined by magnetic resonance imaging (MRI) for other indicated reasons had mucosal thickening in the sinuses as an incidental finding. Glasier et al. *(28)*, in a similar study, evaluated the incidence and significance of radiographic sinus opacification in 100 infants from birth to 12 mo. CT was performed for indications other than sinusitis. Of the 100 infants, 70 had CT sinus opacification, including 67% of those without historical or physical evidence of URI. On the basis of their findings, the authors concluded the radiographic sinus opacification in infants is of uncertain significance and is not diagnostic of sinusitis. Lesserson et al. *(29),* on the basis of their findings, came to the same conclusion.

On the other hand, Kovatch et al. *(30),* in a study to determine also the frequency of abnormal sinus radiographs in unselected children having skull radiographs performed for indications unrelated to respiratory infections, although confirming that abnormal maxillary sinus radiographs were common in children <1 yr of age, found that children older than 1 yr of age infrequently had abnormal maxillary sinus radiographs and, when present, were generally related to inflammation of the upper respiratory tract. Arruda et al. *(31),* in a study of 33 children undergoing surgery for tonsil and adenoid enlargement without a previous diagnosis of sinusitis, were found to have preoperatively complete radiologic opacification of their maxillary sinuses. Puncture of maxillary sinuses was performed and aspirates cultured for pathogens. Seventy percent of those children with maxillary opacification were found to have a significant bacterial infection despite the fact that a diagnosis of maxillary sinusitis had not been considered prior to surgery.

Although done in 31 adults, the results of a recent study by Gwaltney and his coworkers *(32)* using CT scans have shown that the common cold is associated with frequent and variable anatomical involvement of the upper airways, including occlusion and abnormalities in the sinus cavities. After 2 wk, the CT studies were repeated in 14 subjects, none of whom had received antibiotics, and the abnormalities in the infundibula and sinuses had cleared or were markedly improved. Though no similar study has been done in children, it would seem likely that similar findings would be found. Thus, it would seem prudent not to treat patients simply on the appearance of the sinus radiographs or CT scans, but to correlate the abnormal findings with the recent or recurrent clinical symptoms of respiratory infection and to also classify the degree of abnormality of the radiographic findings.

Despite the controversy surrounding the significance of abnormal sinus radiographs as being indicative of sinusitis, my associates and I are convinced of the value of this diagnostic technique in

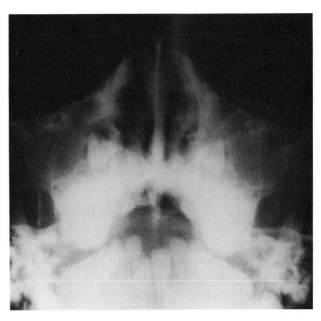

Fig. 4. Water's view of a 13-yr-old cystic fibrosis patient with pansinusitis.

making the diagnosis of sinusitis in children over one yr of age. Significant abnormalities include opacification, air–fluid levels, or mucoperiosteal thickening filling greater than a third of the antrum or >3-mm thickness. In children with the above findings and with symptoms suggestive of acute or subacute sinusitis, Wald et al. *(33)* noted positive bacterial aspirates in 80 and 65%, respectively.

The three widely available diagnostic imaging techniques are the sinus radiograph, CT, and MRI scans. Although the sinus radiograph is safe and rather economical, some authors have questioned its accuracy *(34).* The CT scan is considered "gold standard" for providing images of the sinuses and the best means of making an accurate diagnosis of sinusitis *(35).* However, it has two drawbacks: (1) the amount of radiation exposure and (2) its cost. Recently with the availability of the limited sinus CT, both the amount of radiation and cost have been materially reduced without compromising the reliability of the procedure *(20).* A Water's view of a patient with pansinusitis is shown in Fig. 4, and a CAT scan of this same patient is shown in Fig. 5.

Although the sensitivity of a single Water's view plain radiograph is low and significant, sinus pathology can exist in the absence of maxillary disease; nevertheless, they remain the initial imaging study of choice for children because of the limita-

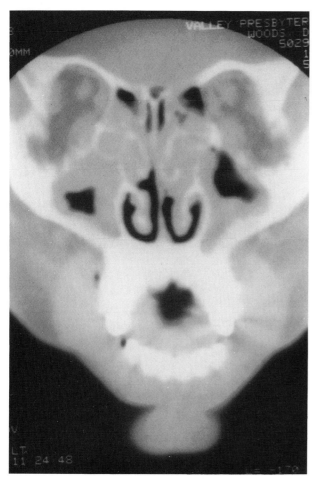

Fig. 5. CAT scan of same patient.

tions of performing CT scans in this age group. It should be kept in mind that it is not universally necessary to perform imaging studies to make the diagnosis of sinusitis in children. If surgery becomes necessary after failure of medical therapy, coronal CT scans are necessary irrespective of the child's age *(36)*. MRI scans are the best technique for evaluating intraorbital or intracranial extension of sinus disease. Because of their cost and technical difficulty in performing MRI scans, they are rarely indicated for the evaluation of sinusitis in children.

Transillumination

Although transillumination has been considered by some to be helpful in older children and adults in diagnosing maxillary and frontal disease, in general, the procedure has been shown to be of limited value in young children. The clinical usefulness of transillumination in children is limited by the thickness of both the soft tissues and bony vault, and

lack of patient cooperation in a dark room. Otten and Grote *(37)* in a study of 52 children between 3 and 9 yr of age with radiographic evidence of maxillary sinusitis, performed preoperative transillumination and compared the results to the drainage findings from a maxillary puncture. They concluded from their results that there is a poor correlation with a positive sinus puncture and considered the transillumination to be an obsolete method for evaluating sinusitis in young children. Even in adults, there is poor intraobserver consistency and the ethmoid and sphenoid sinuses cannot be evaluated *(38)*.

Ultrasound

Sinus ultrasonography has also been found to be of limited value in diagnosing sinusitis, and is only useful if the sinuses show a fluid level or are completely opaque on radiologic examination. However, there are several advantages of ultrasonography:

1. There is no ionizing radiation;
2. It is inexpensive;
3. It has a rapid test time; and
4. Repetitive studies can be performed on the same individual to assess response to treatment.

Studies from the Scandinavian countries have reported a high correlation between positive echoes on ultrasonography and the presence of fluid on maxillary antral puncture *(39–41)*.

These same groups of investigators from Finland in a later study concluded that the initial diagnosis of pediatric maxillary sinusitis in patients older than 3 yr, the reliability of combined sonography, and physical examination compared favorably with Water's view radiography and proved useful for followup resolution of the sinusitis by reflecting a return to normality quicker than radiography *(42)*. On the other hand, Shapiro et al. *(43)*, in comparing Water's view radiographs with ultrasonography in a mainly pediatric population (median age of 10 yr), found the sensitivity and specificity of ultrasound were only 50–60%. In our own studies of 99 adult subjects, we found that both instruments had high specificities in the diagnosis of maxillary sinusitis, but the sensitivities for both were low *(44)*. We also concluded that the ultrasound is of limited value in diagnosing mucosal thickening. In a more recent study comparing CT with A-mode ultrasonography and standard radiography, Pfister et al. *(45)* concluded that A-mode ultrasonography is not suitable for initial screening of patients for sinus disease, but may prove helpful as a follow-up in selected patients. Further studies, especially in children, are necessary before ultrasound is routinely used as a diagnostic tool. Its greatest value relates to its noninvasive nature and its usefulness for serially following an already diagnosed patient with sinusitis.

Rhinoscopy

In older children and adults, fiberoptic rhinoscopy with a flexible endoscope enables one to obtain a detailed examination of the upper nasal cavities, posterior nasopharynx, and sinus ostia. Direct visualization of mucopurulent secretions exuding from the sinus ostia confirms the diagnosis of sinusitis. Unfortunately, complete patient cooperation is required, and success with rhinoscopic examination in children is rarely successful.

Nasal Cytology

Examination of nasal cytology can often provide clues as to the etiology of chronic respiratory symptoms in both children and adults. A large number of polymorphonuclear cells (PMNs), especially with intracellular bacteria, is a frequent finding in patients with sinusitis *(46)*. Although PMNs may predominate during a viral URI, their presence in large numbers in profuse rhinorrhea of several weeks duration suggests sinusitis. Staining the smear with Hansel's stain will enable one to identify eosinophils easily. When present in a concentration >10%, a diagnosis of allergic rhinitis is most likely since nonallergic eosinophilic rhinitis is rare in children. During an acute or chronic sinusitis, eosinophils are temporarily replaced by PMNs, and on recovery from the infection, eosinophils again become evident if the patient has an underlying allergic rhinitis. Although admittedly in only a small series of patients, we observed this reversal of cytological findings of PMN predominance, bacteria pretreatment, and eosinophilia predominance posttreatment in 12 children with chronic maxillary sinusitis confirmed by antral cultures and serial Water's view roetgenograms *(47)*. It should be kept in mind that absence of neither PMNs nor eosinophils in nasal secretions precludes the need for further evaluation of the patient when other signs and symptoms suggest allergic rhinitis or sinusitis.

Sinus Aspiration

Maxillary sinus aspiration is rarely necessary in the pediatric age group for diagnostic or therapeutic purposes. It can be safely performed in an ambulatory setting by a skilled otolaryngologist using a transnasal approach *(17)*. However, sedation or general anesthesia is usually required in young children. Current indications for maxillary sinus aspiration in an immunologic intact child include:

1. Failure to respond to multiple courses of antibiotics;
2. Severe facial pain; or
3. Orbital or intracranial complications.

A diagnostic sinus aspiration should also be considered in immunocompromised cystic fibrosis patients, and nosocomial sinusitis, where there is a high probability of recovering unusual organisms *(48,49)*. Material aspirated from the sinus should be cultured aerobically and anaerobically, and undergo Gram's staining. The recovery of bacteria in a density of at least 10^4 (CFU)/mL is considered significant in implicating a specific pathogen. Microbial sensitivity tests will help in choosing an appropriate antibiotic.

Microbiology

BACTERIA

Studies utilizing maxillary sinus lavage in children have consistently shown that the predominant organisms of acute and subacute sinusitis are *Streptococcus, pneumoniae*, nontypable *H. influenzae*, and *Moraxella catarrhalis* (formerly *Neisseria* and *Branhamella catarrhalis*) *(17,33,50)*. Although similar organisms have been found in adults with sinusitis, Gwaltney et al. *(51)* additionally recovered anaerobes in 7% and *Staphylococcus* species in 3% from 383 aspirates from 339 patients. Anaerobic organisms and *Staphylococci* should be suspected in pediatric patients who have long-standing symptoms or in those whose symptoms are so severe or complicated that sinus surgery is indicated.

Only a limited number of bacteriologic studies have been performed in pediatric patients with chronic sinusitis. Brook *(52)* cultured aspirates from 40 children for anaerobes and aerobes, and obtained growth in 37 patients. Anaerobic organisms were recovered from all of these patients. The predominant organisms were *Bacteroides*,

Table 3
Fungal Sinusitis Syndromes[a]

Disease	Host	Course	Histopathology	Concurrent lung disease	Treatment	Prognosis
Indolent fungal sinusitis	Immunocompetent	Chronic	Granulomatous reaction; acute and chronic inflammation	None	Surgery with or without antifungal therapy	Excellent after surgical resection
Invasive fungal sinusitis	Immunocompromised	Acute	Necrosis; mycelia invasion of vessels	Common	Surgery plus antifungal therapy	Poor
Mycetoma	Immunocompetent, with previous sinus disease, trauma, or foreign body	Chronic	Mycelial mass ("fungal ball")	None	Surgery with or without antifungal therapy	Excellent after surgical resection
Allergic fungal sinusitis	Immunocompetent, with nasal polyps, atopy, or asthma	Chronic	Allergic mucin	Occasional allergic broncho-pulmonary mycosis	Surgery and steroids	Good, but recurrence common

[a]Reproduced with permission from ref. 57.

gram-positive cocci, and *Fusobacterium* species. The predominant aerobic isolates were α-Hemolytic *streptococci, S. aureus,* and *Haemophilus* species. Because quantitative cultures of the sinus secretions were not performed, the results of this study have been questioned by Wald *(50).* In a more recent study, Muntz and Lusk *(53)* cultured the mucosa of the anterior ethmoid cells in 105 children with chronic sinusitis undergoing endoscopic ethmoidectomy. Anaerobic organisms were grown from 6% of the specimens. Because all of these children were treated with appropriate antibiotics until the day before surgery, their findings probably represent residual bacterial flora and organisms usually not etiologic in chronic sinusitis.

We also attempted to evaluate the bacteriology of chronic sinusitis *(47)* in 12 children, ages 3 to 9, with documented allergy and with opacification of one or both maxillary sinuses and chronic respiratory symptoms for 30 or more days. From maxillary sinus aspirations, *M. catarrhalis* was recovered from six patients, and mixed cultures of streptococci were recovered from three patients. Only one patient had anaerobic streptococci mixed with aerobic *streptococci.*

In summary, the usual bacterial isolates associated with sinusitis in children are: *S. pneumoniae, H. influenzae,* and *M. catarrhalis.* In contrast, anaerobic organisms and *staphylococci* should be suspected in severe or complicated sinusitis, and α *streptococci* in patients with pretreated symptoms.

FUNGI

Fungal sinusitis may present as an acute or chronic disorder in both children and/or adults who are immunocompetent and immunocompromised *(54,55).* Although in the immunocompetent patient fungal sinusitis is less common than bacterial sinusitis, it is very recognized increasingly as a cause of chronic sinusitis.

Fungal disease of the paranasal sinuses has been categorized into four distinct forms:

1. Chronic indolent sinusitis;
2. Invasive sinusitis;
3. Mycetoma; and
4. Allergic fungal sinusitis *(56).*

The clinical and histolopathologic features are unique for each form, as are the treatment modalities, as shown in Table 3.

Chronic indolent fungal sinusitis occurs primarily in healthy persons without associated pulmonary manifestations. The clinical presentation is usually that of chronic unilateral maxillary sinusitis resistant to medical therapy. Histopathology is characterized by a granulomatous inflammatory reaction with multinucleated giant cells. Mycelial elements can be identified by special fungal stains. Cultures usually reveal *Aspergillus fumigatus* and other *Aspergillus* species. Typically, these patients are not atopic and respond well to surgical debridement with or without antifungal therapy.

The invasive (or fulminant) fungal sinus infection is characterized histologically by fungal invasion and massive necrosis in mucosal and bony tissue, as well as corresponding vasculature. Typically, it occurs in immunocompromised hosts. Mortality rates are as high as 80%, despite aggressive surgical debridement and antifungal therapy.

Mycetoma is a rare form of a benign fungal sinusitis. Patients usually present with unilateral sinus symptoms and opacified radiographs. Usually patients are healthy and nonatopic. Histologic examination reveals a tangled mass of fungi with little inflammatory reaction. Surgical debridement and aeration cure most patients.

Allergic fungal sinusitis is a relatively newly described clinical entity that is more likely to be encountered in an allergic practice, and is common in the pediatric age group and young adults. Most of the patients have a history of chronic symptomatic rhinosinusitis for months to years, asthma, nasal polyp disease, and roentgenographic evidence of multiple opacified paranasal sinuses. The diagnosis is confirmed histologically by the absence of tissue invasion, distinctive mucinous material containing eosinophils, Charcot-Leyden crystals, cellular debris, and scattered fungal hyphae. Culture results from most cases have revealed *Aspergillus* species, but other fungi—Bipolar, *Exserohilium, Curvularia*, and *Alternaria*—have been implicated as the causative organism (54,58). Most patients tested display positive immediate and late-phase hypersensitivity skin test responses to the pathogenic fungi. Elevated levels of serum fungal IgE and IgG may be found, although usually not to the markedly elevated degree as noted with bronchopulmonary aspergillosis. Peripheral eosinophilia also is usually present. Optimal therapy for allergic fungal sinusitis consists of surgical removal of impacted debris and restoration of mucociliary drainage and ventilation. Daily or alternate-day systemic oral corticosteroids are frequently necessary along with the use of topical intranasal corticosteroids. The issue of antifungal therapy for allergic fungal sinusitis has not been resolved.

Medical Management

The treatment of acute or chronic sinus disease in children should be aimed at promoting drainage, controlling infection, and providing symptomatic relief.

ADJUNCTIVE THERAPY

Decongestants. To improve nasal and sinus ostial patency and to facilitate drainage from the sinus cavities, various agents have been recommended for the management of sinusitis. Oral and/or topical decongestants have been frequently prescribed, but their use remains controversial. Melen et al. (59) demonstrated in adults that the use of oral phenylpropanolamine increased 30–50% the functional diameter of the maxillary sinus ostium. On the other hand, Aust et al. (60), in a study of 20 adult patients with acute sinusitis, were unable to find any differences in symptoms or side effects when comparing the effects of phenylpropanolamine to a placebo. In our own double-blind study evaluating the role of antimicrobials with an antihistamine decongestant combination (carbinoxamine maleate-pseudoephedrine HCl) in 84 children with chronic sinusitis, we demonstrated that the chronic respiratory symptoms were likely to respond clinically and radiographically with antimicrobial therapy, but not to the antihistamine-decongestant combination (61). Oral decongestants are not always well tolerated. Side effects of hyperactivity and insomnia are common in children, whereas hypertension and inhibition of micturition occurs more often in adults.

Topical decongestant use should be limited to a 3–5-d course to achieve decongestion early in the treatment course. Patients should be advised that use of these agents beyond this time limitation will lead to rebound edema of the nasal mucosa and the possible development of rhinitis medicamentosa. Theoretically, topical decongestants, being vasoconstrictors, may worsen disease by decreasing blood flow and, in turn, decreasing local tissue delivery of antibiotics and potentially creating a worsening anaerobic environment. There are no published controlled studies evaluating either the short-term use of topical decongestants or the long-term use of oral decongestants for the prevention or treatment of recurrent or chronic sinusitis.

Antihistamines. The use of antihistamines for the treatment of sinusitis has been controversial. Because the anticholinergic properties of the first-generation antihistamines may lead to reduced nasal secretions and to drying and inspissation of sinus contents, some physicians have advocated that they be avoided in the treatment of sinusitis. However, if an underlying allergic rhinitis is contributing to frequent recurrences or to chronic sinusitis, these agents may have a beneficial effect. In this instance, nonsedating antihistamines should be used owing to their lack of anticholinergic activity.

Anti-Inflammatory Agents. Theoretically, topical corticosteroids, because of their marked anti-inflammatory properties, might increase sinus ostial diameter by decreasing inflammation in the area of the sinus ostia. Several intranasal preparations are available commercially in the US. These include beclomethasone, triamcinolone, flunisolide, budesonide, and dexamethasone. Although these corticosteroids have variable anti-inflammatory activity, they are all highly effective in reducing airway inflammation and symptoms when used in the recommended doses for the treatment of patients with allergic rhinitis *(62)*. To date, there has been no evidence that these agents induce superinfection, encourage development of resistant organisms, or adversely affect mucociliary clearance of secretions. Recently, Meltzer and coworkers *(63)* reported the use of intranasal flunisolide compared to a placebo as an adjunctive treatment to a 3-wk course of amoxicillin/potassium clavulanate. Although the subjective global improvement assessment favored flunisolide, the objective improvement in sinus radiographs and symptoms after 3 wk was comparable in both groups. The flunisolide group also showed a reduced rate of recurrence after completion of antibiotic therapy. Additional studies to assess the value of topical corticosteroids, especially for the prevention or treatment of recurrent or chronic sinusitis, seem warranted. Similar investigations are needed to evaluate the use of bursts of systemic corticosteroids in refractory sinusitis and especially in patients with significant nasal polyposis.

Although less effective than topical corticosteroids in the treatment of allergic rhinitis, cromolyn sodium also has anti-inflammatory properties that could be of benefit in the treatment of chronic sinusitis. Because intranasal and inhaled cromolyn has been used extensively in children without any serious adverse effects, it would seem appropriate to use this preparation initially when treating infants and young children with chronic sinusitis. However, as is the case with corticosteroids, their use for this purpose has not been adequately evaluated and needs further study.

Saline Irrigation. Humidifying the patient's environment, irrigating with normal saline, and applying moist heat to the face several times a day may be helpful in providing symptomatic relief and aiding mucociliary function. Young children, however, are usually intolerant of any device, such as the Grossan's waterpik or bulb syringe, for nasal irrigation. Spray plastic bottles containing sterile saline are available in over-the-counter containers, and can be readily used in this younger age group for loosening and removing purulent secretions and crusts from the nasal passages.

Expectorants. Although guaifenesin frequently is advocated to thin secretions and thereby promotes improved mucociliary clearance, there are no controlled clinical trials proving its efficacy.

Antimicrobial Agents. The key to successful management of acute or chronic sinusitis is the use of a sufficient dosage of an appropriate antimicrobial agent administered for an adequate period of time. For acute sinusitis, 10–14 d of therapy are usually sufficient. Although clinical improvement occurs most often within a 3- to 4-d period, it is important that a full course of the agent be given. Patients responding more slowly or who have a history of recurrent or chronic sinusitis frequently require a more prolonged antimicrobial course of 3–6 wk. Insufficient duration of therapy is one of the common errors in treating patients with recurrent or chronic sinusitis. Because symptoms may transiently improve, therapy is often prematurely stopped, allowing the infection to continue and smolder, and finally results in an exacerbation at a later time.

The choice of antimicrobials is based on an appreciation of the bacteria generally responsible for the infection. In Table 4 are listed the antimicrobial agents, daily dosage, mg of drug/5 mL of its liquid preparation, and times per day the drug should be administered for the treatment of pediatric patients with sinusitis and their cost. In acute

Table 4
Dosage of Antimicrobial Agent for Pediatric Sinusitis

Generic name	Trade name	Dosage (mg/kg/24 h)	Liquid preparations (mg/5 mL)	Regimen (times/day)	Cost[a]
Amoxicillin	Generic Amoxil® (SKB)	40	125	tid	$6.02 $6.10
Amoxicillin (Potassium clavulate)	Augmentin® (SKB)	40–10 (over 40 kg adult dosage of 250 mg)	125	tid	$48.10
Erythromycin + sulfasoxazole	Generic Pediazole® (Ross A)	50–150	200–600	qid	$22.77 $30.08
Trimethoprim-sulfamethoxazole	Generic Bactrim® (Roche) Septra® (BW)	8–40	40–200	bid	$3.43 $12.83 $12.26
Cefaclor	Ceclor® (Lilly)	40	5	tid	$51.78
Cefuroxime axetil	Ceftin® (Glaxo)	30	125	bid	$128.58
Cefixime	Suprax® (Lederle)	8	100	qd or bid	$145.66
Loracarbef	Lorabid® (Lilly)	30	100 and 200	bid	$156.40
Clarithromycin	Biaxin® (Ross-A)	7.5	125	bid	$124.92
Cefprozil	Cefzil® (Bristol)	15	125, 250	bid	$45.59
Cefpodoxime	Vantin® (Upjohn)	10	50, 100	bid	$56.30

[a]Wholesale cost to pharmacist for 10-d treatment of a 15-kg child from *Red Book,* Feb. 1994.

and most cases of subacute and chronic sinusitis, as indicated in the section on microbiology, the predominant organisms are *S. pneumoniae, H. influenzae,* and *M. catarrhalis.* Wald *(4)* has recommended that amoxicillin be initially given to most cases of uncomplicated sinusitis in children, because it is effective most of the time, inexpensive, and safe. She felt that the latter consideration was important, since there is a high rate of spontaneous cure *(64).* Dohlman et al. *(65)* have also recently reported that in children with subacute sinusitis, there was a similar response to treatment with antimicrobials (amoxicillin, amoxicillin-clavulanate potassium, or trimethoprim-sulfamethoxazole) or with just a decongestant and saline spray for 3 wk. Otten and Grote *(66),* after comparing the use of amoxicillin in 141 children, drainage of the sinuses, combination of the two, or a placebo, concluded that maxillary sinusitis in children is a self-limiting disease and recommended a conservative approach to therapy. Additional factors to be considered in making the choice of an antimicrobial are the side effect profile, compliance considerations (dosing schedule and taste), and their likelihood for β-lactamase production as well as the resistance pattern in a given area.

Despite the spontaneous improvement that occurs in some patients with sinusitis and despite abnormal roentgen findings being frequently found in some asymptomatic individuals, the role of antimicrobial agents for the treatment of symptomatic patients with sinusitis has been firmly established. We evaluated the role of antimicrobial agents in the treatment of chronic maxillary sinusitis in allergic children *(61).* Eighty-four children were treated in a double-blind manner with either amoxicillin, erythromycin, trimethoprim-sulfamethoxazole, or an antihistamine/decongestant (carbonoxamine maleate-pseudoephedrine HCl). Radiographic and clinical response was best with amoxicillin, but tremethoprim-sulfamethoxazole was an adequate alternative. On the other hand, there was no improvement with either erythromycin or the antihistamine/decongestant. Wald *(4)* has summarized numerous other studies demonstrating the bacteriologic efficacy and/or cure of sinusitis in both adults and children with sinusitis.

The antimicrobial management of chronic sinusitis has not been as extensively examined as acute sinusitis, with very few studies of adults or children. Nevertheless, when a child's condition fails to respond to amoxicillin, a complication is present, or the sinusitis is recurrent, and then a broader-spectrum antimicrobial agent is indicated. The most comprehensive coverage of the pathogens involved in children are amoxicillin-clavulinate potassium, erythromycin sulfasoxazole, and the second- and third-generation cephalosporins.

Amoxicillin-clavulinate potassium has the advantage that it inhibits β-lactamase enzymes and thus enhances the spectrum of amoxicillin to include β-lactamase producing *H. influenzae, M. catarrhalis, S. aureus,* and many anaerobes. Cure rates of 82–87% have been reported with this agent. Unfortunately, it has the disadvantage of frequently causing abdominal cramping and diarrhea.

The combination of erythromycin and sulfasoxazole was designed to broaden the spectrum of antimicrobial activity rather than to provide syndergistic activity. This combination covers therapy for *S. pneumoniae, H. influenzae, M. catarrhalis,* and group *A. streptococcus,* the most common organisms causing otitis and sinusitis. Additionally, it is effective against chlamydia and *S. aureus.* Disadvantages of this combination are the need for administration four times a day and the frequent side effect of diarrhea.

The second- and third-generation cephalosporins are also useful agents for the treatment of both acute and chronic sinusitis. Cefaclor, a second-generation cephalosporin, has the disadvantage that some strains of *H. influenzae* and *M. catarrhalis* are resistant, and it is occasionally associated with serum-sickness-like reactions. Although the manufacturer claims that with higher doses the drug can be given twice a day, efficacy studies would suggest that it should preferably be given three times daily.

Another second-generation cephalosporin, cefuroxime, appears to have advantages over cefaclor. Both drugs are well absorbed orally, but intake of food actually increases absorption and bioavailability of cefuroxime. It is also more effective against β-lactamase-producing *H. influenzae* as well as *M. catarrhalis,* and has good coverage against *S. aureus* and *Pneumococcus.* Furthermore, it has a longer half-life so that it can be administered twice a day, and it has not been associated with an increased incidence of serum sickness. Recently, it has become available in a liquid form for administration to young children who cannot swallow tablets.

A third-generation cephalosporin, cefixime, has wider coverage against gram-negative organisms than first- and second-generation agents. It is more resistant than other cephalosporins to β-lactamases, but less effective against *Pneumococcus* and *S. aureus.* It has the major advantage of having to be administered orally once a day. Accordingly, cefixime should probably be best used in a child who has previously been treated with an antimicrobial that adequately covered *S. pneumococci.*

Recently, clarithromycin and azithromycin macrolide antibiotics with broad-spectrum coverage have been released. Both of these agents are better tolerated than erythromycin and have broader coverage. Only clarithromycin is available in a liquid form for the treatment of young children. Although clarithromycin has been shown to have some activity against *H. influenzae* and *M. catarrhalis,* it is most effective in sinusitis resulting from *S. pneumoniae.* Although reported to be effective in the treatment of acute maxillary sinusitis, further studies need to be performed to assess the value of these macrolide antibiotics for the treatment of sinusitis in children *(67).*

Loracarbef, a carbacephem class of β-lactam antibiotics, is being extensively evaluated for the treatment of bacterial respiratory infections. It has a good activity profile against a broad spectrum of pathogens that cause sinusitis, has relative stability to β-lactamase hydrolysis, and has a good safety profile. Foshee *(68)* compared loracarbef to amoxicillin-clavulanate in 475 children between the ages of 6 mo and 12 yr in the treatment of bacterial acute otitis media with effusion and found the two drugs to be comparable in efficacy. Two other studies comparing loracarbef to amoxicillin-clavulanate in the treatment of acute maxillary sinusitis in adult patients *(69)* also found the two antibiotics to be comparable in efficacy *(69,70).* Data reported to date that would suggest that loracarbef is going to be a useful agent in treating both acute and chronic sinusitis, but additional studies in children are necessary to assess its place in treating sinusitis in this younger age group.

As previously stated, children with recurrent or chronic sinusitis should be carefully evaluated for possible underlying disorders, such as allergic rhinitis, immunodeficiency, immobile cilial syndrome, cystic fibrosis, or anatomic abnormalities. When appropriate treatment for these disorders fails to alter the pattern of recurrent or chronic sinusitis, we have on occasion used antimicrobial prophylaxis. Although antimicrobial prophylaxis has not been studied in children with recurrent sinusitis, the favorable results in reducing recurrent bouts of otitis media would suggest that this modality of therapy would be useful in recurrent sinusitis *(71)*.

COMPLICATIONS

Although serious complications of acute or chronic sinusitis have become rare since the advent of antimicrobial agents, serious sequelae still occasionally occur that can lead to significant morbidity and rarely death *(72,73)*. Serious complications include orbital cellulitis, abscess formation, cavernous sinus thrombosis, meningitis, subdural empyema, and osteomyelitis. Orbital infection is the most common complication and is manifested by eye swelling, exophthalmos, and impaired eye movements. Intracranial complications are second in frequency to orbital complications. Signs and symptoms of an extradural or subdural abscess include headache, meningeal irritation, fever, somnolence, and seizures. Unexplained focal neurological signs may be the first indication of disease in the paranasal sinuses. In cases presenting as isolated nerve palsies, diseases of the sinuses must be excluded. Osteomyelitis usually occurs in the frontal sinus area because of the venous drainage into the diploic veins of the skull. Because the frontal sinuses are not well developed in children, it is not a problem until the frontal sinuses have become well developed in older children. A CAT scan is essential for the diagnosis of any serious complication of sinusitis, and antibiotic therapy and surgical drainage are usually required for their management.

Sinus infections frequently are complicated by lower respiratory tract infections and asthma *(74–77)*. We and others have observed several patients whose reactive airway disease was thought to occur secondary to chronic sinusitis *(78,79)*. We observed 48 children with "difficult to control" asthma markedly improve when they received adequate treatment for sinusitis. All were treated with antimicrobial agents for 2–5 wk. Thirty-nine children responded both clinically and radiologically. Antral lavage was required in 9 children, whereas 38 (39%) of the subjects were able to discontinue bronchodilators with resolution of their sinusitis. Although a direct cause-and-effect relationship of sinusitis and asthma has been questioned *(80)*, we recommend that sinus disease be

considered in all patients with moderately severe asthma and treated aggressively when it is identified. The mechanisms whereby the sinusitis links asthma are not clearly understood. The most plausible theories include exacerbation of asthma secondary to the presence of eosinophils and inflammatory mediators, or via the sinobronchial reflex *(81)*.

SURGICAL THERAPY

Surgical intervention for the treatment of chronic sinusitis in children is rarely necessary unless the course has been complicated by abscess formation requiring drainage. Before considering surgical intervention for refractory sinus disease, a judgment must be made that optimal and appropriate antimicrobial therapy has been administered. When a child has been deemed to have failed medical management and surgical intervention is being considered, a coronal CT scan should be performed to evaluate the extent and location of disease.

The use of sinus irrigation, as a modality of therapy rather than as a diagnostic tool to determine the offending pathogen, has been controversial. Some investigators have found that it is not significantly more effective than antibiotic therapy alone for chronic pediatric sinusitis *(82,83)*, whereas others have recommended it after failure to respond to multiple courses of antibiotics, for severe facial pain, and for orbital or intracranial complications *(4)*. Sedation or a general anesthetic is usually required for this procedure in younger children.

When adenoidal hypertrophy causes nasal obstruction, which is thought by some to predispose to sinusitis as well as otitis media, Takahashi et al. have claimed adenoidectomy to be effective treatment for chronic sinusitis *(84)*.

The surgical creation of nasal-antral windows (i.e., intranasal inferior meatus antrostomies) was performed in children with chronic maxillary sinusitis for many years without any documentation to support the procedure. Muntz and Lusk *(85)* in a retrospective study of pediatric sinusitis treated by nasal-antral windows and found only a 27% success rate after 6 mo. They concluded that their poor results were attributable to involvement of anterior ethmoid cells and that the procedure did not alter the normal mucociliary clearance function toward the natural middle meatus ostia.

The older Caldwell-Luc operation, frequently performed on adults in the past, although offering better access to diseased maxillary sinus tissue for debridement, has a complication rate that is substantially higher than the nasal-antral window procedure. This procedure has usually been avoided in children because of its potentially deleterious effect on developing tooth buds and facial growth. It is usually reserved for severe sinusitis with polyposis and for treating complications of sinusitis.

The technique of endoscopic sinus surgery, first introduced by Messerklinger (86) in Europe in the late 1970s has radically changed the nature of surgical intervention for chronic sinusitis. Endoscopic sinus surgery has the advantage of restoring the natural function of the sinus by minimal disruption of the sinus mucosa. The procedure is based on the assumption that the osteomeatal complex is the key area in the pathophysiologic development of chronic sinus disease. The orifices of the maxillary, ethmoid, and frontal sinuses open into the osteomeatal complex region, and even a small amount of chronic inflammation may obstruct these ostia. During surgery, the natural ostia of the maxillary and frontal sinuses may be reopened and enlarged to establish mucociliary clearance and ventilation. Several recent publications have reported favorable results from this surgical procedure performed in children with chronic sinusitis (87–90). Others have presented a more cautious and conservative view regarding the value of endoscopic surgery in children (91,92). Although endoscopic surgery for chronic sinusitis in children is promising, it requires expert knowledge and expertise, and should only be performed in those patients who have not responded to a prolonged trial of medical management. A final assessment of the value of this surgical approach in children with chronic sinusitis requires further study.

REFERENCES

1. Rachelefsky GS, Golberg M, Katz RM, Gyepes MT, Shapiro M, Mickey MR, Finegold SM, Siegel SC. Sinus disease in children with respiratory allergy. J Allergy Clin Immunol 1978;61:310–314.
2. Shapiro GG. Role of allergy in sinusitis. Pediatr Infect Dis 1985;4:55–58.
3. Scuderi AJ, Harnsberger HR, Boyer RS. Pneumatization of the paranasal sinuses: normal features of importance to the accurate interpretation of CT scans and MR images. AJR 1993;160:1101–1104.
4. Wald ER. Sinusitis in children. N Engl J Med 1992; 326:319–323.
5. Wald ER. Acute and chronic sinusitis: diagnosis and management. Pediatr Rev 1985;7:150–157.
6. Rachelefsky GS, Katz RM, Siegel SC. Diseases of paranasal sinuses in children. Cur Problems in Pediatr 1982;12:6–57.
7. Aust R, Falck B, Svanholm H. Studies of the gas exchange and pressure in the maxillary sinuses in normal and infected humans. Rhinology 1979;17:245–251.
8. Kaliner MA. Human nasal host defense and sinusitis. J Allergy Clin Immunol 1992;90:424–430.
9. Wald ER, Dashefsky B, Byers C, Guerra N, Taylor F. Frequency and severity of infections in day care. J Pediatr 1988;112:540–546.
10. Fleming DW, Cochi SL, Hightower MS, Broome CV. Childhood upper respiratory tract infections: to what degree is incidence affected by day-care attendance. Pediatrics 1987;79:55–60.
11. Wald ER, Guerra N, Byers C. Upper respiratory tract infections in young children: duration of an frequency of complications. Pediatrics 1991;87:129–133.
12. Reid TE, Shearer WT. Recurrent sinusitis and immunodeficiency. Immunol Allergy Clin North Am 1994; 14:143–169.
13. Hanson IC. Respiratory infections in HIV-infected children. Immunol Allergy Clinics North Am 1993;13:205.
14. Fitzsimmons SC. The changing epidemiology of cystic fibrosis. J Pediatr 1993;122:1–9.
15. Ledesma-Medina J, Osman MZ, Girdnay BR. Abnormal paranasal sinuses in patients with cystic fibrosis of the pancreas: radiologic findings. Pediatr Radiol 1980;9:61–64.
16. Wallace CS, Hall M, Kuhn RJ. Pharmacologic management of cystic fibrosis. Clin Pharm 1993;12:657–674.
17. Wald ER, Milmore GJ, Bowen A, Ledesma-Medina J, Salamon N, Bluestone CD. Acute maxillary sinusitis in children. N Engl J Med 1981;304:749–754.
18. Shapiro GG, Rachelefsky GS. Introduction and definition of sinusitis. J Allergy Clin Immunol 1992;90: 417,418.
19. Bluestone CB. The diagnosis and management of sinusitis in children. Proceedings of a closed conference. Pediatr Infect Dis J 1985;6(Suppl.):549–581.
20. Garcia DP, Corbett ML, Eberly SM, Joyce MR, Le HT, Karibo JM, Pence HL, Nguyen K. Radiographic imaging studies in pediatric chronic sinusitis. J Allergy Clin Immunol 1994;94:523–530.
21. Hoshaw TC, Nickman NJ. Sinusitis and otitis in children. Arch Otolaryngol 1974;100:194,195.
22. Cherry JD, Dudley JP. Sinusitis. In: Feizin RD, Cherry JD, eds. Pediatric Infectious Diseases. Philadelphia: WB Saunders, 1992; pp. 142–148.
23. Lazar RH, Younis RT, Gross CW. Pediatric functional endonasal surgery: review of 210 patients. Head Neck 1992;14:92–98.
24. Grote JJ, Kuijpers W. Middle ear effusion and sinusitis. J Larygol Otol 1980;94:177–183.
25. Silverman FN, Kuhn JP. Caffey's Pediatric X-ray Diagnosis. St. Louis, MO: Mosby-Year Book, 1993; pp. 75–90.
26. Diament MJ, Senac MO, Gilsanz V, Baker S, Gillespie T, Larsson S. Prevalence of incidental paranasal sinus opacification in pediatric patients. A CT Study. J Comput Assit Tomogr 1987;11:426–431.
27. Kihn JP. Imaging of the paranasal sinuses: current status. J Allergy Clin Immunol 1986;77:6–8.

28. Glasier CM, Mallory GB Jr, Steele RW. Significance of opacification of the maxillary and ethmoid sinuses in infants. J Pediatr 1989;114:45–50.

29. Lesserson JA, Kiesserman SP, Finn DG. The radiographic incidence of chronic sinus disease in the pediatric population. Laryngoscope 1994;104:159–166.

30. Kovatch AL, Wald ER, Ledesma-Medina J, Chiponis DM, Bedingfield B. Maxillary sinus radiographs in children with nonrespiratory complaints. Pediatrics 1984;73:306–308.

31. Arruda LK, Mimica IM, Sole D, Wecky LLM, Schoettler J, Heimer DC, Naspitz CK. Abnormal maxillary sinus radiographs in children. Do they represent bacterial infection? Pediatrics 1990;85:553–558.

32. Gwaltney JM, Phillips D, Miller RD, Riker DK. Computed tomographic study of the common cold. N Engl J Med 1994;330:25–30.

33. Wald ER, Byers C, Guerra N, Casselbrant M, Beste D. Subacute sinusitis in children. J Pediatr 1989;115:28–32.

34. McAlister WH, Lusk R, Muntz HR. Comparison of plain radiographs and coronal CT scans in infants and children with recurrent sinusitis. AJR 1989;153:1259–1264.

35. Lazar RH, Younis RT, Parvey LS. Comparison of plain radiographs, coronal CT, and intraoperative findings in children with chronic sinusitis. Otolaryngol Head Neck Surg 1992;107:29–34.

36. April MM, Zinreich SJ, Baroody FM, Naclerio RM. Coronal CT scan abnormalities in children with chronic sinusitis. Laryngoscope 1993;103:985–990.

37. Otten FWA, Grote JJ. The diagnostic value of transillumination for maxillary sinusitis in children. J Pediatr Otorhininolaryngol 1989;18:9–11.

38. Spector SL, Lotan A, English G, Philpot I. Comparison between transillumination and the roentgenogram in diagnosis of paranasal sinus disease. J Allergy Clin Immunol 1981;67:22–26.

39. Revonta M. Ultrasound in the diagnosis of maxillary and frontal sinusitis. Acta Otolaryngol 1980;370(Suppl.):1–54.

40. Levonta N, Suonpää J. Diagnosis and follow-up of ultrasonographical sinus changes in children. Int J Pediatr Otorhinolaryngol 1982;4:301–308.

41. Jannert M, Andreasson L, Holmer N-G, Lorine P. Ultrasonic examination of the paranasal sinuses. Acta Otolaryngol 1982;389(Suppl.):1–51.

42. Revonta M. Kuuliala I. The diagnosis and follow-up of pediatric sinusitis. Water's view radiography versus ultrasonography Laryngoscope 1989;99:321–324.

43. Shapiro GG, Furukawa CT, Pierson WE, Gilbertson E, Bierman CW. Blinded comparison of maxillary sinus radiography and ultrasound for diagnosis of sinusitis. J Allergy Clin Immunol 1986;77:59–64.

44. Rohr AS, Spector SL, Siegel SC, Katz RM, Rachelefsky GS. Correlation between A-mode ultrasound and radiography in the diagnosis of maxillary sinusitis. J Allergy Clin Immunol 1986;77:59–64.

45. Pfister R, Lutolf M, Schapowal A, Glatte B, Schmitz M, Menz G. Screening for sinus disease in patients with asthma: a computed tomography-controlled comparison of A-mode ultrasonography and standard radiography. J Allergy Clin Immunol 1994;94:804–809.

46. Wilson NW, Jalowayski AA, Hamburger RN. A comparison of nasal cytology with sinus x-rays for the diagnosis of sinusitis. Am J Rhinol 1989;3:13–15.

47. Goldenhersh MJ, Rachelefsky GS, Dudley J, Brill J, Katz RM, Rohr A, Spector SL, Siegel SC, Summanen P, Baron EJ, Feingold S. The microbiology of chronic sinus disease in children with respiratory allergy. J Allergy Clin Immunol 1990;85:1030–1039.

48. Caplan ES, Hoyt NJ. Nosocomial sinusitis. JAMA 1982;146:589–593.

49. Tinkelman DC, Silk HJ. Clinical and bacteriologic features of chronic sinusitis in children. Am J Dis Child 1989;143:938–941.

50. Wald ER. Microbiology of acute and chronic sinusitis in children. J Allergy Clin Immunol 1992;90:452–460.

51. Gwaltney JM, Scheld WM, Sande MA, Sydnor A. The microbial etiology and antimicrobial therapy of adults with acute community-acquired sinusitis: a fifteen-year experience at the University of Virginia and review of other selected studies. J Allergy Clin Immunol 1992;90:457–462.

52. Brook I. Bacteriologic features of chronic sinusitis in children. JAMA 1981;248:967–969.

53. Muntz HR, Lusk RP. Bacteriology of the ethmoid bullae in children with chronic sinusitis. Arch Otolaryngol Head Neck Surg 1991;117:179–181.

54. Manning SC, Schaefer SD, Close LG, Vuitch F. Culture-positive allergic fungal sinusitis. Arch Otolaryngol Head Neck Surg 1991;117:174–178.

55. Manning SC. Pediatric sinusitis. Otolaryngol Clinic North Am 1993;26:623–638.

56. Ence BK, Gourley DS, Jorgensen NL, Shagets FW, Parsons DS. Allergic fungal sinusitis. Am J Rhinology 1990;4:169–178.

57. Goldstein MF. Allergic fungal sinusitis: an undiagnosed problem. Hosp Pract 1992;27:73–92.

58. Gourley Ds, Whisman BA, Jorgensen NL, Martin ME, Reid MJ. Allergic Bipolaris sinusitis: clinical and immunopathologic characteristics. J Allergy Clin Immunol 1990;85:583–591.

59. Melen I, Andreasson L, Ivarsson A, Jannert M, Johansson CH. Effects of pheynylpropanolamine on osteal and nasal patency in patients treated for chronic maxillary sinusitis. Acta Otolaryngol 1986;101:494–500.

60. Aust R, Drettner B, Faluk B. Studies of the effect of peroral fenylpropanolamin on the functional size of the human maxillary ostium. Acta Otolaryngol 1979;88:455–458.

61. Rachelefsky GS, Katz RM, Siegel SC. Chronic sinusitis in children with respiratory allergy: the role of antimicrobials. J Allergy Clin Immunol 1982;69:382–387.

62. Siegel SC. Topical corticosteroids in the management of rhinitis. In: Settipane GA, ed. Rhinitis, 2nd ed. Providence: Oceanside Publications, 1991; pp. 231–240.

63. Meltzer EO, Busse WW, Druce HM, Metzger WJ, Mitchell DO, Selmer JC, Shapiro GG, VanBavel JH. Assessment of flunisolide nasal spray vs placebo as an adjunct to antibiotic treatment of sinusitis (abstract). J Allergy Clin Immunol 1992;89:301.

64. Wald ER, Chiponis D, Ledesma-Medina J. Comparative effectiveness of amoxicillin-clavulanate potassium in acute paranasal sinus infection in children: a double-blind, placebo-controlled trial. Pediatrics 1986;77:795–800.

65. Dohlman AW, Hemstreet MPB, Odrezen GT, Bartolucci AA. Subacute sinusitis: are antibiotics necessary? J Allergy Clin Immunol 1993;91:1015–1023.

66. Otten FWA, Grote JJ. Treatment of chronic maxillary sinusitis in children. Int J Pediatr Otorhinolaryngol 1988;15:269–278.

67. Dubois J, Saint-Pierre C, Tremblay C. Efficacy of clarithromycin vs amoxicillin/clavulanate in the treatment of acute maxillary sinusitis. ENT J 1993;72:804–810.

68. Foshee WS. Loracarbef (LY163892) versus amoxicillin-clavulanate in the treatment of bacterial acute otitis media with effusion. J Pediatr 1992;120:980–986.

69. Sydnor TA, Scheld WM, Gwaltney J, Nielsen RW, Huch W, Therasse DG. Loracarbef (LY 163892) vs amoxicillin/clavulanate in bacterial maxillary sinusitis. ENT J 1992;71:225–232.

70. Nielsen RW. Acute bacterial maxillary sinusitis: results of US and European comparative therapy trials. Am J Med 1992;92(Suppl. 6A):70S–73S.

71. Perrin JM, Charney E, MacWhinney JB Jr, McInerny KK, Miller RL, Nazarian LF. Sulfazoxazole as chemophrophylaxis for recurrent otitis media: a double-blind crossover study in pediatric practice. N Engl J Med 1974;291:664–667.

72. Wald ER, Pang D, Milmore GJ, Schramm VL. Sinusitis and its complications in the pediatric patient. Pediatr Clinics North Am 1981;28:777–796.

73. Havas TE. Complications of sinusitis in the paediatric age group. Aust Fam Physician 1986;15:701–705.

74. Friedman R, Ackerman M, Wald E, Casselbrant M, Friday G, Fireman P. Asthma and bacterial sinusitis in children. J Allergy Clin Immunol 1984;74:185–189.

75. Silk HJ. Sinusitis and asthma: a review. J Asthma 1990;27:5–9.

76. Brook V, Englander M. Allergic sinusitis and bronchial asthma in children. Pediatr Asthma Allergy Immunol 1992;6:57–60.

77. Businco L, Feore L, Frediani T, Artuso A, DiFazio A, Bellioni P. Clinical and therapeutic aspects of sinusitis in children with bronchial asthma. Int J Pediatr Otorhinolaryngol 1981;3:287–294.

78. Slavin RG, Cannon RE, Friedman WH, Palitang E, Sundaram M. Sinusitis and bronchial asthma. J Allergy Clin Immunol 1980;66:250–257.

79. Rachelefsky GS, Katz RM, Siegel SC. Chronic sinus disease with associated reactive airway disease in children. Pediatrics 1984;73:526–529.

80. Adinoff AD, Cummings NP. Sinusitis and its relationship to asthma. Am J Asthma Allergy 1988;1:93–99.

81. Corren J, Rachelefsky GS. Interrelationship between sinusitis and asthma. Immunol Allergy Clin North Am 1994;14:171–184.

82. Moes JJ, Clement PA. The usefulness of irrigation of the maxillary sinus in children with maxillary sinusitis on the basis of Water's x-ray. Rhinology 1987;25:259–264.

83. Otten FW, Grote J. Otitits media with effusion and chronic upper respiratory tract infections in children: a randomized, placebo-controlled clinical study. Laryngoscope 1990;100:627–633.

84. Takahashi H, Fujita A, Honjo I. Effects of adenoidectomy on otitis media with effusion, tubal function and sinusitis. Am J Otolaryngol 1989;10:208–213.

85. Muntz HR, Lusk RP. Nasal antral windows in children: a retrospective study. Laryngoscope 1990;100:643–646.

86. Messerklinger W. Endoscopy of the Nose. Baltimore, MD: Urban Schwargenberg, 1978.

87. King V, Moss RB. The role of sinus surgery in chronic sinusitis in children. Am J Asthma Allergy 1992;5:203–208.

88. Derkay CS, St. George M, Poe D. Pediatric endoscopic sinus surgery. AORN J 1991;54:989–1000.

89. Duplechain JK, White JA, Miller RH. Pediatric sinusitis. Arch Otolaryngol Head Neck Surg 1991;117:422–426.

90. Lazar RH, Younis RT, Gross CW. Pediatric functional endonasal sinus surgery: review of 210 cases. Head and Neck 1992;14:92–98.

91. Poole MD. Pediatric endoscopic sinus surgery: the conservative view. ENT J 1994;73:221–228.

92. Manning SC. Surgical management of sinus disease in children. Ann, Rhinol Laryngol 1992;101:42–45.

9

Diagnosis and Medical Management of Recurrent and Chronic Sinusitis in Adults

Howard M. Druce, MD

SYNOPSIS

Diagnosis of sinusitis is based on a history of chronic symptoms suggesting inflammation arising from the paranasal sinuses (purulent nasal secretion, postnasal drainage, facial pain, nasal obstruction) combined with a positive imaging test inferring the location of the pathology. Medical management of recurrent and chronic sinusitis is based on empiric goals. Adjunctive agents are frequently prescribed in addition to antibiotics to aid drainage of retained secretions through the sinus ostia into the nasal cavity. Scientific data to support combination therapy are based on clinical experience. It is unclear how many cases of chronic sinusitis result from incomplete treatment of acute sinusitis.

PATHOPHYSIOLOGY

Chronic sinusitis may follow incomplete resolution of an initial episode of acute sinusitis. Acute

From: *Diseases of the Sinuses* (M. E. Gershwin and G. A. Incaudo, eds.),
©1996 Humana Press Inc., Totowa, NJ.

sinusitis is a secondary bacterial infection following a viral upper respiratory infection *(1)*. The initial episode may have been unrecognized and perceived as a severe head cold. The paranasal sinuses are generally considered to be microbiologically sterile in the absence of active infection. For infectious organisms to reach the sinuses during a head cold, there must be either a failure of the mucociliary clearance system, which conducts surface fluid out of the sinuses into the nasal cavity, or direct cell-to-cell infection. In either case, pyogenic organisms enter the sinus cavities. Pus in the antrum may not completely resorb, and its presence generates inflammation *(2)*. This leads to swelling and possibly hypertrophy of the sinus mucosa with resulting occlusion of the sinus ostia. Accumulation of secretions leads to stasis and impaired mucociliary clearance. There is also histologic evidence of formation of new glands in chronic sinusitis and hyperactivity of the normal seromucous glands *(3)*. A decrease in ciliary beat frequency may also be observed *(4)*. These processes

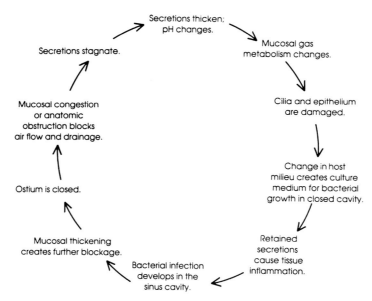

Fig. 1. The sinusitis cycle. Reprinted from ref. *4a* with permission.

have been termed collectively the "sinusitis cycle" and predispose an individual to further infection (Fig. 1). It is difficult to assess the relative contributions of infection, inflammation, and anatomic destruction in most cases of chronic sinusitis. If fever and visible pus persist, an infectious process is active. Chronic symptoms of postnasal drainage, headaches, and pressure may persist after infection is eradicated. Thus, therapy is directed at reversing all aspects of pathophysiology.

CLASSIFICATION AND STAGING

The term "sinusitis" is used to describe clinical syndromes associated with inflammation of the paranasal sinuses. Because the sinus mucosa is contained within a series of irregularly shaped bony cavities that drain into the nose, symptoms vary over time. Classical symptoms associated with the paranasal sinuses are shown in Table 1. The term sinusitis is commonly understood to mean infection of a sinus (or sinuses), but this is not always the case. Active infection, as manifested by nasal pus, with or without fever, is often hard to demonstrate.

A temporal modifier, such as acute or chronic, is usually applied to sinusitis to describe the overall symptom pattern. No definitions for such terms as acute, recurrent, or chronic sinusitis have been widely accepted. This has led to difficulties in interpreting the literature. Each review or interventional study has used a novel set of criteria. One

Table 1
Sinus-Associated Symptoms

Local	Facial pain/pressure
	Head congestion/"stuffiness"
	Purulent nasal discharge
	Headache
	Bad breath
	Toothache (upper jaw)
	Facial swelling
	Sore throat
	Fullness, pain, or popping of ears
Systemic	Fever
	Malaise

Table 2
Sinusitis Syndromes—One Classification[a]

Acute sinusitis
Recurrent or relapsing acute sinusitis
Chronic sinusitis
Acute on chronic (or exacerbation of chronic) sinusitis
Sinus-related headaches or nasal symptoms

[a]Adapted from ref. *5*.

classification of sinusitis was presented by this author *(5)* (Table 2). One problem is that imaging techniques are not routinely obtained after resolution of each individual episode. It is thus hard to separate recurrent acute from chronic sinusitis, especially if there is a background of nonspecific rhinitis symptoms, such as headache, nasal obstruc-

Table 3
Sinusitis Temporal Modifiers

Acute
Recurrent or relapsing acute
Subacute
Chronic
Acute on chronic (or exacerbation of chronic)
Sinus-related syndromes

tion, rhinorrhea, or postnasal drainage. The lack of universal definitions has hampered understanding of pathophysiology and has led to widespread inappropriate patient management *(6,7)*. Table 3 shows different temporal modifiers that have appeared in the literature.

Acute

Acute sinusitis is usually an acute bacterial infection following an unresolved viral upper respiratory infection. Symptoms have usually been present for <2 wk. The symptoms are those of a severe head cold: nasal congestion, purulent rhinorrhea and postnasal drip, headache, and fever. Radiographic findings include characteristic air–fluid levels, opacification, or mucoperiosteal thickening of the affected sinus. Other causes of acute sinusitis include barotrauma, direct trauma, and nosocomial infection.

Recurrent (Relapsing) Acute

Recurrent acute sinusitis may be defined as repetitive episodes of symptoms of sinus infection concurrently with abnormal radiographic findings. Cultures, if taken, would show evidence of infection, but not necessarily with the same organism(s). Radiographs, or other imaging tests, obtained between attacks show no abnormality, but are rarely obtained to confirm that resolution has occurred.

Subacute

This term has been used to indicate the presence of symptoms lasting from 2 wk to 3 mo, but has not gained wide use *(8)*.

Chronic

The time-course of chronic sinusitis is considered to be 3 mo or more. In chronic sinusitis, symptoms and abnormal images both persist. Symptoms that wax and wane may be more suggestive of inflammation within the sinus cavities and ostia than infection.

Acute on Chronic (or Exacerbation of Chronic)

Acute-on-chronic disease may be characterized by reappearance of infective symptoms, such as purulent discharge, on a background of chronic symptoms. The background may be clear or intermittent colored nasal discharge, or may be another sinus-related symptom, such as head pressure or congestion.

Sinus-Related Syndromes

Sinus-related syndromes include isolated vacuum-type headaches referred to the sinuses in the absence of demonstrable pathology. Other possible symptoms that may occur in isolation are listed in Table 1.

A recent paper *(9)* described sinusitis as a disease characterized by "inflammation of the paranasal sinuses and associated with obstruction of the sinus ostia, retention of secretions, and infection." Patients enrolled in this study were considered to have chronic sinusitis based on the combination of one or more of history, roentgenographic appearance, or physical examination. The elements in the history required for a positive diagnosis were not enumerated in the methods section. Thus, a normal radiograph would be compatible with the diagnosis. The authors developed a scoring system for Computed tomography (CT) abnormalities in this paper. "Chronic" patients were defined as having symptoms for more than 3 mo, as opposed to acute sinusitis, defined by the authors as manifested by the signs and symptoms of upper respiratory infection persisting between 7 and 10 d or longer. The pattern of observed symptoms described in the results is typical of similar studies. Relying on abnormal CT data as indicating the presence of sinus pathology without excluding the presence of a common cold requires caution in light of recent data from Gwaltney's group, which showed that coronal CT abnormalities could occur after a common cold *(10)*.

Williams et al. *(11)* attempted to identify the most useful clinical examination findings for the diagnosis of acute and subacute sinusitis. The authors discussed the overlap in symptoms between acute sinusitis and rhinitis, but did not produce a definition. They accepted an abnormal radiograph as indicating presence of sinusitis, as opposed to rhinitis. The patients enrolled were those who presented with nasal discharge of any quality, facial pain unrelated to trauma, or self-suspected sinusitis.

Wald and colleagues *(12)* proposed arbitrary temporal modifiers based on discussions at a closed conference *(13)*. Acute was defined as onset to 2–4 wk; subacute (2–4 wk to 2–3 mo), and chronic (more than 2–3 mo). It has been documented that the radiographic findings of paranasal sinus opacification and mucosal thickening, the "hallmarks" of sinusitis, are also found in children free of symptoms *(14,15)*. Dohlman et al. *(8)* termed "subacute sinusitis" symptoms of mucoid nasal drainage, cough, or poorly controlled asthma for more than 3 wk and <3 mo and to have radiographic evidence of sinusitis, i.e., mucosal thickening of >6 mm of the maxillary sinuses or >33% loss of air-space volume within the maxillary sinuses and/or opacification or air–fluid levels of any of the paranasal sinuses.

Staging

Staging techniques to quantify the extent of disease identified within a sinus cavity have been proposed by several authors, including Friedman et al. *(16,17)* and Kennedy *(18)*, and clinical staging was proposed by Newman et al. *(9)*. However, these are more appropriate for baseline evaluation and/or follow-up for those cases intended for surgery.

DIAGNOSIS OF SINUSITIS

Diagnosis is difficult because the sinus mucosa is hidden. Even the most sensitive imaging technique provides an indirect method of proving presence of disease. There are few studies of mucosal pathology in chronic sinusitis. No consistent pathologic finding has been described that would merit the inconvenience of routine diagnostic biopsy *(2)*. Beyond imaging techniques, direct visualization of the ostiomeatal area has been enhanced by introduction of fiberoptic rhinoscopy with the flexible endoscope *(19)*. This enables pathology that may lead to sinus ostial obstruction to be seen. Pus draining from the ostia may also be seen, but the sinus ostia cannot be cannulated to visualize the sinus cavities. The short rigid endoscope may be used to define ostiomeatal anatomy *(20)*.

Antral aspiration has been used in both acute and chronic sinusitis to obtain cultures for microbiologic analysis. Its place in chronic sinusitis syn-

Table 4
Differential Diagnosis of Chronic Sinusitis

Idiopathic/vasomotor rhinitis/perennial nonallergic rhinitis
Structural rhinitis
Allergic rhinitis
Sinus ostial obstruction
Nasal polyposis
Aspirin/NSAID sensitivity
Foreign body
Dental abscess
Chronic headache
Abnormal visual refraction
Malignancy

dromes in which inflammatory changes are more likely is undetermined. Unless characteristic ultrastructural observations can be identified that correlate well with symptoms, diagnosis will continue to be inferential.

Differential Diagnosis (Table 4)

Chronic sinusitis is frequently incorrectly diagnosed when there is no sinus pathology. This underscores the importance of demonstrating pathology within the sinus cavities (ethmoid and sphenoid) as well as maxillary, in the face of chronic symptoms that could refer to the sinuses or adjacent structures. For example, both chronic sinusitis and nonallergic rhinitis may present with only postnasal drip or mucus pooling in the back of the throat at night, leading to cough. An imaging test that concentrates on the ethmoid sinuses would provide inferential evidence to make this distinction. Nonallergic rhinitis may also present with nasal obstruction and intermittent symptom expression, leading to confusion with chronic sinusitis *(21,22)*.

Structural rhinitis may be caused by a marked nasal septal deflection, nasal septal erosion, ulcer, or perforation. The symptoms of obstruction and rhinorrhea may mimic chronic sinusitis or nonallergic rhinitis. Allergic rhinitis usually presents a distinct pattern with sneezing paroxysms and clear rhinorrhea. However, nasal obstruction or rhinorrhea may present as the only symptom. Coronal CT examination has shown that sinus-related symptoms can occur when the sinus ostia are blocked. In some cases, this occurs without infection or inflammation in the sinus cavities. This may be because of anatomic variation or intranasal inflammation.

Table 5
Differential Diagnosis of Nasal Obstruction

Nasal polyposis
Sinusitis
Deviated nasal septum
Foreign body
Tumors
Hypertrophy of nasal turbinate mucosa
Atrophic rhinitis
Trauma (e.g., nasal fracture)

Nasal polyposis is discussed in more detail in Chapter 14. Nasal obstruction in polyposis may be unilateral or bilateral, may be progressive or intermittent, and may be associated with anosmia. If no obvious cause for nasal obstruction is seen on inspection of the anterior part of the nose, the next logical step is to image the nose directly. The first step should be decongestion of the nasal mucosa. If no obvious cause is seen, then the physician who is competent to perform flexible endoscopy (rhino-laryngo-pharyngoscopy) should do so.

Aspirin or NSAID sensitivity presents with one of two major syndromes: chronic urticaria and rhinosinusitis. It may not be appreciated that chronic sinusitis is the result of repetitive ingestion of these drugs. Patients may not consider these analgesics as "drugs" when giving their medication history.

Dental abscess in the upper jaw produces intermittent or chronic pain, which can mimic maxillary sinusitis. Pressure on the affected tooth may simulate symptoms. Patients who complain of chronic upper facial pain should be examined for abnormal visual refraction. Although tumors of the sinuses are rare, they present late. Any suspicion of a space-occupying or bleeding lesion should prompt urgent referral and evaluation. Nasal obstruction is the major symptom leading to considering a differential diagnosis (Table 5).

IMAGING

A summary of clinical indications to obtain an imaging test is listed in Table 6 (*see also* Fig. 2). The tests available are listed in Table 7.

A patient with typical nasal allergy who presents with the classical symptoms of sneezing, itching, rhinorrhea, and nasal obstruction does not need an imaging test as part of the routine work-up. Visualizing the largest area of nasal mucosa possible is best achieved by anterior rhinoscopy with an otoscope with a large-diameter nasal head, combined with decongestion with a topical decongestant, such as 1% phenylephrine, to shrink the mucosa. This will allow examination of the middle turbinates and give a general indication of the maximal nasal patency that might be obtained after therapeutic decongestion. If it is necessary to view more of the surface area of the nasal mucosa, the use of a flexible or rigid endoscope is indicated. The most common causes of nasal obstruction refractory to this type of treatment are nasal polyposis, deviated nasal septum, and sinusitis.

Imaging Modalities

Various tests have been used to image the sinuses or locate the pathology from which sinus-related symptoms arise.

PLAIN RADIOGRAPHY—
USE AND DECLINE IN SINUSITIS

This is no longer the currently accepted standard for diagnosis of chronic sinusitis, despite its widespread use. The likelihood of detecting the presence of antral fluid increases with the number of views obtained *(15)*, but in screening for chronic sinusitis in which fluid is frequently absent, two or three projections are usually obtained *(23)*. The occipitomental (Water's) view gives the best image of the maxillary sinuses, and the occipitofrontal (Caldwell) view shows the frontal and ethmoid sinuses *(24)*. Studies have compared radiographic abnormalities with the occurrence of fluid in the maxillary antra and recovery of bacteria from antral punctures *(15)*. Some of these studies have specifically addressed acute sinusitis, and others have not distinguished patients with acute and chronic syndromes. In chronic sinusitis, there is no good correlation among symptoms, signs, and prediction of an abnormal radiograph. Moreover, patients with minimal mucosal thickening alone, which on Evans' data would not be expected to have a bacterial infection *(23)*, respond only to antibiotic therapy.

The significant incidence of abnormal radiographic findings in asymptomatic patients makes the continued use of plain radiographs tenuous. In a study of children undergoing sinus radiography for reasons unrelated to respiratory infection, Kovatch et al. found a 53% incidence of abnormal radiographs above the age of one *(24)*. These stud-

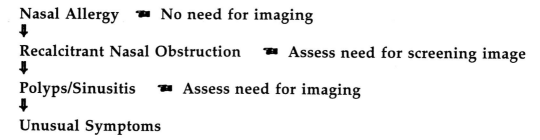

Fig. 2. Simplified flow chart for imaging in suspected chronic or recurrent sinusitis.

Table 6 Indications for Imaging Tests in Patients with Chronic Nasal Symptoms
Recalcitrant nasal obstruction
Unilateral nasal symptoms
Severe or recalcitrant nasal pain
Unexplained bleeding
Concomitant deformity or congenital abnormality

Table 7 Adjunctive Tests in Chronic Sinusitis
Plain radiographs
A-mode ultrasound
CT
MRI
Fiberoptic endoscopy
Maxillary antral aspiration

ies discounted the suggestion that opacification or sinus fluid can be produced by crying. A similar proportion of abnormal sinus images occur using other techniques detailed below.

ULTRASOUND

The advantages of ultrasound include absence of ionizing radiation, rapid test time, and patient convenience. Repetitive studies can be done on the same individual to assess response to treatment. Initial studies reported from Finland *(25,26)* and Germany *(27)* reported a high correlation between positive echoes on A-mode ultrasound and presence of fluid on maxillary antral puncture. Experience in the US with two commercially available instruments has been mixed. In addition to case reports *(28)*, two series were reported. Shapiro et al. *(29)* found a poor correlation between ultrasound and radiographic findings in a mixed population of children and adults, whereas the data of Rohr et al. *(30)* suggested a better correlation. Poor correlation between ultrasound findings and presence of pus in the antra was noted in a Swedish study *(31)*.

No longitudinal data have been presented to date on patients with chronic sinusitis. Two major problems arise with ultrasound. First, only the maxillary and frontal sinuses may be examined. Second, most patients with chronic sinusitis do not have fluid in the sinuses, but have mucosal thickening. No study reported to date has studied this systematically. Our data suggested a poor correlation

between ultrasonographic criteria for mucosal thickening and its detection on plain radiographs *(32)*. We suggested that another parameter needs to be correlated with the ultrasound for it to have any relevance. These data are not available, and ultrasound should be reserved as a screening method to detect presence of maxillary antral fluid. This may be especially useful when the maxillary antra are opacified after previous sinus surgery. Recently, enthusiasm for ultrasound in the US has declined.

CT (LIMITED AND TOTAL CORONAL)

CT produces greater definition of the contents and anatomy of the sinus cavities *(33,34)*. In patients who have had previous surgery, the technique may be useful to distinguish fluid from fibrosis or mucoperiosteal thickening *(35)*. CT is especially useful if sphenoid sinusitis *(36)*, ethmoid sinusitis *(37,38)*, or malignancy *(39)* is suspected. CT has supplanted multidirectional tomography *(40)* and plain radiography to some extent. Coronal view CT without contrast is currently favored as the most reliable test to detect inflammatory sinus disease. Screening protocols involving fewer cuts, and therefore less time and expense, have been introduced. Examples of procedures include screening protocols (5–12 coronal slices, 5-mm thick every 7 mm); limited protocols (24–30 coronal slices; thin cuts through the ostiomeatal complex; 5 5-mm cuts elsewhere), and complete protocols (50 axial and coronal slices. Axial: 5-mm thick every 5 mm; coronal 3-mm thick every 3 mm through the ostiomeatal complex; 5-mm thick every 5 mm elsewhere). Approximate costs of $135, $250, and $450 compare favorably to a typical $100 cost for a three-view plain radiograph series. CT has led to widespread acceptance of functional endoscopic sinus surgical procedures on the ostiomeatal complex. Most otolaryngologists prefer a complete CT examination before surgery. It is still unclear whether a screening protocol (defined as one that shows only the ostiomeatal complex area) is adequate. Timing of the CT scan in relation to the presence of symptoms is critical. Recent data have shown that common colds can cause abnormalities to appear on the CT scan *(10)*. Thus, CT scans should only be obtained in the context of chronic symptoms and, after an adequate therapeutic trial, to allow demonstration of residual disease.

NUCLEAR MAGNETIC RESONANCE (MRI SCANNING)

MRI has a very high definition for soft tissue structures and, like ultrasound, does not involve exposure of the patient to ionizing radiation. In one study, MRI was administered to 272 patients as part of a neurological evaluation *(41)*. As with CT, a high incidence of abnormal images was detected. Sixty out of 272 patients (22%) had abnormal findings. Solitary maxillary disease was found in 37%, and combined maxillary and ethmoid disease occurred in 42%. Two patients had isolated ethmoiditis, two sphenoiditis, and one had combined ethmoid and sphenoid disease. Data such as these make assertions that ethmoid sinusitis and frontal sinusitis are always associated with maxillary disease less tenable *(42)*. In another study, MRI was administered to 1120 patients as part of a neurologic evaluation. As with CT, a high incidence of abnormal images was detected with 13% having abnormal findings *(43)*. MRI is now considered the imaging test of choice to detect fungal disease or cancer in the sinus cavities.

FLEXIBLE ENDOSCOPY

The introduction of flexible endoscopes with a small diameter (3–4 mm) and light bending radius permits detailed examination of the upper nasal cavities and posterior nasopharynx. A variety of pathologies may be seen *(19,44)*. Use of the endoscope involves administration of a topical local anesthetic and decongestant to the nasal mucosa, but should not replace use of the head mirror and posterior pharyngoscopy in those patients who can tolerate it. I use endoscopy for atypical symptoms, recalcitrant symptoms, and to identify structural abnormalities, high in the nasal vault. I have found the instrument useful to detect rostral septal deviations, ethmoid polyps, and residual adenoid tissue in adolescents. Skill is required not in merely passing the endoscope, but in differentiating variations in normal anatomy from pathologic lesions. Guidelines for the use of the flexible endoscopes have been proposed. Even the fiberoptic scope does not reveal the maxillary sinus ostia. Rigid endoscopy, after more extensive topical anesthesia, is a technique well suited for this purpose *(45)*.

RIGID ENDOSCOPY

In cases where there is questionable pathology in the area of the ostiomeatal complex, flexible endoscopes do not give an adequate view. The use of the rigid endoscope can provide a superior image in this area. The rigid endoscope should not be used by the casual user. Considerable skill and training are needed to identify structures through any scope other than with the 0° viewing angle; 30° and 120° endoscopes are used largely by otolaryngologists.

ANTRAL PUNCTURE

Puncture of the maxillary antrum is an office procedure that may be used for diagnostic aspiration or therapeutic lavage. It is more commonly used in Europe than the US. Approaches may be made intranasally through the maxillary antrum or through the canine fossa *(46)*. Therapeutic lavage is indicated in acute sinusitis to relieve pressure symptoms. No systematic data are available to document its efficacy. Its role in chronic disease is undetermined. Diagnostic lavage should be considered in patients with resistant air–fluid levels or when there is a high probability of recovering unusual organisms, such as in immunocompromised patients or malignancy.

OTHER INDIRECT IMAGING MODALITIES

Although not studied systematically, thermography *(47,48)* and positron emission tomography have potential to show active inflammation in the sinus cavities. Radionuclides, such as ^{67}Ga, cannot be currently localized with the precision required to differentiate sinus disease from intranasal pathology. Xenon-enhanced dynamic CT may allow assessment of sinus ventilation *(49)*.

Table 8
A Sample Regimen to Treat Chronic
Sinus-Related Symptoms in the Absence
of Concomitant Allergic Disease

Amoxicillin 500 mg tid or Trimethoprim/Sulfameth-
  oxazole DS bid for 21 d
Beclomethasone aqueous nasal spray 2 sprays bid × 30 d
Guaifenesin 600 mg/pseudoephedrine 120 mg combination
  tablets bid × 30 d
Steam inhalations bid for 30 d
Nasal saline sprays or irrigation

MANAGEMENT

Therapeutic Trials and Algorithms for Management

Treatment of sinusitis is associated with resolution of radiographic abnormalities and improves symptoms of asthma. Yet, scarce data exist on the efficacy of treatment for chronic sinusitis. Medical management should be designed to treat infection in the sinuses effectively, reduce tissue swelling in the region of the sinus ostia, which may block egress of secretions, facilitate drainage of retained secretions, promote ciliary function, and maintain ostial patency, both during and after therapy.

I use treatment protocols such as the example detailed in Table 8. The rationale for this is based on clinical experience rather than formal trials.

MANAGEMENT OF SUSPECTED CHRONIC SINUSITIS (FIG. 3A,B)

The place for a medical therapeutic trial depends on the likelihood of a diagnosis of sinusitis being reached. If the clinician feels confident of the diagnosis from the history and physical examination (Fig. 3A), it is reasonable to proceed to a medical therapeutic trial before obtaining an imaging test. This strategy is not always appropriate for acute symptoms and should not be considered if the acute symptoms are severe. The imaging tests may then be used to define residual disease after optimal medical treatment.

If the trial is successful, no further investigation is needed. Patients may be maintained on empiric medication for selected symptoms, e.g., nasal steroids and oral decongestants. Partial success, e.g., relief of some symptoms, should point directly to the medications that need to be continued. Complete relief, which lasts only for a limited duration, may indicate any of the factors described in Table 9.

If the differential diagnosis is still unclear and the suspicion of sinusitis is weaker, tests to visualize the area may be done sooner (Fig. 3B). It is hard to justify the expense of a complete CT scan for an uncertain diagnosis. Thus, a screening CT as described in CT (Limited and Total Coronal) above may be considered. Failure of a medical therapeutic trial undertaken without evidence of sinus-related pathology should prompt a more intensive search for alternative diagnoses. Often "diagnoses of exclusion," such as nonallergic perennial rhinitis or tension headache, are given as a label for untreatable symptoms.

LATE RECURRENT OR PERSISTENT DISCHARGE OR POSTNASAL DRIP AFTER SINUS SURGERY

Initially, review pre- and postsurgery CT scans. Comparable cuts should be taken. If recurrent or localized disease is apparent, this should be referred back to the operative surgeon. If there is no evidence of disease on the imaging test, endoscopy and microbial cultures should be obtained. Aerobic and anaerobic bacterial, and fungal cultures may be appropriate. Antibiotic treatment should be selected appropriately if cultures suggest presence of an organism that might be producing the symptoms. It is important to realize which organisms may be commensals or colonizing the postsurgical site. Symptomatic treatment should be combined with the antibiotics and used without antibiotics if the cultures are negative or if they persist as positive after an adequate antibiotic course. Such therapy can include lavage, steam and saline instillation, alkylol nasal spray, topical antibiotics and antiseptics, pharmacotherapy, such as guaifenesin and decongestant combinations, and the use of empiric antibiotics known to decrease mucus viscosity, e.g., erythromycin and clarithromycin. Failure of all the above should lead to further consideration of revision surgery.

Symptoms occurring immediately postoperatively include adhesions and the failure to eradicate key ethmoid air cells. Multiple factors need to be considered when treatment failure occurs.

1. Is the diagnosis correct? Multiple diagnoses are appropriate in many cases because of imprecision in defining syndromes (22). For example, a patient may have nasal obstruction and rhinorrhea secondary to perennial allergic rhinitis, nasal polyposis, and chronic sinusitis. Specific elements of treatment may be needed for each com-

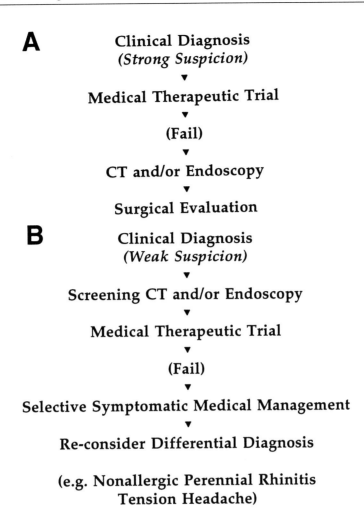

A Clinical Diagnosis
(Strong Suspicion)
▼
Medical Therapeutic Trial
▼
(Fail)
▼
CT and/or Endoscopy
▼
Surgical Evaluation

B Clinical Diagnosis
(Weak Suspicion)
▼
Screening CT and/or Endoscopy
▼
Medical Therapeutic Trial
▼
(Fail)
▼
Selective Symptomatic Medical Management
▼
Re-consider Differential Diagnosis

(e.g. Nonallergic Perennial Rhinitis
Tension Headache)

Fig. 3. Management of suspected sinusitis.

Table 9
Factors Implicated in Treatment Failure

Is the diagnosis correct?
Is there a need for multimodal therapy?
Is the organism sensitive to the antibiotic chosen?
Is the dose of therapy sufficient?
Is the duration of treatment adequate?
Is the patient compliant with medication regimen?
Is the cause of the symptoms environmental?
Is excess mucus physiologic?

ponent, e.g., antihistamines or immunotherapy for the allergic rhinitis.

2. Is there a need for multimodal therapy? This was discussed above. Also, therapy, such as intranasal steroids, may be appropriate for several diagnostic categories.

3. Is the organism sensitive to the antibiotic chosen? Since cultures are rarely obtained in chronic sinusitis, the choice of antibiotic is generally empiric and broad-spectrum. Antibiotic choice is discussed in Antibiotic Choice below. Recalcitrant disease that is clearly infective (persistent pus and/or fever) should mandate appropriate cultures.

4. Is the dose of therapy sufficient? With adjunctive medication, such as guaifenesin, some patients get an adequate therapeutic response at 600 mg bid, whereas others may need double this amount.

5. Is the duration of treatment adequate? There are no good data indicating optimal duration of antibiotic administration in chronic sinusitis.

6. Is the patient compliant with medication regimen? Side effects are common with these medications and may lead to termination of use, e.g., agitation or insomnia with α-adrenergic agonists or nasal burning with topical nasal formulations.

7. Is the cause of the symptoms environmental? If the patient relates symptoms to physical location, e.g., only at home or work, a further search for allergic causes may be appropriate. Alternatively, symptoms may be caused by temperature and/or relative humidity changes. The so-called sick building syndrome with inadequate air exchange may be associated with similar symptoms to chronic sinusitis. Frequent aircraft flights may similarly lead to recurrent respiratory symptoms. Certain foods, particularly dairy products, may cause airway mucus to appear more viscous or increased in volume. The mechanism by which this occurs is unclear, but a trial of reducing dairy product intake may ease symptoms.

8. Excess mucus may be physiologic. When all potential factors have been considered, there is a group of patients who produce more upper airway secretions than might be considered normal. In these individuals, no pathology may be detected, and patients are often told that they have to "live with" the condition. This should not be done without a thorough consideration of the differential diagnosis and a therapeutic trial of appropriate medications (Table 8).

Management of Specific Problems After Therapeutic Trials

PERSISTENT RHINORRHEA

Increased secretions that are not discolored usually suggest rhinitis rather than sinusitis. However, patients often cannot tell the secretion color if they are swallowed. Persistent posterior rhinorrhea may be perceived as nocturnal cough or a gagging sensation as thick secretions pool in dependent areas while recumbent. The source of the secretions may be from infected posterior ethmoidal cells. An empiric clinical trial may be of value followed by a CT scan of the sinuses if no resolution occurs.

THICK MUCUS

Thick mucus does not always indicate infection. Flecks of solid green mucus may occur with reduced hydration of the upper airway, e.g., with exposure to excessive air conditioning. Hydration with topical saline, steam inhalations, or hot showers may provide enough relief. Mucus may be "thinned" by such agents as guaifenesin. Some patients report that they sense an increased volume of secretion. A guaifenesin/decongestant combination may prevent this. For patients with more severe problems without evidence of infection, a course of an antibiotic with mucous viscosity-reducing properties, such as erythromycin or clarithromycin, may be helpful.

NASAL CONGESTION

Isolated nasal congestion has proven to be one of the nasal symptoms most resistant to effective long-term treatment. It is important to consider a wide differential diagnosis, but often no cause is found, and symptomatic treatment is needed. A trial of oral guaifenesin combined with a decongestant, such as pseudoephedrine, is often helpful. After an initial regular regimen, relief may be obtained by prn use. If this fails, intranasal corticosteroids may be effective. Juniper et al. have shown that some patients also derive adequate relief from prn usage *(50)*.

Medical Management— Rationale for Antibiotic Use

Management of sinusitis usually includes an oral antibiotic; but about 45% of acute cases will resolve without the use of antibiotics. In one study of 50 patients with chronic anterior or posterior purulent nasal discharge, 20 patients were treated with topical dexamethasone and decongestant sprays, 20 patients with the above medications and topical neomycin, and 10 with matched placebo sprays or propellants alone. Significantly more patients receiving the active treatments showed improvement in symptoms compared to placebo. The authors concluded that improving sinus draining permitted host mechanisms to recover and that topical antibiotics added no additional benefit. However, systemic antibiotics were not used *(51)*. In another study of 80 allergic children with asthma, 4–14 yr of age, sinus X-ray abnormalities were detected in 55 patients. The observations of mucosal thickening >2 mm, opacification, or air–fluid level were defined as abnormal radiographs. Thirteen children with purulent postnasal drip were treated with ampicillin, phenylephrine, and triprolidine. In 42 children without purulent drainage, the ampicillin was replaced by intranasal beclomethasone spray for 1 mo, together with phenylephrine and triprolidine. In both treatment groups, sinus radiographs improved with a decrease in severity of the asthma. However, the presence of bacterial sinusitis was not adequately documented, and all children received topical decongestant so that the

Table 10
Warning Signs Against Medical Management

Severe headache
Lateralized or focal headache
Headache at vertex
Epistaxis
Eye symptoms
Severe fever
Pain unresponsive to nonnarcotic analgesics

role of the intranasal beclomethasone could not be adequately assessed (52).

These studies suggest that systemic antibiotics are not required. However, the serious complications of sinusitis, such as intracranial extension of infection, have decreased in frequency since the advent of antibiotics, and antibiotics are now generally prescribed as primary therapy. Another recent study has questioned the need for antibiotic therapy in a group of afebrile patients with symptoms from 3 wk to 3 mo (8).

ANTIBIOTIC CHOICE

Many patients have already taken multiple courses of 7- to 10-d antibiotic therapy at doses appropriate for acute upper respiratory infections. This may produce a partial and temporary improvement in symptoms. Many practitioners have found that prescription of larger doses as described in Table 10, for a minimum of 21 d, has a more salutary effect (32). The contents of maxillary antral cavities may be sterilized in 7–10 d, but the dose and duration required to penetrate the ethmoid sinuses and ostiomeatal complex tissues have not been demonstrated. In most adults who yield mixed flora on maxillary sinus aspiration, broad-spectrum antibiotics, such as amoxicillin or sulfamethoxazole-trimethoprim, generally suffice if given at adequate doses (23,53,54). In children and resistant adult cases where *Moraxella catarrhalis* is the predominant pathogen, amoxicillin-clavulanate is currently the antibiotic of choice (55). The temptation to treat recurrent episodes with successive short courses of increasingly potent and expensive single agents should be vigorously resisted. Persistence of frank pus or air–fluid levels should prompt the physician to obtain aerobic, anaerobic, and fungal cultures. The prevalence of chronic fungal sinusitis in immunocompetent hosts is uncertain (56).

OTHER ANTIBIOTICS IN SINUSITIS

Clinical trials for regulatory authority approval have been based mainly on short-term therapy of acute maxillary sinusitis. The end point has usually been taken as improvement or resolution of maxillary air–fluid levels on plain radiographs or, more recently, CT scans. Extrapolation to chronic sinusitis or to disease in the other sinuses is difficult, and may explain poor therapeutic results or treatment failures in practice.

Cephalosporins. Comparative studies of cephalosporins suggest that cefuroxime axetil (250 mg bid) is more effective than cefaclor in acute maxillary sinusitis (54). Cefuroxime had similar efficacy to amoxicillin (57).

Macrolides. Although erythromycin is not recommended for acute sinusitis, recent studies have evaluated modified macrolide molecules azithromycin and clarithromycin. Data suggest comparable efficacy to amoxicillin for acute maxillary sinusitis (58–61).

Ciprofloxacin. This drug has also been tested in sinusitis, and was found to be superior to Penicillin V (62).

Investigational Antibiotics. Third-generation cephalosporins, not yet approved in the USA have been used in sinusitis with good results (63). A variety of agents, such as cefprozil and cefpodoxime, are under study (64). Various other antibiotics have been used in clinical studies (65).

Antibiotics not recommended in sinusitis include tetracycline because of resistant *Pneumococci*, and penicillin, erythromycin, and cefalexin because of resistant *Haemophilus influenzae (66).*

Adjunctive Agents

Adjunctive agents used concurrently with antibiotics to fulfill treatment goals are detailed below (Tables 11 and 12).

PHARMACOLOGIC ADJUNCTS

Decongestants. Oral decongestants are α-adrenergic agonists that produce a reduction in nasal blood flow (67). They increase sinus ostial patency, which is narrowed in chronic sinusitis (68,69). There has been concern that α-sympathomimetics may cause ciliary stasis, which would counteract any beneficial effect. However, the presence of pus in active infection inhibits ciliary activity, so the clinical effects of this are not apparent. Oral preparations are safe for long-term administration. Topi-

Table 11
Efficacy of Selected Antimicrobial Agents for the Common Pathogens in Acute Sinusitis[a]

Staphylococcus antimicrobial agents	Recommended adult dosage	Streptococcus pneumoniae, 30	Haemophilus		Moraxella pyogenes, <5	Streptococcus aureus, <5
			influenzae, 20	catarrhalis, 20		
Ampicillin	500 mg q 6 h	+	±	±	+	±
Amoxicillin	500 mg q 8 h	+	±	±	+	±
Amoxicillin clavulanate potassium (500/120)	1 tablet q 8 h					
Cefaclor	500 mg q 6 h	+	+	±	+	+
Cefuroxime axetil	250 mg q 12 h					
Trimethoprim/sulfa-methoxazole (160/800)	1 DS tablet q 12 h					

[a]Adapted from ref. 7.

Table 12
Adjunctive Therapies for Acute Bacterial Sinusitis[a]

Nonpharmacologic measures	Pharmacologic measures
Steam inhalation	Decongestants, topical (for 3 d)
Astringents (pine oil, menthol)	Decongestants, oral (>3 d)
Spicy foods (garlic, horseradish)	Corticosteroids, topical
Saline sprays	Mucoevacuants/decongestants (guaifenesin, iodinated compounds)
Hot, dry air	Analgesics

[a]Adapted from ref. 76.

cal nasal formulations should not be used for more than three to five consecutive days because of the risk of development of tolerance, rhinitis medicamentosa, and rebound after drug withdrawal. Efficacy of topical preparations may diminish after several days of therapy, but this does not occur with oral formulations. This may be related to downregulation of α-adrenoceptors at high topical doses (70).

These agents are not always well tolerated. Side effects of hyperactivity, insomnia, and inhibition of micturition are common. The safety of these drugs in the presence of hypertension is controversial (71,72). The former two symptoms may be mitigated by prescribing a lower dose or use of a combined decongestant-antihistamine preparation.

Topical Intranasal Corticosteroids. Topical intranasal corticosteroids (beclomethasone, dexamethasone, triamcinolone, flunisolide, budesonide, fluticasone) may theoretically increase sinus ostial diameter by reducing inflammation in the area of the sinus ostia. No evidence has been presented to suggest that they induce superinfection or encourage development of resistant organisms. Data showing their clinical efficacy as adjunctive therapy have recently appeared (73). Use of nasal steroids has been restricted by some practitioners to those patients with overt nasal obstruction, coexisting nasal polyposis, or allergic rhinitis. The rationale for using them more widely is to suppress inflammation of the nasal mucosa at the sinus ostia (74). There is evidence that topical corticosteroids do reach the affected area by ciliary transport and have the capability to suppress inflammation. In patients with severe nasal obstruction, it is not feasible to use topical nasal steroid preparations initially. A topical nasal decongestant, such as oxymetazoline 0.05%, for the first 3 d of treatment will open the nares. The patient takes the topical steroid preparation after decongestion is obtained. The steroid also mitigates the development of rhinitis medicamentosa. For those patients who cannot tolerate any nasal medication, a short course (7–10 d) of prednisone is a possible alternative. Using a combined topical corticosteroid and decongestant, preparation produced symptomatic relief in patients with chronic mucopurulent rhinosinusitis in a British trial (51).

Long-term safety of topical nasal steroids has been demonstrated provided the patient develops no overt symptoms, such as epistaxis, caused by the drug. There is no good reason to restrict use of these drugs to a short course, if the patient is continuing to obtain benefit. Nasal septal perforations have occurred in patients on chronic nasal steroid therapy. These have not been related to a specific steroid molecule or formulation. The perforations have usually been preceded by crusting and ulcer formation. The nasal septum should be examined carefully before initiating topical steroid treatment. I do not prescribe more than a 6-mo supply without an office revisit to check the septum. I instruct patients on correct usage of the spray devices and on how to recognize adverse effects. Topical nasal steroids should not be prescribed for patients with recent nasal septal surgery.

MUCOLYTICS/EXPECTORANTS

Guaifenesin. Guaifenesin (glyceryl guaicolate; 3-[2-methoxyphonoxy]-1, 2-propanediol) is a water- and alcohol-soluble substance used as an expectorant to loosen respiratory secretions. It is indicated for the symptomatic management of coughs associated with the common cold, bronchitis, laryngitis, pharyngitis, influenza, and measles, as well as sinusitis *(75)*, when these conditions are complicated by tenacious mucus and/or mucous plugs and congestion. By reducing viscosity of secretions, guaifenesin increases the efficiency of the cough reflex and of ciliary action in removing accumulated secretions from the trachea and bronchi. There is clinical evidence that guaifenesin is an effective expectorant in that it increases expectorated sputum volume over the first 4–6 d of a productive cough, decreases sputum viscosity and difficulty in expectoration, and improves associated symptoms. There is currently insufficient evidence to support efficacy of the drug as an antitussive or an adjunct in sinusitis despite widespread use *(76)*. High-dose guaifenesin (1200 mg bid) has been used empirically for its ability to thin tenacious respiratory secretions, based on data derived from its effects on sputum. Clinical efficacy was demonstrated in chronic bronchitis *(77)*. No clinical trials have been reported in sinusitis to demonstrate its efficacy.

Guaifenesin has a plasma half-life of 1 h. The major urinary metabolite is β-(2-methoxyphenoxy) lactic acid. Guaifenesin may increase renal clearance for urate and thereby lower serum uric acid levels. Guaifenesin may produce an increase in urinary 5-hydroxyindoleacetic acid and interfere with the interpretation of this test for the diagnosis of carcinoid syndrome. It may falsely elevate the VMA test for catechols. Guaifenesin is considered as pregnancy category C, since animal reproduction studies have not been conducted *(78)*.

Iodine. Iodine-containing compounds, such as potassium iodide or iodinated glycerol, might be expected to have similar empiric effects to guaifenesin. They have not proven as popular in clinical use. This may be because of the potential adverse effects of iodine hypersensitivity or chronic iodine ingestion.

Potassium iodide syrup is considered an expectorant for the symptomatic treatment of chronic pulmonary diseases with tenacious mucus, including bronchial asthma, bronchitis, and pulmonary emphysema. Side effects may include gastrointestinal upset, metallic taste, minor skin eruptions, nausea, vomiting, and epigastric pain *(79)*.

Iodinated Glycerol. Iodinated glycerol (Organidin®) is an isomeric mixture formed by the interaction of iodine and glycerol. The active ingredient is thought to be iodopropylidine glycerol, but structural and chemical formulas have not been precisely established. Iodides are readily absorbed form the gastrointestinal tract after oral ingestion and are concentrated primarily in respiratory tract secretions. Their mechanism of action as mucolytic expectorants is unclear. In some way, the drug is thought to stimulate bronchial and nasal glands to secrete a watery mucus. No studies yet published have addressed the mechanism in the upper respiratory tract. This drug was indicated for adjunctive treatment as a mucolytic expectorant in respiratory tract conditions, such as bronchitis, bronchial asthma, emphysema, cystic fibrosis, chronic sinusitis, or after surgery to prevent atelectasis. Contraindications include history of sensitivity to inorganic iodides, pregnancy, newborns, and nursing mothers. Adverse reactions are rare, but include gastrointestinal irritation, rash, hypersensitivity, thyroid gland enlargement, and acute parotitis. Since the suggested regimen is four times daily, many patients consider this therapy inconvenient. Compared to saturated solution of potassium iodide (SSKI), iodinated glycerol provides approximately nine times less iodine. In addition, the metallic taste of organic iodides is absent *(80)*. In 1993 this drug ceased to be marketed in the US after animal tests revealed possible cancer-causing effects.

Bromhexine. Nebulization with bromhexine, a mucolytic agent that reduces mucous viscosity in vitro, was symptomatically beneficial, but not superior to saline in one study *(81)*. The authors commented that the lack of benefit compared to saline in this study could be owing to the more important effect of humidification on mucous viscosity. Bromhexine was effective in enhancing clearance of secretions in chronic bronchitis *(82)*.

ANALGESICS

Analgesics are usually beneficial in short-term relief of pain. Over-the-counter sinus preparations that contain decongestants as well as acetaminophen or ibuprofen are useful provided there are no contraindications to the decongestants. Avoid the use of aspirin because of the risks of Reye's syndrome in children and of gastrointestinal bleeding in adults.

Sensitivity to aspirin, the nonsteroidal anti-inflammatory drugs, or both occurs in about 10% of patients who have both asthma and sinusitis—particularly in patients who have asthma and nasal polyps *(83)*. Although many patients may obtain pain relief from these drugs, a few patients may compound their symptoms by taking them. Only rarely should a patient with sinusitis require a narcotic analgesic.

ANTIBIOTICS AS MUCOLYTICS

The mucolytic properties of antibiotics have been investigated. Norfloxacin reduced the elastic modulus (G') of mucus in one study of chronic sinusitis patients *(84)*, and erythromycin reduced respiratory glycoconjugate secretion in an in vitro preparation of human airways *(85)*. Current studies are investigating the effects on antibiotics with a more favorable antimicrobial profile for the organisms recovered in chronic sinusitis. At present, antibiotics should be selected primarily on their antimicrobial profile.

ANTIHISTAMINES

Antihistamines and other "allergy" medications are generally withheld unless the patient has a history of concomitant allergic disease, supported by appropriate positive laboratory tests. Antihistamines are only of value in treating conditions associated with histamine liberation. There are two instances in which antihistamines are of value in sinusitis therapy: (1) When a patient has symptoms of allergy in conjunction with acute sinusitis in the allergy season, for example, in the ragweed season from mid-August until the first frost. Typically the patient manifests a clinical picture of thin, watery nasal discharge, sneezing, and itchy nose, nasal obstruction, head pain, and congestion. A sinus radiograph, if taken, would be abnormal. This may indicate sinusitis related to an allergic reaction. In such a situation, it is impossible to say whether the problem is allergic rhinitis or an allergic reaction occurring within the sinus cavities. Nevertheless, it is evident the patient needs therapy with either a topical corticosteroid, an antihistamine, or both to reduce mucosal swelling and to keep the ostia open. This strategy helps prevent escalation of an allergic reaction into the infectious process of acute sinusitis as a result of obstruction of the ostiomeatal complex (2). During allergy season, the patient has signs of infection—fever and purulent discharge. First-line treatment of infection using antibiotic and decongestant therapy is indicated. Once the infection is resolved, antihistamines help prevent recurrence. It would also be sensible to put the patient on antiallergy therapy (e.g., topical corticosteroids) before the start of each allergy season. This would help prevent obstruction of the sinus ostia and progression into the sinusitis cycle, and also inhibit the mast cell-mediated late-phase reaction.

The association of allergy and sinusitis is important. European investigators have studied allergy in association with sinusitis with interesting results. In Finland, Savolainen *(86)*, in a study of 224 young adults with verified acute maxillary sinusitis, found allergy in 25% and probable allergy in another 7%. This is compared with corresponding percentages of 16.5 and 3% in a control group of 103 healthy young adults of comparable age. In Belgium, DeCleyn et al. *(87)* studied 270 patients with asthma, rhinitis, or both for sinus pathology, and found that asthma was significantly more often associated with sinus X-ray film abnormalities (65%) than with rhinitis, or chronic cough, or both (44%).

Whether allergy or sinusitis is the primary event in these cases is unknown. Clinically, however, it is clear that the treatment of sinusitis is an important aspect of the therapy of asthma. It has been suggested that children with chronic allergic asthma may be predisposed to sinusitis *(88,89)*. Many children with asthma fail to respond to appropriate therapy for that disease until their sinusitis is diagnosed and treated *(90)*.

Nonpharmacologic Adjuncts

Many nonpharmacologic measures are advocated for symptomatic relief of acute sinusitis. Because scientific data on efficacy are lacking, research-oriented physicians may dismiss some of these measures as folk medicine. For many patients, however, one or more of these treatments may provide effective relief of distressing symptoms while the infection is resolving. Unfortunately, most of these measures are short-lived in effectiveness and must be repeated as symptoms recur.

WETTING AGENTS

Saline. Steam and saline prevent crusting of secretions in the nasal cavity and around the ostiomeatal complex. By liquefying secretions, they also help mucociliary clearance. Repetitive saline applications also reduce nasal blood flow, and thus act as a mild nasal mucosal vasoconstrictor *(67)*. The combination of steam and saline instillation has a beneficial effect on pressure symptoms and prevents nasal crusting. Saline nebulizations were shown to be clinically beneficial in one pediatric study *(81)*. Nasal instillation of saline spray two or three times a day, between steam treatments, is often found to be beneficial. Irrigation with saline, or antral lavage, is a familiar procedure, but one that is best left to ENT surgeons after aspiration of purulent matter from the sinuses of severely congested patients *(83)*.

Steam. The traditional method of steam inhalation is to instruct the patient to pour boiling water in a pan or basin on a low table; sit at the table with a towel draped over the head to make a tent over the pan of water, hold the face a few inches above the water, and breathe through the nose for approx 10 min.

This procedure liquefies and softens crusts while moisturizing the dry, inflamed mucosa. Many patients find that two such treatments a day, with or without additives discussed in Astringents below, provide effective symptomatic relief. If a patient is unable to perform this simple procedure, using a vaporizer or a facial sauna, or taking long, hot showers may be beneficial, but none of this is a good substitute for the hot water and tent method. The ritual of boiling the kettle, preparing the tent, and relaxing over the steamy brew probably has a good psychologic effect, enhancing the therapeutic benefit. Some patients, however, may need to be reminded not to breathe steam directly from a boiling kettle.

Propylene Glycol. Although propylene/polyethylene glycol and saline have been used in clinical studies as placebos, Spector et al. investigated their possible therapeutic role as wetting agents *(91)*. Eighteen patients with perennial rhinitis

were studied for 4 wk of active treatment. Both agents produced symptomatic improvement and objective improvements in airway obstruction at 2 and 4 wk.

HOT AIR

Some patients report benefit from breathing hot, dry air. This dries secretions and also generates or enhances a feeling of well-being. Air at 41°C has been reported to be virucidal in vitro *(92)*, and some commercially available devices provide heated air. However, maxillary sinusitis is usually bacterial, not viral. Only anecdotal evidence supports the premise that hot, dry air is virucidal in vivo.

Studies with different devices have yielded variable results. Yerushalmi et al. demonstrated symptomatic relief in a group of perennial allergic rhinitis patients 1 wk and 1 mo after treatment *(92)*. Two studies were undertaken by a group in Denver *(93)*. In the first study, patients with chronic nasal symptoms and long-term exposure to a perennial allergen to which they were sensitive underwent 1 wk of baseline observation and treatment with either heated or room-temperature room moisturized air for 30 min twice daily. The effect of treatment was assessed by changes in nasal symptoms and nasal blockage index, and by a global evaluation by the subjects at the end of the treatment period. In the second study, patients with a documented history of grass or weed pollen allergic rhinitis underwent titrated nasal pollen challenges immediately after treatment with either heated or room-temperature moisturized air. The outcome was assessed by the end point of the nasal challenge and change in blockage index at the end point. In both models, there was no significant difference in the response between those treated with heated and those treated with room-temperature moisturized air.

A group from Southampton, England observed 10 subjects with rhinitis treated for 30 min with local hyperthermia or placebo, followed 30 min later by nasal allergen challenge. They observed that local hyperthermia significantly reduced both nasal airway resistance and vascular leakage, but had no significant effect on the number of sneezes, mucous secretion, or tryptase release *(94)*. However, dry air may slow nasal mucociliary clearance, as measured by saccharin transit time *(95)*, and thus, humidification may be necessary as well as the elevated temperature.

ASTRINGENTS

Adding pine oil, mentholated preparations such as Vicks VapoRub®, oil of eucalyptus, or similar aromatics may add to the beneficial effect of the steam treatment. Such additions may help relieve stuffiness or at least give a subjective sensation of increased air flow. Although no scientific data support this view, patients claim efficacy.

SPICY FOODS

Garlic has an active ingredient (*n*-allylthio-sulfinate) that provides short-lived decongestant effects. Eating foods highly seasoned with garlic has been considered therapeutic. Ziment *(96)* included a recipe for his wife's garlic-and-chicken soup in his textbook on treatment of respiratory ailments. Encapsulated garlic powder is sometimes recommended by patients who do not like the flavor of garlic in their food. Chewing horseradish root, which is available from many food markets, is another home remedy reported effective in "clearing the sinuses" by some patients. Again, no scientific data support its reported benefits.

CONCLUSION

There is yet no clear evidence that the use of these adjunctive agents prolongs the symptom-free period or reduces the eventual need for surgery. After patients have obtained relief of symptoms, it is important to maintain ostial patency to prevent recurrence of infection. I maintain nasal steroids and saline sprays as tolerated, and oral decongestants if the patient continues to derive benefit from them. I do not routinely obtain follow-up imaging tests to assess progress, but do so if the pattern of symptoms changes or new ones develop. Surgical referral is indicated if there is any suspicion of malignancy, such as appearance of unilateral nasal polyposis, unilateral symptoms, deep pain behind the eyes, bleeding, or visual disturbance. Medical management is less likely to be effective if anatomic blocks to sinus drainage coexist, if hypertension or glaucoma prevent use of decongestants, if presence of nasal ulcers or perforation precludes administration of topical agents, or if there is significant untreated allergy or intolerance to multiple antibiotics. Patients may simply not accept the inconvenience of multidrug therapy. In chronic cases with anatomic obstruction of sinus drainage, surgery is the ultimate mode of therapy.

There is a need for further research in sinusitis management. Most recent studies have addressed the choice of antibiotic, and generally consist of small comparative study populations with acute maxillary sinusitis. Other studies are now appearing that evaluate the site of adjunctive agents. These studies are difficult to design.

Because patients present with a variety of symptoms, it is hard to conceive a scientifically valid study based on objective parameters. A "sham" surgical procedure to ensure blinding would be unethical. Since the use of adjunctive agents has become the accepted "standard of care," it is hard to withhold them *(97)*.

Appropriate therapy of acute sinusitis today includes measures designed to prevent recurrence of acute disease, development of chronic sinusitis, or both. Although there is a paucity of scientific data to support the addition of pharmacologic and nonpharmacologic adjuncts to appropriate antibiotic therapy, there are still compelling theoretic and practical reasons for doing so. These reasons are backed by clear clinical impressions of favorable effects, not only of pharmaceuticals, but also of popular remedies, such as steam inhalation, the irrigations, and breathing hot, dry air. To determine the precise role of pharmacologic adjuncts—topical and oral decongestants, topical corticosteroids, and mucoevacuants—scientifically validated, double-blind, placebo-controlled clinical studies are indicated.

REFERENCES

1. Weinstein L. Acute sinusitis. In: Petersdorf RG, Adams RD, Braunwald E, et al., eds., Harrison's Principles of Internal Medicine, 10th ed. New York: McGraw-Hill, 1983; p. 1570.
2. Ohashi Y, Nakai Y. Functional and morphological pathology of chronic sinusitis mucous membrane. Acta Otolaryngol suppl 1983;397:11–48.
3. Tos M, Mogensen C. Mucus production in chronic maxillary sinusitis: a quantitative histopathological study. Acta Otolaryngol 1984;97:151–159.
4. Ohashi Y, Nakai Y. Reduction of ciliary action in chronic sinusitis. Acta Otolaryngol Suppl 1983;397:3–9.
4a. Reilly JS. Otolaryngol Head Neck Surg 1990;103: 856–862.
5. Druce HM. Diagnosis and management of chronic sinusitis and its complications. Immunol Allergy Clin North Am 1987;7:117–132.
6. Avant RF, Kennedy DW. Need for a national education program on appropriate care of patients with sinusitis. Otolaryngol Head Neck Surg 1990;103:855.
7. Stafford CT. The clinician's view of sinusitis. Otolaryngol Head Neck Surg 1990;103:870–875.

8. Dohlman AW, Hemstreet MPB, Odrezin GT, Bartolucci AA. Subacute sinusitis: are antimicrobials necessary? J Allergy Clin Immunol 1993;91:1015–1023.

9. Newman L, Platts-Mills TAE, Phillips CD, Hazen KC, Gross CW. Chronic sinusitis: relation of computed tomographic findings to allergy, asthma, and eosinophilia. JAMA 1994;271:363–367.

10. Gwaltney JM Jr, Phillips CD, Miller RD, Riker DK. Computed tomographic study of the common cold. N Engl J Med 1994;330:25–30.

11. Williams JW, Simel DL, Roberts L, Samsa GP. Clinical evaluation for sinusitis: making the diagnosis by history and physical examination. Ann Int Med 1992;117:705–710.

12. Wald ER, Byers C, Guerra N, Casselbrant M, Beste D. Subacute sinusitis in children. J Pediatrics 1989;115:28–32.

13. Bluestone CB. The diagnosis and management of sinusitis in children: proceedings of a closed conference. Pediatr Infect Dis 1985;6(suppl):S49–81.

14. Shopfner CE, Rossi JO. Roentgen evaluation of the paranasal sinuses in children. Am J Radiol 1973;118:176–186.

15. Axelsson A, Grebelius N, Chidekel N, Jensen C. The correlation between the radiologic examination and the irrigation findings in maxillary sinusitis. Acta Otolaryngol 1970;69:302–306.

16. Friedman WH, Katsantonis GP, Sivore M, Kay S. Computed tomography staging of the paranasal sinuses in chronic hyperplastic rhinosinusitis. Laryngoscope 1990;100:1161–1165.

17. Friedman WH, Katsantonis GP. Staging systems for chronic sinus disease. ENT Journal 1994;73:480–484.

18. Kennedy DW. Prognostic factors, outcomes, and staging in ethmoid sinus surgery. Laryngoscope 1992;102, Part 2, 1–18.

19. Selner JC, Koepke JW. Rhinolaryngoscopy in the allergy office. Ann Allergy 1985;54:479–482.

20. Kennedy DW, Zinreich SJ, Rosenbaum AE, et al. Functional endoscopic sinus surgery. Arch Otolaryngol 1985;111:576–582.

21. Druce HM, Rutledge JL. Chronic sinusitis and rhinitis. Am J Rhinol 1989;3:163–166.

22. Druce HM. Chronic sinusitis and nonallergic rhinitis. Am J Rhinol 1988;2:163–168.

23. Evans FO, Sydnor JB, Moore WEC, et al. Sinusitis of the maxillary antrum. N Engl J Med 1975;293:735–739.

24. Kovatch AL, Wald ER, Ledesman-Medina J, et al. Maxillary sinus radiographs in children with non-respiratory complaints. Pediatrics 1984;73:306–308.

25. Revonta M. Ultrasound in the diagnosis of maxillary and frontal sinusitis. Acta Otolaryngol 1980;Suppl 370:13–54.

26. Revonta M, Suonpaa J. Diagnosis and follow-up of ultrasonographical sinus changes in children. Int J Ped Otorhinolaryngol 1982;4:301–308.

27. Mann W, Beck C, Apostolidis T. Liability of ultrasound in maxillary sinus disease. Arch Oto-Rhino-Laryngol 1977;215:67–74.

28. Landman, MD. Ultrasound screening for sinus disease. Otolaryngol Head Neck Surg 1986;94:157–164.

29. Shapiro GG, Furukawa CT, Pierson WE, et al. Blinded comparison of maxillary sinus radiography and ultrasound for diagnosis of sinusitis. J Allergy Clin Immunol 1986;77:59–64.

30. Rohr AS, Spector SL, Siegel SC. Correlation between A-mode ultrasound and radiography in the diagnosis of maxillary sinusitis. J Allergy Clin Immunol 1986;78:58–61.

31. Berg O, Carenfelt C. Etiological diagnosis in sinusitis: ultrasonography as clinical component. Laryngoscope 1985;95:851–853.

32. Druce HM, Heiberg E, Rutledge J. Imaging in chronic sinusitis: disparity between radiographic and ultrasound interpretation. Am J Rhinol 1988;2,61–64.

33. Brant-Zawadki MN, Minagi H, Federle MP. High resolution CT with image reformation in maxillofacial pathology. Am J Radiol 1982;138:477–483.

34. Carter BL, Bankoff MS, Fisk JD. Computed tomographic detection of sinusitis responsible for intracranial and extracranial infections. Radiology 1983;147:739–742.

35. Cable HR, Jeans WD, Cullen RJ, et al. Computerized tomography of the Caldwell-Luc cavity. J Laryngol Otol 1981;95:775–783.

36. Lew D, Southwick FS, Montgomery WW, et al. Sphenoid sinusitis: a review of 30 cases. N Engl J Med 1983;309:1149–1154.

37. Som PM, Lawson W, Biller HF, et al. Ethmoid sinus disease: CT evaluation in 400 cases. Part 1. Nonsurgical patients. Radiology 1986;159:591–597.

38. Som PM, Lawson W, Biller HF, et al. Ethmoid sinus disease: CT evaluation in 400 cases. Part II. Postoperative findings. Radiology 1986;159:599–604.

39. Kondo M, Horiuchi M, Shiga H, et al. Computed tomography of malignant tumors of the nasal cavity and paranasal sinuses. Cancer 1982;50:226–231.

40. Schneider G, Sager WD, Lepuschutz H. Multidirectional tomography and high resolution CT in lesions of the paranasal sinuses and the pharyngeal cavity. Acta Radiologica Diagnosis 1982;23:63–69.

41. Conner BL, Phillips K, Roach ES, et al. Nuclear magnetic resonance (NMR) imaging of paranasal sinuses: frequency of abnormalities. J Allergy Clin Immunol 1986;77:139(abstract).

42. Ludman H. Paranasal sinus diseases. Br Med J 1981;282:1054–1058.

43. Conner BL, Roach ES, Laster W, Georgitis JW. Magnetic resonance imaging of the paranasal sinuses: frequency and type of abnormalities. Ann Allergy 1989;62:457–460.

44. Selner JC, Koepke JW. Rhinolaryngoscopy in the allergy office. Ann Allergy 1985;54:479.

45. Messerklinger W. Endoscopy of the Nose. Baltimore: Urban & Schwartzenberg, 1978.

46. DeWeese DD, Saunders WH. Acute and chronic sinusitis. In: Textbook of Otolaryngology, 6th ed. St. Louis: Mosby, 1982; pp. 223–237.

47. Berman SZ, Mathison DA, Stevenson DD, et al. Maxillary sinusitis and bronchial asthma: correlation of roentgenograms, cultures, and thermograms. J Allergy Clin Immunol 1974;53:311–317.

48. Phipatankul CS, Slavin RG. Use of thermography in clinical allergy. J Allergy Clin Immunol 1972;50:264–275.

49. Kalender WA, Rettinger G, Suess C. Measurement of paranasal sinus ventilation by xenon-enhanced dynamic computed tomography. J Computer Asst Tomogr 1985;9:524–529.

50. Juniper EF, Guyatt GH, Archer B, Ferrie PJ. Aqueous beclometasone dipropionate in the treatment of ragweed pollen-induced rhinitis: further exploration of as needed use. J Alergy Clin Immunol 1993;92:66–72.

51. Sykes DA, Wilson R, Chan KL, Mackay IS, Cole PJ. Relative importance of antibiotic and improved clearance in topical treatment of chronic mucopurulent rhinosinusitis. A controlled study. Lancet 1986;2:359,360.

52. Businco L, Fiore L, Frediani T, Artuso A, Di Fazio A, Bellioni P. Clinical and therapeutic aspects of sinusitis in children with bronchial asthma. Intern J Ped Otorhinol 1981;3:287–294.

53. Hamory BH, Sande MA, Sydnor A Jr, Seale DL, Gwaltney JM Jr. Etiology and antibiological therapy of acute maxillary sinusitis. J Infect Dis 1979;139:197–202.

54. Sydnor A Jr, Gwaltney JM Jr, Cocchetto DM, Scheld WM. Comparative evaluation of cefuroxine axetil and cefaclor for treatment of acute bacterial maxillary sinusitis. Arch Otolaryngol Head Neck Surg 1989;115: 1430–1433.

55. Gwaltney JM. Microbiology of Sinusitis. In: Druce HM, ed., Sinusitis—Pathophysiology and Treatment. New York: Marcel Dekker 1994; pp. 41–56.

56. Washburn RG, Kennedy DW, Begley MG, Henderson DK, Bennett JE. Chronic fungal sinusitis in apparently normal hosts. Medicine 1988;67:231–247.

57. Brodie DP, Knight S, Cunningham K. Comparative study of cefuroxime axetil and amoxycillin in the treatment of acute sinusitis in general practice. J Int Med Res 1989; 17:547–551.

58. Felstead SU, Daniel R. Short-course treatment of sinusitis and other upper respiratory tract infections with azithromycin: a comparison with esythromycin and amoxycillin. J Int Med Res 1991;19:363–372.

59. Casiano RR. Azithromycin and amoxicillin in the treatment of acute maxillary sinusitis. Am J Med 1991;91: 275–305.

60. Karma P, Pukander J, Penttila M, Yeikoski J, Savolainen S, Olen L, Melen I, Loth S. The comparative efficacy and safety of clarithromycin and amoxycillin in the breakthrough of outpatients with acute maxillary sinusitis. J Antimicrob Chemother 1991;27:Suppl A:83–90.

61. Marchi E. Comparative efficacy and tolerability of clarithromycin and amoxycillin in the treatment of outpatients with acute maxillary sinusitis. Curr Med Res and Opin 1990;12:19–24.

62. Falser N, Mittermayer H, Weuta H. Antibacterial treatment of otitis and sinusitis with ciprofloxacin and penicillin V—a comparison. Infection 1988;16:Suppl 1:S51–54.

63. Gauger U, Inoka P, Gesmano G, Kissling M. Cefetamet in the treatment of acute sinusitis in adult patients. J Int Med Res 1990;18:228–234.

64. Gehanno P, Depondt J, Barry B, Simonet M, Dewever H. Comparison of cefpodoxime proxetil with cefaclor in the treatment of sinusitis. J Antimicrob Chemother 1990;26: Suppl E:87–91.

65. Boezeman AJ, Kayser AM, Siemelink RJ. Comparison of spiramycin and doxycycline in the empirical treatment of acute sinusitis: preliminary results. J Antimicrob Chemother 1988;22:Suppl B:165–170.

66. Winther B, Gwaltney JM Jr. Therapeutic approach to sinusitis: anti-infectious therapy as the baseline of management. Otolaryngol Head Neck Surg 1990;103: 876–879.

67. Druce HM, Bonner RF, Patow C, et al. Response of nasal blood flow to neurohormones as measured by laser-Doppler velocimetry. J Appl Physiol: Respir Environ Exercise Physiol 1984;57(4):1276–1283.

68. Melen I, Lendahl L, Andreasson L, et al. Chronic maxillary sinusitis: definition, diagnosis and relation to dental infections and nasal polyposis. Acta Otolaryngol 1986; 101:320–327.

69. Melen I, Friberg B, Andreasson L, et al. Effects of phenylpropanolamine on ostial and nasal patency in patients treated for chronic maxillary sinusitis. Acta Otolaryngol 1986;101:494–500.

70. Mygind N. Pharmacotherapy of nasal disease. N Engl and Regional Allergy Proc 1985;6:245–248.

71. Pentel P. Toxicity of over-the-counter stimulants. JAMA 1984;252:1898–1903.

72. Radack K, Deck CC: Are oral decongestants safe in hypertension? An evaluation of the evidence and a framework for assessing clinical trials. Ann Allergy 1986;56: 396–401.

73. Meltzer EO, Orgel HA, Backhaus JW, Busse WW, Druce HM, Metzger WJ, Mitchell DQ, Selner JC, Shapiro GG, van Bavel JH, Basch C. Intranasal flunisolide spray as an adjunct to oral antibiotic therapy for sinusitis. J Allergy Clin Immunol 1993;92:812–823.

74. Patow CA, Kaliner M. Corticosteroid treatment of rhinologic diseases. Ear Nose Throat J 1983;62:14–27.

75. McEvoy GK, ed. AFHS Drug Information 1992. Bethesda, MD: American Society of Hospital Pharmacists, 1992; pp. 1600,1601.

76. Druce HM. Adjuncts to medical management of sinusitis. Otolaryngol Head Neck Surg 1990;103:880–883.

77. Petty TL. Results of a randomized, double-blind, placebo-controlled study of iodinated glycerol in chronic obstructive bronchitis. Chest 1990;97:75–83.

78. Physicians Desk Reference, 47th ed. Montvale, NJ, Medical Economics 1993; p559.

79. Physicians Desk Reference, 47th ed. Montvale, NJ, Medical Economics 1993; p1023.

80. Anonymous. Compendium of Organidin® data. Wallace Laboratories, Cranbury NJ, 1985.

81. Van Beuer HPS, Bosmans J, Stevens WJ. Nebulization treatment with saline compared to bromhexine in treating chronic sinusitis in asthmatic children. Allergy 1987;42: 33–36.

82. Thomson ML, Pavia D, Gregg I, Stark JE. Bromhexine and mucociliary clearance in chronic bronchitis. Brit J Dis Chest 1974;68:21–27.

83. Slavin RG, Friedman WH. Nasal allergy: medical and surgical treatment. Adv Otolaryngol Head Neck Surg 1987;1:91–108.

84. Majima Y, Hirata K, Takeuchi K, Hattori M, Sakakura Y. Effects of orally administered drugs on dynamic viscoelasticity of human nasal mucus. Am Rev Respir Dis 1990;141:79–83.

85. Goswami SK, Kivity S, Marom Z. Erythromycin inhibits respiratory glycoconjugate secretion from human airways in vitro. Am Rev Respir Dis 1990;141:72–78.

86. Savolainen S. Allergy in patients with acute maxillary sinusitis. Allergy 1989;44:116–122.

87. Cleyn KM, Kersschot EA, De Clerck LS, et al. Paranasal sinus pathology in allergic and non-allergic respiratory tract diseases. Allergy 1986;41:3131–3138.

88. Rachelefsky GS, Shapiro GG. Diseases of paranasal sinuses in children. In: Bierman CD, Pearlman DS, eds. Allergic Diseases of Infancy, Childhood and Adolescence. Philadelphia: WB Saunders, 1980; pp. 526–535.

89. Rachelefsky GS, Goldberg M, Katz RM, et al. Sinus disease in children with respiratory allergy. J Allergy Clin Immunol 1978;61:310–314.

90. Shapiro GG. Role of allergy in sinusitis. Pediatr Infect Dis 1985;4(suppl):55–58.

91. Spector SL, Toshener D, Gay I, Rosenman E. Beneficial effects of propylene and polyethylene glycol and saline in the treatment of perennial rhinitis. Clin Allergy 1982;12:187–196.

92. Yerushalmi A, Karman S, Lwoff A. Treatment of perennial allergic rhinitis by local hyperthermia. Proc Natl Acad Sci USA 1982;79:4766–4769.

93. Oppenheimer J, Buchmeier A, Nelson HS. Double-blind trial of a heated nasal aerosol in the treatment of perennial allergic rhinitis. J Allergy Clin Immunol 1993;92:56–60.

94. Johnston SL, Price JN, Lau LCK, Wells AF, Walters C, Feather IH, Holgate ST, Howarth PH. The effect of local hyperthermia on allergen-induced nasal congestion and mediator release. J Allergy Clin Immunol 1993;92: 850–856.

95. Salah B, Dinh Xuan AT, Fouilladieu JL, Lockhart A, Regnard J. Nasal mucociliary transport in healthy subjects is slower when breathing dry air. Eur Respir J 1988;1:852–855.

96. Ziment I. Respiratory Pharmacology and Therapeutics, 1st ed. Philadelphia: WB Saunders, 1978.

97. Druce HM, Slavin RG. Sinusitis: a critical need for further study. J Allergy Clin Immunol 1991;88: 675–677.

10 Ancillary Medical Approaches to the Treatment of Sinusitis

Christopher Chang, MD, PHD
and Stanley Naguwa, MD

CONTENTS

INTRODUCTION

Acute bacterial sinusitis and chronic bacterial sinusitis are often difficult to treat, especially in the patient with associated allergic disease. In addition to the infective inflammation caused by the bacteria in the sinuses, the presence of allergic rhinitis produces further inflammation both in the sinus mucosa and in the nasal pharynx, which is further complicated by a deficiency in mucociliary clearance, increased nasal secretion, and decreased drainage. Thus, the treatment of sinusitis often requires additional measures other than antibiotics, measures that may also ameliorate the need for surgical intervention *(1)*.

These ancillary measures require an understanding of the features of sinusitis. Sinusitis may be acute, chronic, or subacute. The onset of sinusitis may be heralded by a pre-existing viral infection and exacerbated by a variety of host features *(2)*. These features are listed in Table 1. Several of these

From: *Diseases of the Sinuses* (M. E. Gershwin and G. A. Incaudo, eds.), ©1996 Humana Press Inc., Totowa, NJ.

host features may be present simultaneously. The sinuses should be considered closed structures, since inflammation in the sinus can inhibit optimal drainage. Therefore, although antibiotic therapy is crucial, it alone will not suffice to eradicate a nondraining sinus, which is essentially an abscess. Other measures must be taken and are of equal importance *(3)*. These measures take into consideration improving mucociliary clearance and changing the consistency of mucus, or enlarging the outflow tract to facilitate drainage. Eosinophilic and basophilic reactions in the sinuses often further complicate bacterial sinusitis, and structural defects are known to inhibit drainage of cellular exudates and pus, and therefore delay the effectiveness of antibiotics. Inherent defects in mucociliary clearance are thought to be important pathologic entities that must be corrected to facilitate antibiotic therapy of sinusitis. Optimization of treatment requires that we improve conditions for the host to eradicate the disease. This includes treatment of all pre-existing conditions, such as allergic rhinitis, polyps, immunodeficiency disorders, and if possible, even viral upper respiratory infections (URIs).

Table 1
Host Features Involved in Sinusitis

Allergic causes
  Allergic rhinitis
  NARES
Immune deficiency
  Antibody deficiency
    Bruton's agammaglobulinemia
    Common variable immune deficiency
    Wiskott Aldrich Syndrome
    Selective IgG subclass deficiency
    Ataxia telangectasia
    AIDS
    Selective IgA deficiency
    SCIDS
  Complement abnormalities
    C3b inactivator deficiency
    C3 deficiencies
  Leukocyte abnormalities
    Chronic granulomatous disease
    Hyper IgE syndrome
    Chediak-Higashi Syndrome
Structural defects
  Cleft palate
  Ciliary defects
  Osteopetrosis
  Foreign bodies
Other
  Cystic fibrosis
  Asthma
  Nasal polyposis
  Allergic fungal sinusitis
  Aspirin sensitivity

ANCILLARY MANAGEMENT OF SINUSITIS—PREVENTION

Viral URIs

It is a common practice for primary care physicians to treat runny noses, cough, congestion, and other signs of a simple viral URI with antibiotics. Although this may not be intellectually sound, it may not be as ludicrous as first believed. The number of viral infections that have an associated sinusitis component of either bacterial or viral origin varies between studies, from an average of about 5% (4) to a high of about 21% (5) in a recent study using computerized tomography (CT) scanning in otherwise healthy adults. Although some of these subjects recovered spontaneously without antibiotics, suggesting a viral origin, there is certainly the subset of these patients who do develop

chronic bacterial sinusitis as a result of a viral URI. Early treatment may be a way of preventing a full-blown sinusitis. On the other hand, there are those who would argue that empirical antibiotic therapy would only serve to produce sinusitis caused by bacteria that are even more resistant to treatment.

PREVENTION

Prevention of viral infections therefore does provide benefit both from a clinical standpoint and from a medically cost-effective standpoint, since measures that prevent viral infections are usually less expensive than the treatment of an ensuing bacterial sinusitis. Simple principles that would help to prevent viral infections are reducing the intensity and frequency of exposure by general hygienic measures or vaccinations, or by simple avoidance, especially in children. The latter has been rendered more difficult to achieve because of the increase in families with two working parents and the increased utilization of day-care facilities with high numbers of infants and toddlers. The time of virus shedding by children with respiratory syncytial virus (RSV) is commonly 3–8 d, except in younger children, where it may be as long as 3–4 wk (6).

General Hygiene. Frequent hand washing by personnel who are in contact with small children, especially those who are sick, will help in reducing exposure to viral infections. Hand washing is applicable to children and adult patients as well. Avoidance of contact of nasal or ocular mucosa by unwashed hands is also helpful. Antiviral measures may be implemented by the use of cleansing agents on work or play surfaces both in the home and work environments. The life-span of RSV, for example, on inanimate objects is probably many hours, and inoculation can be accomplished by contact with contaminated infant secretions long after the infant has been removed from the area (6). RSV can be killed using solvents, such as CIDEX (7). RSV is most common in the winter and early spring, and eventually will infect all children during the first 3 yr of life (8). Bronchiolitis is the most common manifestation of RSV in young children, but in older children and adults, the illness usually presents as an upper respiratory tract illness or bronchitis (9,10). This may thus be a trigger for the onset of sinusitis in the latter population. Although RSV is the most common viral pathogen in young children, other viruses, such as picornavirus, parainfluenza virus, or coronavirus, may be more predominate pathogens of viral URIs in older children or adults. Influenza virus, common in the winter months, results in a viral syndrome consisting of malaise, congestion, and cough, and may be also be a trigger for sinus infection.

Vaccinations. Prevention of influenza virus illness in individuals with chronic respiratory diseases, such as asthma, has been conducted for several years during the fall/winter season in the US. This strategy to prevent viral URIs in large numbers of individuals during the winter months has been recommended for all individuals with chronic rhinosinusitic or pulmonary disease (perennial allergic rhinoconjunctivitis, asthma, cystic fibrosis), as well as immune deficiency syndromes, immunosuppressive therapy, sickle-cell anemia and other hemoglobinopathies, significant cardiac disease, diabetes mellitus, chronic renal disease, chronic metabolic diseases, AIDS, and long-term aspirin therapy *(11)*. Household contacts of the above-mentioned individuals, day-care providers, and hospital personnel in contact with pediatric patients should also receive influenza vaccine. The split virus vaccine is recommended for children under 12 yr of age, with a second dose given to children under 8 yr of age. Side effects of the vaccine are uncommon, the most frequent being local reactions in older children and adults.

TREATMENT

Treatment of viral URIs includes the use of antiviral medications, measures that may be toxic to viral replication, as well as a pharmacopoeia of over-the-counter (OTC) medications. Since many of the OTC medications are also utilized by patients with already existing sinusitis, each individual class of these medications will be discussed in a later section. Currently, antiviral medications are not routinely indicated for the chemoprophylaxis or treatment of URIs in older children or adults. Aerosolized Ribavirin is presently being used to treat severe bronchiolitis in hospitalized children *(12,13)*. Amantadine and rimantadine are approved by the Food and Drug Administration (FDA) for use in children and adults for prophylaxis against influenza A infection. There are specific indications for the use of these agents in treatment of influenza because of their potential side effects, including renal toxicity. In addition, these agents are only beneficial in specific strains of influenza

virus infection. Although prevention of influenza in some patients may stall the development of sinusitis, amantadine and rimantadine are not currently recommended in the treatment of routine "viral illnesses," and therefore do not play a role in the treatment of sinusitis in otherwise healthy individuals.

It is a popular notion by both the public and the health care sector that milk causes increased production and viscosity of mucus. Although this association is probably no more than a subjective belief that has not been substantiated in two studies in patients with rhinovirus-2 induced infection and asthmatics *(14,15)*, milk avoidance is practiced by patients who have URIs or chronic respiratory diseases.

HYPERTHERMIA

Hyperthermia may exert physical changes on the consistency of mucus, but its beneficial effects may not end there. Rhinoviral replication has been shown to be inhibited at temperatures at or around 43°C *(16)*. To what degree this in vitro observation can be extrapolated to the clinical setting has yet to be confirmed *(17–21)*. Studies have been inconclusive, although this has not prohibited the manufacture, patent, and selling of devices, such as the Rhinotherm or Virotherm, both of which deliver heated air to the nasal mucosa by various devices *(17,18,20,21)*. The success of the Rhinotherm has been demonstrated in one study, where three 22- or 30-min treatments were able to improve nasal symptoms by 73–81% within 24 h *(22,23)*. These reports have not been confirmed by subsequent studies. Similarly, although the Virotherm has been found to improve symptoms of a treatment group significantly over a group given 30°C air *(17)*, there were enough problems with the design and methodology of the study that the results are still equivocal. One must be careful not to use heated air indiscriminately, since the in vitro effects of air between 40 and 55°C on ciliary beat frequency is one of beat cessation. This has not been proven to be so in vivo, suggesting that the nasal mucosa regulates nasal temperature enough that all this discussion of nasal air temperatures may be academic.

Using Hot Drinks (Tea, Water, or Chicken Soup)—Does It Work (24,25)? On the other hand, it has been common among old wives' tales of various cultures to recommended hot liquids to treat a cold. In China, hot tea has been a remedy for the common cold for many centuries, and in the Western world, chicken soup has been passed down from generation to generation as a mode of treatment for the "flu." The longevity of these beliefs would lead one to conclude that there is indeed some benefit from the administration of hot liquids. More recently, attempts to study this phenomenon have revealed that hot liquids have improved mucociliary clearance without having much effect on nasal airway resistance (26).

Allergies and Environmental Exposure

ALLERGIC RHINITIS

Allergen-induced inflammation of the nasal mucosa is known to lead to decreased sinus clearance and drainage owing to the swelling around the nasal osteomeatal complex (27). Skin testing or radioallergosorbent (RAST) assay may improve identification of specific environmental or food triggers in allergy-prone individuals. This would subsequently allow for the avoidance of such triggers, if possible, and if not, by desensitization. Immunotherapy and sinusitis are discussed further below.

BAROTRAUMA

Swimming, diving, working in tunnels, and playing wind or brass instruments all increase intranasal, intrasinus, and intrapharyngeal pressures (28). There are no studies to confirm that these activities will cause sinusitis, but to the extent that such activities may reduce clearance of secretions, they do have the potential to exacerbate already existing problems with sinus drainage, such as in those people with allergic rhinitis, polyps, and so forth.

CIGARET SMOKE, POLLUTION, AND OTHER IRRITANTS

Passive smoking is known to increase the incidence of upper and lower respiratory infections in children and adults (29–32). Exposure to other irritants, such as air pollution (33), as well as odors and perfumes in susceptible individuals can cause edema of the nasal, conjunctival, and airway mucosa, and thus increase the risk for developing sinusitis. Passive cigaret smoking, in particular, causes an increased incidence of nasal congestion and irritation in both atopic and nonatopic children, but also increases the incidence of middle ear effusions, tympanostomy tubes, and tonsillectomy and

adenoidectomies. There are no studies attempting to relate passive smoking with sinusitis, but considering the similarities in pathogenesis between otitis media and sinusitis (34), it is reasonable to postulate that a connection does exist.

Anatomic Obstruction

Septal deviation, nasal polyps, sinus polyps, sinus mucous retention cysts, tumors, and foreign bodies are all fixed conditions that inhibit sinus drainage. CT scan imaging (35) and rhinoscopy (36) have been invaluable in making the diagnosis of underlying structural abnormalities that may decrease sinus ostia diameter and subsequently decrease drainage. In addition, it has been shown that a sinus ostia diameter of <2.5 mm leads to a decrease in sinus paO_2, which is associated in turn with an increased incidence of sinusitis (37). The use of corticosteroids to reduce the size of such obstructions will be discussed later.

ANCILLARY MANAGEMENT OF SINUSITIS—TREATMENT

Ancillary treatment of sinusitis begins at home, where most people will employ a variety of medical and nonmedical measures to relieve the symptoms of sinusitis. These modes of therapy are possible because of the wide variety of medications and nonmedical equipment available to the public without a prescription. Decongestants, antihistamines, expectorants, mucolytics, and combinations of these make up the major revenue generated business for pharmaceutical manufacturers. Clearly, not all of the above are safe or even medically indicated for the treatment of sinusitis. In addition, vaporizers, humidifiers, air filters, special vacuum devices and so on, are examples of the equipment that may be purchased in any general merchandise store.

Nonmedical Approaches to the Treatment of Sinusitis

HUMIDIFICATION

The rationale behind the use of humidification of surrounding air is that moisture tends to facilitate mucociliary clearance, partly by changing the consistency of the mucus. There are many techniques available to accomplish this, ranging from simple saline nose drops (38,39) to the use of (relatively) expensive equipment (40) to increase the humidity in the nasal passages. In patients with chronic sinusitis, nasal saline irrigation has resulted in clinical improvement in 11 of 13 patients, primarily as a result of removal of the obstructing media. Nasal saline nose drops are available in any drugstore. They may also be prepared at home by mixing 1/4 teaspoon of salt with one small cup of warm water, and agitating until all the saline is dissolved. The saline can then be administered with a standard medicine dropper or by irrigation of the sinuses with a bulb syringe. Although this mode of therapy appears safe and there are no documented cases of sinusitis caused by the use of saline made from tap water, one must realize that tap water may contain contaminants, as evidenced by Acanthamoebic eye infections in contact lens wearers who have prepared their saline in the above fashion *(41)*.

The use of warm, humidified air delivered via controlled delivery devices, such as the Rhinotherm and Virotherm, has been extensively studied in the treatment of allergic rhinitis and viral URIs, as described above. Whether these devices have any role in treatment of sinusitis has yet to be determined.

Improving the humidity of environmental air also has been proposed to have an effect on mucociliary clearance. The use of either vaporizers or humidifiers has been recommended by various specialists, including allergists, pediatricians, and otolaryngologists. Occasionally, patients may achieve symptomatic relief from a hot washcloth placed over the face.

EXERCISE AND SINUSITIS

Exercise has been beneficial in reversing ostial obstruction in patients with allergies *(42)*. The reason for this may be the stimulation of systemic catecholamine release or by an increase in sympathetic release at the local level *(43)*. This effect appears to be transient and does not occur in patients with concurrent sinus disease *(44)*. Since the effect is not persistent after cessation of physical exertion, the use of exercise in the treatment of sinusitis or even to treat allergic rhinitis in an attempt to circumvent sinusitis is not recommended at this time.

Ancillary Medications Used in Sinusitis

DECONGESTANTS

α-Adrenergic decongestants are commonly found in OTC medications for colds, sinuses, and other ailments. They are frequently used for symptomatic relief and make up much of the revenue

Table 2
Nonantibiotics Used in Sinusitis—Oral Decongestants

Pseudoephedrine
  Onset of action 15–30 min
  Duration of action—variable
  Typical dosage—120 mg a day in divided doses
  Side effect: raises blood pressure
Phenylpropanolamine
  Onset of action 15–30 min
  Duration of action—variable
  Typical dosage—100 mg qid in divided doses
  Side effect: raises blood pressure

generated by the pharmaceutical industry. The rationale behind the use of these agents is that they decrease edema in the nasal mucosa, and thereby maintain or widen ostea patency via their vasoconstrictive effects. There are both nasal (topical) and oral (systemic) decongestants.

Nasal Decongestants. Nasal decongestants are widely sold in drugstores, supermarkets, and large discount stores. Both α_1- and α_2-adrenergic agents are available (Table 2). The advantage of the α_1-adrenergic topical decongestants is that they have less action on nasal resistance vessels and thus cause less compromise of mucosal blood flow. In general, however, the use of nasal decongestants is not recommended because of its potential for overuse or abuse, its addictive nature, and a condition known as rhinitis medicamentosa. In addition to rhinitis medicamentosa, prolonged use of nasal decongestants (especially the α_2 class) results in atrophy of the nasal mucosa owing to vasoconstriction. Vasoconstriction may theoretically lead to decreased delivery of antibiotics to the sinuses and thereby compromise antibiotic therapy. Rhinitis medicamentosa appears to occur predominately in patients with pre-existing chronic nasal disease. In these patients, tolerance to the topical agent develops and increased use of the drug ensues. A rebound interstitial edema results, leading to a rebound congestion, whereupon most patients who use this type of medication enter into a viscous cycle, with progressive edema complicated by continued overuse of topical α-adrenergic decongestants. In a controlled trial in patients with uncomplicated vasomotor rhinitis, the prolonged (3 wk) use of topical xylometazoline resulted in decreased effectiveness of the medication, but did not cause tolerance in any of the subjects *(45)*.

There are specific instances in which topical adrenergic agents may be indicated. They may be used just prior to the use of anti-inflammatory nasal sprays to improve delivery during administration of the latter, or they may be used for short-term therapy of acute viral and bacterial sinusitis. In addition, they may be beneficial in improving mucociliary clearance. However, in any event, we do not recommend topical α-adrenergic agents for long-term therapy under any circumstances.

Oral Decongestants. Unlike nasal decongestants, several studies have not clearly shown untoward effects of oral decongestants on nasal mucosa and turbinate edema. In contrast, oral decongestants have clearly been shown to be able to decrease nasal airway resistance. The two oral decongestants used are pseudoephedrine, in doses of 60–120 mg, and phenylpropanolamine, dosage 30–100 mg. Clinically, these agents are effective in reducing symptoms of congestion, and multiple studies have demonstrated a significant increase in the ostial openings from the sinuses in patients who are treated with oral decongestants. The effects of oral decongestants generally have their onset within 30 min and last anywhere from 4–12 h, depending on the manufacturing methodology. The nonregulated use of these medications alone or in combination speaks for its low adverse effect rate. However, oral decongestants do have potential to cause hypertension at fairly low dosages, and safety issues with regard to the frequent use by patients are yet to be fully resolved. There is some evidence that high-dose oral decongestants may be of additional benefit in the treatment of sinusitis.

Antihistamines

First-Generation Antihistamines. Although use of antihistamines is generally not recommended for the treatment of sinusitis alone, they are beneficial when the sinusitis occurs in atopic individuals *(39)*. Most of the earlier antihistamines had significant anticholinergic effects, and this may play a role in drying out secretions, which generally makes them more difficult to clear.

Second-Generation Antihistamines. Currently, there are three nonsedating antihistamines available. All are prescription medications. These are astemizole, terfenadine, and loratadine. Two of the three, terfenadine and loratadine, have recently been combined with an α-adrenergic decongestant.

Table 3
Nonantibiotics Used in Sinusitis—
Mucoactive Agents

Mucolytics
Expectorants
Mucokinetics
Mucoregulators
Mucorrheics
Ciliary stimulants
Detergents

Antihistamine use should be reserved for those patients with allergic rhinoconjunctivitis.

Combination Products

There are numerous combination products on the market. These products attempt to combine the beneficial effects of decongestants, antihistamines, and expectorants. Often an agent with cough-suppressant activity or an analgesic is added. Most of these products are OTC. Most manufacturers provide a variety of combinations for the public to choose from. Unfortunately, this strategy of treating sinusitis is scientifically unsound and essentially adheres to the "shotgun" approach to medicine. Most people who purchase these medications from their local supermarket have little knowledge of the actions of each of the ingredients. Much of the beneficial effects are psychological in nature. Clearly, should there be tighter restrictions on the use of these medications, a decrease in unwarranted medical costs would be seen.

Mucoactive Agents

Mucoactive agents may include expectorants, mucolytics, mucorrheics, mucokinetic agents, and other mucoregulatory agents *(46)* (Table 3). In addition, there are also detergents and ciliary stimulants available. Many products have multiple activities. The most commonly used mucolytic agent is *N*-acetylcysteine *(47–49)*, which is not available in the United States for treatment of upper respiratory conditions. However, its experience in Europe and Asia both in nebulized and oral liquid form has shown that it is an effective agent in decreasing sputum viscosity in chronic bronchitis. Other activities of *N*-acetylcysteine include normalization of mucoprotein secretion, stimulation of gastropulmonary vagal reflexes, and stimulation of mucosal secretions. In addition, *N*-acetylcysteine also acts as a chelator and an antioxidant.

Table 4
Nonantibiotics Used in Sinusitis—Nasal Steroids

Medication	Made by	Topical potency relative to hydrocortisone	Systemic potency	µg/spray	Adult dosage	µg/d/relative daily topical potency	Delivery method
Flunisolide (Nasalide)		3000	12.8	25	2 sp bid	100/300,000	Freon
Beclomethasone dipropionate (Beconase AQ, Vancenase AQ)		5000	3.5	42	2 sp bid	168/840,000	Freon or aqueous
Triamcinolone (Nasacort)	Rhone Poulenc Rorer	1000	5.3	55	2 sp qid	110/110,000	Freon
Budesonide (Rhinocort)		10,000	1.0	50	2 sp bid	200/2,000,000	Freon
Fluticasone propionate		20,000		50	1 sp bid	100/2,000,000	Aqueous

Its use as an antidote for acetaminophen poisoning is based on its antioxidant properties. Similar derivatives of L-cysteine include S-carboxymethyl cysteine (SCMC), which has also been shown to be effective in the treatment of bronchitis when given in oral dosages of 3 or 2.25 g daily over placebo (50). Improvement in sputum volume and viscosity, forced expiratory volume in 1 s, and overall clinical symptomatology were noted. Both N-acetylcysteine and SCMC have been extensively studied, and their safety has been clearly demonstrated. However, like other OTC medications available in the US, their use in chronic sinusitis has not been clearly demonstrated, although one study with SCMC did show an improvement in mucociliary clearance (51). Serratio peptidase and L-cysteine ethyl ester also improved the viscoelastic properties of mucus. Improvement in symptoms was also noted in patients with chronic bronchitis (52).

A double-blind, placebo-controlled study was done to investigate the effectiveness of the mucolytic iodoglycerol in relieving symptoms of chronic bronchitis in adults (53). Iodoglycerol is a potent mucolytic with a long history of widespread use for upper respiratory disease. It is also a significant ciliary excitatory agent. Iodoglycerol in 60 mg qid dosaging resulted in subjective clinical improvement in cough frequency and productivity, chest pain, and number of days of illness. There are, however, no controlled studies on the use of iodoglycerol in chronic sinusitis, and it has been taken off the market by the FDA.

Guaifenesin has an even longer history, and is a common component of cold and cough formula-

tions. It is reputed to have significant expectorant effects, owing to its ability to change sputum adhesiveness, although it has no effect on the amount of secretions and their viscosity (54). However, its clinical efficacy in the treatment of sinusitis is not scientifically proven, and, like other OTC medications, is of dubious value for this indication.

Other mucoregulatory agents include bromhexine, 2 mercaptoethane sulfonic acid, and ambroxol. Most of the medications have been studied for chronic bronchitis, and any benefit in chronic sinusitis is speculative at the present time. However, there are similarities between the two diseases, and there is preliminary evidence that decrease in mucoviscosity with improvement in mucociliary clearance may result from SCMC, L-cysteine ethyl ester, and N-acetylcysteine (NAC) use.

ANTI-INFLAMMATORY AGENTS

Steroids: Topical. Nasal steroids are now the mainstay of therapy for allergic rhinitis (Table 4). The effectiveness of nasal steroids in treating sinusitis is less clear. The rationale behind the use of nasal steroids in sinusitis is based on the observation that sinusitis, whether infectious or not, involves a significant inflammatory process. Patients with seasonal allergic rhinitis demonstrate an increase in sinus mucosa activity during allergy seasons, as shown by single-photon emission CT scanning. Pathologic findings in patients with allergic rhinitis-related sinus disease include increased levels of nasal eosinophils, as well as sinus mucosa damage similar to the inflammation seen in asthma. Neutrophilic and basophilic cell

Table 5
Nonantibiotics Used in Sinusitis—Nasal Decongestants

Sympathomimetic agents
　　Phenylephrine
　　Neosynephrine, NS, Dristan
Imidazoline derivatives
　　Naphazoline
　　Tetrahydozoline
　　Oxymetazoline
　　Xylometazoline

infiltrates are also seen. Increased levels of eosinophilic cellular secretions are found in patients with allergy-related sinusitis. Eosinophilic cationic protein and major basic protein exert opposite effects on respiratory glycoconjugate and lactoferrin release from respiratory epithelium.

A placebo-controlled multicenter study in which flunisolide was evaluated as an adjunct to antibiotics in sinusitis patients revealed that the flunisolide-treated group did better clinically, according to global assessment evaluation. The flunisolide-treated group also showed a significant improvement in the degree of radiologic involvement. Both groups went into remission after 3 wk of antibiotics, but in neither group was the remission long-standing and relapses occurred in 1/4 to 1/3 of patients (55).

In a double-blind study using maxillary sinus irrigation with neomycin alone or in conjunction with the topical steroid tixocortal pivalate, there was a significantly better rate of ostia patency in the steroid-treated group (56). Clinical symptomatology was not studied. In another study, dexamethasone with or without tramazoline was associated with a higher improvement rate of sinus drainage, mucociliary clearance, and nasal airway resistance over placebo. There was no significant difference between the two study groups (57).

Topical corticosteroid therapy is considered safe as an ancillary treatment of sinusitis. Human ciliary function and mucociliary clearance is not adversely affected by topical steroid therapy (58,59). The nasal steroids currently commercially available are shown in Table 5. Beclomethasone dipropionate sprays are provided both as an aqueous solution and as a Freon powder, whereas flunisolide, triamcinolone, and budesonide are available only as Freon powder. In contrast, fluticasone propionate is provided only in aqueous solution

form. Some patients prefer one delivery mode over the other. In general, topical corticosteroids only need to be administered once or twice a day, so patient compliance is fairly good.

Steroids: Systemic. Systemic steroids can be given orally, intramuscularly, intravenously, or intraturbinate. There are no controlled trials of systemic corticosteroids in sinusitis. However, in a comparative study of 53 adults with nasal polyps, it has been shown that a single dose of oral steroids had at least an equivalent improvement in smell and nasal airway resistance over surgical polypectomy after 1 yr and an even greater short-term improvement (60). Both groups also received intranasal beclomethasone sprays twice daily during the year-long trial. In addition, a single dose of methylprednisolone was shown to be able to decrease nasal obstruction for 4 wk in patients with allergic rhinitis (61,62). Systemic steroids may be indicated in patients in whom nasal obstruction is so severe that nasal sprays are ineffective in penetrating the nasal mucosa. Intraturbinate injections of steroids are an unproven mode of delivery in sinusitis. The safety of intraturbinate injections is also not yet established.

Cromolyn Sodium—Is There a Role? Cromolyn is widely used as an anti-inflammatory in asthmatic patients. It is also used for allergic rhinitis. Cromolyn inhibits immediate- and late-phase allergic reactions. Controlled studies have failed to demonstrate any significant improvement in the clinical symptomatology in patients with URIs and documented maxillary sinusitis (63). Cromolyn has also not been found to be effective for treatment of the so-called nonallergic rhinitis with eosinophilia syndrome (NARES) (64). Cromolyn is therefore not recommended as an ancillary measure for prevention or treatment of sinusitis.

ANTICHOLINERGICS

Ipratropium bromide (Atrovent) is currently the only anticholinergic agent used topically to treat nonallergic or vasomotor rhinitis. Although its effectiveness in the treatment of nonallergic forms of rhinitis has been clearly demonstrated (65), there are no good studies on its use in chronic sinusitis. However, it may also have some usefulness in sinusitis, because of its ability to reduce methacholine hyperactivity, thereby indirectly modulating secretion volume and edema of the sinus and nasal mucosa. Ipratropium bromide is a derivative

Table 6
Nonantibiotics Used in Sinusitis—Intravenous Immunoglobulins

Nonantibiotic	Distributor	Concentration	IgG content	IgA content, μg/mL	Shelf-life, mo	Half-life, d
Polygam	American Red Cross	5% (10%)	>90%	<3.7	24	24
Venoglobulin-I	Alpha	5% (10%)	>97%	24–38	24	29
Venoglobulin-S	Alpha (solution)	5%	>99%	10–27	24	33.5
Gammar-IV	Armour	5% (10%)	>98%	20	36	25
Gammagard S/D	Baxter/Hyland	5% (10%)	>90%	<3.7	27	24
Gamimune N	Cutter/Miles	5%, 10%	>98%	<270	5%: 36, 10%: 27	21–35
Iveegam	Immuno-US	5%	100%	<2	24	23–29
Sandoglobulin	Sandoz	3, 6, 9, 12%	>96%	<970	36	23

of noratropine, and acts to inhibit nasal glandular secretion, but, in contrast to atropine, has no effect of lacrimal gland, goblet cell, or sinus secretions. Atropine, therefore, is not recommended for the treatment of sinusitis, since decreased mucociliary clearance may result from its use.

IV γ-GLOBULIN

Patients who present with recurrent bouts of sinusitis or pneumonia often have an underlying immune deficiency, which usually lies in B-cell function. This usually presents as IgA deficiency or IgG subclass deficiency. Encapsulated organisms like *Haemophilus influenzae* are the most commonly seen pathogens. In these patients, monthly infusions of iv γ-globulin, given to keep the trough level of serum IgG within a normal range, have been effective in preventing further episodes of sinusitis. A typical dose of immunoglobulin may be 200 mg/kg/mo. Several different preparations of immunoglobulin are available, as shown in Table 6.

IMMUNOTHERAPY AND SINUSITIS

There are no controlled studies on the use of immunotherapy in sinusitis. Immunotherapy may be beneficial in patients whose sinusitis is secondary to increased mucosal edema and secretions caused by allergic rhinitis.

PAIN MANAGEMENT

Control of headache and facial pain in sinusitis must not be de-emphasized, since many patients are often debilitated by a bout of sinusitis. Acetaminophen, aspirin, or ibuprofen is often sufficient to alleviate pain of sinusitis. Since drug sensitivity to

aspirin and other nonsteroidal anti-inflammatory medications may occur in patients with asthma, nasal polyps, and sinusitis, acetaminophen is generally safer. Desensitization to aspirin in this small group of patients, who comprise about 3–4% of all asthmatics with sinusitis, may be performed. Sinusitis, along with allergic rhinitis and nasal congestion may play a trigger role in migraine headaches.

OTHERS

Furosemide is beneficial in patients with asthma. However, its efficacy in rhinitis and sinusitis has not been uniformly demonstrated (66,67). Although astringents are frequently recommended, again they have not been subjected to controlled studies (68). Posture has been shown to affect nasal patency, and it is recommended that the patient attempt to lie on the side opposite to a unilateral sinusitis since nasal patency decreases on the "down" side, presumably owing to gravitational shifting of the turbinates (69). As our understanding of the mediators involved in the inflammatory response increases, we anticipate future promising areas of study to include the modulation of the inflammatory response in sinusitis by platelet-activating factor antagonists, leukotriene antagonists, protease inhibitors, and tachykinins. As our understanding of gene regulation and our ability to control bodily functions at a DNA level increases, mucin gene regulation may become one of the mechanisms by which we may control the consistency and volume of secretions during an episode of sinusitis and thereby facilitate treatment.

CONCLUSIONS

Despite exciting advances in medical research, the ancillary treatment of sinusitis is still limited to a few very popular age-old therapies. From the above discussion, we are able to formulate a plan to reduce the incidence of sinusitis and to treat sinusitis that does not involve, or is complementary to the use of antibiotics and surgery. This recommendation takes into account the known causes or exacerbating factors of sinusitis in a wide range of patients.

Avoidance

1. Identify known host factors;
2. Identify environmental factors;
   a. Avoid allergens;
   b. Avoid passive smoking;
   c. Avoid contact with URIs;
3. Immunotherapy.

Treatment

1. Hot liquids (potential indirect benefit);
2. Nasal saline irrigation and hydration;
3. Topical nasal steroids;
4. Oral decongestants (not nasal decongestants);
5. Antihistamines (may help in allergic patients);
6. Mucoactive agents;
7. IV γ-globulin (in patients with immunodeficiency).

REFERENCES

1. Dohlman AW, Hemstreet MPB, Odrezin GT, Bartolucci AA. Subacute sinusitis: are anti-microbials necessary? J Allergy Clin Immunol 1993;91:1015–1023.
2. Kaliner MA. Human nasal host defense and sinusitis. J Allergy Clin Immunol 1992;90:424–430.
3. Sykes DA, Chan KL, Wilson R, MacKay IS, et al. Relative importance of antibiotic and improved clearance in topical treatment of chronic mucopurulent rhinosinusitis. Lancet 1986;2:359,360.
4. Wald, ER, Guerra N, Byers C. Upper respiratory tract infections in young children: duration of and frequency of complications. Pediatrics 1991;87:120–133.
5. Gwaltney JM, Phillips CD, Miller RD, Riker DK. Computed tomographic study of the common cold. N Engl J Med 1994;330: 25–30.
6. Peter G, Halsey NA, Marcuse EK, Pickering LK, eds. 1994 Red Book: Report of the Committee on Infectious Diseases, 23rd ed., Elk Grove Village, IL: American Academy of Pediatrics, 1994; pp. 396–398.
7. Cidex Activated Dialdehyde Solution package insert. Arlington, TX: Johnson and Johnson Medical Inc., 1994.
8. Lewis FA, Rae ML, Lehmann NI, et al. A syncytial virus associated with epidemic disease of the lower respiratory tract in infants and young children. Med J Aust 1961; 2:932,933.
9. Hall CB, Douglas RG. Respiratory syncytial virus and influenza. Practical community surveillance. Am J Dis Child 1976;130:615–620.
10. Glezen WP, Denny FW. Epidemiology of acute lower respiratory tract disease of children. N Engl J Med 1973;288:498–505.
11. Peter G, Halsey NA, Marcuse EK, Pickering LK, eds. 1994 Red Book: Report of the Committee on Infectious Diseases, 23rd ed., Elk Grove Village, IL: American Academy of Pediatrics, 1994; pp. 275–283.
12. Hall CB, McBride JT, Walsh EE, et al. Aerosolized ribavirin treatment of infants with respiratory syncytial virus infections: a randomized double-blind study. N Engl J Med 1983;308:1443–1447.
13. Rodriguez WJ, Kim HW, Brandt CD, et al. Aerosolized ribavirin in the treatment of patients with respiratory syncytial virus disease. Pediatr Infect Dis J 1987;6:159–163.
14. Pinnock CB, Graham NV, Mylvagnanam A, Douglas RM. Relationship between milk intake and mucus production in adult volunteers challenged with rhinovirus-2. Am Rev Resp Dis 1990;141:352–356.
15. Haas F, Bishop MC, Salazar-Schicchi J, Axen KV, et al. Effect of milk ingestion on pulmonary function in healthy and asthmatic subjects. J Asthma 1991;28:349–355.
16. Lowff A. Death and transfiguration of a problem. Bacteriol Rev 1969;33:390–403.
17. Tyrrell D, Barrow I, Arthur J. Local hyperthermia benefits natural and experimental common cold. Br Med J 1989;298:1280–1283.
18. Macknin MC, Mathew S, Medendorp SV. Effects of inhaling heated vapor on symptoms of the common cold. JAMA 1990;264:989–991.
19. Forstall GJ, Macknin ML, Yen-Leiberman BR, Medendorp SV. Effects of inhaling heated vapor on symptoms of the common cold. JAMA 1994;271:1109–1111.
20. Yerushalmi A, Karman S, Lwoff S. Treatment of perennial allergic rhinitis by local hyperthermia. Proc Natl Acad Sci 1981;79:4766–4769.
21. Ophir D, Elad Y, Dolev Z, Geller-Bernstein C. Effects of inhaled humidified warm air on nasal patency and nasal symptoms in allergic rhinitis. Ann Allergy 1988;60:239.
22. Shim C, King M, Williams MH. Lack of effect of hydration on sputum production in chronic bronchitis. Chest 1987;92:679–682.
23. Ophir D, Elad Y. Effects of steam inhalation on nasal patency and nasal symptoms in patients with the common cold. Am J Otolaryngol 1987;3:149–153.
24. Yerushalmi A, Lwoff A. Traiteniente du coryza infectieux des rhinities persistantes allergiques par la thermothérapie. CR Acad Sci (D) Paris 1987;281:957–959.
25. Bang BC, Mukherjee AL, Bang FB. Human nasal mucous flow rates. Johns Hopkins Med J 1967;121:38–48.
26. Ingels KJAO, Kortman MJW, Nijziel MR, et al. Factors influencing ciliary beat measurements. Rhinology 1991;29:17–26.
27. Sakethoo K, Januszkiewicz A, Sackner MA. Effects of drinking hot water, cold water and chicken soup on nasal mucus velocity and nasal airflow resistance. Chest 1978;74:408–410.

28. Spector SL. The role of allergy in sinusitis in adults. J Allergy Clin Immunol. 1992;90:518–520.

29. Slavin RG. Nasal polyps and sinusitis. In: Middleton E, Reed CE, Ellis EF, Adkinson NF, et al., eds., Allergy: Principles and Practice. St. Louis: Mosby-Yearbook, 1993; pp. 1455–1470.

30. Kreaemer MJ, Richardson MA, Weiss NS, et al. Risk factors for persistent middle-ear effusions. JAMA 1983; 249:1022–1025.

31. Said G, Zalokar J, Lellouch J, Patois E. Parental smoking related to adenoidectomy and tonsillectomy in children. J Epidemiol Community Health 1978;32:97–101.

32. Iversen M, Birch L, Lundqvist GR, Elbrond O. Middle ear effusions in children and the indoor environment: an epidemiological study. Arch Environ Health 1985;40: 74–79.

33. Forastiere F, Corbo GM, Michelozzi P, Pistell R, et al. Effects of environment and passive smoking on the respiratory health of children. Int J Epidemiol 1992;21:66–73.

34. Joakkola JJK, Paunio M, Virtanen M, Heinonen OP. Low-level air pollution and upper respiratory infections in children. Am J Pub Health 1991;81:1060–1063.

35. Otten FWA, Grote JJ. Otitis media with effusion and chronic upper respiratory tract infection in children. Laryngoscope 1990;100:627–633.

36. Corren J, Rachelefsky GS. Interrelationship between sinusitis and asthma. Immunol Allergy Clin North Am 1994;14:171–184.

37. Sinreich SJ. Imaging of chronic sinusitis in adults: X-ray, computed tomography and magnetic resonance imaging. J Allergy Clin Immunol 1992;90:445–451.

38. Aust R, Drettner B. Oxygen tension in the human maxillary sinus under normal and pathological conditions. Acta Otolaryngol (Stockh) 1974;78:264–269.

39. Druce HM. Adjuncts to medical management of sinusitis. Otolaryngol Head Neck Surg 1990;103(Suppl.):880–883.

40. Mabry RL. Therapeutic agents in the medical management of sinusitis. Otolaryngol Clin North Am 1993; 26:561–570.

41. Zeiger RS. Prospects of ancillary treatment of sinusitis in the 1990s. J Allergy Clin Immunol 1992;90:478–495.

42. Stapleton F, Seal DV, Dart J. Possible environmental sources of *Acanthamoeba* species that cause keratitis in contact lens wearers. Rev Infect Disease 1991;13(Suppl. 5):5892.

43. Okki M, Hasigawa M, Kurita N, Watanabe I. Effects of exercise on nasal resistance and nasal blood flow. Acta Otolaryngol (Stockh) 1987;104:328–333.

44. Juto JE, Lungberg C. Nasal mucosal reactions, catecholamines and lactate during physical exercise. Acta Otolaryngol (Stockh) 1984;98:533,534.

45. Melen I, Andreasson L, Ivarsson A, et al. Effects of phenylpropanolamine on ostial and nasal airway resistance in healthy individuals. Acta Otolaryngol (Stockh) 1986;102:99–105.

46. Akerlund A, Bende M. Sustained use of xylometazoline nose drops aggravates vasomotor rhinitis. Am J Rhinol 1991;5:157–160.

47. Wanner A. The current status of mucolytic drugs. Contemp Int Med 1991;3:29–37.

48. Hirsch SR, Kory RC. An evaluation of the effect of nebulized N-acetylcysteine on sputum consistency. J Allergy 1978;39:265–273.

49. Ziment I. Acetylcysteine: a drug with an interesting past and a fascinating future. Respiration 1986;50(Suppl. 1):26–30.

50. Boman G, Backer U, Larsson S, et al. Oral acetylcysteine reduces exacerbation rate in chronic bronchitis: report of a trial organized by the Swedish Society for Pulmonary Diseases. Eur J Respir Dis 1983;64:405–415.

51. Edwards GF, Steel AE, Scott JK, Jordan JW. S-carboxymethylcysteine in the fluidation of sputum and treatment of chronic airway obstruction. Chest 1976;70:506–513.

52. Sakakura Y, Majima Y, Ukai SS, Miyoshi Y. Reversibility of reduced mucociliary clearance in chronic sinusitis. Clin Otolaryngol 1985;10:79–83.

53. Majima Y, Hirata K, Takeuchi K, Hattari M, et al. Effects of orally administered drugs on dynamic viscoelasticity of human nasal mucus. Am Rev Respir Dis 1990;141:79–83.

54. Petty TL. The National Mucolytic Study: results of a randomized, double-blind, placebo-controlled study of iodinated glycerol in chronic obstructive bronchitis. Chest 1990;97:75–83.

55. Hirsch SR, Viernes PF, Kory RC. The expectorant effect of glycerol guaiacolate in patients with chronic bronchitis (a controlled in vitro and in vivo study). Chest 1973;63:9–14.

56. Meltzer EO, Orge HA, Backhaus JW, Busse WW, et al. Intranasal flunisolide spray as an adjunct to oral antibiotic therapy for sinusitis. J Allergy Clin Immunol 1993;92: 812–823.

57. Cuenant G, Stipon JP, Plante-Longchamp G, et al. Efficacy of endonasal neomycin-tixocortol pivalate irrigation in the treatment of chronic allergic and bacterial sinusitis. ORI. J Otorhinolaryngol Relat Spec 1986; 48:226–232.

58. Sykes DA, Chan KL, Wilson R, et al. Relative importance of antibiotic and improved clearance in topical treatment of chronic mucopurulent rhinosinusitis: a controlled study. Lancet 1986;2:159,160.

59. Lildholdt T, Fogstrup J, Gammelgaard N, et al. Surgical versus medical treatment of nasal polyps. Acta Otolaryngol (Stockh)1988;105:140–143.

60. Holmberg K, Pipkorn U. Influence of topical beclomethasone dipropionate suspension on human nasal mucociliary activity. Eur J Clin Pharmacol 1986;30: 625–627.

61. Dechateau GSMJE, Zuidema J, Merkus HM. The in vitro and in vivo effect of a new non-halogenated corticosteroid-budesonide aerosol on human ciliary epithelial function. Allergy 1986;41:260–265.

62. Brown E, Seideman T, Siegelaub AB, Popvitz C. Depomethylprednisolone in the treatment of ragweed hay fever. Ann Allergy 1960;18:1321–1330.

63. Sederberg-Olsen JF, Sederberg-Olsen AE. Intranasal sodium cromoglycate in post-catarrhal hyperreactive rhinosinusitis: a double-blind placebo controlled trial. Rhinol 1989;27:251–255.

64. Nelson BL, Jacob RL. Response of the nonallergic rhinitis with eosinophilia (NARES) syndrome to 4% cromolyn sodium nasal solution. J Allergy Clin Immunol 1982;70:125–128.

65. Roszko R, Bornsky E, Druce H, Findlay F, et al. Ipratroprium bromide nasal spray 0.03%. Assessment of

efficacy and safety in non-allergic perennial rhinitis. J Allergy Clin Immunol 1993;91:196.

66. El-Mallah ME, Abul-Khair MM, El-Hadidi SS, Fouda EE, et al. Furosemide spray in inhalation allergic rhinitis. J Allergy Clin Immunol 1993;91:260.

67. Prat J, Mullal J, Ramis I, Rosello-Catafan J, et al. Release of chemical mediators and inflammatory cell influx during early allergic reaction in the nose: effect of furosemide. J Allergy Clin Immunol 1993;92:248–254.

68. Druce HM. Medical management of sinusitis in the adult. In: Druce HM, ed. Sinusitis. New York: Marcel Dekker 1994; pp. 73–85.

69. Cole P, Haight JS. Posture and nasal patency. Am Rev Respir Dis 1984;129:351–354.

11

Orbital and Intracranial Complications of Sinusitis in Children and Adults

Katherine A. Kendall, MD and Craig W. Senders, MD

CONTENTS

INTRODUCTION

Intracranial and intraorbital complications are often the first indication of untreated or partially treated sinus disease. All patients presenting with an intracranial or orbital infection must be evaluated for the presence of occult sinus disease. Successful treatment of intracranial and intraorbital complications of sinusitis requires the recognition and successful treatment of the initial focus of infection within the sinuses.

ETHMOID SINUSES

Introduction

The ethmoid sinuses are present at birth. Thus, patients of any age may be subject to complications arising from infection of the ethmoids. Orbital cellulitis is secondary to ethmoid sinusitis in 75% of cases *(1)*. Approximately 85% of the patients presenting with orbital complications of sinusitis are in the pediatric age group *(2,3)*.

From: *Diseases of the Sinuses* (M. E. Gershwin and G. A. Incaudo, eds.), ©1996 Humana Press Inc., Totowa, NJ.

Orbital Complications

ANATOMY AND PHYSIOLOGY

The orbit is located directly adjacent to the ethmoid sinuses and is divided from them by the thin lamina papyracea. The lamina is often congenitally dehiscent, and contains ostia for the passage of the anterior and posterior ethmoid arteries and nerves. These openings in the bone allow the direct extension of infection from the ethmoid sinuses into the orbit. More importantly, valveless veins drain directly from the sinuses into the orbit. The lack of valves allows the flow of septic thromboemboli through these vessels from the sinuses into the orbit. The superior ophthalmic vein is in continuity with the nasofrontal vein and the angular vein of the face. In the posterior portion of the orbit, it drains the anterior and posterior ethmoid veins, passes between the two heads of the lateral rectus muscle, and then through the superior orbital fissure to empty into the cavernous sinus. The inferior ophthalmic vein drains a number of small veins that originate along the medial wall and floor of the orbit. It courses through the inferior orbital fissure to drain into the pterygoid plexus, or it drains directly into the cavernous sinus *(4)*.

The periosteum of the orbit is called the periorbita. It is easily elevated from bone, except in the area of the suture lines between the bones of the orbit, which include the ethmoid, frontal, maxillary, sphenoid, lacrimal, and palatine bones. The extension of an orbital subperiosteal abscess is partially limited by the suture lines. Further extension of infection may progress directly through the periorbita and into the orbital contents rather than beyond bony suture lines *(4)*.

The periorbita becomes the orbital septum as it is reflected from the orbital rims and extends within the eyelid to the tarsal plates. The orbital septum acts as a relative barrier to infection. Infections anterior to the orbital septum do not usually extend into the orbit and must be distinguished from orbital infections with eyelid edema. Similarly, abscesses forming within the orbit and posterior to the orbital septum rarely perforate anteriorly through it. The orbital septum can thus act to maintain increasing pressure within the orbits owing to space-occupying lesions, such as abscesses. Occasionally, a medially located subperiosteal abscess of the orbit will drain through the skin near the medial canthus of the eye.

CLASSIFICATION

Chandler's classification (1970) *(4a)* describes the progression of orbital infection owing to sinusitis. Modifications of the classification were made by Schramm et al. in 1982, who distinguished patients with periorbital cellulitis and chemosis from patients otherwise in the periorbital cellulitis group. He felt that patients with periorbital cellulitis and chemosis had a more severe form of the disease and were more likely to require surgical drainage of the infection *(5)*. The original classification as described by Chandler is:

1. Inflammatory edema: Inflammatory edema of the eyelids and orbit without infection results from impedance of orbital venous drainage into the thrombosed sinus veins. The absence of valves in this entire complex permits the transmission of elevated pressure in the sinus veins resulting from infection to the vascular bed of the orbit and the eyelids.
2. Orbital cellulitis: The same venous continuity allows the migration of bacteria into the orbit and eyelids via the extension of septic phlebitis and periphlebitis. If the infection is posterior to the orbital septum, true orbital cellulitis results.

3. Subperiosteal abscess: Although venous continuity plays a role in the development of subperiosteal abscess, the accumulation of pus directly adjacent to the infected sinuses may also occur by extension of organisms through neurovascular foramina and bony dehiscences, or as a result of osteitis and necrosis of the thin shared bony walls. Subperiosteal abscess can occur early in the course of disease and may be present before diffuse orbital cellulitis develops.
4. Orbital abscess: Orbital abscesses typically result from progression and organization of diffuse orbital cellulitis or from extension of a subperiosteal abscess into the orbit.
5. Cavernous sinus thrombosis: Thrombosis of the cavernous sinus occurs when orbital thrombophlebitis spreads distally via the veins that drain the orbit into the cavernous sinus. Bilateral orbital involvement rapidly develops as a consequence of the cavernous sinus thrombosis.

The ordering of the classification should not be taken as a rigid chronology for the development of orbital complications resulting from sinusitis. A subperiosteal abscess often is not associated with orbital cellulitis (Fig. 1).

DIAGNOSIS

Many patients with orbital complications of sinusitis present with a history of a recent upper respiratory tract infection (URI) followed by rapid development of eyelid edema and pain *(6)*. Sinusitis and orbital infection may be accompanied by fever, purulence from the middle meatus, changes in visual acuity, decreased extraocular mobility, and proptosis.

The first sign of orbital cellulitis is edema of the eyelid. Chemosis of the sclera may occur at this point. The edema is thought to result from impairment of orbital venous drainage, and usually begins in the upper lid and progresses to involve the lower eyelid. Ecchymotic discoloration of the lids is known to occur with *Haemophilus influenzae* periorbital infections *(1,2)*. Involvement of the orbital contents posterior to the orbital septum leads to the development of proptosis. The globe may protrude in an axial direction with orbital cellulitis *(2)*, and down or out in the case of a subperiosteal abscess or an orbital abscess. Decreased extraocular mobility accompanies proptosis. Selective limitation of ocular mobility suggests a localized collection of pus, such as a subperiosteal abscess.

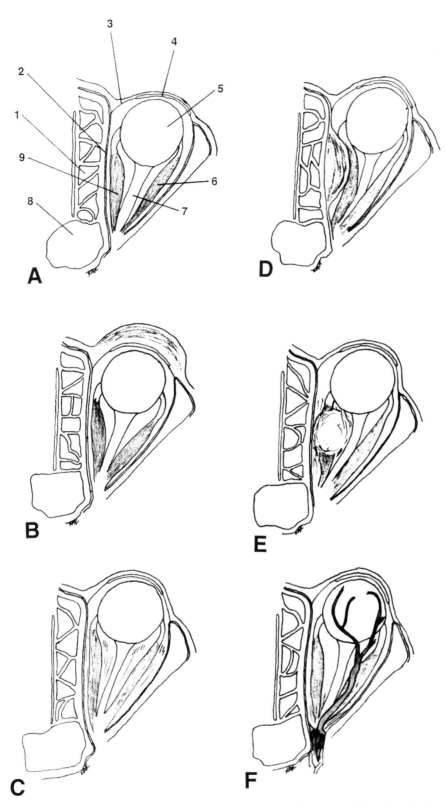

Fig. 1. Categories of orbital infection. **(A)** normal orbit (1, ethmoid air cells; 2, periorbita; 3, orbital septum; 4, tarsal plate; 5, globe; 6, lateral rectus muscle; 7, optic nerve; 8, sphenoid sinus; 9, medial rectus muscle); **(B)** preseptal cellulitis; **(C)** orbital cellulitis; **(D)** subperiosteal abscess; **(E)** orbital abscess; **(F)** cavernous sinus thrombosis.

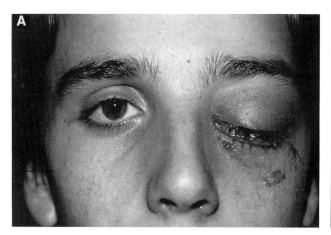

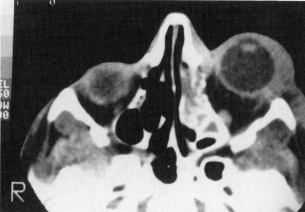

Fig. 2. (A) Photograph showing patient with subperiosteal abscess. **(B)** CT scan of patient with subperiosteal abscess.

Complete ophthalmoplegia is more likely to develop with orbital abscess or cavernous sinus thrombosis than with orbital cellulitis (Fig. 2A).

Visual loss, in addition to decreased acuity, may present as a Marcus-Gunn pupil, which is an ipsilateral afferent pupillary defect, decreased color vision, or as visual field defects. Ideally, a thorough examination by an ophthalmologist is performed in all patients with periorbital infection. Decreased visual acuity is thought to be related to the increased intraorbital pressure. The orbital fat and extraocular muscles become edematous owing to inflammation caused by the infection. The superior ophthalmic vein may be compressed as it passes through the heads of the rectus muscles and exits the superior orbital fissure. Loss of venous drainage from the orbit further increases the intraorbital pressure. Eventually, when intraorbital pressure is high enough, retinal artery occlusion results. In cases of subperiosteal abscess and orbital abscess, traction on the optic nerve resulting from forward displacement of the globe by the expanding abscess directly compromises the blood supply to the nerve and the retina.

CT scans and orbital ultrasound are the most useful tools currently available to aid in the diagnosis of an orbital abscess. If CT is not possible, ultrasound can distinguish between orbital abscess and cellulitis. However, there is poor resolution of the orbital apex with ultrasound, and an abscess in this region can be missed *(1,5)*. When using CT scanning to rule out an orbital abscess, it is important to use thin (2–4 mm) sections with high-resolution capabilities for viewing soft tissue and bone detail. Scans should be obtained in both the axial and coro-

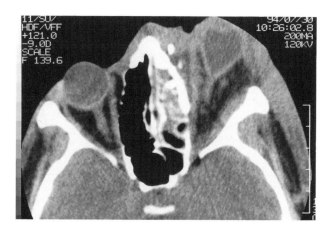

Fig. 3. CT scan of patient with orbital abscess originating from ethmoid sinus infection.

nal plane with proper window settings to evaluate both bone and soft tissue. The presence of an orbital abscess is suggested on CT by a low-density mass effect, with or without rim enhancement (Figs. 2B and 3). An air–fluid level within a mass is very specific for an abscess. Lateral displacement of the medial rectus muscle with associated edema is an indication of subperiosteal inflammation, but subperiosteal abscess can only be identified with certainty by very low density or gas adjacent to the lamina papyracea and evidence of displacement of the periosteum away from the lamina papyracea (Fig. 4). Edema of the medial rectus alone is consistent with orbital cellulitis.

There is a small but significant incidence of false-negative results on CT scan performed to evaluate for intraorbital or subperiosteal abscess. Difficulty in delineating cellulitis from an abscess arises when the scans demonstrate areas of post-

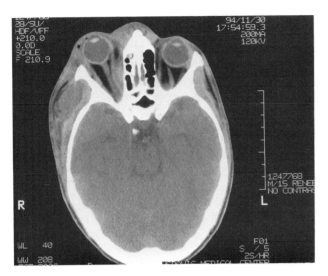

Fig. 4. Right orbital subperiosteal abscess on CT scan.

septal mass effect, contrast enhancement, or both without definite tissue necrosis. In a study by Gutowski et al. *(3)*, 33 patients with orbital complications of sinusitis were reviewed. All patients underwent CT scan for diagnostic purposes that demonstrated an 84% accuracy in distinguishing abscess from cellulitis. The clinical exam had established the correct diagnosis in 70% of patients. In cases of periorbital cellulitis with chemosis, the diagnosis was established 100% of the time by CT scan or physical examination. The diagnosis of other orbital complications by either modality tended to underestimate the severity of the disease especially in the group of patients given a diagnosis of orbital cellulitis. Forty percent of cases initially diagnosed as periorbital cellulitis progressed to require surgery where an abscess was found.

Patt and Manning reported from a 10-yr review from Parkland Memorial Hospital including 38 patients that the four cases resulting in permanent blindness all had CT scans that did not definitely demonstrate an orbital abscess. They concluded that the CT reading contributed to a delay in surgical drainage and thus the blindness in these patients. Vision changes eventually prompted surgical exploration in these cases, and it is important to recognize that such findings may not be apparent until permanent visual loss has occurred *(7)*.

Timing of the CT scan is somewhat controversial, since there may be a question regarding what constitutes an adequate therapeutic trial before entertaining the diagnosis of abscess and the need for surgical drainage. In general, a CT scan is rec-

ommended if the patient shows no signs of clinical improvement within 48 h of the initiation of antibiotic therapy. Axial and coronal sections are recommended, since they will have less likelihood of missing an abscess near the orbital roof and give a full evaluation of the sinuses to aid in planning of the surgical approach should an abscess be diagnosed. In patients who present with visual changes or a clinical picture consistent with orbital abscess, a CT scan should be performed immediately.

MRI of the orbit is excellent for delineating orbital abscesses when fat saturation is used to decrease the signal from orbital fat. The test, however, is generally more expensive than a CT scan, takes longer to obtain, and may require sedation or general anesthesia for pediatric patients since movement during the longer scanning times will compromise the study. The environment of the MRI scanner is not conducive to adequate monitoring of patients under sedation. For these reasons, MRI has not been used commonly for the evaluation of orbital infections.

Cultures of infected material should be obtained to direct appropriate antibiotic therapy. The question arises regarding the best source of fluid for culture of an infected tissue deep within the structures of the face. Blood cultures are positive in 33% of children <4 yr of age, but are usually not helpful in older children and adults. Cultures of purulent material draining from the middle meatus are more useful and should be done if possible. Fluid aspirated or swabbed from the skin of the eyelid has been unreliable in determining the organisms responsible for the orbital infection *(2,4,5)*. Purulent material taken directly from the abscess yields the most accurate results, but frequently can be negative owing to partial treatment of the infection with antibiotics *(1)*. The use of lumbar puncture to obtain cerebral spinal fluid (CSF) for culture in patients with periorbital cellulitis is not warranted unless the patient exhibits clear signs of central nervous system (CNS) involvement *(5,8)*.

In general, blood cultures should be drawn in children <4 yr of age presenting with periorbital cellulitis. In all patients, an attempt to obtain fluid from the middle meatus should be made, keeping in mind that a swab of fluid from elsewhere in the nose is not accurate because of contamination with normal nasal flora. In those patients who require surgical exploration, orbital cultures should always be taken.

Preseptal cellulitis must always be included in the differential diagnosis of orbital infection. It usually results from a break in the skin, such as an insect bite, or it can develop from a stye. Preseptal cellulitis involves the orbital structures anterior to the orbital septum. Both preseptal and orbital cellulitis present with chemosis, conjunctival injection, pain, erythema, and eyelid swelling. In addition to these signs, orbital cellulitis presents with proptosis, decreased extraocular mobility, and decreased visual acuity, which distinguish it from preseptal cellulitis. Preseptal cellulitis rarely involves postseptal anatomy, and treatment consists of the administration of broad-spectrum antibiotics covering the common skin pathogens that results in rapid resolution of symptoms. Most investigators agree that CT is unnecessary for evaluation of simple preseptal periorbital cellulitis unless there is evidence of proptosis or gaze restriction, and the possibility of orbital involvement must be ruled out. Surgery is not indicated unless there is progression to lid abscess.

Several other space-occupying lesions affect the orbit and must be differentiated from an orbital abscess. Orbital pseudotumor, which presents as a mass in the orbit without fever or sinusitis, is treated with steroids. Neoplasms of the orbit are similar in presentation to an abscess, but signs develop more gradually. Orbital neoplasms include rhabdomyosarcoma in children, leukemia, lymphoma, and metastatic neuroblastoma. Hematoma of the orbit is difficult to distinguish from an abscess on CT scan, but is usually accompanied by a history of trauma.

The progression of an orbital infection owing to sinusitis is not the only cause of cavernous sinus thrombosis, and patients presenting with cavernous sinus thrombosis may be suffering from other sources of infection, such as a superficial skin infection. The Tolusa Hunt Syndrome is a nonspecific granulomatous inflammation involving the cavernous sinus, orbital apex, and granulomatous periarteritis of the cavernous carotid. The clinical criteria characterizing the syndrome are:

1. Steady, gnawing retro-orbital pain;
2. Paresis in the third, fourth, sixth, or the first branch of the fifth cranial nerve with less common involvement of the optic nerve or sympathetic fibers around the cavernous carotid artery;
3. Symptoms lasting days to weeks;
4. Occasional spontaneous remission;

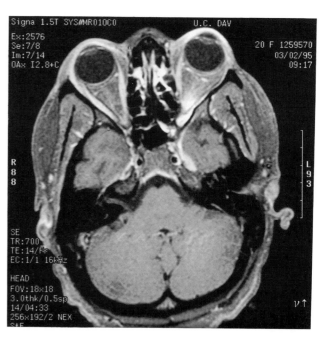

Fig. 5. T1-weighted MRI scan using fat saturation and gadolinium showing findings of Tolusa-Hunt Syndrome.

5. Recurrent attacks; and
6. Prompt response to steroid therapy *(9)*.

CT and MRI may show asymmetric enlargement of the cavernous sinus by a soft tissue mass with convex lateral margins *(10)*. A cavernous sinus abnormality that is isointense with muscle on T_1-weighted images and isointense with fat on T_2-weighted images is found on MRI (Fig. 5) *(9)*.

Dacryoadenitis is an infection of the lacrimal gland and presents with preseptal cellulitis. There is no orbital involvement with this condition *(2)*. A ruptured dermoid cyst can also present with eyelid swelling and is usually located on the superolateral bony margin of the orbit. Again, a dermoid cyst presents with minimal involvement of the globe.

TREATMENT

The organisms usually cultured from infections of the orbit are those organisms most commonly involved in sinusitis. In children, the most common pathogen grown from blood cultures is *H. influenzae* followed by *S. pneumoniae (4,5)*. The cultures of orbital purulence from adults have most often grown *Streptococcus* species and *Staphylococcus aureus.* Other organisms involved include: *Klebsiella pneumoniae, Esherischia coli, Pseudomonas,* and anaerobes. In cases of chronic sinusitis in older patients, anaerobes play a larger role *(2,4)* (Table 1).

Table 1
Most Common Organisms
Involved in Complications of Sinusitis

Orbital infection
    Children
        H. influenzae
        S. pneumoniae
    Adults
        Streptococcal species
        S. aureus
    General
        K. pneumoniae
        E. coli
        P. aeruginosa
        Anerobes
Meningitis
    S. aureus
    S. pneumoniae
    H. influenzae
    Anerobes
Spenoid sinusitis
    S. aureus
    Streptococcal species
    H. influenzae
    P. aeruginosa
    K. pneumoniae
    Enterobacter species
Frontal osteomyelitis
    Anerobic *Streptococci*
    Staphylococci
Cerebral abscess
    Staphylococcal species
    S. pneumoniae
    H. influenzae
    Anerobes
Epidural and subdural abscess
    Streptococcal species
    S. aureus
    Fusobacterium species
    Bacteroides fragilis
    H. influenzae
    Lactobacillus species
Cavernous sinus thrombosis
    S. aureus

Drugs selected to treat orbital complications of sinusitis should be able to cross the blood–brain barrier because intracranial complications are the sequelae of both intraorbital infection and ethmoid sinus infection *(1)*. Broad-spectrum antibiotics known to be effective against the most commonly involved organisms should be chosen. Treatment should be continued for a total of 14 d. Oral antibi-otics can replace the iv antibiotics when the patient has improved and has been afebrile for 48 h. Steroids should be avoided in the presence of active infection when there is no evidence of concurrent meningitis.

The production of β-lactamase by many of the organisms involved in these infections has resulted in an increasing problem with antibiotic resistance. The incidence of penicillin-resistant *S. pneumoniae* in the United States from 1990 to 1991 was 20%. Thirty percent of *H. influenzae* type B, 15% of non-type B *Haemophilus* species, and >85% of *Moraxella catarrhalis* produce β-lactamase. These penicillin-resistant organisms have been found to be sensitive to some of the cephalosporins, including cefotaxime, ceftriaxone, cefuroxime, cefpodoxime, cefdinir, and cefprozil. When choosing antibiotics for empiric therapy of infections originating in the sinuses, the possibility of antibiotic resistance must be taken into consideration *(11)*.

Surgical exploration of the orbit with simultaneous drainage of the affected sinuses is indicated when there is no clinical improvement or a progression of symptoms, such as a decrease in visual acuity, after 24–48 h of antibiotics, or when there is clear evidence of abscess on presentation, such as air–fluid levels seen on CT of the orbit. Visual checks every 2 h are recommended during the first 48 h of iv antibiotic therapy, and decreasing visual acuity is an absolute indication for immediate surgical exploration. Some authors recommend that a lateral canthotomy be performed at the bedside when there are signs of worsening visual acuity. This is done in an attempt to decrease intraorbital pressure rapidly while the patient is being prepared for surgery *(1)*. In patients who are immuno-compromised (diabetes, HIV), it is recommended that surgical exploration be performed with decreases of visual acuity to 20/60, since these patients tend to progress rapidly to serious complications, such as blindness *(7)*. Controversy exists over whether a CT scan showing an apparent abscess is always an indication for immediate surgery. Some authors have reported that such patients may clear with antibiotic therapy alone *(2)*. We recommend surgery in these cases to avoid the potentially serious complications of an undrained abscess and believe that patients who resolve with antibiotics alone most likely did not have a true orbital abscess (Fig. 6).

Treatment Algorithm for Orbital Cellulitis

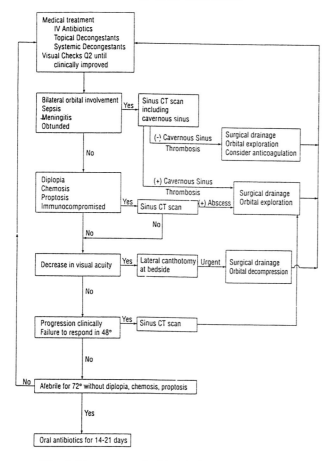

Fig. 6. Treatment of orbital infection algorithm.

The traditional approach to the orbit is via an external ethmoidectomy incision, which allows for a simultaneous drainage and exenteration of the involved ethmoid sinuses prior to exploration of the orbit. With advances in endoscopic instrumentation and surgical technique, some surgeons feel comfortable approaching the orbit endonasally. The lamina papyracea can be removed under visualization through the ethmoid air cells with the use of an endoscope. This approach is effective in draining limited subperiosteal abscesses, but is not appropriate for draining an orbital abscess. The technique avoids an external scar, but is more limited in its exploration and requires a highly experienced endoscopic sinus surgeon *(12)*.

OUTCOME

Long-term sequelae of orbital complications of sinusitis include permanent visual loss and cavernous sinus thrombosis. Loss of retinal blood flow for 90 min will result in permanent blindness. Cavern-

ous sinus involvement presents with multiple cranial nerve defects, proptosis, involvement of the contralateral eye, and altered mentation. Many of these neurologic complications may not resolve even after the infection has been eradicated.

Intracranial Complications

ANATOMY AND PHYSIOLOGY

The roof of the ethmoid cavity is formed by the fovea ethmoidalis. Adjacent to the fovea in the cribriform plate that is perforated by the olfactory foramina for the passage of the olfactory nerves. The pathway for direct intracranial spread of infection from the ethmoid cavities is along the perineural sheaths of the olfactory nerves and by direct vascular extension within the vessels that accompany the olfactory nerves *(13)*.

CLASSIFICATION

The brain and spinal cord are covered by three membranes. The tough outer layer is the dura mater, which is attached to the inner surface of the cranial bones much like periosteum. Beneath the dura is the spider web-like arachnoid mater. Adherent to the brain is the fibrous membrane known as the pia mater. The dura mater is also called the pachymeninx, whereas the arachnoid and pia mater are collectively called the leptomeninges. Intracranial infections are classified according the their location in relation to the brain coverings. Epidural abscess refers to a collection of infected fluid between the cranial bones and the dura. If infection spreads beneath the dura into potential space between the arachnoid and the dura, it is classified as a subdural empyema. Because the arachnoid mater is not adherent to the dura, there is no impedance to the spread of infection in this space, and purulent material can spread over the entire surface of the brain. Beneath the arachnoid is the subarachnoid space in which cerebral spinal fluid flows. Infection in this space is meningitis. An understanding of the layers covering the brain is also pertinent to the intracranial spread of infections from the sphenoid and frontal sinuses (Fig. 7).

MENINGITIS

Meningitis accounts for 70% of all intracranial complications of sinusitis. Rhinogenic meningitis may also occur after cranial or facial trauma in which a bony dehiscence or mucocele resulted. The intracranial infection may not occur for years after

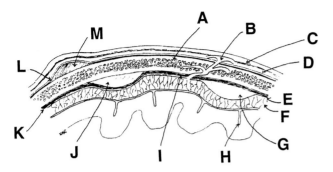

Fig. 7. Cranial skin and bone and meninges. Spaces typically involved in infection: **(A)** cranial bone; **(B)** diploic vein; **(C)** skin and subcutaneous tissue; **(D)** galea aponeurotica; **(E)** arachnoid; **(F)** subarachnoid space (CSF); **(G)** subdural abscess; **(H)** pia mater; **(I)** subdural space; **(J)** epidural abscess; **(K)** dura; **(L)** pericranium; **(M)** subperiosteal abscess.

the injury so it is important to obtain a trauma history in patients with meningitis or intracranial abscess.

The symptoms of meningitis include fever, progressive severe headache, irritability, somnolence, and delirium. In meningitis associated with sinusitis, the clinical presentation may be atypical *(14)*. Since partial antibiotic treatment can mask other signs and symptoms, mild headache, retro-orbital pain, or subtle changes in sensorium are often the only presenting complaints. Early in the course of disease, a high index of suspicion is required to make the diagnosis.

Signs of meningeal irritation are Brudzinski's Sign (flexion of the neck causes flexion at the knees) and Kernig's Sign (the knee cannot be extended while the hip is flexed). These signs are produced by meningeal irritation, which causes muscle splinting throughout the paravertebral musculature radiating out into the extremities.

The lumbar puncture (LP) is the most important study in the evaluation of meningitis, and typically reveals elevated white count, elevated protein, and decreased glucose. CSF should be sent for culture. A CT scan should be obtained prior to LP to rule out the presence of an intracranial mass lesion commonly accompanied by increased intracranial pressures and an increased risk of brain herneation during the LP. On a nonenhanced CT scan, meningitis produces increased density of the usually black CSF spaces. On a normal enhanced CT scan, the blood vessels on the surface of the brain and the meninges are enhanced. Meningitis must, therefore, be diagnosed on enhanced CT by an increased

degree of enhancement and thickening of the meninges beyond the normal range. On MRI, there is usually minimal dural enhancement in the patient without a meningeal abnormality. When meningitis is present, enhancement is easy to see.

The most common organisms involved in meningitis originating from sinusitis are similar to those organisms most commonly cultured from the sinuses themselves. Anaerobes are common, as are *S. aureus* and other *Staphylococcal* species, *S. pneumoniae* and *H. influenzae* (Table 1).

When culture results are not available, a cephalosporin known to be effective against the common pathogens, including those that produce β-lactamase, is a good empiric antibiotic to use initially, and it should be continued for at least 1 wk. These agents penetrate well into the CSF and produce levels much higher than their minimum bactericidal concentrations. They sterilize the CSF more rapidly than do traditionally used antibiotics, such as Chloramphenicol and Ampicillin. Further advantages of second-and third-generation cephalosporins include safety, no need to monitor plasma concentrations (as with chloramphenicol), and a low incidence of side effects *(15)*.

Surgical drainage of the infected sinuses may be required as an adjunct to iv antibiotics and is indicated if the patient fails to improve clinically within the first 48 h of therapy. Some would recommend surgical drainage immediately if the patient presents with significant changes in mental status.

Although the importance of the host inflammatory response in the pathophysiology of bacterial meningitis has been demonstrated, the use of steroids to treat meningitis is still controversial. In the CSF, bacterial cell-wall particles stimulate the local release of proinflammatory cytokines and thereby initiate an inflammatory response. The concentration of the cytokines in the CSF correlates with the severity of meningitis both experimentally and clinically. The cytokine-induced inflammatory response leads to cerebral edema and impaired cerebral blood flow, as well as increases intracranial pressure and abnormalities of cerebral metabolism *(15)*. It is thought that because steroids block the cytokine release, they may be effective in modulating the inflammatory response within the meninges to reduce tissue damage.

Antibiotic treatment of meningitis leads to rapid bacterial lysis. Endotoxins produced by the bacteria are released within the CSF during bacterial

lysis and result in the production of cytokines by
the meningeal tissues. Steroids, in order to be
effective, must therefore be administered before or
with the first dose of antibiotics. In clinical trials,
the concurrent administration of steroids with
antibiotics is associated with lower CSF pressure,
less cerebral edema, and lower mortality than treatment with antibiotics alone. There is a more rapid
resolution of fever, associated with a return of the
CSF cell count and metabolic abnormalities to
normal, and a lower frequency of seizures. The rate
of CSF sterilization is the same in steroid-treated
patients as it is in patients who have not received
steroids *(15)*. Studies of children with bacterial
meningitis, most frequently owing to *H. influenzae,*
showed a beneficial effect of steroids on the incidence of hearing loss and neurological sequelae
(16). In a prospective randomized study of 115
children with bacterial meningitis, Schaad et al.
found a decrease in the long-term neurologic
sequelae in the patients who received both antibiotics and steroids as compared to those who were
treated with antibiotics alone (*p* < 0.06) *(17)*.

Steroids have also been shown to reduce mortality of meningitis in adults with *pneumococcal*
meningitis *(16)*. Controlled clinical studies in
adults with bacterial meningitis secondary to
sinusitis have not been carried out. However, concurrent steroid administration in the treatment of
adults with meningitis resulting from sinusitis
holds promise.

Additional measures to treat increased intracranial pressure include elevating the head of bed to
30°, hyperventilation to maintain a carbon dioxide
concentration between 25 and 30 mm Hg, and the
administration of hyperosmolar agents *(16)*. Fluid
restriction is controversial and is not generally recommended *(15)*.

Overall mortality rate from meningitis is about
10%. Neurologic sequelae from meningitis are fairly
common in children, with an estimated 28% having
focal neurologic deficits, seizures, motor abnormalities, or mental retardation. Meningitis remains the
single most common cause of acquired sensorineural
hearing loss in childhood, and this complication
occurs in up to 10% of survivors. Early recognition
and treatment help to minimize morbidity.

INTRACRANIAL ABSCESS

Although a possible complication of ethmoid
sinusitis, intracranial abscess is more commonly

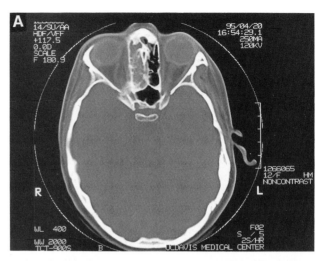

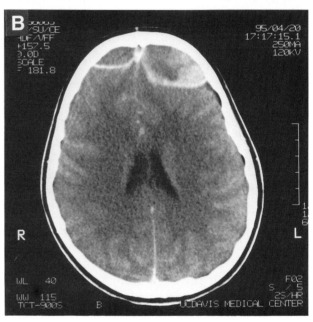

Fig. 8. (A) CT of ethmoid sinusitis and a 12-yr-old girl
whose frontal sinus has not developed. **(B)** CT of bifrontal
cerebral abscesses in patient from Fig. 8A.

the result of frontal and sphenoid sinusitis, and
will be discussed in detail under those sections
of this chapter. The ethmoid and sphenoid spaces
do not usually cause subdural or epidural
abscess, because adjacent to these sinuses, the
brain is intimately attached to the skull and the
subdural and epidural spaces are not present *(13)*.
In a review of 24 intracranial complications of
sinusitis of every type, Clayman reported that
only 27% of frontal lobe abscesses were caused
by isolated posterior ethmoid sinusitis (Fig.
8A,B) *(18)*.

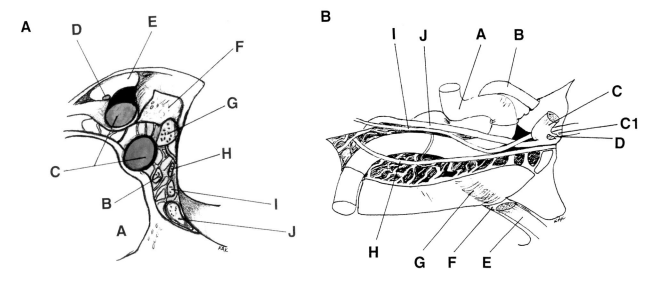

Fig. 9. **(A)** Coronal view: relationship of the cavernous sinus contents to the sphenoid sinus. A, sphenoid sinus; B, abducens nerve (VI); C, carotid artery; D, ophthalmic artery; E, optic canal; F, anterior clinoid process; G, oculomotor nerve (III); H, trochlear nerve (IV); I, ophthalmic nerve (V1); J, maxillary nerve (V2). **(B)** Lateral view of cavernous sinus with dura and trigeminal nerve and ganglion removed. A, carotid artery; B, optic nerve (II); C, ophthalmic nerve (V1); C1, frontal nerve; D, lacrimal nerve; E, maxillary nerve (V2); F, foramen rotundum; G, meckel's cave; H, abducens nerve (VI); I, trochlear nerve (IV); J, ophthalmic nerve (III).

CAVERNOUS SINUS THROMBOSIS

Cavernous sinus thrombosis is the second most common intracranial complication of ethmoid sinusitis. It develops via the orbit with retrograde progression of septic thrombophlebitis in the valveless inferior and superior ophthalmic veins.

The cavernous sinus lies between the layers of the dura on either side of the pituitary fossa, posterior to the optic chiasm, just over the thin roof of the sphenoid sinus, and extends from the superior orbital fissure to the apex of the petrous portion of the temporal bone. The right and left sinuses are connected by the anterior and posterior intercavernous, or circular, venous sinuses and by the larger basilar venous sinus located posterior to the dorsum sella. Flow within the cavernous sinus occurs as a result of pressure gradients, gravity, and carotid pulsations *(10)*. The horizontal portion of the internal carotid artery, surrounded by a plexus of sympathetic nerves, passes forward through the cavernous sinus. The abducens nerve passes through the sinus between the artery and the lateral wall of the sinus. The oculomotor nerve, trochlear nerve, and maxillary and ophthalmic branches of the trigeminal nerve are contained in the lateral wall, separated from the venous blood by a thin

fibrous sheath. Only the ophthalmic division of the trigeminal nerve traverses the length of the cavernous sinus to the superior orbital fissure. The maxillary division has a short course in the cavernous sinus before leaving by the foramen rotundum. The mandibular division of the trigeminal nerve exits the skull base via the foramen ovale before entering the cavernous sinus (Fig. 9A,B).

Veins afferent to the cavernous sinus drain the anterior portion of the face, oral cavity, tonsils, pharynx, nasal cavity, orbit, eye, and paranasal sinuses via the pterygoid plexus. Veins from the middle ear, mastoid region, cerebral cortex, and pituitary also drain into the cavernous sinus. Efferent flow from the cavernous sinus drains via the superior petrosal sinus to the transverse sinus, and via the inferior petrosal sinus into the internal jugular vein.

The signs and symptoms of cavernous sinus thrombosis evolve according to which of the surrounding structures are affected. These signs may be categorized according to the following etiologies: venous obstruction, involvement of adjacent nerves, and generalized sepsis and meningitis. The early symptoms of cavernous sinus thrombosis are headache, eyelid edema, and chemosis. Proptosis, photophobia, and diplopia follow shortly *(19)*. Ptosis and paralysis of extraocular muscles occur as a consequence of adjacent nerve involvement. Ophthalmoplegia may be the result of cranial nerve damage within the cavernous sinus or within the orbit owing to increased orbital pressure. Depending on the involvement of the orbital apex, there may be variable retinal signs of increased retrobulbar pressure and changes in vision. The pupils generally become fixed and dilated with the loss of parasympathetic control, but if there is involvement of the carotid sympathetic plexus, the pupils will be small and fixed. Bilateral orbital involvement usually develops within 24–48 h. Any patient who presents with bilateral orbital symptoms of eyelid edema, proptosis, or decreased visual acuity must be assumed to be suffering from cavernous sinus thrombosis until proven otherwise.

In addition to orbital symptoms, thrombosis of the facial veins leads to facial edema. There may be edema over the mastoids, cerebral edema, and tonsillar and pharyngeal edema. Paresthesia of the ophthalmic and maxillary divisions of the trigeminal nerve may exacerbate retrobulbar pain and headache.

Systemic signs owing to infection in the cavernous sinus include spiking fever, chills, nausea, vomiting, tachycardia, and signs of toxemia. Mental status changes quickly follow the onset of eye complaints. Signs of meningeal irritation may be present. Thatai et al. reported that meningitis was present in 85% of patients who presented with cavernous sinus thrombosis *(20)*. Seizures, lethargy, and coma are also symptoms of venous sinus thrombosis.

In most cases, a diagnosis of sinus thrombosis can be made on the basis of CT findings. Clot formation within the cavernous sinus appears as multiple filling defects on high-resolution CT, making CT the diagnostic modality of choice for demonstrating cavernous sinus thrombosis (Fig. 10) *(21)*. Diagnosis can be confirmed by cerebral angiography or venography, but this is rarely required. The majority of the findings are seen on a contrast-enhanced CT. Other signs indicating the presence of venous thrombosis include gyral enhancement, intense tentorial enhancement, and edema with enhancement. Small ventricular size is a finding in 32% of patients with venous thrombosis. The "empty delta sign" represents a clot within the sinus and is present on over 35% of cases *(22)*. MRI findings include enlargement of the cavernous sinuses and engorgement of the orbital veins. A clot within the sinus appears hyperintense on T1-weighted images, and heterogeneously hyperintense on T2-weighted images (Fig. 11) *(21)*. Magnetic reso-

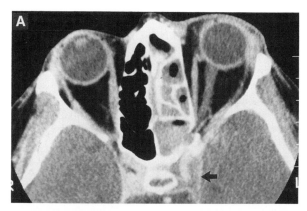

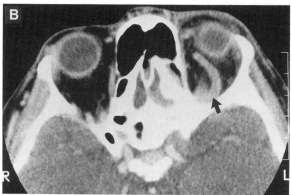

Fig. 10. (A) CT scan of patient with cavernous sinus thrombosis. Arrow points to the distended and thrombosed cavernous sinus. **(B)** Superior cut from the same CT scan showing the venous thrombosis of the superior orbital vein (arrow).

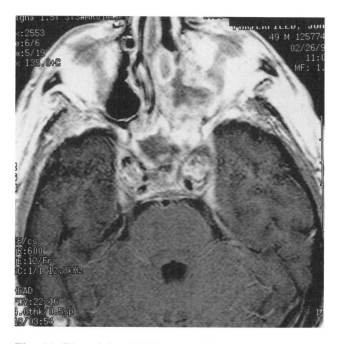

Fig. 11. T1-weighted MRI scan with gadolinium from patient with cavernous sinus thrombosis.

nance angiography can be performed with flow rates specified for the cavernous sinus to confirm the diagnosis of thrombosis. MRI angiography is somewhat difficult in this region, however, because there is normally some variation in flow rates between the two sides.

The diagnosis of cavernous sinus thrombosis is more difficult when only one eye is involved. The differential diagnosis includes neoplasms of the orbit, nasopharynx, lacrimal gland and optic nerve, orbital pseudotumor, cerebral vascular accidents, superior orbital fissure syndrome, arteriovenous fistulas, and aneurysms. The presence of sepsis and the patient's history should help focus the differential diagnosis on an infection of the cavernous sinus.

S. aureus is the most commonly involved organism in cavernous sinus thrombosis (Table 1). Blood cultures are usually positive in patients with cavernous sinus thrombosis and can be an aid in directing the choice of antibiotics for treatment. The mainstay of therapy is early aggressive antibiotic treatment and surgical drainage of the infected sinuses. Surgery on the cavernous sinus itself is not recommended. Broad-spectrum antibiotic therapy is instituted until the results of cultures are known. Antibiotics should be continued for 2–4 wk after local and general signs have subsided.

The use of anticoagulants in the treatment of cavernous sinus thrombosis is controversial, but most recent literature supports their use unless there is a specific contraindication. The theory behind anticoagulation is that it prevents further propagation of the clot with extension into the other venous sinuses and it inhibits the dissemination of septic emboli. Anticoagulants are also thought to aid in recanalization of the clot, which allows earlier antibiotic penetration.

Corticosteroids are recommended in cases that do not appear to be responding to antibiotic therapy. Steroids are thought to decrease the incidence of adrenal insufficiency and collapse, and to reduce orbital congestion.

Although mortality of cavernous sinus thrombosis has decreased, the morbidity remains high. Thirty percent of patients with cavernous sinus thrombosis had permanent neurologic sequelae in a study reported by Thatai et al. in 1992 *(20)*. Associated cranial nerve palsies may not resolve after treatment. Fifty percent of those who survive cavernous sinus thrombosis suffer from partial or complete cranial nerve palsies *(23)*.

MAXILLARY SINUSES
Introduction

At birth, the maxillary sinus is 7 × 4 × 4 mm in size. The growth rate is estimated to be 2 mm vertical and 3 mm anteroposteriorly each year. The size of the sinus depends on the dentition, since as the teeth erupt into the alveolus, the space left by the tooth bud becomes pneumatically expanded by the developing sinus lumen. Thus, the sinus becomes a significant structure during the second year of life coincidental with the development of oral dentition. The tooth roots remain in close proximity to the sinus and are often involved in maxillary sinus infection. In patients with an isolated maxillary sinusitis, the presence of a dental infection must be ruled out.

Complications of Maxillary Sinusitis

The maxillary sinus is rarely involved in direct intracranial spread of isolated infection because of its distance from the cranial cavity. It is more often involved as part of a global pan-sinusitis. The inferior orbital vein could, however, become thrombosed because of a solitary maxillary sinus infection, leading to spread of the infection into the cavernous sinus. Intraorbital spread from the maxillary sinus is also less common than from the ethmoid air cells, but can occur via the floor of the orbit. Treatment of intraorbital or intracranial spread of maxillary sinusitis is the same as the treatment of these conditions when they arise from sinusitis in the ethmoid cavity.

SPHENOID SINUS
Introduction

Sphenoid sinusitis is commonly seen as part of a more generalized pan-sinusitis. In this situation, it responds well to the usual therapy appropriate for the treatment of sinusitis. Isolated sphenoid sinusitis, however, is an indication of a significant impedance of drainage of the sinus and carries an increased risk of serious complications.

The sphenoid sinus begins significant development at approx 3 yr of age. Thus, it is rare to see complications from sphenoid sinusitis prior to this time. The radiographic appearance of the developing sphenoid sinus could be mistaken, however, for a fluid-filled space on CT or MRI. At birth, the hematopoietic bone marrow of the presphenoid region is low signal intensity relative to brain on MRI in most individuals. The region is normally isointense to muscle on T1-weighted MRI in children younger than 6 mo of age because of the presence of red marrow (24). After 1 yr of life, some of the marrow is replaced by fat, so the signal becomes patchy with areas of increased enhancement. All individuals show some fatty replacement of the marrow in this space by age 7 (25). These patchy areas of high signal intensity occur prior to pneumatization. With iv gadolinium, there is variable uptake in this region prior to pneumatization. After age 2, pneumatization begins, and the hyperintense fat is replaced by the signal void of air. Pneumatization of the sphenoid sinus begins by bilateral invagination of nasal mucosa into paired sphenoid concha (bones of Bertin) located at the cranial end of the basisphenoid and incorporated into the sphenoid bone at birth. Beginning around age 4, the sinus extends into the anterior sphenoid bone and, by age 10, extends posteriorly into the basisphenoid. The sinus reaches maturity by age 14.

ANATOMY AND PHYSIOLOGY

The sphenoid sinus lies in the body of the sphenoid bone. The walls of the sinus are in contact with the pituitary gland, optic canals, dura mater, and cavernous sinuses. Within the cavernous sinuses are found the thin-walled internal carotid arteries, and the oculomotor, trochlear, and abducens nerves. The maxillary division of the trigeminal nerve may indent the bony walls of the sphenoid sinus. The sphenoid walls can be extremely thin or dehiscent, and these vital adjacent structures may be separated from the cavity by only a thin mucosal barrier (26) (Fig. 9B). The spread of infection intracranially from the sphenoid sinus can be by direct extension, but is also owing to the progression of septic thrombophlebitis, this time via the carotid venous plexus. Temporal lobe abscess may be a result of sphenoid sinusitis.

DIAGNOSIS OF SPHENOID SINUSITIS

Solitary sphenoid sinus pathology is difficult to diagnose on the basis of symptomatology alone and must be considered part of the differential diagnosis of headache. Retro-orbital, occipital, or bitemporal headaches are considered characteristic of sphenoid sinusitis. The condition mimics trigeminal neuralgia, migraine, carotid artery aneurysm, and brain tumor. Commonly, infection of the sphenoid is not suspected until complications occur. In a report by Lew et al., only 6 of 15 patients with sphenoid sinusitis were correctly diagnosed at the time of admission to the hospital. Headache was the most common presenting symptom in this group, and most of the patients reported pain in more than one location (26). The headache of sphenoid sinusitis is severe, worsens with head movements, interferes with sleep, and is not relieved by aspirin (27).

Nasal complaints may be absent in patients with isolated sphenoid sinusitis, which is why the diagnosis of sphenoid sinusitis is not entertained immediately on presentation. In addition, patients may complain of facial, nasal, mandibular or dental pain, or facial paresthesia, and may describe nasal congestion, abnormal perceptions of smell, or even complete anosmia. Visual complaints, including blurred vision or diplopia, as well as cranial nerve deficits suggest extension of infection and involvement of contiguous structures.

The presentation of sphenoid sinus infection may include fever, but this is not always present. On physical examination, purulent drainage may be seen from the sphenoid recess. The most frequent neurologic deficit is paresthesia of the ophthalmic or maxillary divisions of the trigeminal nerve. Lew et al. noted this finding was present in one-third of their patients (26).

The diagnosis of sphenoid sinusitis is made on CT scan. Plain radiographs can help in the diagnosis of sphenoid sinusitis, but because of the presence of overlying structures in these films, it is often difficult to determine either sinus opacification or air–fluid levels by this method. CT scan is the most useful study for demonstrating sphenoid sinus pathology and has the added advantage of detecting associated complications, such as bone erosion, cavernous sinus thrombosis, or abscess formation.

The white cell count may be elevated or normal, but the erythrocyte sedimentation rate is usually at least mildly elevated (above 25 mm/h). Many authors recommend the monitoring of the erythrocyte sedimentation rate as a method of following the response to therapy.

CSF cultures are positive in 40% of patients and grow the same pathogens found on sphenoid sinus aspirates (27). *S. aureus* and *Streptococci* were the most common organisms found at operation in acute and chronic sphenoid sinusitis (26). In cases of chronic sphenoiditis, gram-negative organisms were also cultured, and anaerobes were cultured in approx 25% of cases (Table 1).

Tumors of the sphenoid should be included in the differential diagnosis of sphenoid sinusitis and are now seen with increasing frequency *(28)*. Fibrous dysplasia of the sphenoid bone can also present with symptoms similar to those of a complicated sphenoid sinusitis.

TREATMENT

The most common organisms in community-acquired sphenoid sinusitis are *S. pneumoniae* and other streptococcal species. *S. aureus* and *H. influenzae* are also frequently reported. Nosocomial sinusitis secondary to nasal packing or indwelling nasotracheal or nasogastric tubes usually produces a polymicrobial infection that may include *Pseudomonas aeruginosa, Klebsiella pneumoniae,* or *Enterobacter* species.

Any delay in treatment of acute sphenoid sinusitis can result in serious or fatal sequelae. In all nine patients in which there was a delay in diagnosis, Lew et al. noted serious neurologic deficits that persisted after the infection resolved, and four patients died *(26)*. Some authors might consider the use of oral antibiotics with close follow-up of the patient as initial therapy in acute, uncomplicated sphenoid sinusitis. Others believe that treatment of sphenoid sinusitis with iv antibiotics as a minimum is indicated. Regardless of the initial choice of therapy, should the patient's clinical picture fail to improve within 24–48 h, iv antibiotics along with prompt surgical drainage are required.

Failure to respond to treatment with antibiotics considered to be effective in combating the most common infecting organisms must raise the suspicion of a fungal sinusitis. Treatment of fungal sinusitis is primarily surgical with opening of the sinus, removal of the fungus ball, and may include irrigation of the sinus with antifungal agents. Systemic antifungal agents may also be added to the regimen, but are not always required if adequate surgical drainage of the sinus has been achieved. In immunocompromised patients, an invasive fungal infection must be treated promptly with surgical removal of involved tissues, or blindness or death is likely to result. (*See* Chapters 16 and 17.)

Complications of Sphenoid Sinusitis

SPHENOID SINUS MUCOCELE

The incidence of mucoceles in the posterior ethmoids and sphenoid sinus is low. They are more common, however, in patients who have previously undergone surgery on the paranasal sinuses *(29)*.

In general, a postoperative mucocele develops 15 or more years postsurgery. Scarring of the surgical site, repeated infections, and incomplete treatment all contribute to the development of an obstruction to drainage of the sinus. As pressure builds within the sinus owing to the mucus and debris collecting there, the sinus expands, and may cause bone expansion or erosion and pressure on the surrounding structures, such as the optic nerve. In addition to pressure, the mucocele may become infected, and the surrounding inflammation may affect the nearby structures. The relatively sparse vascular supply to the optic nerve as it passes through the optic canal is thought to contribute to frequency with which visual disturbances develop. Rothfield et al. found that of 13 patients with isolated sphenoid sinus disease, mucoceles and other space-occupying lesions within the sphenoid were more likely to cause visual changes than cases of acute sinusitis without complications. Both conditions presented with headache as a major component of the symptom complex *(28)*.

Once a mucocele develops, visual disturbances may be the primary symptom of the disease, although more commonly, mucoceles present with subtle or vague symptoms that contribute to delay in diagnosis. Headache with occipital, vertex, or deep nasal pain may accompany various ophthalmological complaints, such as diplopia, visual field disturbance, and globe displacement. Symptoms may also result from involvement of other nearby structures, including cranial nerves II–VI and the pituitary gland, although these symptoms are rare. Patients will often not have any presenting nasal complaints.

The diagnosis of a mucocele is made on CT scan, which is necessary to determine the extent of the lesion and involved structures (Fig. 12). MRI is helpful in differentiating mucoceles from tumors, but is not able to demonstrate bony anatomy well enough to be used alone. Sinonasal mucoceles show a variable appearance on MRI depending on the water content of the debris within them (Fig. 13A,B) *(10)*.

Surgical drainage is the treatment for sphenoid sinus mucoceles. The approach to the sinus is traditionally via a sublabial, transeptal approach that was initially developed to gain access to tumors of the pituitary. This approach has the advantage of avoiding external surgical scars and provides excellent surgical exposure. It also has a decreased incidence of damage to vital structures surround-

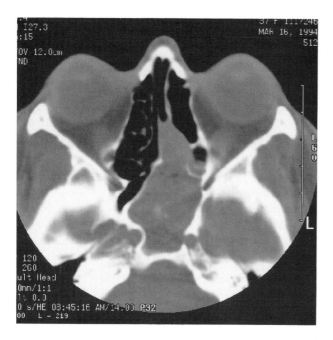

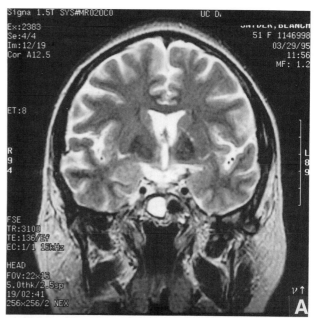

Fig. 12. CT scan of patient with sphenoid sinus mucocele.

ing the sinus laterally and superiorly because it is directed anteriorly and in the midline *(28)*. Recent advancements in endoscopic techniques have popularized this modality as a tool for use in the draining of both frontal sinus and sphenoid sinus mucoceles. If septal deviation is present, it must be corrected prior to opening the sphenoid sinus in order to allow adequate endoscopic visualization *(30)*.

The prognosis for return of vision lost as a result of a sphenoid sinus mucocele is poor in cases of sudden onset where there tends to be an increased incidence of accompanying severe visual disturbance. In cases of mild to moderate visual disturbance of gradual onset, the chance for return of visual function with surgical drainage of the mucocele depends on how soon after the onset of the visual changes the surgery is done. Prompt surgical intervention has the best chance of restoring visual function *(29)*.

MENINGITIS, CAVERNOUS SINUS THROMBOSIS, AND INTRACRANIAL ABSCESS

Meningitis is the most common intracranial complication of sphenoid sinusitis. Although subdural and cerebral abscesses can occur, they are rare *(19,31)*. Sphenoid sinusitis has been the most common cause of cavernous sinus thrombosis in some series *(32)*. Thrombosis of the cavernous sinus is thought to occur via direct extension of the infection through the thin sphenoid walls into the

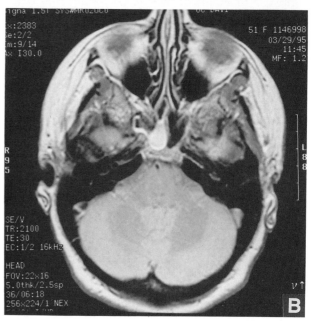

Fig. 13. (A) Coronal T1-weighted MRI scan in patient with a sphenoid sinus mucocele. **(B)** Axial view of scan from Fig. 13A.

cavernous sinus or by retrograde thrombosis via the veins that drain the sinus (Fig. 14).

SUPERIOR ORBITAL FISSURE AND ORBITAL APEX SYNDROME

The superior orbital fissure syndrome results from pathological involvement of the nerves passing through the superior orbital fissure (III, IV, VI, V_1), and results in paralysis of the extraocular

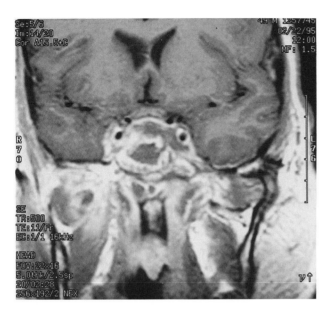

Fig. 14. T1-weighted MRI scan with gadolinium in a patient with sphenoid sinusitis, cavernous sinus, and pituitary abscess.

muscles and loss of parasympathetic control to the globe. Additional involvement of the optic nerve and associated visual impairment is known as the orbital apex syndrome *(33)*. Marked visual loss and ophthalmoplegia are present, but with minimal proptosis or signs of anterior segment inflammation. A patient with orbital apex syndrome mandates evaluation of the sphenoid sinus to rule out sinusitis as an underlying cause. The close relationship of the optic nerve to the sphenoid sinus becomes even closer if there is extension of pneumatization into the greater wing of the sphenoid.

FRONTAL SINUS

Introduction

Infection of the frontal sinus carries with it the highest risk of intracranial complications. The frontal sinuses develop by the expansion of a superior ethmoid air cell into the vertical portion of the frontal bone. The frontal sinus is separated from the orbit by the orbital portions of the frontal bone, which may be very thin.

ANATOMY AND PHYSIOLOGY

The vascular supply of the frontal sinus originates in the dura mater for the inner table, in the periorbita for the orbital plate, and in the cranial periosteum for the outer table. The membranous cranial bones are formed from both dura and galea,

and derive their blood supply from both structures. Frontal sinusitis leads to focal osteitis involving the inner table of the frontal bone and thrombophlebitis in the sinus mucous membranes. A layer of compact bone as thin as 100–300 μ thick separates the sinus from the diploic space *(13,34)*. Infection, thus, has easy access to the marrow space. With spread of thrombosis into the diploic veins (Veins of Brechet) of the marrow space, osteitis becomes frontal bone osteomyelitis owing to thrombophlebitic avascular necrosis. The valveless diploic veins empty into veins in the dura mater and from there empty into the superior sagittal sinus. A purulent infection between bone and dura results in an epidural abscess. Further extension of infection in the diploic veins results in involvement of the subdural space. Infection of the subdural space spreads widely over the cerebral surface. Eventually thrombosis extends into the sagittal sinus, and cerebral abscess or meningitis may ensue (Fig. 7).

An actual nasofrontal duct from the frontal sinus is unusual, and the sinus usually drains through variable pathways in the anterior ethmoid air cells and from there into the middle meatus. The sinus narrows inferiorly to form the os through which it drains into the ethmoids *(30)*.

DIAGNOSIS OF FRONTAL SINUSITIS

Persistent pain and tenderness over the frontal area is suggestive of frontal sinusitis, but CT scan is required to confirm the diagnosis. When performed with contrast, CT scan can also detect the presence of osteomyelitis of the adjacent frontal bone.

Infection of the frontal sinus and the adjacent tissues more commonly involves anaerobes than infections of the other sinuses. This may be explained by the relatively lower oxygen concentration in the frontal sinuses and the often more chronic nature of frontal sinus disease.

Orbital Complications

Although the ethmoid sinus is the most common sinus involved in the production of orbital complications, frontal sinus infections spreading to the orbit may entail a more complicated course and more frequently require surgical intervention *(6)*.

Intracranial Complications

Many authors feel that adolescent males are at higher risk for developing intracranial complications of frontal sinusitis, although no anatomical explanation for this tendency has been identified *(31,34)*. One theory suggests that there is increased vascularity of the diploe during adolescence and continued expansion of the frontal sinus *(18)*. Other predisposing factors to the development of frontal sinusitis include drug abuse, immunocompromise, trauma, and chronic sinusitis. Ten percent of patients hospitalized for frontal sinusitis develop intracranial complications *(31)*.

Infection from the frontal sinus invades the cerebral parenchyma by two routes. Occasionally, direct extension may occur through necrotic areas of posterior table osteomyelitis. The underlying dura, which is adherent to the inner surface of the bone, becomes thickened, an intense inflammatory reaction occurs, and a purulent exudate results in the subsequent development of an epidural abscess. The dura becomes further involved by extension of the infection along the vessels that penetrate it. By this means, infection is able to enter the space deep to the dura. A subdural empyema often results, which in turn induces an inflammatory reaction in the subarachnoid space *(31,34)*.

The more classical pathophysiologic route of intracranial infectious spread from the frontal sinus is via the valveless diploic venous system as discussed in the Anatomy and Physiology section. Focal osteitis of the posterior table results in a septic retrograde thrombophlebitis directly along the veins that penetrate into the dura and, from there, drain into the sagittal sinus *(31,34)*.

Epidural Abscess

Epidural abscess is also known as pachymeningitis and is often associated with osteomyelitis of the posterior table of the frontal sinus. Epidural abscess usually presents as an insidious process. Increased intracranial pressure results in unremitting headache and occasionally causes vomiting. If the infection remains extradural, then the patient usually remains alert. CT scan and MRI are the best tools for diagnosing an epidural abscess. The abscess may be small, but an adjacent bony defect seen on CT scan is a clue to the presence of an epidural abscess. Epidural abscess occurs almost exclusively as a complication of frontal sinusitis and is the second most common complication of frontal sinusitis after osteomyelitis.

Subdural Empyema

Subdural empyema is a collection of purulent material between the dura and the arachnoid.

Empyema refers to an infection in a pre-existing potential space and is thus the most appropriate term for infection in the subdural space. It usually results from retrograde thrombophlebitis of the valveless veins draining the mucosa of the infected frontal sinus. Unrestricted access owing to the few attachments between layers in the supratentorial subdural space allows a thin layer of purulent material to be deposited diffusely over the cerebral convexity and in the parafalcine and paratentorial regions. This complication of sinusitis is most common in the 10–20 yr age group *(35)*. Sinusitis is considered the cause of 80% of subdural empyemas in children older than 18 mo of age and in adults *(36)*. In children <18 mo old, meningitis is the most common cause of subdural empyema. When infection spreads to the subdural space, stupor and coma may develop after initial complaints of intense headache. The arachnoid acts as a relative barrier to infection, and although signs of meningeal irritation, such as nuchal rigidity and photophobia, may be present, this can be explained by inflammation secondary to increased pressure rather than actual involvement of the CSF by infection *(34)*. Seizures, muscle weakness, dysphagia, aphasia, and visual disturbances are among the focal neurologic deficits that are thought to result from a combination of local brain compression, cortical venous thrombosis, and cerebral infarction *(31)*. Without treatment, progression of thrombophlebitis ensues to involve the cortical veins and major dural sinuses with edema, ischemia, and infarction of the subjacent cortex.

CT scanning is used to confirm the diagnosis of subdural empyemas. Concurrent bone and sinus involvement is also delineated with this diagnostic modality. Early in the course of disease, however, CT findings can be subtle and easily overlooked. Hoyt and Fisher reported a series of 17 cases in which CT scans were positive in only 82% of subdural empyemas *(36)*. The presence of osteomyelitis or a subgaleal abscess on a CT scan favors the diagnosis of epidural abscess over subdural empyema. Without osteomyelitis, these two lesions look similar by CT *(37)*. If forced to differentiate between the two on CT scan, a localized fluid collection of low density within the epidural space assumes a biconvex shape. A crescentic configuration over a larger area indicates that the fluid collection is within the subdural space *(38)*. The administration of contrast produces enhancement of the meninges surrounding the empyema on CT scan, but this finding can be obscured by the proximity of overlying bone.

MRI may be superior in evaluating early epidural abscess and subdural empyemas by enabling more sensitive detection, more accurate localization, and more complete delineation of disease. Frequently, loculations of pus are imaged on MRI that cannot be appreciated on CT. Superficial lesions are more conspicuous on MRI than CT owing to the absence of bone artifact (contrast enhancement of the meninges is obscured on CT by the adjacent bony skull), multiplanar imaging capability, and excellent contrast between brain and CSF. MRI also demonstrates greater specificity than CT in differentiating a subdural empyema from an epidural abscess and from a parenchymal abscess. A hypointense rim, representing inflamed dura, is seen on MRI in the case of an epidural abscess, but not in the case of a subdural empyema. Fluid collections appear relatively gray on T1-weighted images and are hyperintense on a T2-weighted scan. Involved meninges are enhanced with gadolinium and are more easily seen by MRI than they are by CT scan.

CSF cultures are often sterile in subdural empyema (36). When organisms have been cultured from the abscess, Streptococci are found most commonly (70%). Staphylococci, Fusobacterium, Bacteroides, Haemophilus, Lactobacillus, and aerobic gram-negative bacilli have also been cultured from subdural empyemas (32) (Table 1).

Treatment of subdural empyema involves prompt surgical evacuation, usually via a frontal craniotomy. Concurrent drainage of the frontal sinus and debridement of necrotic bone should be performed to remove the original focus of infection. Systemically administered antibiotics do not penetrate the subdural space in therapeutic amounts, but decrease spread to adjacent areas and should be used concurrently with prompt surgical drainage. Prophylactic antiseizure medication is indicated because the incidence of postoperative seizures is >80%. Other persistent focal neurologic deficits are common. Despite aggressive medical and surgical therapy, three of seven patients diagnosed with subdural empyema in Magnilia et al.'s series died (39). Hoyt and Fisher reported a 12% mortality rate and a 59% incidence of permanent neurologic sequelae, including hemiparesis, aphasia, seizures, ptosis, and hyperopia (36).

After surgical drainage, those patients who fail to improve neurologically or improve initially, but then regress or continue to spike fevers should undergo repeat CT scan to evaluate for undrained collections of fluid (36). Reaccumulation of fluid necessitates re-exploration and drainage.

VENOUS SINUS THROMBOSIS

Venous sinus thrombosis of the superior sagittal sinus is most commonly associated with frontal sinusitis. Retrograde thrombosis from the diploic veins draining the sinus is the mechanism by which the venous sinus thrombosis occurs. Drainage of the focus of infection within the sinuses and any associated intracerebral purulent collections along with the administration of antibiotics is the therapy of choice for this condition.

CEREBRAL ABSCESS

Some 13–15% of all brain abscesses are secondary to sinusitis (40). There is an increased incidence of brain abscesses from all causes between the ages of 10 and 30 yr (41). Brain abscesses secondary to sinusitis can occur anywhere in the brain, but are most common in the frontal lobe. They are usually located superficially within the brain and are solitary (42).

Fever and headache are the most common presenting signs of an intracranial abscess (18). Nausea and vomiting occur in up to 50% of patients owing to increased intracranial pressure. Seizures occur in 50% of patients prior to surgical drainage of the abscess (42). The frontal lobes are typically neurologically silent, and an abscess may present with no focal signs. Subtle mood or behavioral changes may be all that is noted (31). Once encapsulation of the site of initial encephalitis occurs, intracranial pressure increases, and the classic symptomatology may become apparent, including projectile vomiting, focal seizures, cranial nerve dysfunction, slowing of the pulse, and coma. One-third of the patients studied by Yang and Zhao presented with hemiparesis (43).

The mechanism of cerebral abscess formation is not clear. Some feel that longitudinal sinus thrombosis or a subdural empyema must precede the development of a rhinogenic cerebral abscess (34). Infection is then spread into the cerebral parenchyma by thromboembolic phenomenon or by direct seeding. Seeding is most likely to occur at the junction of the gray and the white matter where blood flow is sluggish. The initial stage of brain abscess formation is that of an encephalitis. A wall of granulation tissue and collagen forms around the infection in an attempt to contain it. During this phase, the abscess is undergoing localization and encapsulation. Eventually, symptoms progress as the abscess enlarges or ruptures into the ventricles. The stages of brain abscess have been categorized as:

1. Early cerebritis (1–3 d) during which there is bacterial seeding of a necrotic area accompanied by a local inflammatory response resulting in marked edema (the lesion is not demarcated from surrounding brain);
2. Late cerebritis (4–9 d) in which pus formation leads to enlargement of the necrotic center, which is surrounded by inflammatory cells and fibroblasts and at which time surrounding edema is at its maximum;
3. Early capsule formation (10–13 d) when the capsule around the necrotic center becomes more developed; and
4. Late capsule formation (14 d or more) characterized by distinct capsule formation (42).

The virulence of the infecting organism and the immunocompetence of the host both affect the timing of these stages (44).

Diagnosis of intracranial abscess is made by CT scan, which defines both the abscess and the extent of cerebral involvement. Breakdown of the blood–brain barrier in the region of the abscess allows contrast material to move across that barrier. Using contrast enhancement, diagnostic accuracy of CT scans is reported to be 92–100%. CT scans differentiate between the stages of encephalitis and abscess formation (45). During the early encephalitis stage, the CT scan may show a poorly defined zone of nonenhancing lower density that corresponds to a region of cerebral edema. A CT scan during the late cerebritis stage may show solid enhancement of the lesion, incomplete ring-shaped enhancement, or a complete thick-walled ring enhancement depending on the amount of capsule formation (43). CT scans obtained up to an hour after the infusion of contrast show diffusion of contrast into the center of abscesses in the cerebritis stage (42).

MRI has been shown to be more sensitive in the early detection of cerebritis in animal models, but superiority over CT in a clinical setting has not yet been demonstrated (46). Paramagnetic contrast agents, such as gadolinium, cross the blood–brain

barrier in areas of cerebritis or abscess. During the encephalitis stage, T1-weighted images show hypointensity signals, and T2-weighted images show high-intensity signals, both with indistinct margins between the areas of inflammation and the surrounding edema.

When the abscess is encapsulated, a CT scan shows an area of radiolucency in the abscess cavity and density in the capsule on contrast enhancement (Fig. 8B). Encapsulated abscesses continue to show ring enhancement with no central diffusion of contrast an hour after the contrast has been injected (42,44). On MRI, the central necrotic region shows a low-intensity signal on T1 and a high-intensity signal on T2. The capsule is mildly hyperintense on T1, with low signal intensity on T2.

The differential diagnosis of a ring-enhancing abscess on imaging studies is primary tumor, such as glioblastoma multiforme, metastatic tumor with central necrosis or breakdown of the blood–brain barrier on the perimeter of an infarct or a hemorrhage (38,47). The conditions that may mimic cerebritis on an imaging study include cerebral infarction and noninfectious inflammatory disease (38).

Results of lumbar puncture in cases of intracranial abscess are nondiagnostic, and the risk of brainstem herniation outweighs any potential benefits. The serum white count and erythrocyte sedimentation rate may or may not be elevated in patients with brain abscess, and thus cannot be relied on in making the diagnosis (18).

The most commonly reported organisms during brain abscess are *Staphylococcus, S. pneumoniae, H. influenzae,* and β-hemolytic *Streptococci.* Anaerobic bacteria usually play a role (grown in 74% of isolates) (48), but may remain undetected owing to the difficulties in collecting specimens properly for anaerobic culture (18). In many series, anaerobic organisms are the most common cause of brain abscess (Table 1). Treatment with broad-spectrum antibiotics should be initiated and continued until surgical decompression of the abscess and infected sinus can be achieved. Once the offending organisms are identified, appropriate antibiotics should be continued for 4–6 wk (42).

Several reports claim success in treating intracranial abscesses with antibiotics alone, but the majority of the literature supports surgical drainage of loculated intracranial infections followed by the administration of antibiotics as the treatment of choice *(18,44,48)*. Medical therapy alone is recommended only for specific cases when the abscess is <2 cm in diameter on CT scan *(42)*, when the lesion is high-density (indicating the cerebritis stage) *(41)*, when multiple abscesses are present, when the abscess is surgically inaccessible, and only if the patient is in a good clinical state without any deterioration of the level of consciousness. This approach can be considered only when blood cultures are positive, allowing for identification of the causative organisms without aspiration of fluid from the abscess itself *(44)*. It must be kept in mind that blood cultures often are not an accurate reflection of the infecting organisms inhabiting a brain abscess *(47)*.

Drainage of the abscess is usually required in order to obtain fluid for accurate cultures to direct antibiotic coverage. Surgery is always necessary when a focal intracranial infection enlarges on CT despite medical treatment *(49)*. Simultaneous drainage of the infected sinus, and thus removal of the inciting focus, is a key to successful outcome. The choice between complete excision of the abscess and aspiration is controversial, and may be dictated by the depth of the abscess.

Aspiration immediately reduces the mass effect, confirms the diagnosis of abscess, and is less traumatic to surrounding tissues, but has a higher incidence of recurrence *(42)*. Image-directed stereotactic techniques now allow accurate aspiration of deeply located abscesses. According to Seydoux and Francioli, there was no detectable difference in outcome for patients who underwent either aspiration or excision of brain abscesses *(46)*, but other studies have observed an increased rate of sequelae after complete or partial excision of the abscess. These were not prospective, randomized trials, and it is difficult to extrapolate conclusions from studies in which treatment methods are determined by the clinical presentation of the individual patient (which may itself be the actual determinant of outcome).

Other studies have shown a higher incidence of postoperative seizures when the abscess capsule was not excised *(49)*. Excision is not appropriate for abscesses in the cerebritis stage, during which time, aspiration can be performed with relative ease *(42)*. When aspiration is used as a primary modality of abscess drainage, repeat CT scan may demonstrate reaccumulation of fluid. In such cases, repeat aspiration is recommended. Multiple aspirations

may be needed to clear an abscess completely. Serial CT scans are recommended to follow the progress of all types of therapy (Fig. 15).

Steroid therapy for the treatment of intracranial abscesses is also controversial. It may inhibit collagen deposition and, thus, capsule formation by stabilizing capillary permeability and the chemotaxis of inflammatory cells and fibroblasts. Delayed encapsulation of the abscess theoretically allows the area of infection to become larger. Steroids may interfere with antibiotic penetration and may inhibit the host's immune response, but the cerebral edema and mass effect that accompany an abscess have also been clearly shown to be reduced by the administration of steroids *(42)*. Experimental work shows no effect of steroid administration during the acute phase of the brain abscess on late sequelae from brain abscess *(48)*. Obana and Rosenblum recommend, however, that steroids should be avoided in the cerebritis and early encapsulation phase, and should be withdrawn as soon as the mass effect of the abscess has subsided *(44)*. In a retrospective study reported by Seydoux and Francioli, 28 patients with brain abscess were treated with corticosteroids, and no detectable difference in outcome was observed between those patients who received steroids and those who did not. Seydoux and Francioli concluded that steroids are not contraindicated and recommend their use in cases of massive cerebral edema *(46)*. Mannitol is also helpful in decreasing intracranial pressure and probably should be used where pressure reduction is a necessity *(50)*.

Death rates reported from cerebral abscess in the late 1970s were as high as 65%, despite the use of modern antibiotic regimens. Since then, CT scanning has allowed earlier diagnosis and more accurate localization, and can indicate whether the abscess is in the cerebritis stage or is encapsulated. Improved bacteriologic techniques, particularly for the culture of anaerobic organisms, have resulted in more appropriate use of antibiotics. Recent reports estimate mortality to be between 5 and 10% *(18)*. Seizures occur in 30–50% of survivors, and other neurologic sequelae are common (42). The prognosis is clearly linked to the condition of the patient when presenting to the hospital, and those patients with lowered levels of consciousness on admission are more likely to die from the infection or to have permanent neurologic sequelae irrespective of the modality of treatment *(50)*.

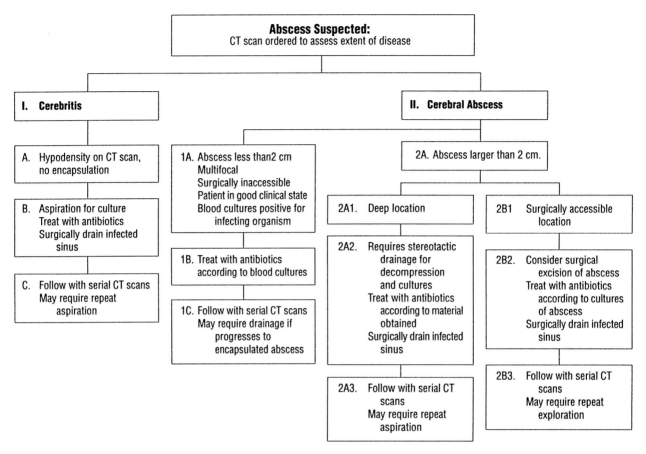

Fig. 15. Brain abscess treatment algorithm.

OSTEOMYELITIS

An infection of the frontal sinus readily spreads to the marrow space of the frontal bone via the valveless veins that drain the sinus through the marrow space. The result is osteomyelitis. This type of infection can spread beyond the suture lines that would otherwise be a barrier to the spread of bone infection. The infection moves from the bone to the adjacent epidural space and thus strips the dura off the inner surface of the bone beyond the suture lines. The loss of dural covering essentially devascularizes the bone beneath it, because the bone derives its blood supply from the dura. A vascular necrosis of the bone results and infection readily moves into the devascularized tissue *(13)*.

Osteomyelitis is characterized by a mottled appearance of the normal bone architecture on CT scan with a loss of sharpness of the inner and outer tables of the calvarium. On MR images, there is a decrease in the intensity of the fatty marrow signal on a T1-weighted image, with the area of infection being relatively isointense to brain tissue.

Complete excision of all diseased bone combined with obliteration of the frontal sinus is required for treatment of frontal osteomyelitis *(13)*. Antibiotics should be continued for 4–6 wk postsurgical debridement. The organisms typically cultured from frontal osteomyelitis are similar to those cultured from chronic frontal sinusitis, and include anaerobic *Streptococci, Staphylococci* and/ or a mixture of organisms *(32)* (Table 1).

POTT'S PUFFY TUMOR

Pericranial abscess may develop as infection spreads from the diploe of the anterior table of the frontal sinus under the periosteum of the frontal bone and eventually into the soft tissues of the forehead. Pott's Puffy Tumor is a subperiosteal abscess of the frontal bone that presents as a localized swelling of the forehead overlying the frontal sinus. This disease entity was first described by Percival Pott in 1775, thus the name Pott's Puffy Tumor. The typical clinical presentation is that of erythema, edema, tenderness, and doughy swelling of the forehead.

Pott's Puffy Tumor occurs in both acute and chronic frontal sinusitis. In cases of acute sinusitis, osteomyelitis and abscess are more likely to occur in patients with a history of antecedent frontal sinus trauma. The pathological process is the same for epidural abscesses as it is for pericranial abscess, and these patients are at high risk of concurrent intracranial complications of frontal sinusitis. CT scans should be performed in all patients with Pott's Puffy Tumor to rule out concurrent intracranial abscesses.

Aggressive surgical management is the mainstay of successful therapy for Pott's Puffy Tumor. The subperiosteal abscess, the affected sinus, and intracranial foci should be drained, and infected bone debrided. Cultures should be obtained from each site of involvement. Intravenous antibiotic therapy should be instituted to cover the typical organisms found in frontal sinusitis and then adjusted based on the intraoperative culture results. *Staphylococcus* is the pathogen that most often produces frontal osteomyelitis, but other aerobic and anaerobic organisms have been implicated. The antibiotics chosen should have good CNS penetration. Selected second- and third-generation cephalosporins have good CNS penetration and are active against the majority of organisms involved in frontal sinusitis, but should be used in combination with an antibiotic that provides better anaerobic coverage. Antibiotics should be continued for 4–6 wk as in the treatment of osteomyelitis. Reconstruction of surgical defects should be delayed for 1 yr posttreatment to rule out recurrence. Long-term follow-up is required, since osteomyelitis has been known to recur up to 20 yr after the initial infection *(14)*.

MUCOCELE

Mucoceles are most common in the frontal sinus. Unlike mucoceles in the sphenoid sinus, which erode into the orbital apex, frontal sinus mucoceles erode into the anterior orbit and the anterior cranial fossa. They occur with equal frequency in males and females. Mucoceles commonly present with frontal headache and proptosis. Downward and outward displacement of the globe may result in diplopia (Fig. 16).

Diagnosis is by CT scan, which is necessary to determine the extent of the lesion and involved structures (Fig. 17). MRI is helpful in differentiating mucoceles from tumors, but is not able to dem-

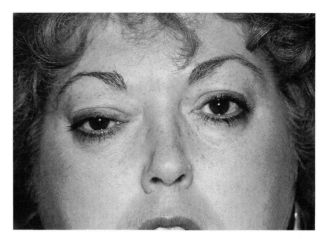

Fig. 16. Photograph of patient with frontal sinus mucocele.

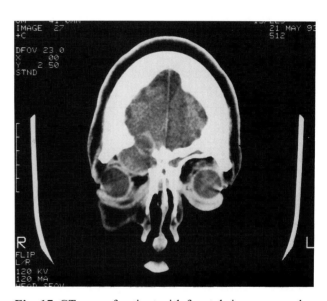

Fig. 17. CT scan of patient with frontal sinus mucocele.

onstrate bony anatomy well enough to be used as a sole radiographic modality.

This condition is traditionally treated by surgical removal of the mucoceles and ablation of the sinus. Ablation by any technique has disadvantages, and the development of endoscopic sinus surgery instruments allowing better intranasal visualization, has lead to controversy over the best surgical approach in the treatment of the frontal sinus mucoceles continues.

In the approach used most commonly, an osteoplastic flap is raised, and the sinus mucosa and mucocele are removed. The sinus is then obliterated by a fat graft. This procedure avoids a cosmetic deformity of the forehead since the bone of the sinus is left in place, but has the drawback of making the frontal sinus opaque on CT scan, possibly masking recurrent disease. This makes postoperative follow-up by CT scan difficult. Mucoceles grow very slowly and ultimately, and it is difficult to really know the efficacy of this treatment method because such long-term follow-up is required to determine it.

The Riedel procedure ablates the sinus completely by removing the anterior table of the sinus and allowing the soft tissue of the forehead to collapse against the posterior table of the sinus. The procedure is very successful in treating mucoceles and allows for early detection of recurrent disease, but results in a significant cosmetic deformity. After a period without evidence of disease, patients may undergo a secondary procedure to correct the cosmetic defect using methyl methacrylate or split calvarial bone to re-create the forehead contour.

The Lynch procedure was designed to remove the floor of the frontal sinus and the anterior ethmoid air cells, and allow good drainage of the frontal sinus and mucocele. Difficulty arose with restenosis of the neo-naso frontal duct thus created, and recurrence of frontal sinus disease was common. Modifications have been designed to line the new drainage channel with mucosa, but the bony framework of the duct is removed by the approach through the medial wall of the orbit, and the problem of mucosal collapse and restenosis has not been eliminated. Long-term success appears to be higher with osteoplastic flap and fat obliteration of the sinus.

Some authors have advocated the use of endoscopic sinus surgery to drain the sinus and mucocele while preserving the sinus anatomy and allowing postoperative follow-up with CT scanning. This type of treatment does not include removal of the mucocele, but incorporates its lining into the roof of the opened sinus. The majority of frontal sinus mucoceles involve the frontal recess of the ethmoids, and this area is approachable through the nose using endoscopy. Theoretically, one could widely marsupialize a frontal sinus mucocele via the anterior ethmoids. Kennedy et al. reported on 11 frontal sinus mucoceles treated this way. None of the patients had complications related to the procedure, such as a CSF leak. Three of the patients could not be adequately treated by this approach and required a different procedure to remove the

mucocele. None of the patients had evidence of recurrent disease on follow-up of 2–48 mo *(30)*. This technique is not yet widely practiced. Long-term results remain unknown.

REFERENCES

1. Goodwin WJ. Orbital complications of ethmoiditis. Otolaryngol Clin North Am 1985;18(1):139–147.
2. Moloney JR, Badham NJ, McRae A. The acute orbit—preseptal (periorbital) cellulitis, subperiosteal abscess and orbital cellulitis due to sinusitis. J. Laryngol Otol 1987;12(Suppl.):1–18.
3. Gutowski WM, Mulbury PE, Hengerer AS, Kido DK. The role of CT scans in managing the orbital complications of ethmoiditis. Int J Pediatr Otolaryngol 1988;15:117–128.
4. Schramm VL, Myers EN, Kennerdell JS. Orbital complications of acute sinusitis: evaluation, management, and outcome. ORL J Otolaryngol Related Specialties 1987;86:221–230.
4a. Chanoller JR, Langenbrunner DJ, Stevens ER. The pathogenesis of orbital complications in acute sinusitis. Laryngoscope 1970;80:1414–1428.
5. Schramm VL, Curtin HD, Kennerdell JS. Evaluation of orbital cellulitis and results of treatment. Laryngoscope 1982;92:732–738.
6. Shahin J, Gullane PJ, Dayal VS. Orbital complications of acute sinusitis. J Otolaryngol 1987;16(1):23–27.
7. Patt BS, Manning SC. Blindness resulting from orbital complications of sinusitis. Otolaryngol Head and Neck Surg 1991;104(6):789–795.
8. Antoine GA, Grundfast KM. Periorbital cellulitis. Int J Pediatr Otorhinolaryngol 1987;13:273–278.
9. Yousem DM, Atlas SW, Grossman RI, Sergott RC, Savino PJ, Bosley TM. MR Imaging of Tolusa-Hunt syndrome. Am J Radiol 1990;154:167–170.
10. Larson T. Petrous apex and cavernous sinus: anatomy and physiology. Semin Ultrasound, CT, and MRI 1993; 14(3):232–246.
11. Baquero F, Loza E. Antibiotic resistance of microorganisms involved in ear, nose and throat infections. Pediatr Infect Dis J 1994;13(Suppl. 1):S9–S13.
12. Elverland H, Melheim I, Anke I. Acute orbit from ethmoiditis drained by endoscopic sinus surgery. Acta Otolaryngol 1992;492(Suppl.):147–151.
13. Fairbanks DNF, Milmoe GJ. Complications and sequelae: an otolaryngologist's perspective. Pediatr Infect Dis 1985;4(6):S75–S78.
14. Parker GS, Tami TA, Wilson JF, Fetter TW. Intracranial complications of sinusitis. South Med J 1989;82(5): 563–568.
15. Nathavitharana KA, Tarlow MJ. Current treads in the management of bacterial meningitis. Br J Hosp Med 1993;50(7):403–407.
16. Pfister HW, Feiden W, Einhaupl KM. Spectrum of complications during bacterial meningitis in adults. Arch Neurol 1993;50:575–581.
17. Schaad UB, Lips U, Gnehm HE, Blumberg A, Heinser I, Wedgwood J. Dexamethasone therapy for bacterial meningitis in children. Lancet 1993;342:457–461.

18. Clayman GL, Adams GL, Paugh DR, Koopmann CF. Intracranial complications of paranasal sinusitis: a combined institutional review. Laryngoscope 1991;101: 234–239.

19. Deans JA, Welch AR. Acute isolated sphenoid sinusitis: a disease with complications. J Laryngol Otol 1991;105: 1072–1074.

20. Thatai D, Chandy L, Dhar KL. Septic cavernous sinus thrombophlebitis: a review of 35 cases. J Indian Med Assoc 1992;90(11):290–292.

21. Ellie E, Houang B, Louail C, Legrain-Lefermann V, Laurent F, Drouillard J, Julien J. CT and high-field MRI in septic thrombosis of the cavernous sinuses. Neuroradiology 1992;34:22–24.

22. Rao KCVG, Knipp HC, Wagner EJ. Computed tomographic findings in cerebral sinus and venous thrombosis. Radiology 1981;140:391–398.

23. Karlin RJ, Robinson WA. Septic cavernous sinus thrombosis. Ann Emer Med 1984;13(6):449–455.

24. Kuta AJ, Laine FJ. Imaging the sphenoid bone and basiocciput: anatomic considerations. Semin Ultrasound, CT, and MRI 1993;14(3):146–159.

25. Appelgate GR, Hirsch WL, Appelgate LJ, Curtin HD. Variability in the enhancement of the normal central skull base in children. Neuroradiology 1992;34:217–221.

26. Lew D, Southwick FS, Montgomery WW, Weber AL, Baker AS. Sphenoid sinusitis. N Engl J Med 1983; 309(19): 1149–1154.

27. Goldman GE, Fontanarosa PB, Anderson JM. Isolated sphenoid sinusitis. Am J Emer Med 1993;11(3): 235–238.

28. Rothfield RE, de Vries EJ, Rueger RG. Isolated sphenoid sinus disease. Head and Neck 1991;13:208–212.

29. Moriyama H, Hesaka H, Tachibana T, Honda Y. Mucoceles of ethmoid and sphenoid sinus with visual disturbance. Arch Otolaryngol Head and Neck Surg 1992;118:142–146.

30. Kennedy DW, Josephson JS, Zinreich SJ, Mattox DE, Goldsmith MM. Endoscopic sinus surgery for mucoceles: a viable alternative. Laryngoscope 1989;99:885–895.

31. Daya SS. A "silent" intracranial complication of frontal sinusitis. J Laryngol Otol 1990;104:645–647.

32. Baker AS. Role of anaerobic bacteria in sinusitis and its complications. Annals of Otol, Rhihol, and Laryngol 1991;(Suppl 154):17–22.

33. Abramovich S, Smelt GJC. Acute sphenoiditis, alone and in concert. J Laryngol Otol 1982;96:751–757.

34. Wenig BL, Goldstein MN, Abramson AL. Frontal sinusitis and its intracranial complications. Int J Pediatr Otorhinolaryngol 1983;5:285–302.

35. Rosenbaum GS, Cunha BA. Subdural empyema complicating frontal and ethmoid sinusitis. Heart and Lung 1989;18(2):199–202.

36. Hoyt DJ, Fisher SR. Otolaryngologic management of patients with subdural empyema. Laryngoscope 1991; 101:20–24.

37. Weingarten K, Zimmerman RD, Becker RD, Heier LA, Haimes AB, Deck MDF. Subdural and epidural empyemas: MR imaging. Am J Radiol 1989;152:615–621.

38. Latchaw RE, Hirsch WL, Yock DH. Imaging of intracranial infections. Neurosurg Clin North Am 1992;3(2):303–322.

39. Magnilia AJ, Goodwin WJ, Arnold JE, Ganz E. Intracranial abscesses secondary to nasal, sinus, and orbital infections in adults and children. Arch Otolaryngol Head and Neck Surg 1989;115:1424–1429.

40. Bradley PJ, Manning KP, Shaw MDM. Brain abscess secondary to paranasal sinusitis. J Laryngol Otol 1984; 98:719–725.

41. Bagdatoglu H, Ildan F, Cetinalp E, Doganay M, Boyar B, Uzuneyupoglu Z, Haciyakupoglu S, Karadayi A. The clinical presentation of intracranial abscesses: a study of seventy-eight cases. J Neurol Sci 1992;36(3):139–143.

42. Osenbach RK, Loftus CM. Diagnosis and management of brain abscess. Neurosurg Clin North Am 1992;3(2): 403–420.

43. Yang S, Zhao C. Review of 140 patients with brain abscess. Surg Neurol 1993;39:290–296.

44. Obana WG, Rosenblum ML. Nonoperative treatment of neurosurgical infections. Neurosurg Clin North Am 1992;3(2):359–373.

45. Kraus M, Tovi F. Central nervous system complications secondary to otorhinologic infections. An analysis of 39 pediatric cases. Int J Pediatr Otolaryngol 1992;24:217–226.

46. Seydoux C, Francioli P. Bacterial brain abscesses: factors influencing mortality and sequelae. Clin Infect Dis 1992;15:394–401.

47. Lunardi P, Acqui M, Ferrante L, Mastronardi L, Fortuna A. Non-traumatic brain abscess. Neurosurg Rev 1993;16: 189–196.

48. Johnson DL, Markle BM, Wiedermann BL, Hanahan L. Treatment of intracranial abscesses associated with sinusitis in children and adults. J Pediatr 1988;113(pt1): 15–23.

49. Leys D, Christiaens JL, Derambure P, Hladky JP, Lesoin F, Rousseaux M, Jomin M, Petit H. Management of focal intracranial infections: is medical management better than surgery? J Neurol, Neurosurg, and Psychiatry 1990;53: 472–475.

50. Bidzinski J, Koszewski W. The value of different methods of treatment of brain abscess in the CT era. Acta Neurologica 1990;105:117–120.

12 Mucosal Swellings, Mucoceles, and Polyps in Paranasal Sinuses

Pathophysiological Implications

Michel R. Wayoff, MD

CONTENTS

INTRODUCTION

There is a large and progressive spectrum in the inflammatory changes of the sinus mucosa from a localized swelling to a mucosal cyst, a deforming mucocele, or a major polyposis. All these terms represents different clinical pictures, easily recognized by the rhinologist, but sometimes intriguing for other practitioners. Intrasinusal chronic inflammatory changes are often discovered on routine radiographs *(1,2)*. If the CT scan offers invaluable pictures, they are often difficult to interpret by the radiologist without more sophisticated imaging. In fact, in most cases, the diagnostic accuracy of a major sinus opacity is limited before an invasive injection with a contrast medium or an MRI can be performed. Common sense calls for a true partnership between the radiologist and the rhinologist *(3)*.

From: *Diseases of the Sinuses* (M. E. Gershwin and G. A. Incaudo, eds.),
©1996 Humana Press Inc., Totowa, NJ.

Since so many specialists are interested today in "sinus problems," it is necessary to outline certain points:

- Physicians have to treat living patients, and not just pictures;
- Modern nasal and sinus endoscopy is the first mandatory step before deciding on any complementary investigation; and
- The clinical aspects of each patient have to be integrated into his or her more or less complex history.

For example, there are no apparent links between a silent swelling of the floor of the maxillary sinus and nasal polyposis. However, these two mucosal changes often have the same histological picture, and in clinical practice, I have observed some patients going slowly, year after year, from the first to the second condition.

The unity of this chapter consists of the chronic noninfectious inflammatory response of the sinus mucosa considered from a realistic point of view.

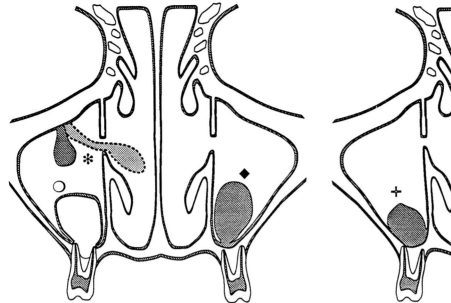

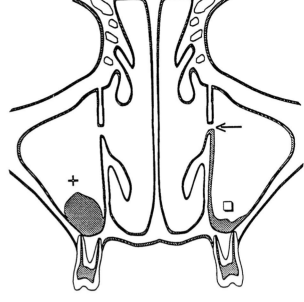

Fig. 1. Cysts (○) or pseudocysts (◆) appear on conventional radiographs as "sun-rise" pictures. They are generally asymptomatic and without proximate periodontitis. (○) Radicular cyst secondary to the development of an apical granuloma. For a time, a thin osseous shell separates the cyst lining membrane from the sinus mucosa. (*) Mucosal pseudocysts hanging on the roof of the maxillary sinus frequently occur. They may evolve into a solitary antro-choanal polyp by passing through the ostial area.

Fig. 2. (❑) Inflammatory mucosal swelling related to a periapical chronic infection. As the clinical significance of such mucosal changes may be discussed, they may also explain sinusitis recurrencies of apparently rhinogenic seasonal etiology, regarding a permanent subliminal ostiomeatal impairment. (+) Cysts or pseudocysts of the maxillary sinus mucosa are difficult to differentiate. They may be a response to dental foci, often difficult to demonstrate without a Denta-scan®.

As a practical guide to help all categories of physicians, I have chosen the following topics:

1. Intrasinusal mucosal swellings;
2. Chronic inflammatory mucosal pathology with deformities of the sinus walls; and
3. Nasal polyps and diffuse polyposis.

INTRASINUSAL MUCOSAL SWELLINGS

Every modification of the sinus mucosa of whatever etiology may be a combination of areas of hyperplastic, edematous, polypoid, atrophic, and fibrotic changes. Moreover, the consistency of secretions varies greatly according to protein concentration and degree of desiccation. The precise analysis of any intrasinusal mucosal modification may require all the modern imaging armamentarium: axial and coronal CT examination, and MRI studies with contrast material to obtain T_1 and T_2 relaxation times *(3)*.

In daily practice, such expensive investigations are rarely justified. It must be outlined that the radiologist cannot differentiate between acute and chronic

inflammation, and that he or she can easily underestimate the thickness of the mucosa. By way of compensation, clinical manifestations, nasal endoscopy, and sinus endoscopy are complementary studies.

Intrasinus Benign Mucosal Cysts (BMCs) and Pseudocysts

The intrasinus BMCs are usually asymptomatic, and incidentally discovered by conventional radiography or CT scan as rounded shadows in otherwise clear maxillary sinuses. Generally, such cysts, or pseudocysts, appear as so-called sun-rise pictures merging from the lower part of the maxillary sinus. Occasionally, these cysts or pseudocysts may produce mild and mainly subjective nonspecific symptoms. It could be difficult to establish a causal relationship between such symptoms and the intrasinus lesion. Too rapid and/or aggressive therapeutic decisions must be avoided (Figs. 1 and 2).

PATHOPHYSIOLOGY

The pathogenesis of such BMCs is uncertain. This condition can be differently designed as nonsecreting cyst, mucosal or mucous cyst, retention cyst, pseudocyst, interstitial or mesothelial cyst, or even polypous cyst. Each designation is related to different and generally hypothetical pathophysiological mechanisms based on histological studies:

- Blockage of glandular duct with secondary retention of mucus and acini dilatation;
- Result of a mild or silent infection promoting the scaling of many little glands, near one another, and forming a series of little cysts that may coalesce in a larger one, without any more identifiable epithelial-limiting membrane;
- Submucosal circumscription of extravased fluids; and
- Occlusion of a lymphatic vessel producing a nonsecreting cavity, bordered by a flattened, condensed "mesothelium," and containing a yellow and translucid liquor.

INCIDENCE

The BMC is common, and its incidence varies widely between 2 and 9%. Its growth rate is not known and, very often, different pictures taken over a period of months or years do not show demonstrable modifications in size. The size of these cysts commonly varies from 10 mm to 30 or 40 mn. The sinus cavity may be completely filled on rare occasions.

CLINICAL IMPLICATIONS

The BMC may sometimes induce a sensation of heaviness located on the same side as the cyst. It is debatable to assume a causal relationship with a functional ipsilateral nasal obstruction or a posterior nasal drip.

The spontaneous rupture of such cysts may produce a sudden and copious anterior or posterior nasal discharge of yellow fluid, relieving the pre-existing symptoms. More commonly the cysts are incidentally found on a panoramic dental radiograph and are unrelated to local signs or symptoms. It is conceivable that these formations may herniate into the nasal fossa through the ostium, and therefore appearing as a solitary antrochoanal polyp (*see* Solitary Choanal Polyps Section).

RADIOLOGIC EXAMINATION

The bone adjacent to BMC always remains intact. The CT scan demonstrates only the morphological shape, and a BMC cannot be differentiated from a solitary polyp or from a pseudocyst. Their relationships with dental apices may be clarified

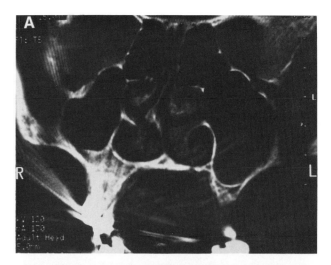

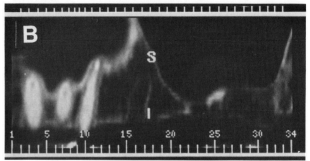

Fig. 3. Conventional picture of a cyst or pseudocyst on the floor of the left maxillary sinus **(A)**. The dental origin by a sequestrated tooth debris was demonstrated only by Denta-scan® **(B)**.

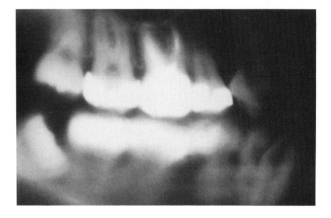

Fig. 4. Polytomographs in lateral view showing great probability of dental origin of a round-shaped swelling, cyst, or pseudocyst.

by a Denta-scan®. In rare cases, MRI sequences are necessary to distinguish them from tumors. Sinus endoscopy may be a preferred approach to this question (Figs. 3–6).

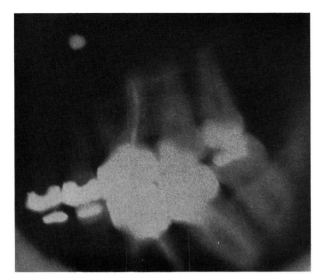

Fig. 5. Foreign body of dental origin associated with a mucosal irregular swelling in the floor of the maxillary sinus. This patient presents an aspirin triad associated.

TREATMENT

The treatment of these reputedly innocent cysts consists mainly of reassuring the patients. Large cysts may be evacuated through a diameatic or transcanine puncture.

Dental Implications in the Maxillary Sinus

Taking into account the fact that the normal adult size of the maxillary sinus is not reached until about 20 yr, there is a relatively large scale of individual variations. Some patients possess very large antral cavities. The two upper premolars and the two first upper molars (so-called sinusal teeth) may be only separated from the antral cavity by a mucoperiosteum. This is especially the case with the palatal apex of the upper first molar *(4)*. Sometimes the apices are projected into the sinus cavity. Even if the apices are not in close relation with the sinusal cavity, the main blood supply of the dental and periodontal structures anastomose reciprocally, with the vessels going in the sinus mucosa through the marrow spaces of the basal portion of the maxillary bone *(5)*. It has been demonstrated that successful periodontal treatment may result in normalization of the sinus mucosa in most cases *(6)*. In the literature, a very large scale between 4.6 and 47% estimates the dental origin of chronic maxillary sinusitis *(7,8)*.

Periodontis is an intermittently evolving disease in which bursts of inflammatory infiltrate progress

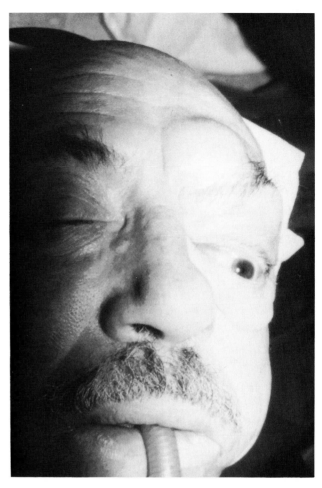

Fig. 6. A 63-yr-old patient with previous multiple polypectomies and developing a large frontal mucocele with a "toad-eye" aspect.

through intra-alveolar vessels with a slow and long-lasting bone resorption. The bone reactivity, variable among each patient, explains the manner in which the host is dealing with this disease. In such a way, positive correlations can be demonstrated between the degree of hyperplasia of the sinus mucosa and the severity of periodontis.

DENTAL EXTRACTION

When particular anatomical situations are present, such as when the osseous floor of the sinus is very thin or even dehiscent, a fracture may occur as a result of forces applied during a molar or premolar extraction. Minor fissures remain unknown and heal silently. When the lining mucosa is torn, some blood collects in the sinus floor. A radiological cloudiness of the antrum may be demonstrated, but will disappear in 2 wk. In some cases, a complete communication may be established between the air-containing sinus and the oral cavity. An awkward maneuver or, more frequently, an unavoidable fatality may result in the dislodgment of a root's fragment or of the entire tooth in the sinus air space.

The evolution of such complications depends on many factors: size of the oro-antral fistula, nature and importance of the periodontic or periapical infection, and size of the dental fragment. Exceptionally little debris may be spontaneously evacuated through the ostium. Failure of the tooth debris to move (demonstrated by successive radiographs) implies that it is trapped in the edematous reactive mucosa. Sometimes, apices fragments remain in the bony wall, where they may be quite well tolerated (Fig. 3).

Acute or subacute sinusitis may develop after such difficulties. A systemic antibiotherapy with or without ancillary antral punctures gives generally good results.

A chronic oro-antral fistula may require invasive intra-alveolar maneuvers. The sinus infection may have an adequate drainage through the fistula, but it must be controlled before the closure procedure. Different techniques for such fistula closure (with buccal or palatal flaps) are useful.

COMPLICATIONS OF ENDODONTAL TREATMENT

In many patients, either the floor of the sinus cavity slips down between the roots of molars or the apices of premolars may protrude through the quite indistinguishable bony floor of the antrum. In such conditions, when a tooth devitalization is necessary, the amalgam used by the dentist to fill the dental canal may pass into the sinus cavity, even if the filling was cautiously done.

Most of the amalgam can be evacuated through the ostium. The filling contains mercury or zinc, which may promote the installation and growth of *Aspergillus fumigatus*. Generally, the fungal sinusitis of dental origin is nonallergic and noninvasive. In the presence of radiologically dense intrasinusal opacities (Fig. 5), the diagnosis of fungal sinusitis should be considered *(9)*.

ACUTE MAXILLARY SINUSITIS

The clinical picture is quite the same as in a rhinogenic acute sinusitis, with its aching pain, often more intense in the morning or in the evening, associated with more or less purulent discharge. In spite of those symptoms, there is a minimal general disturbance and pyrexia remains moderate. The

diagnosis of dental origin is evident in the presence of a recent tooth extraction with or without signs of oro-antral communication, as well as a recent endodontic treatment.

The palpation over the cheek usually causes more tenderness than in rhinogenic acute sinusitis, and the pain is generally proportionate to the pus retention. The acute sinusitis of dental origin is always unilateral, and a careful endoral examination reveal that a molar or premolar is abnormal and exquisitely reacts by pressing the tip index in the jugal vestibule as well as in the palatal side, or by an instrumental axial percussion.

In rare cases, the discussion rises to differentiate an odontalgia of sinus origin from a sinusalgia by dental mechanism. It would be a pity if an unmerited suspected tooth were extracted under such conditions. The acute maxillary sinusitis of dental origin represents 5–10% of the acute sinusitis *(4)*.

CHRONIC MAXILLARY SINUSITIS OF DENTAL ORIGIN

The chronic maxillary sinusitis of dental origin is properly named "hypocritical." It develops insidiously, as a more or less long delay following the early lesions of periodontic infection. The dental responsibility is often denied by the patient who wishes to conserve, for example, an expensive dental prosthesis, or by the dentist, who feels anger at having the quality of his or her care questioned. It must be explained that the close relationship of the sinus cavity with the molar and/or premolar apices constitutes a fatality in itself, independently of an insufficient tooth devitalization or the possibility of the antral penetration of an excess of amalgam material. A major argument against the dental origin to sinus disease is that a lot of people are carrying chronic apical or periodontic pathologies without any noticeable symptoms. There are no epidemiological studies describing the silent evolution of this process. It is very difficult to appreciate the importance of dental infection in chronic maxillary sinusitis at a time when modern sinus surgery focuses on ostial dysfunction as the main target of the therapeutic strategy *(8)*.

PATHOPHYSIOLOGY

There could be an explanation for the less frequent appearance of classical forms of chronic sinusitis with pyogenic hyperplasia of the sinus mucosa. As a result of the antibiotic era, and sometimes of associated corticoids abuses, the clinical aspects of chronic sinusitis switch more often toward edematous and polypous changes of the mucosa than would be the case in the natural development of such primarily infectious lesions.

The healthy sinus mucosa is reputed to be sterile, but some studies demonstrated recently the presence of normal flora, aerobic and anaerobic in the uninfected sinus. Classically, it is admitted that aerobe species are predominant in the initial course of acute sinusitis, with secondary apparition of anaerobes when the ostium obstruction creates a hypoxic state within the sinus. Anaerobes are cultured in more than 50% of the patients with chronic or dentogenic sinusitis.

The discussion is not closed about the role of anaerobic bacteria in chronic sinus disease. They certainly more easily develop in a hypoxic sinus cavity, but, in many cases, they may migrate from deep periodontal pockets. Since the same types of anaerobes are obtained in sinus secretions as in periodontal diseased tissues, there is some support for linking the periodontitis and the sinus involvement. The clinical significance of the sinus mucosa swellings caused by advanced periodontal disease is not always clear. They can be silent for long periods, but may also be an important factor of sinus mucosa weakness for other causative or etiological factors (5–7).

The dental origin of chronic sinusitis remains controversial for many reasons. Overall, it will be outlined that many people present asymptomatically with advanced periodontal and apices lesions, coexisting with localized swellings of the near sinus mucosa.

There are no extensive epidemiological studies to appreciate the incidence and prevalence of the hyperplastic of edematous modifications of the "dental gutter" of the maxillary sinus. Several recent publications indicate a positive correlation between the degree of hyperplasia of the sinus mucosa and the severity of periodontis (12). With clinically controlled studies, Engstrom et al. further tested this hypothesis by the effects of periodontal therapy on the thickening of the sinus mucosa, which was reduced by about 80% (13).

Reviewing the dissection of 350 block specimens of jaws, Moskow demonstrated that human periodontis is much more widespread and pervasive than previously thought (5). In a serially sectioned group of 20 blocks, this author showed a very good correlation between the advancement of periodontal lesions and the importance of pathologic changes of the sinus mucosa. The histological modifications include edema, all types of inflammatory cells infiltration, interstitial cyst formation, and polyps. A similar osseous inflammatory response was noted in the marginal portion of the periodontium.

In humans, destructive periodontic lesions are commonly associated with anaerobes, and it should be noted that aspirations, methodically taken from the sinus secretions and pus in patients with maxillary sinusitis, also contain anaerobes in 80–90% of the cases (10). Mainly located near the dental foci, the inflammatory changes in the antral mucosa are often widespread, at least microscopically: presence of many goblet cell glandular structure proliferations, obstruction of gland ducts, hyaline degeneration of the connective tissue, and vascular microthrombosis.

DENTAL OSSEO-INTEGRATED IMPLANTS

The technology of osseo-integrated implants for edentulous patients is not really new, but always in progress and generally well supported (14). In fact, very few papers deal with the long-term results and tolerance from the sinus cavity toward the implanted material. When molars and premolars are extracted, the sinus cavity may prolapse inferiorly in an expansion increasing with age. We can thus imagine that the implant roots, depending of their more or less complicated design, may enter the sinus cavities, and provoke edematous and polypous changes.

The patient may forget to report having had dental implantation. All physicians interested in sinus problems must have some notions about these modern aspects of dental prosthesis. Recently, to increase the indications of dental implantation, a technique was proposed to raise the floor of the sinus cavity by osseous grafting after sinus mucosa elevation. An implant should not be done without having an osseous support of at least 10 mm high and 6 mm thick (15).

CHRONIC MUCOSAL PATHOLOGY WITH DEFORMATION OF THE SINUS WALLS

Many pathological processes may extend beyond the limits of the osseous frame of the paranasal sinuses, such as fulminating acute sinusitis, fungal invasive chronic sinusitis, nonhealing granulomas, and malignant tumors. Nonspecific inflammations of the sinus mucosa are responsible for some insidiously exteriorization evolutions that are easily recognized by the clinician. Their prognosis is much better than with the first group of pathologies, although some cases of mucoceles may have aggressive behavior.

Mucoceles of the Paranasal Sinuses

DEFINITION

Strictly speaking, a mucocele is a mucus-containing formation, with or without a proper limiting membrane. In paranasal pathology, a mucocele consists of an accumulation of sterile inspissated mucoid secretions within the sinusal cavity *(16)*:

- A limiting membrane made of the sinusal mucosa is always present. Contrary to a simple pseudocyst, as a rule, the mucocele eventually fills the sinus cavity obstructing the sinus ostium.
- A mucocele is characterized by progressive thinning and distension of one or more of the sinus bony walls, either endonasally or more remarkably by deforming the facial projection area of the sinuses, particularly in the orbitofrontal region.

PATHOLOGY

Sinus mucoceles were identified by Langenbeck in 1818, and named by Rollet in 1896. It is difficult to estimate their incidence. The published series are limited and scattered among the literature of some specialities: ENT, neurosurgery, ophtalmology, and radiology. As the diagnosis results mainly in osseous deformation or oculo-orbitary complications, the first steps of the mucoceles remain difficult to observe. There are four classical theories to explain the development of that pathology *(16)*:

1. Primary ostial obstruction followed by retention of mucus;
2. Endosinusal hypersecretion of mucus with secondary ostial impairment;
3. A particular form of "blocked sinusitis" with slow and mild persisting inflammation; and
4. Accidental or surgical traumatization of the ostial area.

The literature is in general agreement with the association of two main factors: ostial obstruction and insidious inflammation. Noting that such conditions are frequent, it remains difficult to explain the relative rarity of the "mucocelic syndrome." It is not known why some patients are prone to mucocele formation in otherwise common clinical conditions. In about 30% of the cases, there are no supposed etiological factors or evident associated lesions. The biochemical interactions between the facial skeleton and the pneumatizing properties of the sinus mucosa are not well known even in normal conditions. Moreover, during chronic inflammatory processes, the action of biochemical mediators and the switching of cytokine production may be subjected to great individual variations with differing effects on osseous metabolism. Lund found PGE_2 in higher concentrations in the mucocelic membrane than in normal mucosa *(17)*.

The nature of the lesions associated with the "mucocelic syndrome" pleads for the predominant role of a slow but severe ostia obstruction. The cases reported in most publications often present various chronic conditions: allergy, cystic fibrosis, long-standing sinusitis. Nasal polyps were noted in 11 patients in a series published by Canalis et al. *(18)*. The authors quoted that, in 7 cases (out of 20), intranasal operations preceded the mucocele development. In this author's department, we observed frontal mucoceles after endonasal ethmoidosphenoidectomies in four cases of nasal polyposis with ASA triad. Experimentally, investigators have tried to demonstrate the role of the nasofrontal duct obstruction in mucocele formation. Schenk et al. failed to provoke mucocele formation in dogs. However, this study has been criticized due to possibly too short a delay of observation *(19)*.

CLINICAL ASPECTS

The onset of the mucocele formation passes generally unnoticed. The first symptoms are included with those of the associated pathology: sinusalgia and facial heaviness. Rhinorrhea and/or nasal obstruction may not be seen before the evidence of external deformities. Sometimes, the diagnosis may be made earlier on a CT scan indicated because of ophthalmologic symptoms. When the mucocele develops in the posterior ethmoid and sphenoid area, the proper diagnosis is delayed until orbital and visual complications appear. When the mucocele is infected, a skin fistula may be formed or, in rare cases, infection may spread intracranially.

TOPOGRAPHIC FORMS

Mucoceles of the paranasal sinuses are relatively uncommon. A very active ENT department observes no more than a few cases each year. The interval between primary surgery and the first clinical or radiological presentation of the mucocele can extend from <2 yr to >20 yr. Bilateral cases are extremely rare. The frontoethmoidal localization is the most frequent, followed by the sphenoid occasionally, and the maxillary sinus very rarely.

Frontal Mucoceles. As the expansion of the mucocele (Fig. 6) provokes a progressive bone resorption, lacrimal drainage impairment is frequently one of the first symptoms, accompanied by a variable degree of swelling in the medial orbitofrontal region. A displacement of the eye inferiorly and laterally may follow progressively. Diplopia is frequent. The mucocele expansion may be midline, lateral with eye displacement, or lateral without eye displacement.

The clinical examination shows the classical "egg shell cracking" or a fluctuation sensation by palpation. Endoscopically, the nasal fossa may be normal or show evidence of nasal polyps or surgical scars.

Rarely, the mucocele may rupture spontaneously and be drained by the nasal fossa. More frequently, after an infectious episode, a discharging fistula forms in the upper eyelid. Some cases of giant mucoceles extended posteriorly and connecting the dura have been described.

Ethmoidal Mucoceles. Each ethmoidal cell represents a quite independent sinusal cavity with its own ostium. Every cell may be the starting point of a mucocelic development, which quickly resorbs and presses the surrounding lamellae. The anterior ethmoidal mucoceles are more frequently seen. Five anterior types can be distinguished:

1. Localized anterior *(20)* ethmoidal type has limited swelling in the external canthus area, associated with epiphora, often without ocular displacement;
2. Frontoethmoidal mucocele may reach an important volume depending on the initial size of the frontal sinus;
3. Total ethmoidal mucocele starts anteriorly as a rule and presses back the ethmoidal ground lamella, reaching the sphenoid fissure, and even the dura. The oculo-orbital symptoms are always present with diplopia and chemosis, accompanying sometimes an important external displacement of the eyeball ("toad eye" aspect);
4. Multiple ethmoidal mucoceles are uncommon; and
5. Middle turbinale mucocele is diversely admitted to be an entity. As the concha bullosa arise from the ethmoidal pneumatization process, they may originate as a true mucocelic syndrome developing internally against the nasal septum.

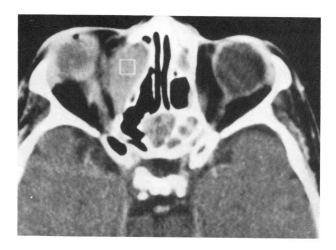

Fig. 7. Multiple mucoceles in a 40-yr-old female, having undergone a sinus surgery at 10 yr. On the right side: large ethmoido-frontal mucocele with exophtalmy. On the left: multiloculated ethmoidosphenoidal mucocele.

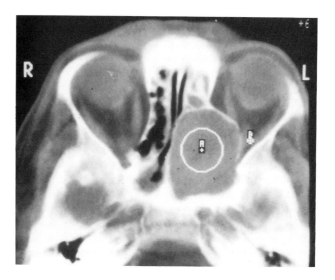

Fig. 8. Large sphenoidal mucocele with exophtalmia and visual loss.

Posterior Ethmoidosphenoidal Mucoceles. They are uncommon and tardily diagnosed. They may start from the Onodi cell, pressing the sphenoid wall back. The sphenoidal mucocele is perhaps more frequent, generally invading the two sinuses before extending toward the sellar area. The anterior ethmoidal extension is relatively well tolerated in such cases *(20)*. After a long asymptomatic period, the symptoms are mainly (Figs. 7 and 8) permanent orbital and retro-ocular pains; optic nerve compression with visual loss; oculo-motor palsies; and, surprisingly, for moderate exophtalmy.

Maxillary Sinus Mucoceles. The total antral form and the localized forms developing in the malar recess of the sinus cavity are very uncommon. They must be distinguished from anatomical variations (bipartite sinus, abnormal intrasinusal osseous septum), as well as from the rounded swellings of the sinus roof (pseudocyst or glandular retention true cyst).

The clinical findings are the sinus wall bulging deformation with the ping-pong ball or fluctuating consistency according to the degree of osseous lysis. The differential diagnosis is antral carcinoma, odontogenic cysts, or even the exceptional sinus cholesteatoma.

RADIOLOGICAL FINDINGS

Before the mucocele provokes any bone erosion, their identification may sometimes be disputable on conventional sinus films. Its homogeneous regularly hemispheric density within a sinus cavity may be difficult to differentiate from a polypoid thickening or a retention cyst. The CT gives a homogenous appearance isodense to the brain tissue or with a mucoid attenuation. MRI contributes to a better differentiation of fluid-filled structures from benign and malignant tumors.

When the sinus contours are regularly expanded, a mucocele is most likely to be present. The MRI is very significant with a high-intensity signal on the T_1 and T_2 images, except in old lesions where these signals became dark (Fig. 9). The CT gives better information on any bone changes present.

DIFFERENTIAL DIAGNOSIS

The clinical presentation creates suspicion of infection complications in pyo-mucocele or the risk of cutaneous fistulization. Cholesterol granuloma can occur in sinus cavities, as in mastoid air cells, by retentive bleedings of an inflammatory granulomatous reaction. As in otology, the term keratoma seems to be more adapted to designate extremely rare cases of sinus cholesteatoma, which are epidermal cysts. The MRI signals may give some orientations, but the final diagnosis is made during surgery *(20)*.

TREATMENT

The treatment of all forms of mucoceles is surgical. Considering their frequent pathological associations, the results have to be assessed after a long follow-up. Current practice favors endoscopic surgical marsupialization as often as possible.

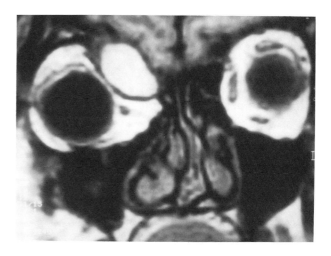

Fig. 9. MRI picture of a fronto-ethmoidal mucocele with enhanced signals.

In many cases, the frontal mucoceles necessitate external approaches, with osteoplastic flap procedures or even sometimes bone grafts, depending on the degree of sinus expansion and bone destruction. As much as possible, the sinus cavity must be left intact or reconstructed, avoiding stripping too much mucosa, thereby allowing the reconstitution of a well-drained sinus cavity. The drainage may be improved by local mucosal flaps or even by largely reuniting the two frontal sinuses to obtain a cavity draining medially after associating an adapted septal resection. When severe mucosal degeneration is present and when the posterior wall of the frontal sinus is dehiscent on the dura. Sinus obliteration or sinus cranialization is to be used.

Maxillary Sinus Atelectasis

Asymmetric developments of the maxillary sinus are common in normal subjects. When they are noted in pathological conditions, the question of their independent pre-existence or their secondary character arises. With modern CT and MRI imaging, such cases are better documented. In 1966, Montgomery reported two cases of complete opacity of the maxillary sinus with enophthalmy that he considered to be caused by mucoceles (cited in ref. *21*). Two recent papers give a review of the literature pleading for a new syndrome they called "atelectasis of the maxillary sinus" *(21,22)*.

The CT scan shows a generalized collapse of the antral cavity with inward bowing of the sinus limits without evidence of bone destruction. When they remain moderate, such findings are generally neglected or anecdotal. In some cases, this sinus intussusception mechanism may produce enophthalmia with some retreat of the infraorbital region plane. The sinus residual cavity contains a thickened and pale mucosa, associated with banal nonspecific inflammatory histological pictures, whereas the ostium blockage is not always present *(22)*.

Pneumosinus Dilatans (or Pneumocele)

This is a rare condition of unknown mechanism producing an evolutive hyperpneumatizing process of one or more sinuses. As a rule, the frontal sinus is always involved, and mainly unilaterally. Its name was given by Benjamin in 1918. The reported cases are rare and sporadic *(16)*.

This pathology involves most commonly males, between 20 to 40 yr. Very insidiously the patient becomes aware that his supraorbital region stands out more and more. If bilateral, this aspect may be considered a personal feature by a young male, terminating with his growth. Intermittent and short localized pain, with a lightly congestive aspect of the overlying skin are seen. A Neanderthalian aspect is rare. When the bony wall is thinned, fractures may be provoked by minimal traumas.

Some cases of maxillary pneumoceles were described with frequent intrasinus pressure changes from airplane decompression or incessant nose blowing *(23)*. The posterior ethmoidosphenoidal localization is exceptional and may be revealed by oculo-orbital symptoms.

The pathophysiology of the pneumocele remains unexplained. Inside the sinus, the mucosa is normal and there is no ostial obstruction or checkvalve mechanism.

The diagnosis is easily assumed with modern sinus imaging, demonstrating air-filled cavities, and extremely thin osseous contours. Surgical corrections are sometimes wished by patients, or even necessary in major cases. Osteoplastic procedures with or without contour modeling bone grafts are used.

Cystic Cavities of the Upper Jaw

CLASSIFICATION

It is mandatory to keep in mind a general sketch of the pathologic conditions that may invade or encroach on the maxillary sinus.

Bony Dysplasia. This belongs to the properly osseous pathology: fibrous dysplasia, ossifying fibroma, and Paget disease.

Odontogenic Cysts. The term "odontogenic tumors" is used to describe a group of lesions that include extreme morphological variants from odontomas to hamartomas or cementomas. In this group, there are four types of cystic lesions that are of interest:

1. Fissural cysts: of dysembryoplastic origin, medial or paramedially sited, they are not likely to encroach the maxillary sinus;
2. Dentigerous cysts arise from the enamel organ enveloping symmetrically the crown of the tooth;
3. Odontogenic cysts form a group, the varieties of which need to be appreciated by the oral surgeon. The odontogenic keratocyst may be multiple or multilocular, and is more frequent in young patients. Lined by a squamous keratinizing epithelium without cholesterol precipitation, it possesses an aggressive behavior;
4. Periodontic cysts are the most frequent and start from periodontic vestigial debris activated by a chronic periodontic infection (periapical and radicular cysts) or by extended caries (Fig. 1). Beginning as a granuloma, the developed cyst is lined by a squamous cell epithelium without keratin, but with the presence of giant cells and cholesterol deposits. From their early beginning, such granulomas may encroach the antral limits.

CLINICAL ASPECTS

Whatever the nature of a lesion arising from the upper jaw, the clinical presentation appears usually as a hard bony swelling in the buccal sulcus. When its size increases, palpation may give a crackling egg shell or a fluctuating sensation. The presence of a dead tooth or the absence of a tooth is to be verified. The modern radiological imaging (dentascan) permits a better expertise than existed in the past.

In general, the behavior of a cyst that has encroached on the maxillary sinus follows two main courses: (1) the bone covering the cyst toward the sinus cavity resists for some time and the cyst develops laterally, is diagnosed, and treated without sinus implication; or (2) the bony layer separating the cyst from the sinus mucosa may be thin and then disappears. In such a way the cyst expands intrasinusally (Figs. 1 and 4) and should be difficult to differentiate from an intrasinusal cyst, particularly if the responsible tooth had been extracted earlier, and the bulging is absent in the buccal vestibule.

Three findings are an invaluable aid for the diagnosis:

1. The aspiration puncture of a cyst of dental origin demonstrates very numerous cholesterine crystals. In more advanced cases, aspiration brings keratin debris or inspissated mucous, but not malodorous material;

2. During surgery, the limiting membrane of the radicular cyst is easily dissected from the sinus mucosa even if a limited communicating breakdown exists when the cyst is infected. This is never the case in a sinusal cyst; and

3. The histological verification shows a rather thick stratified squamous epithelium in the cyst of periodontic origin. However, apical cysts have been reported to be lined by both ciliated and squamous epithelium areas. In such rare cases, the other differential criteria prevail.

Nasal Polyposis with Osseous Deformities

The more classic and histologically benign polyposis *(see below)* shows, in rare cases, the capacity to provoke bony resorption of the midfacial skeleton with subcutaneous deformation. In 1988, Parker *(24)* reported three cases and proposed the name of "aggressive sinonasal polyposis," with bony erosion of the frontal, the maxillary, and the ethmoid sinuses, without findings consistent with the presence of a mucocele and no evidence of osteomyelitis. Multiple small mucous retention areas may act as so many micromucoceles. In fact, we observed some cases without important retention of mucus. Immunological factors are assumed, but not demonstrable.

In adults, these forms of "deformans polyposis" are mainly associated with aspirin intolerance triad (Fig. 10). In children, an enlargement of the nasal bones may be observed, generally in cystic fibrosis cases. Such a condition was labeled in European countries in the early 1990s as the Woakes syndrome, related to a chronic necrotizing ethmoiditis.

NASAL POLYPS
AND NASAL POLYPOSIS (NP)

In daily practice, the chronic inflammatory sinus pathology is truly a "melting pot" where the different clinical conditions are hardly differentiated by the physicians, difficult to treat, and difficult to explain to the patients. Among these conditions, the NP deserves its enigmatical reputation. With the

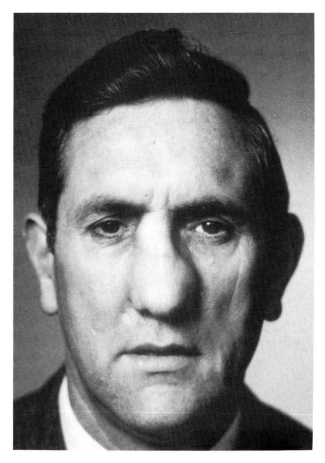

Fig. 10. Deforming nasal polyposis with nasal bones erosions (case of ASA triad).

improved knowledge concerning the regulation of the inflammatory response, a better understanding of the singular, diffuse, and recurrent forms of NP may evolve.

Definition

The term "polyp" is commonly used by patients as well as by medical practitioners to describe a mass of tissue projecting from a mucous membrane and supported by a stalk-like attachment. Therefore, much confusion exists concerning the location, nature, and evolution of such features. The name itself is often semantically misunderstood and compared, for example, with a polypod or vegetating tumor. A true polyp does not have many feet, but just one. Frequently, there are many polyps near each other. These are designated polyposis. In clinical practice, there are two main groups of nasal polyps: the solitary polyp originating, as a rule, in the maxillary sinus, which is the classic antrochoanal polyp described by Killian; and the multiple degenerative polyposis of the sinusal mucosa. In the nasal fossae, some neoplastic masses may have a pedunculated appearance. The clinician must be able to differentiate a polyp from inverted papillomas, angiofibromas, and other tumors (*see* Chapter 13). In unilateral conditions, a common reactional polyp may mask a genuine tumoral growth as "a sentry polyp."

Rhinologically, a nasal polyp represents an inflammatory, edematous pseudotumoral and pedunculated formation, regularly inserted in the middle meatus and originating from the paranasal sinuses system. Nasal polyposis represents a clinical entity characterized by the accumulation of polyps mainly inserted in the ethmoidal cells and the middle meatus. It is typically bilaterally and has a great tendency to recur.

In its early stages, a nasal polyp may be quite asymptomatic. Its limiting membrane eventually grows thicker with superficial metaplastic changes, expanding toward the nostril anteriorly or occupying the choanal area posteriorly.

Histological Aspects

The microscopic aspect of nasal polyps is relatively stereotyped, whereas their microscopic features lack specificity. Though they appear in different etiological processes, their histologic study does not today provide any precise indication of their true pathogeny.

Preliminarily, it is necessary to remember, from a medicolegal point of view, that every polyp removed from a nasal fossa must be histologically examined to avoid misdiagnosis. For example, a wood worker may present simultaneous common polyps with an adenocarcinoma of the ethmoid, or an inverted papilloma may be misleading.

According to Hellquist *(25),* four histological types of polyps may be described. All these types are more or less pedunculated or translucent. When the membrane is sectioned, a yellow, pale liquor escapes in beginning forms, or a relatively dense parenchyma is exposed in old recurrent superinfected polyps. Since edema is constant, the infiltration of the stroma by the pool of the effector cells of the inflammatory process provides differentiation.

The So-Called Allergic Type

About 90% of nasal polyps belong to this category. Until about 1960, it was believed that the predominant presence of eosinophils was the sig-nature of allergy. This variety is histologically characterized by:

- A normal epithelium with a more or less important activity of goblet cells;
- A thickened basement membrane that is in reality a pseudothickening line, as can be shown by special colorations (PAS-negative silver staining);
- Abundant eosinophils, frequently clustered around vessels along with plasmocytes and histiocytes; and
- Many mast cells being widespread in the stroma.

It should be stressed today that the pure allergic origin of polyposis is relatively infrequent, and that associated factors are often seen. The allergic component in nasal polyps may occur in about 20% of cases. In fact, the local eosinophil attraction depends on the modulation by which the mediators and cytokines are released. In many cases, eosinophils are so abundant that they represent more than 50% of the infiltrated cells.

The Chronic Inflammatory Type

- The epithelium shows some modifications as cuboidal stratification or squamous transformation;
- The pseudothickening of the basal membrane is irregular or absent;
- The cellular infiltration consists of a mixture of neutrophils, lymphocytes, and plasma cells; and
- Eosinophils are not much greater in number than in other types, and neutrophils may be predominant.

The Glandular Type

In several cases, the seromucous glands are so numerous and hyperplastic that the diagnosis of tubulocystic adenoma was sometimes reported in past literature. In fact, the cellular infiltration looks like the polyps, so-called allergic polyp with predominant eosinophil infiltration.

Nasal Polyp with Stroma Atypia

This type of nasal polyp is infrequent and must be known by the pathologist to avoid misinterpretation. In a generally very edematous stroma, the presence of active fibroblasts is localized in some areas of the polyp. These fibroblasts show an unusual aspect: they are stellate, and hyperchromatic without mitoses, but, also, sometimes plumped and irregular. If necessary, special immunocytochemical reactions may be used to rule out a suspicion of malignancy.

Pathophysiology

Obviously, nasal polyps represent a nonspecific inflammatory reaction of the sinonasal mucosa. There are neither animal models nor experimental production techniques in humans. They are frequently encountered in clinical practice at different stages of development.

During systematic necropsies, Larsen and Tos *(26)* found nasal polyps in the middle meatus in 2% of cases, whereas Hosemann et al. *(27)* noted a 1.6% incidence. Nasal polyps are frequently asymptomatic when strictly limited to the middle meatus and estimated at 0.2 or 0.5% in a population of living adults. There is a male predominance of 65%, except in the special group with ASA triad.

In this author's experience, the nasal polyps account for 5% of ENT clinic referrals, and 3–4% of allergy clinic referrals. They are present in 10% of chronic inflammatory rhinitis, 40% of a population of atopic asthma, and 70% in an ASA hypersensitive group *(26)*. Among a nasal polyp patient sample, Patriarca et al. found 16.8% to be atopic patients *(28)*. Settipane discovered 6.7% of nasal polyps in a nonselected series of asthmatic patients *(29)*.

Whatever the initiating mechanisms, the inflammatory responses seem grossly stereotyped. On the other hand, the way by which the chronic phase progresses and perpetuates is much more intriguing. It is in the field of cytokine regulation that more explanations may be found.

Mode of Formation of Nasal Polyps

Nasal polyps may be unique or many. Each polyp originates from a more or less elongated and sometimes even sessile stalk at different sites; most commonly the uncinate process, any ethmoidal cell, and meatal side of the middle turbinate.

In the particular case of the solitary polyp described by Killian, the insertion is located on the roof of the maxillary sinus or infrequently limited in a sphenoidal cell. Larsen and Tos *(26)* reviewed the classical theories attempting to explain the mechanisms by which the thin and relatively loose sinus mucosa may produce such a "belly pendulous sac."

More simply, owing to its structural features, the ethmoidal mucosa is likely to swell easily when the inflammatory modifications of the vascular bed permeability lead to fluid and cellular leakage. Chronic or recurrent proinflammatory biochemical events facilitate a "vicious circle" of volume augmentation by blood and lymphatic vessel compression. Recently, Bernstein et al. *(30)* advocated modifications of the transepithelial ionic transfer, supported by those existing in mucoviscidosis. Whatever the source, the sacculate form of nasal polyps depends also on mechanical factors, such as gravity, combined with intranasal aerodynamic powers. In the early stage when inflammatory changes are limited to the middle meatus, the mucosal edematous sac is submitted to high air-stream acceleration and to vortex. The expansion of the polyp membrane may be explained also by internal pressure during further stages of nasal obstruction. The size augmentation rate of nasal polyps varies greatly among patients, often following a "there and back" mode depending on the chronicity of the causal inflammatory process itself. Since the strong edematous polyps may be emptied when undergoing ruptures, some scars are seen on the glistened surface of the polyps, but they are quite few. An extruding process of the glandular epithelium has been advocated to explain the surface enlargement during the growth of the polyps.

Immuno-Cellular Aspects

A complete pathogenic overview is not now discernible. However, there are some data to help understand the inflammatory cell continuous attraction and accumulation in the mucosa. Cultures of fibroblasts and epithelial cells from nasal polyps demonstrate that these cells both produce cytokines perpetuating the inflammatory process: GM-CSF, IL 6, and IL8. Other hemopoietic factors support the differentiation of the migrant myeloid cells: basophils and eosinophils *(31)*. In fluids from nasal polyps, eosinophil survival-prolonging factors were obtained, such as GL-CSF, IL3, or IL5.

Many patients with nasal polyps may have, at least intermittently, significant blood hypereosinophilia. The circulating eosinophils, as well as the eosinophils sitting in polyps, are positive for TGF-β1-mRNA *(31)*. The relationship between mast cells and eosinophils play an evident role in nasal polyps, but the pathogenesis is unclear. Beyond their activation and infiltration in the nasosinusal mucosa, we need more fundamental research to understand the origin of the immune response.

Solitary Choanal Polyps

Among nasal polyps, the so-called antrochoanal polyp occupies a special place because it is usually unilateral and solitary. It was originally described by Killian in 1906.

ORIGIN

The more common choanal polyp arises from the maxillary sinus. There are relatively few choanal polyps pedunculated in a posterior ethmoidal cell or in the sphenoid sinus itself.

THE ETIOLOGY

This is not known. They are usually solitary and not associated with other paranasal sinus or systemic diseases. An immediate allergic mechanism may be suspected to take part in a few cases. They represent <5% of all the removed nasal polyps.

PATHOLOGICAL ASPECTS

Anatomically, two parts can be distinguished in a typical Killian antrochoanal polyp. Its attachment lies most often on the roof of the maxillary sinus (Fig. 1).

1. The endosinusal part of the polyps consists generally of a large cyst with a very thin and translucent limiting membrane, and filled with a yellow, clear, watery fluid. When the cystic wall collapses after incision and fluid evacuation, the membrane is found to form the stem inserted on the sinus wall itself. Sometimes, the endosinusal part of the polyp forms just a stalk reaching directly to the sinus ostium.
2. The nasochoanal part occupies the posterior part of the middle meatus and grows caudally. This part of the antrochoanal polyp is more fleshy and may extend in the nasopharynx, causing displacement of the soft palate inferiorly. Advanced cases are to be viewed in the oropharynx. In such conditions, the covering mucosa appears to be thick and red.
3. A constricted part always separates the two belly portions of the solitary antrochoanal polyp, passing through the accessory ostium, which may be widely enlarged.

In its early stage, the choanal polyp appears as a focal antral inflammatory pedunculated edema of the sinus mucosa. Occasionally, perhaps as a result of blowing the nose, part of this simple antral polyp finds its way through a wide accessory opening in the middle meatus. This supposed developmental mechanism leads back to the origin of this lesion.

Its histological patterns do not give any orientation and do not differ significantly from other inflammatory changes. Inflammatory cells are more concentrated near the mucosal surface, which is of a respiratory type, except in the front of the nasal portion or in the nasopharyngeal expansion, where it is often metaplastic or ulcerated. There are a few glands here and there in a stroma containing relatively few cells. The more characteristic feature is the edematous myxoid appearance of the stroma, with a fibrous tendency in the peripheral parts of the polyp.

CLINICAL IMPLICATIONS AND HISTOLOGICAL ASPECTS

The solitary choanal polyp occurs in all ages, mostly in young adults and children, with equal sex incidence. A progressive nasal obstruction with more or less mucopurulent rhinorrhea may be seen. There may be repeated episodes of mild acute sinusitis in the patient history.

The rhinoendoscopic aspects are quite characteristic, showing the same regular mass present in the nasal fossa anteriorly, as well as in the choanal area posteriorly. The anterior part is classically grayish and edematous, but may be pale red when the polyp completely occupies the nasal fossa. Sometimes, the speculum does not give valuable information, and the rigid or fiberoptic endoscope is mandatory to detail the middle meatus occupation and, even in some cases, the constricted intermediate portion of the polyp may be seen. The nasopharyngeal expansion varies widely.

THE DIAGNOSIS

This is generally easy but considering the age of the patient, some differential diagnoses are to be considered: sarcomas or angiofibroma in children and inverted papilloma or carcinomas in adults. Rare bilateral or successive cases are reported in the literature. Choanal polyps arising from the sphenoid sinus or from a posterior transitional ethmoidal cell are not exceptional.

The precise identification of the site of origin of a choanal polyp is suitable to determine the surgical approach. The CT scan aspects demonstrate the sinus occupation as well as the ostium enlargement (Fig. 11). For the evaluation of particular cases, MRI can be used when malignancy is suspected and, in any case, will demonstrate the continuity of the choanal part from the intrasinusal part of the polyp.

TREATMENT

The simple snare removal is devoted to recurrence.

• The implantation site on the mucosa must be removed.

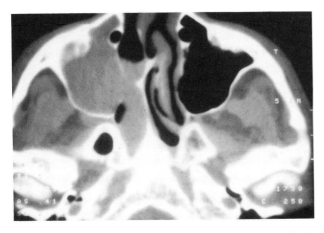

Fig. 11. Solitary antro-choanal polyp (Killian's polyp): This conventional radiograph shows perfectly the two parts of this formation with its intermediate segment going through the enlarged ostium area.

- Endoscopic surgery is the best indication, especially in young patients where the transcanine fossa is contraindicated.
- In spite of that, recurrences are possible for which this classical approach is not yet obsolete.

Nasal Polyposis

The suffix "osis" specifies a frequent clinical condition characterized by a generalized and chronic degenerative process of the paranasal sinuses mucosa. Many stems or stalks are present by which sacciform edematous formations are hanging bilaterally in the middle meatus.

Generally, this process starts from the anterior ethmoidal cells and extends progressively to the entire ethmoidal labyrinth and further to other sinuses. In advanced cases, the intercellular laminae are extremely thinned, as well as the middle turbinate, which may be completely surrounded and laminated. Sometimes, the adjacent area of the septal mucosa may present sessile swellings.

NP is not a disease. It is the inflammatory response of the entire nasosinusal mucosa, depending on the nature of extrinsic agents, but also much more on individual biological characteristics belonging to each patient. NP may be the only problem in some patients, but, since the nasal mucosa represents the first line of the respiratory tract, the incidence of asthma and/or bronchitis in more than one-third of the patients is an understandable association.

CLINICAL FEATURES

NP is a lifelong evolving syndrome, generally well developed in about 40 yr. Quite rare before 20 yr of life, the initial diagnosis is generally made in the presence of different nasal functional symptoms: recurrent mild sinusitis, facial pain or heaviness, anosmia, posterior nasal drip, more or less nasal obstruction.

The history of these patients may give some valuable information, the significance of which will be discussed: allergic manifestation during infancy, nasal hyperreactivity syndrome preceding a progressive anosmia and/or obstruction, late onset of asthma, recurrent bronchitis, manifestations of drugs or chemicals intolerance, infertility in men, and familial history of analogous cases.

The incidence of all these clinical signs in parents is to be noted. Contrary to former beliefs, the incidence of allergy is hardly more important in NP than in the general population. However, the frequency of pseudoallergic reactions in NP parentage is far from negligible. Unfortunately, we lack significant data concerning the familial proneness to NP and associated conditions. If a genetic incidence does exist, it is certainly multifactorial and deals probably with the genetic variations controlling the complex array of inflammatory response in each individual.

In general medical practice, the demarcation lines among allergy, recurrent sinusitis, and chronic hyperplasic sinusitis are somewhat confusing. Before the diagnosis of NP, most of the patients experience temporary relief with multidirectional treatments, which are too often prescribed without preliminary reflections on the etiological signification of clinical data.

Since 1950, the incidence of purely infectious sinusitis decreased considerably, while new antibiotics targeted more microbe varieties. As most cases of acute sinusitis are cured quite easily, it is important to question how recurrence or chronicity occurs. There are three main possibilities:

1. Anatomical variations and anomalies: narrowed sinus ostia, concha bullosa, deviated septum;
2. Dysfunctions of the mechanical first line of local defenses (innate or acquired): mucus anomalies, ciliary pathologies; and
3. Abnormal immune responses: common immunodeficiencies, autonomic imbalance, genetic predisposition *(32)*.

Drake-Lee *(33)* observed that "nasal polyps have not become less frequent" in contrast with the dramatic decrease in acute bacterial sinusitis. In NP,

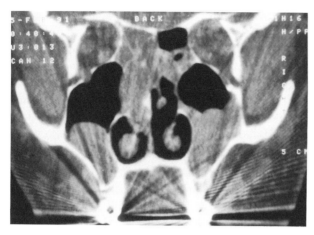

Fig. 12. Bilateral ethmoidal polyposis is more important on the left side. As verified in endoscopic surgery, the maxillary sinus contain a very thick inspissated mucus as currently seen in ASA triad (like in this patient).

pus cells and bacteria are cultured together in under 15% of the maxillary sinuses. Moreover, in classical bilateral NP, the striking feature consists of the role of the eosinophils and the mastocytes.

By itself, NP is a nonspecific inflammatory condition whose macroscopic aspects are mainly related with the nasosinusal skeletal framework, where it developed. It is more important to emphasize that NP develops only in some patients out of many, whose predictive identification is not possible. On a clinical basis, it could be tempting to distinguish two situations with different pathological implications.

Sinusitis where infection plays the first role may give rise to edematous changes in the sinusal mucosa and, then, to nasal polyps after invading the middle meatus. When unilaterally developed, such cases are promoted by the irreversibility of mucosal modifications, insufficient medical treatments, and persistent infections of dental origin. When infection persists and recurs repeatedly on bilateral NP, particularly in children or young adults, the following conditions must be suspected: mucoviscidosis, ciliary anomalies, Young syndrome, or common immunodeficiencies. In all these circumstances, bacteria are easily cultured from sinusal lavages: neutrophils are largely predominant in nasal secretions as well as in polyp biopsies.

Classical nasal polyposis is usually characteristic from the first patient presentation. Generally, the mucosal modifications start from the ethmoids

(Fig. 12). In some cases, the patient relates an old history of mild recurrent infection, and shows a series of X-rays demonstrating a variable and irregular thickening of the sinusal mucosa, before the lesions merge into the middle meatus. Such hyperplastic sinusitis responds very well to corticosteroid treatment, and biopsies show a very important eosinophil stroma infiltration currently up to 50%.

ETIOLOGICAL FACTORS

Despite the evidence that NP is a multifactorial syndrome whose pathophysiology is not yet clear, some specific etiologies or extranasal disturbances are frequently associated. Knowledge of them may be helpful in understanding this disease process.

Cystic Fibrosis. Nasal polyps may be the first manifestation of the disease in 10% of cases, and its incidence reaches 30% of the patients having the disease. A sweat chloride test is necessary in all patients with NP from 5 to 20 yr of age with or without associated digestive or pulmonary symptoms.

Immotile Cilia Syndrome. This is a rare inherited condition with a prevalence of 1/200,000. Infertility is constant in men and as a rule in women. There are large interindividual differences in the symptoms' importance of chronic airways infection, present in early childhood. Ultrastructural studies are the key to the diagnosis and demonstrate that, in fact, the anomalies of the cilia proteins constitute a heterogenous polygenic group. In some cases, anomalies of the cilia motility may exist without identifiable ultrastructural anomalies.

Young's Syndrome. This condition was described in humans with intermittent obstructive azoospermia associated with chronic mucositis of the entire airways. Large and recurrent nasal polyps are often associated with bronchectasies.

An interesting recent paper *(34)* shows some evidence that the toxic effects of mercury (calomel) may have delayed long-term irreversible effects on the ciliated epitheliums (nose, bronchi, head of the epididymis). Young's syndrome is only sporadic in the United States where sale of calomel has been discouraged since 1933. In the UK and Australia, the dramatic decline of its incidence starts with the withdrawal of products containing calomel since 1955, similar to pink disease.

IgE-Type Allergy. In the relatively recent past, there were many controversies concerning the role of allergy in NP. Today, a better diagnosis of IgE reactions shows that allergic diseases seem to be no more common in NP patients than in the general population.

However, since the modifications of the mucosal permeability in mucositis may facilitate the antigen's penetration, it is frequently observed that patients with NP present a relatively high rate of positive skin test toward pneumallergens as well as toward microbial antigens. As a result of disturbed inflammatory mediator release, allergic mechanisms may act as a cofactor in polyp formation.

Common Variable Immunodeficiencies. IgA insufficiency, isolated or associated with IgG deficit, is well known as a predisposing factor to recurrent and chronic airways mucositis. The notion of IgG subclass deficits coexisting with a normal total IgG level affords new interest in patients with chronic rhinosinusitis. In the same way, it is interesting to note the significantly high incidence of allergic patients in series with IgG subclasses insufficiency. Such conditions may represent cofactors of hyperplastic sinusitis with polyps, especially in children.

Asthma with or Without Aspirin Intolerance. NP and asthma are frequently associated. About 30% of patients with asthma and 50% with bronchospasm and ASA intolerance present with typical NP. There seems to be a continuum between the isolated NP and the complete ASA triad. The staggering order of the different components of the triad varies with each patient. The completion of the syndrome may last 5–30 yr or more. For many authors, a methacholine bronchial provocation test seems wise before surgical treatment of NP to detect any subclinical asthma if not evident by history or physical exam.

Treatment

In the last 20 yr, sinus surgery concepts have undergone an evolution under endoscopic guidance. Until now, the technical requirements and adaptation of the surgeons' performances have resulted in so many waves of enthusiasm that the problems of therapeutic indications were often covered.

In good hands, in the presence of the most frequent forms of polyposis, endoscopic surgery of the paranasal sinuses system as described by Messerklinger or Wigand is the most valuable technique.

Nevertheless, the local medical management with topical steroids must be preferred in begin-

ning forms. The routine simple polypectomy allows the topical treatment to reach the mucosa.

Even through a permanent and large meatotomy, the sinus mucosa may remain swollen and secreting. There are no clinical criteria to judge the possible reversibility of the mucosal changes. It appears doubtful that a "radical eradication" of the sinus mucosa will be therapeutic by fundamentally altering the inflammatory responses. If the preeminence of the ostium dysfunction seems to be verified in many surgical results, we have to recognize that the physiology of the ostium is not completely clear *(35)*. What are, for example, the signals attracting the ciliary clearance toward the natural ostium? Is a large meatotomy without adverse consequences on this attraction phenomenon?

Certainly, all the "half-measured" and apprehensive procedures are to be avoided, because they may worsen drainage and ventilation by creating bad scars and synechiae. Naturally, the therapeutic indications depend on an accurate etiological diagnosis. The "neutrophils" polyps are discussed differently from the "eosinophils" polyps, with or without associated asthma.

In children with cystic fibrosis, some publications give encouraging results, but they must be verified in the long term. Before undertaking ethmoidectomies in children with infectious polyposis, a complete immunological investigation must be done first because the surgery itself cannot give good results without an adjuvant immunotherapy. The reader is invited always to remember that NP is still a medical–surgical concern!

REFERENCES

1. Gwaltney JM, Phillips D, Miller D, Riker D. Computed tomographic study of the common cold. N Engl J Med 1994;330:25–30.
2. Havas TE, Motbey JA, Gullane PJ. Prevalence of incidental abnormalities on CT scans of the paranasal sinuses. Arch Otolaryngol 1988;114:5–10.
3. Roithmann R, Shankar L, Hawke M, Kassel E, Noyek A. CT Imaging in the diagnosis and treatment of sinuses disease: a partnership between the radiologist and the otolaryngologist. J Otolaryngol 1993;22:4,253–260.
4. Killey HC, Kay LW. The Maxillary Sinus and Its Dental Implications. Bristol: J. Wright, 1975.
5. Moskow BS. A histomorphologic study of the effects of periodontal inflammation on the maxillary sinus mucosa. J Periodontol 1992;63:674–681.
6. Flack H, Ericson S, Hugoson A. The effects of periodontal treatment on mucous membrane thickening in the maxillary sinus. J Clin Periodontol 1986; 13:217–222.

7. Dzink JL, Socransky SS, Haffajee AD. The predominant cultivable microbiota of active and inactive periodontal lesions. J Clin Periodontol 1988;15:316–323.

8. Melen I, Lindahl L, Andreasson L, Rundcrantz H. Chronic maxillary sinusitis. Acta Otolaryngol (Stockh) 1986;101: 320–327.

9. Legent F, Billet J, Beauvillain C, et al. The role of dental canal fillings in the development of aspergillus sinusitis. Arch Otorhinolaryngol 1989;246:318–320.

10. Wen-Yang Su, Chen Liu, Shuian-Yeng Hung. Bacteriologica study in chronic maxillary sinusitis. Laryngoscope 1983;93:931–934.

11. King JM, Caldarelli DD, Petawnick PP. Denta-scan®: A new diagnostic method for evaluating mandibular and maxillary pathology. Laryngoscope 1992;102:379–387.

12. Moskow BS, Polson AM. Histologic studies on the extension of the inflammatory infiltrate in human periodontitis. J Clin Periodontol 1991;246:318–320.

13. Engstrom H, Chamberlain D, Kiger R, Egelberg J. Radiographic evaluation of the effect of initial periodontal therapy on thickness of the maxillary sinus mucosa. J Periodontol 1988;59:604–608.

14. Branemark PI, Adell R, Albrektsson T. An experimental and clinical study of osseointegrated implants penetrating the nasal cavity and maxillary sinus. J Oral Maxillo-Fac Surg 1984;42:492–506.

15. Kent JN, Block MS. Simultaneous maxillary sinus floor bone grafting and placement of hydroxylapatite-coated implants. J Oral Maxillo-Fac Surg 1989;47:238–242.

16. Rivron A, Bourdinière J. Mucocèles et pneumosinus dilatans. In: Encyclo. Medico-Chirurgicale Oto-Rhino-Laryngologie. Paris: Editions Techniques, 1990; p. 6(20465A10).

17. Lund VJ. Anatomical considerations in the aetiology of fronto-ethmoidal mucoceles. Rhinology 1987;25:83–88.

18. Canalis NL, Zajtchuk JT, Jenkins HA. Ethmoidal mucoceles. Arch Otolaryngol 1978;104:286–294.

19. Schenk NL, Rauchback E, Oguar JH. Frontal sinus disease. Laryngoscope 1974;84:1233–1240.

20. Moriyama H, Nakajima T, Honda Y. Studies on mucoceles of the ethmoid and sphenoid sinuses: analysis of 47 cases. J Laryngol Otol 1992;106:23–27.

21. Antonelli PJ, Duvall AJ, Teitelbaum SL. Maxillary sinus atelectasis. Ann Otol Rhinol Laryngol 1992;101: 977–981.

22. Blackwell KE, Goldberg RA, Calcaterra YC. Atelectasis of the maxillary sinus with enophtalmos and midface depression. Ann Otol Rhinol Laryngol 1993; 102:429–432.

23. Meyer AD, Burtschi T. Pneumocele of the maxillary sinus. J Otolaryngol 1980;9:361.

24. Parker GS, Tami TA, Wilson JF. Aggressive sinonasal polyposis. Am J Rhinol 1988;2:1–6.

25. Hellquist HB. Pathology of the Nose and Paranasal Sinuses. London: Butterworths, 1990.

26. Larsen PL, Tos M. Origin of nasal polyps. Laryngoscope 1991;101:305–312.

27. Hosemann W, Göde U, Wagner W. Epidemiology, pathophysiology of nasal polyposis and spectrum of endonasal sinus surgery. Am J Otolaryngol 1994;15:85–98.

28. Patriarca G, Schiavino D, Nuchera E, et al. Prevention of relapse in nasal polyposis. Lancet 1991;337:1488.

29. Settipane GA. Nasal polyps: Epidemiology, pathology, immunology and treatment. Am J Rhinol 1987;1:119–126.

30. Bernstein JM, Cropp GA, Nathanson I, et al. Bio-electric properties of cultured nasal polyp and turbinate epithelial cells. Am J Rhinol 1990;4:45–49.

31. Gleich GF, Kay AB. Eosinophils in Allergy and Inflammation. New York: Marcel Dekker, 1994.

32. Drake-Lee AB. Nasal polyps in identical twins. J Laryngol Otol 1992;106:1084,1085.

33. Drake-Lee AB. Medical treatment of nasal polyps. Rhinology 1994;32:1–4.

34. Hendry WF, A'Hern RP, Cole PJ. Was Young syndrome caused by exposure to mercury in childhood? Br Med J 1993;307:1579–1582.

35. Perko D, Karin RR. Nasoantral windows: an experimental study in rabbits. Laryngoscope 1992;102:320–326.

13 Tumors of the Paranasal Sinuses

Valerie J. Lund, MS, FRCS, FRCSED
and David J. Howard, FRCS, FRCSED

CONTENTS

INTRODUCTION

This chapter is based on a distillation of the literature and personal experience of over 500 patients with sinonasal neoplasia. These rare, but fascinating tumors pose significant problems of management in that they frequently commence with innocuous symptoms that are often ignored by both patient and clinician for considerable periods of time and are thus extensive lesions when diagnosed. The sinonasal area is also one of greatest histological diversity, including tumors of idiosyncratic behavior that may recur after 20 yr. These factors limit the usefulness of the TNM classification and may invalidate 5-yr survival rates. Add to this the difficulties of oncological resection and cosmetic rehabilitation in an area closely related to the cranial cavity and orbit, and one of the most challenging areas of paranasal disease emerges.

It is clearly beyond the scope of this chapter to cover all aspects of sinonasal neoplasia. Rather an overview of the disease is offered with consideration given to a few of the unusual and fascinating lesions encountered in this area.

HISTORICAL ASPECTS

Surgery for maxillary cancer has a relatively long history, although up to 1825, it consisted largely of as much piecemeal removal as could be tolerated in a preanesthetic era *(1)*. In the English

From: *Diseases of the Sinuses* (M. E. Gershwin and G. A. Incaudo, eds.),
©1996 Humana Press Inc., Totowa, NJ.

literature, the first recorded partial removal was performed by Wiseman, surgeon to Charles II in 1676. In 1826, Lizars proposed subtotal maxillectomy, which he attempted in December 1827. This was abandoned owing to bleeding, but successfully undertaken on August 1, 1829. A comparable procedure had been performed by Syme in May 1829, thus making Syme the first to do the operation, but not the first to describe it.

Similar confusion concerns the description of the incision for maxillectomy, where the classical "Weber-Fergusson" incision should more accurately be referred to as "Blandin-Gensoul."

Between 1830 and 1880, 160 maxillectomies were reported, of which only 50 were performed for "cancer." The rest included various fibro-osseous lesions, angiofibroma, and cysts, but the precise pathology is unclear, since the diagnosis relied primarily on gross description without the benefit of formalized histology. Refinements of the surgery could be seen around the end of the 19th and early 20th centuries, for example with the introduction of lateral rhinotomy by Moure (2) in 1902, and thereafter during the late 1950s and early 1960s, two other landmark procedures, midfacial degloving approach (3) and craniofacial resection (4,5), entered clinical practice.

ETIOLOGY AND EPIDEMIOLOGY

It is clear that regional differences exist in the incidence and histology of sinonasal neoplasia. The link between this and occupation was first made in 1968 when Acheson et al. (6) observed a high frequency of adenocarcinoma of the ethmoids in the wood workers of the High Wycombe area. Since then, similar reports have come from many parts of the world that have wood-working industries. The association appears to be with jobs involving hard woods, such as mahogany, producing fine dust of a sufficient diameter to be deposited in the middle meatus (>5 μm). The exact component of the dust responsible for dysplastic change is still unclear, but some elegant studies have been performed in Scandinavia, in experimental models and cohorts of wood workers (7,8).

The development of adenocarcinoma has also been associated with the manufacture of chrome pigment, isopropyl alcohol, and working in the textile, clothing, leather, and shoe industries. The relative risk for wood working is estimated at 70 times

normal, but it is equally possible to develop the condition without such predisposing factors. Only 10 in a series of 46 adenocarcinomas were wood workers (9).

Occupations implicated in the development of squamous cell carcinoma include: radium dial painting, mustard gas manufacture (both now defunct), nickel refining, and exposure to soft wood dust (Table 1) (10). Cigaret smoking and alcohol have less impact in this area than elsewhere in the head and neck, but should not be entirely discounted.

It has been estimated that some external etiological factors may be relevant in 5–20% of sinonasal malignancy, but it may require up to 20 yr of exposure to manifest it. With changing patterns of work practice, improved working conditions, and an increasingly mobile population, the effects of such occupational factors will become increasingly difficult to discern, despite continued vigilance.

INCIDENCE

Determining the exact incidence of sinonasal neoplasia can be difficult. Under the International Classification of Disease, ICD160 covers not only malignancy in the sinonasal area, but also the middle ear. Although this latter category does not constitute a large proportion, it is often impossible to disentangle it from global statistics, leading to inaccuracy. Notwithstanding this, sinonasal neoplasia and, specifically, malignancy are rare conditions, constituting approx 3% of head and neck cancer (excluding tumors of the external nose). Less than 1% of cancer deaths in the US between 1950 and 1969 were attributed to sinonasal cancer, and there is no suggestion of an increase in numbers. A similar picture emerges in England and Wales (Fig. 1). Global figures suggest an incidence of <1/100,000 people/yr in most countries, but there are some striking local differences (Fig. 2) that probably reflect local predispositions and environmental factors.

SEX, AGE, AND ETHNIC VARIATION

The male-to-female ratio for sinonasal malignancy is approx 2 to 1, except in areas where occupational factors impact heavily. Although the disease can occur at any age, in our own patients, the age range for malignancy was 5–88, the major-

Table 1
Occupational Agents Correlated with Sinonasal Cancer *(10)*

Occupation	Relative risk	Suspected carcinogen	Latent period	Histology	Other assoc. cancers
Wood workers	70	Dust 5-μ diameter Tar Aldehyde Aflatoxin	35 yr	Adenocarcinoma (hardwood) Squamous (softwood)	Lung, testis, brain
Leather/shoe	87	Dust Tar Aldehydes Aflatoxin Tannins	55 yr	Adenocarcinoma	Rectum, bladder
Chrome pigment manufacturers	>21	Calcium chromate Zinc potassium Chromate	—	Adenocarcinoma	Lung
Isopropyl alcohol	>21	Isopropyl oil	<20 yr	Adenocarcinoma	Larynx
Textile and clothing	5.8	Wool dust and dyes	—	Adenocarcinoma Malign. melanoma	Tongue, mouth, pharynx
Nickel refining	>100	Nickel subsulfide, oxide	24 yr (5–40)	Squamous cell Anaplastic	Lung, larynx
Dial painting	—	Radium	15 yr	Squamous	Osteosarcoma, carcinoma mastoid
Mustard gas manufacturer	>30	BB dichloroethyl sulfide	25 yr	Squamous	Tongue, pharynx, larynx, lung

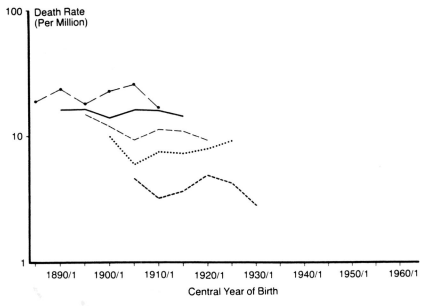

Fig. 1. Graph showing death rate/million owing to malignant neoplasms of the nose in men of different age groups. Age group: ·——·, 65–69 yr; ———, 60–64 yr; — — —, 55–59 yr; ··········, 50–54 yr; - - - - - -, 45–49 yr.

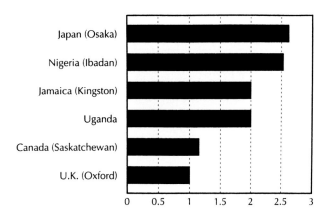

Fig. 2. Histogram showing areas of "high" age-adjusted incidence of sinonasal malignancy in males/100,000.

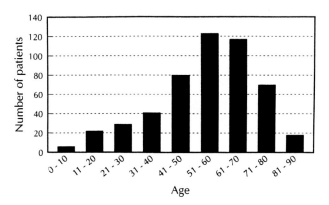

Fig. 3. Histogram showing age distribution of patients with sinonasal malignancy in personal series of 500 cases.

ity presenting between 50 and 69 (Fig. 3). A number of benign tumors can present in children of 2 and 3 yr, and there have been reports in the literature of newborn infants with malignant lesions in this area.

In women, a slight increase in incidence has been noted in association with menopause, similar to Clemmensen's hook observed in breast cancer, which may relate to the presence of estrogen receptors in the nasal cavity.

It is difficult to discern any specific ethnic variation other than that which might be explained by occupational factors. However, the incidence of squamous carcinoma of the maxilla in the Japanese population exceeds that encountered elsewhere.

SITE

Because of late presentation, it is often difficult to distinguish the exact origin of sinonasal malig-

Table 2
Distribution by Anatomical Site (%)
of Sinonasal Malignancy

	Maxilla	Nose	Other sinuses
Japan	93	3	4
Canada	63	26	11
Sweden	48	35	13
United Kingdom			
England and Wales	41	43	16
Oxford	61	13	26
Institute of Laryngology	55	35	10

nancy, and this is reflected in the literature. Overall the maxilla is the most common, although since lesions frequently arise in the middle meatus, the ethmoids, nasal cavity, and antrum are often involved. The distribution of site will show some variation, dependent on environmental factors, e.g., in wood-working communities, and will be skewed by histology (Table 2). Although the ICD classification does not separate the individual paranasal sinuses, the contribution made by the frontal and sphenoid is extremely small, where primary mucosal malignancy is exceptional. Benign tumors more often arise in the nasal cavity, e.g., inverted papilloma or angiofibroma, and spread into the adjacent sinuses.

HISTOLOGY

As in the rest of the aerodigestive tract, squamous cell carcinoma is the most common malignancy in the sinonasal area, and epithelial tumors predominate. However, this region is also one of greatest histological diversity, and every tumor type, both benign and malignant, can be encountered (Table 3). Because of their rarity, sinonasal tumors are often referred to head and neck centers, and these referral patterns may skew figures (Table 4). Modern immunohistochemistry may further differentiate tumors previously categorized as "anaplastic" into olfactory neuroblastomas, malignant melanomas, or lymphomas, so uncorroborated pooled data may contain significant inaccuracies.

The concept of benign and malignant is indistinct in this area where the proximity of vital structures may render a benign tumor as potentially life threatening as its malignant counterpart, and

Table 3
Range of Sinonasal Neoplasia

	Benign	Malignant
Epithelial		
Epidermoid/squamous	Papilloma	Carcinoma (spindle-cell, verrucous, transitional)
Nonepidermoid	Adenoma	Adenoid cystic carcinoma
	Monomorphic	Adenocarcinoma
	Pleomorphic	Mucoepidermoid carcinoma
	Oncocytoma	Acinic cell carcinoma
		Metastases
Neuroctodermal	Meningioma	Malignant melanoma
		Olfactory neuroblastoma
	Neurofibroma	Neurofibroma
	Glioma	Neuroendocrine carcinoma
		Melanotic neuroectodermal tumor of infancy
Odontogenic tumors	Ameloblastoma	
	Calcifying epithelial odontogenic tumor	
Mesenchymal		
Vascular	Hemangioma	Angiosarcoma
	Capillary	Kaposi's sarcoma
	Cavernous	Hemangiopericytoma
	Angiofibroma	
	Angiomyolipoma	
	Paraganglioma	
	Glomus tumors	
Muscular	Leiomyoma	Leiomyosarcoma
	Rhabdomyoma	Rhabdomyosarcoma
Cartilaginous	Chondroma	Chondrosarcoma (mesenchymal)
	Chondroblastoma	
Osseous	Fibro-osseous lesions	Osteogenic sarcoma
	fibrous dysplasia	
	ossifying fibroma	
	Giant cell tumor	
	"Brown" tumor of hyperparathyroidism	
	Osteoma	
	Osteoblastoma	
Lymphoreticular		Burkitt's lymphoma
		Non-Hodgkin's lymphoma
		Extramedullary plasmacytoma
		Midline destructive lesions
Chordoma		
Eosinophilic granuloma	Fibroma	Fibrosarcoma
	Lipoma	Liposarcoma
	Myxoma	Malignant fibrous histiocytoma
		Ewing's sarcoma
		Alveolar soft part sarcoma

where death owing to local spread of a malignant tumor often occurs long before its metastatic capacity is manifest.

CLASSIFICATION

A number of attempts have been made to apply classification systems to the sinonasal region

Table 4
Distribution of Histology (%) of Malignant Tumors

	IARC, n = 3574		ILO, n = 506	
	n	%	n	%
Epithelial				
Squamous	2108	(59)	210	(43)
Adenocarcinoma	321	(9)	46	(9)
Adenoid cystic and salivary gland	72	(2)	55	(11)
Malignant melanoma	40	(1)	60	(12)
Olfactory neuroblastoma	31	(<1)	20	(4)
Mesenchymal				
Sarcoma	110	(3)	52	(10)
Lymphoma	72	(2)	53	(10)
Other	820	(23)	8	(1)

IARC: International Agency for Research on Cancer.
ILO: Professorial Unit, The Institute of Laryngology and Otology.

Table 5
TNM Classification Systems

Lederman et al. *(11)*
    T1 Tumor to one sinus or a tissue of origin, e.g., turbinate, septum, vestibule
    T2 Tumor limited in horizontal spread to the same region or to adjacent vertically related regions
    T3a. Tumor involving three regions, with or without orbital involvement
        b. Extension of the tumor beyond the upper jaw, e.g., nasopharynx, cranial cavity, pterygopalatine fossa
Harrison *(12)*
    T1 Tumor limited to the antral mucosa, with no evidence of bone erosion
    T2 Bony erosion without evidence of involvement of the skin, pterygopalatine fossa or ethmoidal labyrinth
    T3 Bony erosion with involvement of the skin and ethmoidal labyrinth
    T4 Tumor extension to the nasopharynx, sphenoid sinus, cribriform plate, or pterygopalatine fossa
AJC *(13)* (based on Sisson et al. *[14]*)
    T1 Tumor confined to the antral mucosa of the infrastructure without bone erosion
    T2 Tumor confined to the suprastructure and mucosa without bone destruction, or to the infrastructure with destruction of medial or inferior bony walls only
    T3 Massive tumor, invading the skin of the cheek, the orbit, the posterior ethmoids, sphenoid sinus, nasopharynx, pterygoid plates, or base of skull

(Table 5) *(11–14)*. However, it should be remembered that any tumor arising within the bony confines of a paranasal sinus must break out to present clinically. Thus, most tumors are T4 at presentation, but a tumor arising close to the cranial cavity will inevitably have a different prognosis from one arising, for example, in the floor of the maxillary sinus. In addition, the apparently low incidence of metastatic spread significantly undermines the usefulness of the conventional TNM classification. As a consequence, it has been suggested that a more meaningful approach is to base classification on spread of disease *(12)*. None of these classifica-

tions, however, take into account information derived from modern imaging or the prognostic impact of improved oncological resection by a craniofacial approach.

TUMOR SPREAD

Local Spread (Fig. 4)

MAXILLARY SINUS

Tumors generally follow the route of least resistance. From the maxilla, this is via the natural ostium and infundibulum, or by breakdown of the membranous fontanelles, into the middle meatus.

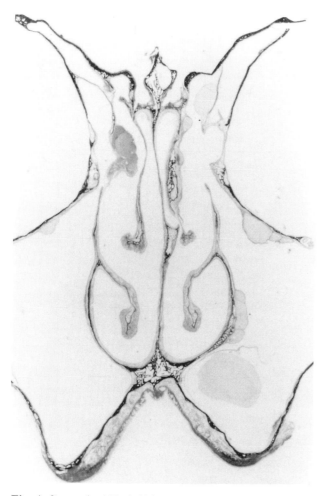

Fig. 4. Coronal midfacial block showing sinonasal region.

The roof is naturally thin and may be dehiscent in the region of the infraorbital canal, so entry into the orbit readily occurs. Similarly, the infraorbital foramen provides a route onto the face of the maxilla. The lateral wall, superolateral corner adjacent to the zygoma, and the floor of the antrum are reasonably thick bone, although the floor may be thin or dehiscent in relation to the roots of the fourth, fifth, and sixth upper dentition. Like the lateral wall, the posterior wall is thinner, separating the sinus from the pterygomaxillary and infratemporal fossae. Once this wall is breached, tumor infiltration of the pterygoid and infratemporal region is associated with an extremely poor prognosis.

ETHMOID SINUS

The ethmoid sinus is a labyrinth of cells and clefts, intimately related to the anterior cranial cavity and orbit. Tumors that probably arise from dysplasia within the middle meatus may easily spread throughout the labyrinth, sometimes crossing the midline to the opposite complex, entering the nasal cavity and the maxilla, and may spread into the frontal and sphenoid sinuses. These latter sinuses more often contain secretions because of ostial obstruction rather than tumor itself. However, once the sphenoid is involved, the patient is at risk of cavernous sinus and middle cranial fossa involvement.

The lamina papyracea offers a convenient route of spread into the orbit, often having areas of natural dehiscence, and although the orbital periosteum provides a significant barrier for some time, ultimately infiltration of orbital structures occurs. The tumor can track posteriorly in the extraperiosteal plane toward the orbital apex or may spread directly from the posterior ethmoids (or sphenoid if the intervening bone is thin) and from there into the middle cranial fossa. Anteriorly, infiltration of the agger nasi region can impinge on the nasolacrimal system.

The roof of the ethmoid is primarily completed by thick frontal bone, but there is a variable amount of ethmoid lying medially above the level of the cribriform plate. This presents a natural area of weakness increased by the passage of ethmoidal vessels and nerves. The tumor may therefore readily enter the anterior cranial fossa. The dura, like orbital periosteum, resists tumor spread for some time, but once breached, infiltration of the frontal lobes can occur, which is invariably fatal. The base of the skull may be specifically involved by tumors, such as meningioma and chondrosarcoma, with obvious consequences for the cranial nerves traversing it.

NASAL CAVITY

All paranasal sinuses may be involved by tumors arising in the nasal cavity. Superiorly, the tumor can extend through the cribriform plate, particularly along the preformed pathways of the olfactory system. Lesions can extend into the nasopharynx posteriorly and even enter the eustachian tube, occasionally presenting in the middle ear cleft. Inferiorly, lesions can spread around the maxillary spine to affect the hard palate. Anteriorly, the nasal bones can be infiltrated, eroded, and/or splayed, and infiltration of the soft tissues of the glabella, which is classically associated with adenocarcinoma, can occur. If malignancy infiltrates the external skin and vestibule, the prognosis is particularly poor and can be associated with bilateral lymphatic spread.

Lesions such as angiofibromas, arising in the region of the sphenopalatine foramen, fill the nasal cavity, nasopharynx, and sphenoid, but also spread laterally, widening the pterygomaxillary fissure and presenting ultimately in the infratemporal fossa.

PTERYGOPALATINE AND INFRATEMPORAL FOSSAE

The extensive blood and nerve supply of these areas facilitates rapid infiltration by malignant tumors. This has significant prognostic consequences both for local and metastatic spread. The orbit and middle cranial fossa are also accessible from these areas, in particular via the inferior and superior orbital fissures, or the foramen lacerum. An extensive mass may grow anteriorly to present in the gingivobuccal sulcus.

Distant Spread

Metastatic spread, the *sine qua non* of malignancy, often appears to be absent in the sinonasal region owing to the rapid demise of the patient from local disease. In most studies, the incidence of cervical lymphadenopathy is around 10%. The submandibular, jugulodigastric, prefacial, and postfacial nodes are mainly involved, and can be bilateral from central facial lesions. Involvement of the retropharyngeal nodes is less evident. Lymphadenopathy is always associated with a very poor prognosis.

Hematological spread to bone, brain, lung, and liver appears to be relatively uncommon, being most often associated with uncontrolled local disease. However, if local disease is controlled in the long term, e.g., by craniofacial resection, the incidence of metastatic disease may be increased and is certainly more frequently associated with certain tumor types. In general, mesenchymal malignancy has a greater propensity to manifest secondary spread either at presentation or during follow-up, but epithelial tumors, such as neuroblastomas and malignant melanoma, not infrequently disseminate widely. Adenoid cystic carcinoma, which is well known for its ability to spread along perineural lymphatics, is also capable of embolization along adjacent cranial nerves.

DIFFERENTIAL DIAGNOSIS (TABLE 6)

A number of lesions may present in the nose and sinuses, simulating neoplasia and obfuscating

Table 6
Benign Conditions Simulating Neoplasia

Cholesterol granuloma
Nasal polyps
Mucoceles
Fungal infections
Dermoid cysts
Meningocele, encephalocele

Table 7
Frequency of Symptoms in Sinonasal Malignancy (%)[a]

Nasal obstruction	56%
Epistaxis	35
Nasal discharge	20
Facial pain/headache	23
Swelling of cheek	24
Visible lesion	12
Epiphora	12
Proptosis	16
Diplopia/visual loss	11
Paraesthesia of face	8

[a]Several symptoms experienced by some patients.

diagnosis. When an individual presents with a mass in the nose, particularly in a child, the possibility of a meningo-encephalocele should always be considered and eliminated by imaging before proceeding to biopsy. Neoplastic lesions may resemble "ordinary" nasal polyps, and it should also be remembered that pathologies, such as inverted papillomas and nasal polyps, can coexist, so it is important that all material removed at surgery be submitted to histology.

EVALUATION AND DIAGNOSIS

History and Clinical Features (Table 7)

Patients frequently present with extensive disease, although symptoms may have been present for a considerable period, neglected by patient or physician. Initial complaints may be made to a dental surgeon or optician. In the nose and sinuses, initial symptoms will be relatively innocuous with only their unilaterality to alert the clinician of a sinister cause. Nasal obstruction, discharge (possibly blood-stained), hyposmia, and slight discomfort may all be readily attributed to chronic rhinosinusitis. A mass may be visible within the nasal cavity. In contrast, extensive destruction of the midline structures can be observed in what frequently proves to be T-cell lymphoma.

The orbit is often affected at an early stage. Anteriorly, the nasolacrimal apparatus can be involved producing unilateral epiphora and occasionally a mass. Displacement of the globe is associated with diplopia, chemosis, and ultimately visual loss, depending on the speed of tumor growth. Infiltration of the infraorbital nerve can produce pain and/or paraesthesia in its distribution and a mass in the cheek.

Involvement of the upper alveolus may loosen teeth, leading to a malignant oro-antral fistula or present as a gingival or palatal mass. Pain, contrary to patient expectation, is an uncommon feature, although it is associated with infiltration of the pterygopalatine region where it also results in trismus. Extension into the anterior (or middle cranial fossa) is relatively "silent." Personality change is subtle if it occurs at all, cerebrospinal fluid leaks and meningitis are exceptional, and the occasional headache is far from specific. Cranial nerve involvement is a late and particularly poor prognostic clinical sign.

Examination

A general ear, nose, and throat (ENT) examination, including anterior and posterior rhinoscopy, will reveal gross masses or ulceration, swelling of the cheek and gingiva, cranial nerve involvement, and lymphadenopathy. Subtle changes in the eye may only be revealed by an ophthalmic examination. Flexible and rigid endoscopy can be helpful in early detection of neoplasia and particularly aid biopsy.

Laboratory Tests

Apart from the usual laboratory investigations to assess the patient's general fitness, these have a limited role to play in the assessment of sinonasal neoplasia. They can be of use in lymphoreticular disorders and an HIV test should be performed in patients with lesions of the head and neck, such as lymphomas, cervical lymphadenopathy, or Kaposi's sarcoma. In midline destructive lesions, other ulcerating conditions, such as Wegener's granulomatosis and sarcoid, must be excluded by antineutrophil cytoplasmic antibodies (ANCA), erythrocyte sedimentation rate (ESR), angiotensin converting enzyme (ACE), creatinine clearance, and so on.

Table 8
Imaging Protocol
for the Investigation of Sinonasal Malignancy

CT scanning
Coronal, axial
Contrast-enhanced
MRI
Coronal, axial, sagittal
T1 (± gadolinium-DTPA), T2-weighted sequences
± fat suppression, FEER, subtraction

Radiology

The details of the various imaging techniques have already been outlined, but a few points specific to the evaluation of sinonasal neoplasia are worthwhile. Although some tissue characteristics are apparent with particular tumors, the primary aim of imaging is to determine extent. This is most accurately achieved by a combination of CT and MRI. The protocol employed in our own unit is shown in Table 8. CT with contrast enhancement provides essential information on bone detail and best demonstrates early cribriform plate enhancement. However, MRI (three planar with gadolinium-DTPA) allows soft-tissue differentiation between tumor, inflammation, retention of mucus, and fibrosis as confirmed by studies comparing histological findings at craniofacial resection with preoperative imaging (15). The three-plane multislice facility using a head coil gives total coverage of the head and neck, so that both the primary tumor and any direct or metastatic cervical involvement can be recognized. MRI can also be of particular use in postoperative follow-up to indicate recurrence (Fig. 5). Indeed, all patients are submitted to regular postoperative imaging, either CT or more usually MRI, in particular after craniofacial resection.

A variety of new techniques are being used to enhance tumor definition, including fat suppression, subtraction GdMR, and field even echo rephasing (FEER) "angiography." These have largely replaced the need for conventional angiography. Imaging of the rest of the body may be appropriate if distant spread is suspected, but is generally not cost-effective in every case unless there is some specific indication.

Biopsy

Endoscopy has greatly facilitated obtaining a biopsy by an intranasal route. Indeed, the use of a

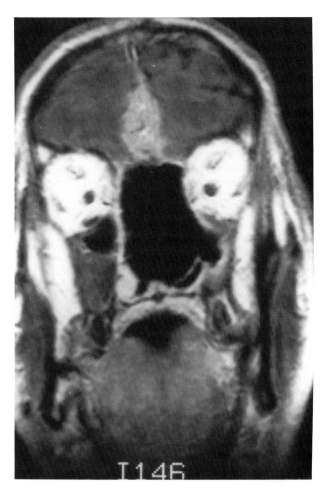

Fig. 5. Coronal MRI (T1-weighted with gadolinium-DTPA) showing recurrent adenocarcinoma in anterior cranial fossa following craniofacial resection.

Caldwell-Luc approach is positively contraindicated, since it can create a route for the exit of the tumor. Although it is perfectly possible to obtain tissue without general anesthesia, it can be a considerable advantage in obtaining representative tissue and to assess tumor extent more accurately. Representative tissue should be taken from the nasal cavity and adjacent sinuses if affected. If a lymphoma is suspected, fresh tissue should also be sent. Conversely, if an angiofibroma is suspected, biopsy is contraindicated. Fine-needle aspirate of cervical masses for cytology has a high yield, generally avoiding excisional biopsy.

SQUAMOUS CELL CARCINOMA

The respiratory mucosa of the sinonasal region gives rise to two basic types of epithelial neoplasms, those arising from metaplastic epithelium (squamous cell carcinoma), which is by far the most common form of tumor, and those arising from mucous glands. The latter constitute the nonepidermoid epithelial tumors. Squamous cell carcinoma may be graded on histologic differentiation and mitotic activity as elsewhere in the body, which can be broadly indicative of prognosis. Variants of squamous cell carcinoma are found in the sinonasal tract—verrucous carcinoma (an extremely well-differentiated lesion associated with limited invasion) and spindle-cell carcinoma or carcinosarcoma (an aggressive tumor with carcinomatous and spindle-cell components, reminiscent of a fibrosarcoma). Transitional carcinoma should also be regarded as a nonkeratinizing squamous cell carcinoma.

Squamous cell carcinoma may occur anywhere within the sinonasal tract, but is associated with a particularly bad prognosis when it arises in the nasal vestibule or anterior nasal septum, largely owing to a propensity for local soft tissue extension and bilateral cervical lymphadenopathy. Late presentation and undertreatment may also in part explain poor results, but even with aggressive combined radiotherapy and radical surgery, nodal metastases are common. Whether additional chemotherapy will improve matters remains to be demonstrated in the long term *(16)*.

Management of Squamous Cell Carcinoma of the Antrum or Antroethmoidal Region

Occasionally with a small lesion, it may be possible to determine the exact site of tumor origin, but generally an extensive lesion is found at presentation (Fig. 6). A combination of modern imaging (CT and MRI) and examination under anesthesia to obtain histology will determine the extent of the tumor with a reasonable degree of accuracy. An optimal treatment plan comprises combined radical surgery and radiotherapy, unless these are contraindicated by previous treatment or the general health of the patient. The choice of surgery will be determined by tumor site and size, and includes:

Lateral rhinotomy/medial maxillectomy;
Radical maxillectomy; and
Craniofacial resection.

In addition, the close proximity of the orbit to many of these tumors necessitates orbital clearance in a proportion of cases. Occasionally, a total rhinectomy is employed.

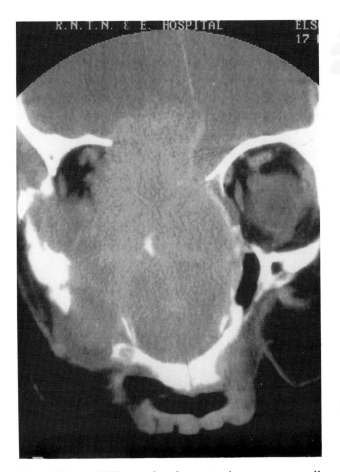

Fig. 6. Coronal CT scan showing extensive squamous cell carcinoma.

The lateral rhinotomy approach offers excellent access to the nasal cavity, and a considerable amount of ethmoid and maxilla (medial maxillectomy) may be resected with excellent cosmetic results *(17)*. However, squamous cell carcinoma arising in the antrum has frequently breached the other walls of the maxilla, for which a radical maxillectomy is indicated with prosthetic obturator repair *(18)*. This may be accomplished via a conventional Weber-Fergusson incision or with greater cosmetic advantage via a midfacial degloving approach *(19)*, and may be accompanied by orbital clearance. Since lymphatic drainage of the orbit does not compromise the lids, these can be preserved to line the socket, which will ultimately receive an orbital prosthesis.

Prior to the advent of craniofacial resection, it was not possible to perform an *en bloc* oncologic excision of lesions that had breached the cribriform plate or ethmoidal roof. Originally described by Smith et al. in 1954 *(4)* and subsequently improved

by Ketcham et al. *(5)*, this operation has now become the standard approach for lesions involving the ethmoidal block, be they malignant or benign *(20)*. It combines access with excellent cosmesis and low morbidity, with postoperative stay averaging 16 d. In the anterior cranial fossa, dura adjacent to disease may be resected and repaired with fascia lata, one of a variety of repair techniques described.

In addition to resection of disease within the anterior cranial fossa, a craniofacial approach allows orbital invasion to be accurately assessed, particularly in relation to the orbital apex. Imaging gives a good indication of gross involvement, but does not reveal microscopic spread. Thus, the orbital periosteum may be examined by frozen section assessment peroperatively, and if not invaded by disease, in selected cases, may be resected and repaired rather than sacrificing the eye.

Whether radiotherapy or surgery is given first has been subject to some discussion, but may be of little clinical relevance *(21)*. It should, however, be remembered that when surgery is performed after radiotherapy, the extent of the resection must encompass the original extent of the tumor irrespective of the apparent response. The dose and fractionation of radiotherapy vary—a radical dose of 55 gy in 20 fractions or 65 gy in 30 fractions is generally accepted.

Although relatively large series of squamous cell carcinomas in this area exist, obtaining accurate survival figures is surprisingly difficult. It would seem that in the majority of cases treated by combined therapy, including radical surgery, such as total maxillectomy, 5-yr survival is on the order of 30% for T3 and T4 lesions, representing the majority of cases. In those rare early lesions (T2), over two-thirds may expect to be alive at 5 yr. Spectacular results from Japan and Holland have been claimed for a combination of debulking, radiotherapy, and topical 5-fluorouracil, though it has not been possible to reproduce these results in other centers *(22*, p. 99). Similarly, the role of induction chemotherapy remains controversial and of unproven benefit.

SPECIAL CONSIDERATIONS OF OTHER EPITHELIAL TUMORS

Papillomas

Papillomas are the most common benign epithelial tumors of the sinonasal region, comprising in

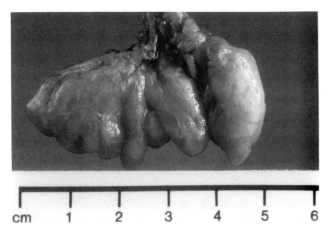

Fig. 7. Photograph of inverted papilloma removed from middle meatal region.

the literature an incidence of between 0.01 and 10% of all neoplasms in this area. They may be classified as:

1. Inverted;
2. Everted; or
3. Cylindric.

The median age range varies from 35 to 60 yr with a male-to-female ratio of 3.5:1. The male preponderance is more marked in everted lesions, whereas the cylindric papillomas affect both sexes equally. Inverted and cylindric papillomas generally arise from the lateral wall of the nose, in the middle meatus from where the adjacent sinuses can be affected. Everted lesions more often arise from the septum. A viral etiology has been suggested *(23)*.

Inverted papillomas present as firm, bulky, red and vascular masses, which may be mistaken for nasal polyps (Fig. 7). A 2.7% association has been reported with nasal polyps *(24)*, and 5% can be bilateral. The length of history varies from 2 wk to 20 yr. In 20%, symptoms have been present for more than 5 yr, this being usually unilateral nasal obstruction. As the tumor enlarges, it produces a well-defined bone defect in the lateral nasal wall, and spreads into the antrum and ethmoids. On CT, areas of apparent calcification are seen within the tumor, and there is frequently some sclerosis of adjacent bone, appearances that are quite characteristic of the condition *(25)*.

Two features of this lesion, recurrence and malignant transformation, have been extensively discussed. Recurrence can occur with all three forms of papilloma. Rates of up to 74% have been

reported for inverted papilloma, although "persistence" would be a better term since this is largely related to inadequate excision. Multiple recurrences are common, up to seven or more in some series *(26)*, and the time interval to recurrence varies from 10 wk to 24 yr, although most occur within the first 2 yr. Malignant transformation in inverted papilloma varies from 0 to 53% in the literature. It is quite clear that, in the majority of cases, carcinoma was present from the outset, and the true incidence of malignant change was <2% *(27)*.

As a consequence of the above, much discussion has centered on the best surgical approach. Local intranasal excisions were associated with a recurrence rate of 75% in the past, but more recently an endoscopic approach has been advocated *(28)*. Only if a localized lesion can be confirmed endoscopically and on CT scan should this be contemplated by an experienced endoscopic surgeon. For the majority of lesions, a more radical approach is required, which is usually best achieved by a midfacial degloving or lateral rhinotomy (medial maxillectomy) *(19,29)*. With long-term follow-up, recurrence rates of between 0 and 33% have been reported. Neither radiotherapy nor oncologic chemotherapy has any role. However, because of the possible viral origin, interferon has been advocated for the more aggressive lesions.

Nonepidermoid Epithelial Neoplasms (Table 9)

ADENOID CYSTIC CARCINOMA

Adenoid cystic carcinoma is an infiltrating malignant tumor with a characteristic cribriform appearance, derived from minor seromucinous salivary glands, which can occur throughout the upper jaw mucosa. However, it is rare in the sinonasal region, constituting 1.3% of all tumors and mainly affecting the maxilla. However, adenoid cystic carcinoma accounts for 24% of all palatal tumors *(31)*, predominantly affecting, the hard palate. Males and females are equally affected, and the age range is 13–84 yr, with the majority occurring in the fourth to sixth decades.

The tumor has a unique natural history, characterized by frequent local recurrence, and early spread by perineural infiltration and hematogenous spread. Consequently, patients may describe neurological symptoms, such as facial pain or tingling and paraesthesia, especially in the distribution of the infraorbital nerve. They may develop local

Table 9
Nonepidermoid Glandular Tumors in the Upper Respiratory Tract *(30)*

Origin of tumor	
Salivary type	*Surface mucosa*
Benign	
Adenoma	Papillary adenoma
Monomorphic	
Pleomorphic	
Oncocytoma	
Malignant	
Adenoid cystic	Adenocarcinoma
Mucoepidermoid	Papillary
Acinic cell	Sessile
Carcinoma ex pleomorphic	
Adenocarcinoma	Alveolar mucoid
Adenosquamous carcinoma	"Colonic" or "colloid"
Clear-cell adenocarcinoma	Undifferentiated
Undifferentiated	

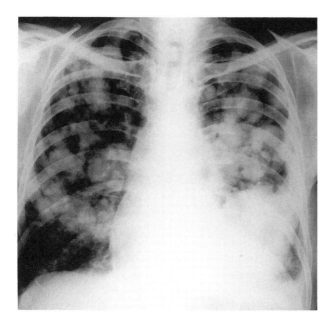

Fig. 8. Chest X-ray showing multiple metastases in a patient with adenoid cystic carcinoma.

recurrences at any point during their remaining lifetime, invalidating the concept of 5-yr survival and frequently manifest systemic metastases (20–50%), especially to the lung, although cervical lymphadenopathy is unusual (Fig. 8). However, in this condition, metastases do not necessarily imply a rapid demise, and patients may live for 6 or 7 yr with pulmonary disease.

Because of the above, radical excision is rarely curative, but although primary surgery may not be curative or affect the frequency of metastases, the number and speed of local recurrences are considerably reduced. Two-thirds of patients can be expected to be alive at 5 yr, but this will fall to 10% or less at 20 yr. Neither radiotherapy nor chemotherapy seems to improve this situation.

ADENOCARCINOMA

Adenocarcinoma is a tumor characterized by the presence of glandular structures, constituting between 4 and 9% of sinonasal malignancy. Because of the importance of occupational factors in the etiology of this tumor, there is a male preponderance of between 4:1 and 11:1. The average age at presentation is usually 50–60 yr, slightly earlier than for squamous cell carcinoma. The lesion probably arises within the middle meatus, affecting the adjacent ethmoids, and spreading into the anterior nasal vault and maxillary antrum. There may be mucosal spread into the nasopharynx, and the contralateral ethmoids may be involved. There is little specificity in the clinical symptomatology or radiology, other than the propensity to expand the nasal bones, producing a mass at the glabella and to affect the orbit and anterior cranial fossa at an early stage. Adenocarcinoma has been classified in a number of ways, and attempts have been made to correlate histological differentiation with prognosis. Low-grade differentiation appears to confer a better prognosis than high-grade tumors. Other descriptions include papillary, sessile, and alveolar-mucoid. The latter group includes a "colloid" or "colonic" subgroup. Prognosis seems to be best in papillary and worse in alveolar-mucoid tumors. The possibility of a metastasis from another site should always be considered.

Adenocarcinoma is particularly suitable for craniofacial resection, being relatively resistant to both radiotherapy and chemotherapy. In our own series, this treatment was associated with a 62% actuarial survival rate, but again the need for long-term follow-up cannot be emphasized too strongly (*22*, pp. 115–121). Only 2–3% develop cervical metastases, but distant secondaries may increase with long-term survival.

METASTASES

The possibility of a secondary tumor should be considered, particularly when a histologic report of clear-cell adenocarcinoma or "anaplastic" carcinoma is given. The kidney is by far the most common primary source, followed by bronchus, breast, and pancreas. Both maxilla and ethmoid can be affected, and a general examination and history may lead to appropriate special investigations. The presence of a secondary deposit in this area is rarely an isolated event, usually signifying disseminated disease, although solitary metastases are possible from the kidney. Consequently, treatment is essentially palliative, but a radical resection that does not disable the patient may be associated with a reasonable symptom-free period. However, generally metastatic disease to the sinonasal region has a poor prognosis, with two-thirds dead within 1 yr. In the literature, radiotherapy and chemotherapy have also been used alone or in combination with surgery (22, pp. 124–128). It is possible for secondaries from organs, such as the pancreas, to precede the primary presentation by several years. This, combined with the rarity of the condition, renders generalized screening of all patients with sinonasal malignancy "cost-ineffective."

Neuroectodermal Tumors

Primary neurogenic tumors of the sinonasal tract are rare. They cover a range of activity and may pose difficulties of management owing to their intimate relationships with intracranial structures. They include:

1. Nasal meningoencephalocele and glioma;
2. Neurofibroma (benign and malignant);
3. Extracranial meningioma;
4. Neuroendocrine carcinoma;
5. Olfactory neuroblastoma;
6. Malignant melanoma; and
7. Melanotic neuroectodermal tumor of infancy.

OLFACTORY NEUROBLASTOMA

This malignant tumor arises from the olfactory epithelium and is composed of undifferentiated neuroectodermal tissue. The increasing number reported in the literature is probably related to a greater awareness of the condition and the use of immunohistochemistry techniques for diagnosis, rather than a genuine rise in numbers (32). The tumor arises in the anatomical distribution of the olfactory mucosa, and all lesions must be regarded as potentially extending intracranially owing to the contiguity of the olfactory fibrils, bulbs, and tracts, irrespective of radiological and macroscopic appearances (33). The gross extent of the anterior

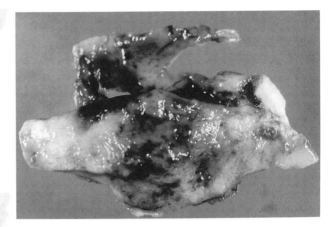

Fig. 9. Surgical specimen of nasal mucosa showing malignant melanoma, with pigmented, amelanotic, and satellite lesions.

cranial fossa extension, however, may be well demonstrated by MRI. Thus, it is ideally suited for craniofacial resection, which enables a genuine oncological excision in many cases. The use of radiotherapy, either pre- or postoperatively, is advisable in all but the most localized lesions (34). Regional and systemic metastases are uncommon at initial diagnosis, but increase with local recurrence and have been treated with a range of chemotherapy regimens with limited response. Survival has been doubled by the replacement of limited resection by craniofacial surgery (from 37.5 to 82% at 4 yr) (34), but disease may recur more than 10-yr later, again invalidating short-term expression of "cure."

MALIGNANT MELANOMA

This tumor arises from melanocytes, which are of neural crest origin and are found throughout the sinonasal mucosa. The tumor is exceptionally rare and generally occurs in the nasal cavity, spreading into the sinuses secondarily (35). It is a most capricious disease, which may be initiated by certain chemical contact and will invariably kill the patient unless another event intervenes. Its capacity for submucosal spread, satellite lesions, and amelanotic areas compromise excision (Fig. 9), and prognostic indicators for skin melanoma, such as depth of invasion, are not applicable to mucosal disease. Between 10 and 18% of patients present with cervical lymphadenopathy, and 4% with systemic metastases. Despite this, some patients survive for long periods of time, punctuated by local or regional disease, whereas others die within a few weeks of overwhelming dissemination. It is unclear what factors determine an individual's natural history, but an event such as a viral infection can adversely affect the immune balance with fatal results. Consequently, most patients are advised to undergo the most radical local surgery that does not encompass significant cosmetic and functional disability, most often a lateral rhinotomy. The tumor is not specifically radiosensitive, but since long-term survivors in the largest series had received combined treatment, it may be worthy of consideration (35). Craniofacial resection is contraindicated in this disease, since it removes physical barriers to tumor spread, enhancing intracranial extension. Cervical nodes have been locally excised or removed by formal neck dissection, without any obvious difference in benefit. As yet the benefit of chemotherapy, including the use of interferon and interleukin, is unproven.

Odontogenic Tumors

AMELOBLASTOMA

A vast array of lesions related to the dentition have been described, of which the most common is the ameloblastoma. This is a benign tumor originating from epithelial components of the embryonic tooth, arrested developmentally prior to enamel formation. Clinically, it is locally invasive, potentially lethal, and occasionally shows malignant features with systemic metastases. The majority occur before the age of 50 and, in the maxilla, are most commonly situated posterior to the canine tooth. They most commonly present as a painless swelling of the cheek, gingiva, or palate, and are often large. There are no pathognomonic features on imaging, since erosion of the tooth roots in the region of the third molar and loculated lesions in this area can be caused by a large range of lesions. Radical surgical excision is the most reliable treatment, since curettage and radiotherapy are almost invariably associated with "recurrence."

MESENCHYMAL NEOPLASMS

Vasoform Tumors

These cover a wide range of benign and malignant conditions, some of which cannot be clearly defined as neoplasms (Table 10).

JUVENILE ANGIOFIBROMA

Although morphologically benign, this tumor can exhibit aggressive local growth with signifi-

Table 10
Vasoform Neoplasms and Other Lesions (36)

Benign
  Localized
    Hemangiomata (capillary, cavernous, or mixed)
    Angiofibroma
    Aneurysmal bone cyst
    Angiomyolipoma
  Inflammatory
    Granuloma pyogenicum
    Granuloma graviderum
  Angiomatous syndromes
    Familial hemorrhagic telangiectasia
Malignant
  Angiosarcoma
  Kaposi's sarcoma
  Hemangiopericytoma
Pericyte-like
  Paraganglioma
  Glomus

cant consequences. Prior to the development of sophisticated radiological techniques, the site of origin was confidently placed within the nasopharynx, the region were it was most easily detected, but it is now clearly established that its site of origin is the margin of the sphenopalatine foramen. Erosion of the base of the medial pterygoid plate with enlargement of the foramen is thus a constant and pathognomonic radiological feature (37). From there, the tumor fills the nasal cavity, nasopharynx, and sphenoid, and extends laterally into the pterygopalatine fossa and infratemporal space (Fig. 10). As a consequence, it may present with swelling of the cheek or blindness in addition to unilateral nasal obstruction and epistaxis. Extension into the middle cranial fossa can occur, but is almost always extradural.

The tumor has excited interest because of its exclusive presentation in young males and the problems of management. Biopsy has frequently been associated with life-threatening hemorrhage, but is actually unnecessary since the diagnosis may be confidently made with imaging, in particular by a combination of CT and MRI. Angiography has traditionally been recommended both for diagnosis and performance of preoperative embolization.

Although the tumor may cease growing or occasionally involute, surgical excision is generally undertaken. A variety of approaches have been described. Of these, the transpalatal approach

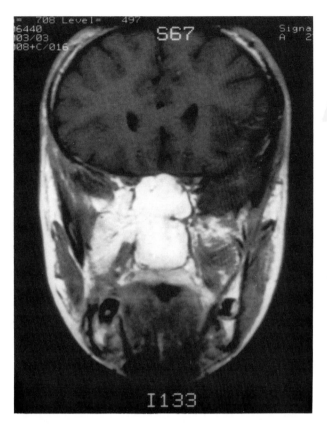

Fig. 10. Coronal T1 MRI with gadolinium showing high-signal mass with signal voids in areas of large vessels in a large angiofibroma.

offers least control of hemorrhage, and most authors agree that either a lateral rhinotomy or, more recently suggested, midfacial degloving approach should be used in most cases *(19)*. Radiotherapy has been used as a primary modality or for recurrent tumors and good results have been reported, but concerns related to malignant transformation or induction as well as the effects on facial growth and the pituitary have been expressed. Because of the tumor's predilection for young men, a variety of hormonal treatments have been proposed, although they have been generally abandoned. Despite radical treatment, the recurrence rate even in the larger series may be up to 30% *(38)*.

KAPOSI'S SARCOMA

Some debate surrounds the exact origin of this lesion, although Batsakis and Rice *(36)* concluded that it arose from vasoformative cells. Originally a dermatological curiosity confined to selected ethnic groups and associated with an indolent course, it gained notoriety for its appearance in a much more aggressive form in immunosuppressed individuals, most recently in those with AIDS. Although preferentially affecting the mouth or pharynx, it is occasionally observed in the sinonasal mucosa. Chemotherapy (vinblastine or α-interferon) and radiotherapy can produce partial or total remission.

HEMANGIOPERICYTOMA

This unusual tumor derives its name from pericytes associated with capillaries, from which it was originally thought to arise. It can occur throughout the sinonasal tract and varies in its aggression, with local recurrence reported at between 25 and 40% and systemic metastases as 5–10% *(22,* pp. 178–181*)*. Five-year follow-up is of little value, and final mortality may be as high as 50%. Wide local excision offers the best option, which may include maxillectomy or craniofacial resection, with radiotherapy reserved for inoperable or residual lesions following surgery.

Tumors of Muscular Origin

Tumors of smooth and skeletal muscle origin are exceptionally rare in the sinonasal region, although the head and neck, and the orbit in particular are common sites. They include: (1) leiomyoma, leiomyoblastoma, and leiomyosarcoma, and (2) rhabdomyoma and rhabdomyosarcoma.

RHABDOMYOSARCOMA

This is a neoplastic analog of embryogenesis of skeletal muscle that can occur at any age, but generally affects the young. Approximately 8% of rhabdomyosarcomas in the head and neck affect the sinonasal region, where the nasal cavity and maxilla are most frequently involved. Four histological varieties have been described: pleomorphic, embryonal, alveolar, and botryoid, of which embryonal is the most common in the head and neck. The tumor is locally aggressive with early hematogenous spread to lungs, bone, brain, skin, pleura, and abdominal viscera. Lymph node involvement is also moderately common compared to other sarcomas, being reported in up to 50% of cases. Fortunately, the previously uniformly poor prognosis has been transformed by the use of triple therapy: surgery, radiotherapy, and multiple-agent chemotherapy. A large number of chemotherapy agents have been used, of which vincristine, actinomycin D, and cyclophosphamide (VAC) are most popular, but many others, including adriamycin and dimethyltrizenoimidazole (DTIC), are reported. Prior to these regimens, only 12% were alive at 5-yr, whereas figures of up to 70% have been published more recently (*22*, pp. 190–195). However, once again this lesion may recur many years later, and if initial treatment fails, survival is usually <12 mo.

Cartilaginous Tumors

A variety of cartilaginous tumors occur in the sinonasal region, some of which are histologically well differentiated accompanied by an apparently slow growth pattern. All should, however, be regarded as having malignant potential and may well cause death by skull base infiltration before manifesting metastatic spread.

They include:

1. Chondroma;
2. Benign chondroblastoma;
3. Chondrosarcoma; and
4. Mesenchymal chondrosarcoma.

CHONDROSARCOMA

Chondrosarcoma arises from hyaline cartilage, and in the sinonasal area is estimated to constitute 1.25% of all chondrosarcomas, where it is less common than osteosarcoma. The anterior maxilla is an area of predilection, as is interestingly the posterior nasal septum, ethmoids, and sphenoid from where the skull base is infiltrated. The inexorable spread of tumor in this region causes cranial nerve damage, frequently resulting in bilateral blindness. The majority of lesions show mottled calcification within a soft tissue mass on CT scanning, although this may range from one or two punctate areas to multiple confluent plaques. This, combined with MRI findings of a high signal on T2-weighted sequences and differential enhancement after gadolinium-DTPA, is diagnostic. Radical surgery offers the primary modality of treatment, and craniofacial resection offers the most oncologically satisfactory approach. Recurrence is relatively common, and although 5-yr survival rates of 62% have been reported, observation over the patient's lifetime is required.

Mesenchymal chondrosarcoma is a rare and very malignant variant occasionally affecting the maxilla.

Tumors of Bony Origin

A considerable range of conditions, developmental, reactive, and genuinely neoplastic, occur

Table 11
Neoplasms and Other Lesions Related to Bone

Fibro-osseous disease
    Ossifying fibroma
    Fibrous dysplasia
Reactive-reparative lesions
    Giant cell granuloma
    "Brown tumor"
    Paget's disease
Neoplasms
    Osteoma
    Osteoid osteoma
    Osteoblastoma
    Osteogenic sarcoma

in the sinonasal region associated with a range of clinical activity (Table 11).

OSTEOMA

This slow-growing benign tumor of bone is relatively common in the sinuses. It may be an incidental finding in up to 1% of sinus X-rays. Genetic factors may play a role, as in Gardner's syndrome, an autosomal dominant condition characterized by intestinal polyps, osteomas, and pigmented skin lesions, but the vast majority of cases are of unknown etiology and would perhaps be best regarded as osseous hamartomas. Osteomata are asymptomatic until they cause a mass effect and are easily diagnosed radiologically. The point at which surgical removal is undertaken and the extent of the surgical approach will depend on clinical features, the tumor's position, and evidence of continued growth. It can therefore range from an external ethmoidectomy to craniofacial resection in exceptional cases.

OSTEOGENIC SARCOMA

This malignant bony tumor affects the upper jaw at a later age than elsewhere in the body, with a mean age of 38 yr. It occasionally occurs in pre-existing lesions, such as Paget's disease or following irradiation. It is characterized by relatively rapid local growth with regional and systemic metastases occurring late. The characteristic "sunburst" appearance seen on imaging elsewhere in the body is uncommon in the paranasal sinuses. Despite triple regimens of radical surgery, radiotherapy, and chemotherapy, survival rates are low with 10-yr figures of around 30% (*22*, pp. 245–249). However, once again, patients are always at risk of recurrence.

Tumors of Lymphoreticular Origin

Tumors of lymphoreticular origin have been among the greatest sources of confusion and diagnostic contention. Improved histopathology techniques have improved matters and have led to the realization that many midline destructive lesions are T-cell lymphomas, leading to more appropriate treatment and consequently better prognosis. The conditions fall into four main groups:

1. Burkitt's lymphoma;
2. Non-Hodgkin's lymphoma;
3. Extramedullary plasmacytoma; and
4. Midline destructive granuloma.

Non-Hodgkin's Lymphoma

Non-Hodgkin's lymphoma is found in both nodal and extranodal forms, and the incidence is increased in association with AIDS. Extranodal disease can occur within the sinonasal region, originating from the maxillary or ethmoid sinuses, lateral wall of the nose, or occasionally nasal septum, but the condition is still relatively rare. Robbins et al. *(39)* reported 38 cases in a 36-yr period with an overall 5-yr survival rate of 56%. It is important that fresh tissue be provided for histology, and once diagnosis is established, a generalized lymphoma screen should be undertaken. If confined to the sinonasal region, irradiation alone is successful. For more extensive local or disseminated disease, additional chemotherapy is employed using agents, such as cyclophosphamide, vincristine, doxorubicin, and procarbazine.

Midline Destructive Granuloma

This condition, which presents as a progressive unrelenting ulceration and necrosis of the midline facial tissues, posed considerable problems to clinicians before the recognition that the majority were T-cell lymphomas *(40)*. Although originally called Stewart's granuloma, it was actually first described by McBride in 1897 *(41)*. Inadequate treatment with limited courses of radiotherapy or steroids invariably leads to death from localized destruction or disseminated lymphoma. Full-course radiotherapy is mandatory in these cases, often combined with chemotherapy.

Other Mesenchymal Neoplasia

A number of other rare tumors of mesenchymal origin are encountered in the sinonasal region. These include:

1. Fibroma and fibromatosis;
2. Fibrosarcoma;
3. Lipoma and liposarcoma;
4. Myxoma;
5. Malignant fibrous histiocytoma;
6. Ewing's sarcoma; and
7. Alveolar soft part sarcoma.

Fibrosarcoma

The maxilla is the most frequent site for this tumor, which exhibits a range of aggression, although death usually results from local intracranial spread. Metastases are more often hematogenous than lymphatic, affecting at least a fifth of patients during the course of the disease. There have been a few reports on the use of adjuvant radiotherapy and chemotherapy, but wide local excision is generally employed. A 20-yr survival of 25% or less is seen in the few large series *(22,* pp. 136–139).

REHABILITATION

The oncologic surgeon is faced with the difficult task of reconciling complete excision of disease with maximal preservation of appearance and function. This is particularly pertinent in the sinonasal region, where any disfigurement is difficult to hide and where both ends of the age spectrum can be affected *(42,43)*. Physical and psychological rehabilitation is therefore of considerable importance when the principal criterion of cure has been satisfied and must be a primary consideration when only therapeutic palliation can be achieved. In a study designed to assess perception of relative severity of 11 common facial surgical disfigurements, orbital exenteration and radical maxillectomy scored highest with total rhinectomy, only outweighed by mandibulectomy *(44)*.

In those patients undergoing radical maxillectomy, close collaboration with the maxillofacial prosthodontist is required. The patient must be assessed preoperatively to obtain dental impressions, modify existing dentures, and discuss the likely extent of excision.

The surgical cavity may be modified to facilitate the design and construction of the most appropriate prosthesis, thus allowing the immediate placement of a temporary obturator at the end of the operation. This can be done using gutta percha molded to the self-retaining preprepared denture base. This allows the patient to eat, drink, and speak immediately after the procedure. A permanent hard acrylic or soft polymer obturator can be made once the cavity has healed.

Rehabilitation in this area has been greatly advanced by the introduction of osseo-integrated techniques, which have improved the retention of both intraoral and facial prostheses, such as the nose or eye, which previously had to be attached to spectacles or to the socket using tissue glues. The Branemark system of osseo-integrated implants uses titanium screws, which become an integral part of the skeleton, to which the prosthesis can be firmly attached for long periods of time *(45)*. The screws can be implanted at the time of the primary surgery or as a secondary procedure. Three to four millimeters depth of bone is needed for implantation, and radiotherapy may slow integration. In the orbit, it is advisable to wait 6 mo or even up to 1 yr if radiotherapy has been given before exposing the fitments for prosthesis attachment, since integration is slower in this region. A temporary orbital prosthesis can be offered during the interim.

The availability of these specialized techniques has dramatically improved the postoperative rehabilitation of our patients, but we should never underestimate the impact of our efforts to cure *(46)*.

REFERENCES

1. Stell P. History of surgery of the upper jaw. In: Harrison DFN, Lund VJ, eds. Tumours of the Upper Jaw. London: Churchill Livingstone, 1993; pp. 1–15.
2. Moure EJ. Traitment des tumeurs malignes primitives de l'ethmoide. Rev Hebdo Laryng 1902;2:401–412.
3. Price JC, Holliday MJ, Johns ME. The versatile midface degloving approach. Laryngoscope 1988;98:291–295.
4. Smith RR, Klopp CT, Wiliams JM. Surgical treatment of cancer of the frontal sinus and adjacent areas. Cancer 1954;7:991–994.
5. Ketcham AS, Wilkins RH, Van Buren JM, Smith RR. A combined intracranial approach to the paranasal sinuses. Am J Surg 1963;106:698–703.
6. Acheson ED, Cowdell RH, Hadfield E, Macbeth RG. Nasal cancer in woodworkers in the furniture industry. Br Med J 1968;2:587–596.
7. Wilhelmsson B, Drettner B. Nasal problems in wood furniture workers. A study of symptoms and physiological variables. Acta Otolaryngol 1984;98:548–555.
8. Drettner B, Wilhelmsson B, Lundh B. Experimental studies on carcinogenesis in the nasal mucosa. Acta Otolaryngol 1985;99:205–207.
9. Lund VJ. Malignancy of the nose and sinuses: epidemiological and aetiological considerations. Rhinology 1991;29:57–68.
10. Roush GC. Epidemiology of cancer of the nose and paranasal sinuses, current concepts. Head Neck Surg 1979;2:3–11.
11. Lederman M, Busby ER, Mould RF. The treatment of tumours of the upper jaw. Br J Rad 1969;42:561–581.
12. Harrison DFN. A critical look at the classification of maxillary sinus carcinomata. Ann Otol Rhinol Laryngol 1978;87:3–9.
13. Chandler JR, Guillamondegui OM, Sisson GA. Clinical staging of cancer of the head and neck: a new system. Am J Surg 1976;132:532–538.
14. Sisson GA, Johnson NE, Amir CS. Cancer of the maxillary sinus: clinical classification and management, Ann Otol Rhinol Laryngol 1963;72:1050–1059.
15. Lund VJ, Howard DJ, Lloyd GAS, Cheesman AD. Magnetic resonance imaging of paranasal sinus tumours from craniofacial resection. Head Neck Surg 1989;11:279–283.
16. Barzan L, Franchin G, DePaoli A. Carcinoma of the nasal vestibule: a report of 12 cases. J Laryngol Otol 1990;104:9–11.
17. Lund VJ. Lateral rhinotomy. In: McGregor IA, Howard DJ, eds. Rob & Smith's Operative Surgery. Head and Neck Surgery, Part 2. Oxford: Butterworth-Heinemann, 1992; pp. 551–554.
18. Lund VJ. Radical maxillectomy. In: McGregor IA, Howard DJ, eds. Rob & Smith's Operative Surgery. Head and Neck Surgery, Part 2. Oxford: Butterworth-Heinemann, 1992; pp. 565–570.
19. Howard DJ, Lund VJ. The midfacial degloving approach to sinonasal disease. J Laryngol Otol 1992;106:1056–1062.
20. Cheesman AD, Lund VJ, Howard DJ. Craniofacial resection for tumours of the nasal cavity and paranasal sinuses. Head Neck Surg 1986;8:429–435.
21. Beale FA, Garrett PG. Cancer of the paranasal sinuses with particular reference to the maxillary sinus. Laryngoscope 1983;99:143–150.
22. Harrison DFN, Lund VJ. Tumours of the Upper Jaw. London: Churchill-Livingstone, 1993; (a) 99; (b) 115–121; (c) 124–128; (d) 178–181; (e) 190–195; (f) 245–249; (g) 136–139.
23. Weber RS, Shillitoe EJ, Robbins KT, Luna MA, Batsakis JG, Donovan DT, et al. Prevalence of human papilloma virus in inverting nasal papillomas. Arch Otolaryngol Head Neck Surg 1988;114:23–26.
24. Batsakis JG. The pathology of head and neck tumors: nasal cavity and paranasal sinuses. Part 5. Head Neck Surg 1980;2:410–419.
25. Lund VJ, Lloyd GAS. Radiological changes associated with inverted papilloma of the nose and paranasal sinuses. Br J Rad 1984;57:455–461.
26. Trible WM, Lekagul S. Inverting papilloma of the nose and paranasal sinuses. Laryngoscope 1971;81:663–668.
27. Woodson GE, Robbins T, Michaels L. Inverting papilloma. Considerations in treatment. Arch Otolaryngol 1985;111:806–811.
28. Wigand ME. Endoscopic Surgery of the Paranasal Sinuses and Anterior Skull Base. Stuttgart, New York: Georg Thieme Verlag, 1990; pp. 116,117.
29. Sacks ME, Conley J, Rabuzzi DD. Degloving approach for total excision of inverted papilloma. Laryngoscope 1984;94:1595–1598.
30. Hyams VJ, Batsakis JG, Michaels L. Tumors of the upper respiratory tract and ear. Atlas of Tumor Pathology, 2nd ser. Fascicle 25, Washington, DC: Armed Forces Institute of Pathology, 1988; pp. 85–88.

31. Eneroth CM. Salivary gland tumors of the parotid gland, submandibular region and the palate region. Cancer 1971;27:1415–1418.
32. Lund VJ, Milroy CM. Olfactory neuroblastoma; clinical and pathologic aspects. Rhinology 1993;31:1–6.
33. Harrison DFN. Surgical pathology of olfactory neuroblastoma. Head Neck Surg 1984;7:60–64.
34. Levine PA, McLean WC, Cantrell RW. Esthesioneuroblastoma: the University of Virginia experience. Laryngoscope 1986;96:742–746.
35. Lund VJ. Malignant melanoma of the nasal cavity and paranasal sinuses. J Laryngol Otol 1982;96:347–355.
36. Batsakis JG, Rice DH. The pathology of head and neck tumours. Vasoformative tumors. Head Neck Surg 1980;3:231–239.
37. Lund VJ, Lloyd GAS, Howard DJ. Juvenile angiofibroma—imaging techniques in diagnosis. Rhinology 1989;27:179–185.
38. McCombe A, Lund VJ, Howard DJ. Recurrence in juvenile angiofibroma. Rhinology 1990;28:1–6.
39. Robbins KT, Fuller LM, Osborne B. Primary lymphomas of the nasal cavity and paranasal sinuses. Cancer 1985;56:814–819.
40. Harrison DFN. Midline destructive granuloma. 1987; 97:1049–1053.
41. McBride P. Photographs of a case of rapid destruction of the nose and face. J Laryngol Otol 1897;12:64,65.
42. Lund VJ, Howard DJ. Head and neck cancer in the young: a prognostic conundrum? J Laryngol Otol 1990;104:544–548.
43. Harries M, Lund VJ. Head and neck cancer in the elderly—a maturing problem. J Laryngol Otol 1989; 103:306–309.
44. Dropkin MJ, Malgady RG, Scott DW, Oberst MT, Strong EW. Scaling of disfigurement and dysfunction in postoperative head and neck patients. Head Neck Surg 1983;6:559–570.
45. Tjellstrom A. Osseointegrated systems and their application in the head and neck. Arch Otolaryngol Head Neck Surg 1989;3:39–70.
46. Jones E, Lund VJ, Howard DJ, Greenberg MP, McCarthy M. Quality of life of patients treated surgically for head and neck cancer. J Laryngol Otol 1992;106: 238–242.

14 Nasal Polyposis
Clinical Spectrum and Treatment Approaches

Guy A. Settipane, MD and Russell A. Settipane, MD

CONTENTS

INTRODUCTION

Nasal polyps and high recurrence rate in patients after treatment have always been an enigma. Despite many new drugs and various surgical procedures, the recurrence rate is unacceptably high. Various factors appear to be related to nasal polyps and their high recurrence rate. These factors include age of onset, asthma, aspirin intolerance, bacterial sinusitis, fungal sinusitis, other disease states, acute upper respiratory infections, and allergens. The classical tetrad syndrome associated with nasal polyps is aspirin intolerance, asthma, chronic sinusitis, and nasal polyps. Part of this tetrad was first described by Widal et al. in 1922 (1,2). They described the triad of nasal polyps, asthma, and

aspirin intolerance, but not chronic sinusitis. Frequently, polyps are associated with chronic sinusitis for three main reasons. First, polyps may disrupt or entirely block the ostiomeatal complex, leading to chronic sinusitis on a mechanical basis. Second, the eosinophilia associated with most polyps is toxic to the ciliated membranes producing a decrease in flow of mucus, and this stasis could result in sinusitis (3). This mechanism is thought to be through the toxic effect of the major basic protein associated with eosinophilia. Finally, polyps can occur within the paranasal sinus causing a mechanical and toxic obstruction (eosinophilia) from within the sinus. Also, pressure on the intrasinus membranes and bone can actually cause destruction of bone, Woakes disease (4), or midfacial expansion. Facial deformation occurring with juvenile nasal polyposis is well described (frog face). The tetrad of nasal polyps, asthma, aspirin

From: *Diseases of the Sinuses* (M. E. Gershwin and G. A. Incaudo, eds.),
©1996 Humana Press Inc., Totowa, NJ.

311

intolerance, and rhinosinusitis is a more realistic grouping of this pattern of classic symptoms.

Nasal polyps also are associated with many systemic diseases. They are as follows: cystic fibrosis, Kartagener's syndrome *(5,6)* (chronic dyskinetic cilia syndrome), Young's syndrome *(7,8)* (sinopulmonary disease, azoospermia) Churg–Strauss syndrome (allergic vasculitis), and allergic fungal sinusitis *(9)*. In some cases, nasal polyps may be visualized only with the use of the rhinoscope. In many situations, the nasal polyp may present as a minor symptom, but in reality may represent the "tip of the iceberg" with the major associated syndromes often being severe manifestations of systemic disorders. In this chapter, nasal polyps will be evaluated historically, epidemiologically, anatomically, histopathologically, by using differential diagnosis, in association with systemic diseases, by chemical mediators, pathogenesis, relationship to atopy, relationship to aspirin intolerance, and finally treatment.

HISTORY

Nasal polyps were known as far back as 1000 BC Vancil *(10)* has presented an excellent historical survey of treatment for nasal polyps. In about 400 BC, Hippocrates developed two surgical methods for nasal polypectomy: extraction by pulling a sponge through the nasal canal and by cauterization. Cato the Censor (234–149 BC) developed the first known medical management of nasal polyps using the local application of herbs. Other ancient authors who have written about nasal polyps through the centuries are as follows: Celsus (42 BC–37 AD), Paulus of Aegina (625–690 AD), Avicenna (980–1037 AD), Saliceto (1210–1270 AD), Fallopius (1523–1562 AD), Petros Forestus (1522–1597 AD), Fabricius ab Acquapendente (1537–1619 AD), Aranzi (1530–1589 AD), and Juncker, who in 1721 wrote: "According as the moon fills or wanes, the polypi of the nose increase or decrease in size"— an excellent clinical observation of remissions and exacerbations of polyps but certainly a faulty lunar correlation. Thus, it appears that nasal polyps have been a medical problem as far back as humans can remember.

EPIDEMIOLOGY

Nasal polyps are most commonly found in nonatopic asthmatic patients over 40 yr of age,

Table 1
Frequency of Nasal Polyps in Various Conditions

Diagnosis	Frequency, %
Aspirin intolerance	36
Adult asthma	7
Intrinsic asthma	13
Atopic asthma	5
Chronic rhinosinusitis	2
Nonallergic rhinitis	5
Allergic rhinitis	1.5
Childhood asthma/rhinitis	0.1
Cystic fibrosis	20
Churg–Strauss syndrome	50
Allergic fungal sinusitis *(9)*	85
Kartagener's syndrome	?
Young's syndrome	?

especially in those patients with severe, steroid-dependent asthma. The overall frequency of nasal polyps in asthmatics between the ages of 10 and 50 yr is 7% (Table 1). In a subgroup of asthmatics over 40 yr old with negative skin test, the frequency ranges from 10 to 15% (Table 2) *(11)*. In patients with aspirin intolerance, the frequency of nasal polyps may be as high as 36% *(12,13)*. Slavin's group *(14)* reported on 33 patients with severe asthma and sinusitis. Fifteen of these patients were receiving corticosteroids: 10 who received continuous corticosteroids and 5 who required intermittent bursts. Of these 33 patients, 30 (or 90%) had a diagnosis of nasal polyps and 17 (52%) had aspirin intolerance. The data demonstrate that the nasal polyps as well as aspirin intolerance found in asthmatic patients usually indicate the presence of a severe asthmatic state. In children, the frequency of nasal polyposis is extremely low, about 0.1% *(11,15)*. Any child 16 yr or younger with nasal polyps should be evaluated for cystic fibrosis.

ANATOMY

Nasal polyps are frequently bilateral, multiple, and have a characteristic appearance (Fig. 1). They are glistening, semitranslucent, pale gray, smooth, soft, freely movable, attached by a pedicle, and they rise from the surfaces of the middle turbinates, the hiatal semilunaries, or ostia of the ethmoid and maxillary sinuses. Most commonly they are found in the middle meatus extending to the nasal cavity filling the nose and finally protruding from the anterior nares. If the polyp projects posteriorly into

Table 2
Frequency of Nasal Polyps in Various Age Groups of Asthmatic Patients

Age when first seen, yr	No. with asthma	No. with nasal polyps	%	p
10–19	491 ⎫	9 ⎫	1.8 ⎫	
20–29	465 ⎬ 1374	18 ⎬ 43	3.9 ⎬ 3.1	
30–39	418 ⎭	16 ⎭	3.8 ⎭	<0.01[a]
40–49	410 ⎫ 854	41 ⎫ 106	10.0 ⎫ 12.4	
50 and over	444 ⎭	65 ⎭	14.6 ⎭	
Total	2228	149	6.7	

[a]The difference between the 10–39-yr-old group (43/1374), 3.1% compared to the 40-yr-old and over group (106/854), 12.4% is statistically significant.

Reprinted from ref. *11.*

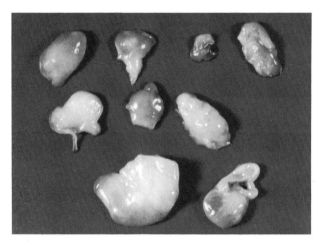

Fig. 1. Gross photograph of multiple nasal polyps from a 64-yr-old male (scale is in centimeters). Reprinted with permission from ref. *16.*

the nasopharynx, it is called a choanal polyp and may not be seen by routine examination through the anterior nares. Choanal polyps may be single, usually occur during the first two decades of life, and are classified in three groups:

1. Antrochoanal polyps arising from the antrum;
2. Polyps arising from other sinuses; or
3. Polyps that are the posterior part of multiple ethmoidal polyps *(17).*

Polyps are one of the most common types of mass found in the nasal passage.

HISTOPATHOLOGY

Nasal polyps have pseudostratified columnar epithelium and cellular constituents of normal nasal mucosa (Fig. 2). Polyps from patients who do not

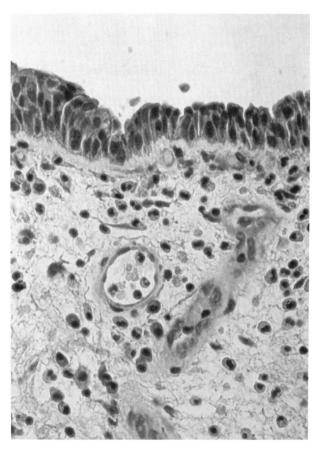

Fig. 2. Nasal polyp (H & E stain, ×400). This high-power view shows orderly pseudostratified columnar epithelium overlying an intact basement membrane. The stroma is edematous, vascular, and contains eosinophils. Reprinted with permission from ref. *16.*

have cystic fibrosis have extensive thickening of the epithelial basement membranes with extension into the submucosa as an irregular hyaline membrane, high stromal eosinophil count, and mainly

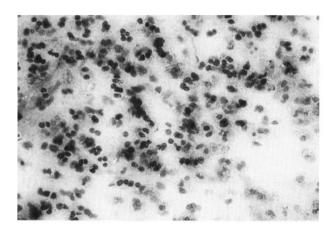

Fig. 3. Smear of nasal secretions from a patient with nasal polyps reveals eosinophils. Reprinted with permission from ref. *16*.

neutral mucin in mucous glands, cysts, and mucous blanket *(18)*.

Glands are few and denervated. Polyp tissue is essentially free of nerve endings, except for nerve terminals in the base of the polyps associated with blood vessels. In most cases, the cells consist of a mixture of lymphocytes, plasma cells, and eosinophils (Fig. 2). Occasionally, neutrophils are numerous. Nasal smears from these patients usually reveal "sheets" of eosinophils (Fig. 3). In contrast, polyps from patients with cystic fibrosis have a delicate, barely visible basement membrane of surface epithelium without submucosal hyalinization, lack of extensive infiltration of eosinophils, and a preponderance of acid mucin in glands, cysts, and surface mucous blanket. Polyps from patients with Kartagener's and Young's syndromes usually lack an eosinophilic component and have neutrophils as the predominant cell.

As for noncystic fibrosis polyps, one report *(19)* demonstrated that all polyps showed evidence of epithelial damage, either ulceration or marked desquamatizatlon. In another study *(20)*, a small proportion of polyps showed a focal dysplastic change of the surface lining of the mucosa with no related changes in the immediately underlying stroma. On follow-up, in none of these patients did an invasive feature supersede, and these changes appear to constitute a local reaction to recurrent irritation.

DIFFERENTIAL DIAGNOSIS

The differential diagnosis of nasal polyps includes chordoma, chemodectoma, neurofibroma, angiofibroma, inverting papilloma, squamous cell carcinoma, sarcoma, and encephaloceles or meningoceles. Most of these lesions present as unilateral lesions. Meningoceles enter the nasal cavity via the cribriform plate. They increase in size with straining, lifting, or crying, and may have a pulsating characteristic. The other lesions included in this differential diagnosis are immobile, bleed easily, and may be sensitive to manipulation. Nasal polyps are characteristically mobile, rarely bleed, are not sensitive to manipulation, and are frequently bilateral and multiple. Malignant tumors frequently are associated with bony, destructive changes. In rare cases, benign paranasal sinus cysts or polyps may also produce bone destruction (Woakes disease) *(4)* (Fig. 4A,B). Diagnostic procedures for the differential diagnosis include angiography, tomographic X-rays, computerized tomography scan, magnetic resonance imaging, and nasal scraping for eosinophils, nasal-pharyngeal circulation time with saccharine, and biopsy done with caution.

ASSOCIATION WITH SYSTEMIC DISEASES

The most common systemic disease associated with nasal polyps is nonallergic asthma, followed by aspirin intolerance (Table 1). The tetrad of nasal polyps, asthma, aspirin intolerance, and rhinosinusitis will be discussed in a separate category later on in this chapter. Patients with cystic fibrosis have a high frequency of nasal polyps (20%). Children age 16 or younger who have nasal polyps should be evaluated for cystic fibrosis. Similar to cystic fibrosis, the polyps associated with the chronic dyskinetic cilia syndrome and Young's syndrome have the neutrophil as the predominant cell. Primary ciliary dyskinesia is classically manifested in Kartagener's syndrome, which is an uncommon genetic condition with an estimated incidence of 1 in 20,000 births *(5,6)*. It appears to be inherited as an autosomal recessive trait and is characterized by bronchiectasis, chronic sinusitis, and situs inversus (complete reversal of internal organs with heart on the right, liver on the left, and so forth). The ciliary abnormality in these cases usually involves the entire body including the respiratory tract and sperm cells. The disorder is in the cilia itself in which the dynein arms are missing and the cilia remains completely immotile. Situs

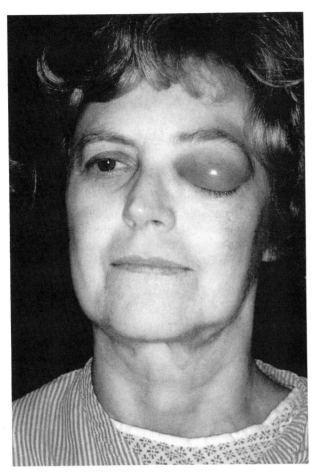
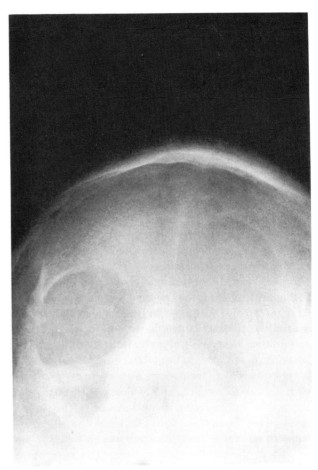

Fig. 4. (A) Severe periorbital edema preoperatively. **(B)** Sinus film showing erosion of the orbital rim. Reprinted with permission from ref. *21*.

inversus is found in only 50% of patients with this syndrome. Infections caused by *Pseudomonas aeruginosa* are often found in patients with Kartagener's syndrome or cystic fibrosis *(22)*.

Young's syndrome consists of recurrent respiratory diseases, azoospermia, and nasal polyposis. The respiratory disease consists of severe chronic sinusitis, which may be associated with bronchiectasis *(7,8)*. These patients have normal sweat chloride values and pancreatic function and, therefore, do not have a variant of cystic fibrosis. Cilia structures are normal in sperm tails taken from testicular biopsy specimens and in the cilia from tracheal biopsy specimens; therefore, these patients do not have a chronic form of immotile cilia syndrome. The azoospermia in Young's syndrome is the result of a block in the epididymis that is distinguishable from the defect in the vas deferens associated with cystic fibrosis. However, spermatogenesis is normal. The prevalence of Young's syndrome is considerably higher than that of cystic fibrosis or Kartagener's syndrome. It is responsible for 7.4% of cases of male infertility. In Churg–Strauss syndrome (allergic vasculitis), 50% of these patients have nasal polyps. Thus, it is apparent that the presence of nasal polyps may be a sign that a basic generalized disease may be present and that nasal polyps may represent just the tip of a deep iceberg. The systemic diseases that are associated with nasal polyps are listed in Table 3 and are in the order of frequency found in the general population.

CHEMICAL MEDIATORS

Chemical mediators found in nasal polyps are histamine, serotonin, leukotrienes (slow reactive substance of anaphylaxis), LTC4, LTD4, LTE4, LTB4, eosinophilic chemotactic factor of anaphylaxis (ECF-A), norepinephrine, kinins, TAME-esterase, and possibly prostaglandin PGD *(23,24)*.

Table 3
Nasal Polyps Associated with Systemic Diseases[a]

Asthma (nonallergic)
Aspirin intolerance (bronchospastic type)
Tetrad of asthma, aspirin intolerance, nasal polyps, and
 chronic rhinosinusitis
Allergic fungal sinusitis *(9)*
Churg–Strauss syndrome (vasculitis)
Young's syndrome (sinopulmonary disease, azoospermia,
 nasal polyps)
Cystic fibrosis
Kartagener's syndrome (bronchiectasis, chronic sinusitis,
 and situs inversus)

[a]The first five diseases are associated with tissue eosinophilia, whereas in the latter group of diseases, the predominant cell is the neutrophil.

Kaliner et al. *(25)* reported that the release of chemical mediators in nasal polyps is modulated by agents affecting the intracellular concentrations of cyclic nucleotides. These authors also stated that the quantity of SRS-A released in relation to the amount of histamine released from nasal polyps is considerably less than that released from the human lung. Bumsted et al. *(24)* reported that there is more histamine in nasal polyps than in normal nasal mucosa and that norepinephrine is present in greater concentration in the base of nasal polyps than in normal nasal mucosa. However, there is no difference in serotonin levels in nasal polyps and normal nasal mucosa. In addition, there is no difference in levels of histamine, serotonin, and norepinephrine in nasal polyps from groups of patients with or without inhalant allergies or asthma.

An interesting finding is that patients with aspirin intolerance have levels of histamine in nasal polyps that are much lower than all other types of patients with nasal polyps, approximating the histamine levels found in normal mucosa. Chandra and Abrol *(26)* reported that polyp fluid contains albumin and immunoglobulins (IgA, IgE, IgG, IgM, and macroglobulins). The concentrations of IgA and IgE and, in some cases, IgG and IgM were greater in the polyp fluid than in the serum. Using the Prausnitz-Kustner procedure, Berdal *(27)* in 1952 reported that skin sensitivity antibody in polyp fluid was many times more concentrated than that found in sera. An explanation for these increased concentrations of serum components found in polyp fluid may be that the polyp may act as a dialyzing membrane with water evaporating through the mucosa.

This causes an increased concentration of large substances in the polyp sack.

PATHOGENESIS

A current theory on the pathogenesis of polyps has been presented by Bumsted et al. *(24)*. Their theory is based on data that norepinephrine is present in greater concentration in the base of nasal polyps than in normal mucosa. They stated that this norepinephrine at the base of the polyp could produce excessive adrenergic receptor-mediated vasoconstriction that might lead to rebound mucosal congestion and edema potentiating the effects of histamine and kinins. Norepinephrine through adrenergic receptor activation would lower the effects of cyclic adenosine monophosphate, which would enhance the release of histamine, SRS-A, and ECF-A. These mediators would cause an increased vascular permeability, edema, and the leakage of macromolecules out of the vascular system eventually causing the polyp formation. They explained the lower levels of histamine found in polyps of aspirin-intolerant patients by stating that these patients have an increased sensitivity to histamines.

Mygind *(28)* believes that polyp formation is related to denervation of blood vessels and degranulation of mast cells in the nasal mucosa. This process leads to increased vascular permeability, edema, and finally polyp formation. He lists causative factors for denervation to be infection, cystic fibrosis, and aspirin intolerance. He lists contributing factors to be mast cell degeneration and IgE-dependent reactions.

An old theory *(29)* on polyp formation deals with Bernoulli's theorem, which states that gases or fluid passing through a constrictor results in an area of negative pressure in its vicinity. Weakened, denervated tissue, such as polyps, may theoretically be sucked out by this negative pressure, leading to edema and enlargement of the polyp.

Other theories of polyp formation have been postulated. Tos and Mogensen's *(30)* theory is based on rupture of the epithelium with protrusion of the subepithelial tissue through the epithelial defect and the epithelization of the prolapsed tissue.

A new theory from Bernstein et al. *(31)* is that a greater rate of transepithelial ion transport occurs in nasal polyps. They suggest that this increased rate may have an effect on the movement of water

Table 4
Nasal Polyps (211 Cases): Characteristics

Clinical categories	No.	%
Males	106	50.2
Females	105	49.8
Asthma	149	70.6
Rhinitis (alone)	62	29.4
Positive allergy shin tests	117	55.5
Total aspirin intolerance	30	14.2
Subtypes of aspirin intolerance		
Bronchospasm	21	70.0
Urticaria	4	13.3
Both bronchospasm and urticaria	2	6.7
Rhinitis	3	10.0

Reprinted from ref. *11*.

Table 5
Patients (167) with Verified Polyps and Polypectomies

Total patients	No. of polypectomies	No. of patients	%
167	1 or more	143	86
143	2 or more	57	40
143	3 or more	34	24
143	4 or more	22	15
143	5 or more	17	12
143	6 or more	11	8

Reprinted from ref. *40*.

Table 6
Frequency of Polypectomies
in Patients with Positive Allergy Skin Tests

Total patients[a]	No. of polypectomies	No. with positive allergy skin tests	%
24	0	12	50
143[b]	1 or more	81	57
57	2 or more	33	53
34	3 or more	20	59
22	4 or more	15	68
17	5 or more	12	71
11	6 or more	8	73

[a]Total patients = 167.
[b]One patient did not have a skin test.
Reprinted from ref. *40*.

into the cell and interstitial tissue, causing edema and formation of nasal polyps. They base their theory on the transepithelial bioelectric potential difference and resistance of nasal polyps and turbinate epithelial cells.

None of these theories appear adequate to account for all of the known facts involving nasal polyps. It has recently been shown by Tos that a rupture of the epithelial layer and basement membrane occurs before the polyp emerges *(31a)*. This rupture of the epithelial layer and basement membrane may occur with chronic subepithelial infections and toxic effects of eosinophils. The fact that nasal polyps are frequently associated with systemic diseases indicates that the underlying cause of polyposis may be related to a basic generalized biochemical disorder. At the present time, the pathogenesis of polyp formation is unknown.

RELATIONSHIP TO ATOPY

Nasal polyps are more frequently found in asthmatic/rhinitis patients who have negative skin tests rather than those with positive skin tests *(11–13)*. There is a relationship to asthma in that over 70% of patients with nasal polyps have an associated asthma (Table 4) *(11)*. Some patients with nasal polyps not only do not have a history of asthma, but also have negative methacholine challenge tests *(32,33)*. Therefore, not all patients with nasal polyps have an associated lower respiratory disease *(34,35)*. Whiteside et al. *(36)* reported that in five of six cases of nasal polyps in nonatopic patients, no IgE-bearing lymphocytes were detected in the polyp tissue. However, in atopic patients, IgE-bear-

ing lymphocytes in nasal polyps correlated well with serum IgE levels.

We reviewed *(37)* 167 patients with nasal polyps of which 143 (86%) of these had one or more polypectomies (Table 5). A number of these patients had a verified history of two, three, four, or even five or more polypectomies. Our data suggest that patients with positive allergy skin tests (pollen, animal dander, or molds) have a progressively higher rate of repeated polypectomies (Table 6).

The frequency of one or more possible allergy skin tests (pollens, danders, or molds) in our patient population with nasal polyps is 56% *(11)*. However, this population was obtained from an allergy-biased practice, both in private practice and in the allergy clinic at Rhode Island Hospital where the overall frequency of one or more positive allergy skin tests was 77% *(11)*. Therefore, the 56% positive allergy skin tests in patients with nasal polyps is lower than that found in our allergy practice and is not directly related to polyp formation.

Table 7
Characteristics of the Bronchospastic Type
of Aspirin Intolerance

Found in asthmatic patients
Correlated with nasal polyposis
Similar age onset as asthma
Severe rhinorrhea with aspirin reactions
Increased frequency in older age groups
Familial occurrence
Eosinophil in nasal smear
Elevated total (blood) eosinophil count
Nonsteroidal anti-inflammatory drug crossreaction
No specific IgE (antiaspiryl)
Normal total IgE
Desensitization possible to aspirin
Pathogenic mechanism: leukotrienes

Table 8
Nonsteroidal Anti-Inflammatory Drugs

Cyclo-oxygenase inhibitors	
Aminophenazone	Indomethacin
Aspirin	Mefenamic acid
Benzydamine	Naproxen
Diftalone	Nictindole
Ditazole	Noramidopyrine
Fenoprofen	Piroxicam
Flumizole	Sulindac
Ibuprofen	Tolmetin

It appears that atopy or IgE-mediated disease is not a cause of nasal polyps, but once polyp formation occurs, atopy or IgE-mediated disease may aggravate and increase the risk of nasal polyp formation. Acute upper respiratory infections are also known to cause an exacerbation or enlargement of nasal polyps *(35)*.

RELATIONSHIP
TO ASPIRIN INTOLERANCE

The full-blown tetrad of asthma, aspirin intolerance, chronic sinusitis, and nasal polyps usually is associated with a severe type of asthma that is frequently steroid dependent. The type of aspirin intolerance associated with nasal polyps is the bronchospastic type, not the urticaria/angioedema type. In many cases, only two components of the tetrad are present, asthma and aspirin intolerance, which usually have onset within 1 yr of each other. However, nasal polyps may occur about 10 yr later *(37)*. The mean age of onset of the asthma and aspirin intolerance part of the tetrad is about 31 yr *(38)*. However, the cumulative frequency increases with age, so that in asthmatic patients older than 40, the frequency of nasal polyps is 10% and above (Table 2).

Other characteristics of this tetrad are listed in Table 7. It is most commonly associated with nonallergic or negative skin test asthma, and with a normal serum IgE level. Specific IgE against aspirin has not been found. During acute bronchospasm produced by aspirin challenge, histamine levels, neutrophil chemotactic activity, and com-

plement activation were not found to be significantly different from baseline levels *(39)*. Elevated blood eosinophils and a marked eosinophilia in the nasal secretions are also characteristic of this syndrome. There is a hereditary disposition of aspirin intolerance in that clusters of this syndrome are found in certain families *(38)*.

The frequency of aspirin intolerance increases with age, especially over 40. However, it is the bronchospastic type of aspirin intolerance, not the urticaria/angioedema type, that increases with age.

It is apparent that there are many similarities between aspirin intolerance and nasal polyps. In addition to being associated together in the triad of asthma, aspirin intolerance (bronchospastic type) and nasal polyps both are associated with chronic sinusitis and nasal eosinophilia. Both conditions increase in frequency with age, both are commonly associated with negative skin test or nonallergic asthma, and both conditions are associated with a high frequency of steroid-dependent asthma as stated.

It is important to remember that nonsteroidal anti-inflammatory drugs (NSAID) crossreact with aspirin and cause a similar acute bronchospasm in aspirin-intolerant asthmatics (Table 8). These drugs are cyclo-oxygenase inhibitors. Some of these NSAID, such as indomethacin and ibuprofen, crossreact with aspirin in intolerant individuals about 100% of the time. Other NSAID crossreact with aspirin in intolerant individuals at a somewhat decreased rate, depending on the dose used and degree of inhibition of cyclo-oxygenase.

The pathological mechanism of aspirin intolerance is unknown. A suspected pathogenic hypothesis for aspirin intolerance is based on the association between prostaglandin and SRS-A. It is possible that in certain individuals, inhibition of the cyclo-oxygenase pathway may cause a shunting toward the lipoxygenase pathway, resulting in increased production of leukotrienes LTC4, LTD4, and LTE4 (SRS-A), which will produce bronchospasm. In addition, products of the lipoxygenase system, such as 5-HPETE, 5-HETE, and LTB4, are chemotactic for eosinophils. Both aspirin intolerance and nasal polyps are associated with eosinophils. A similar mechanism including arachidonic acid and prostaglandins for the formation of nasal polyps has not been developed at this time, but further research is needed in this area.

TREATMENT—NASAL POLYPS

Polypectomy is not the treatment of choice for routine nasal polyposis. We reviewed 167 patients with verified nasal polyps (Table 5) *(40)*. Eighty-six percent (143) had polypectomies. Of these 143, 57 (40%) required 2 or more polypectomies, 34 (24%) required 3 or more polypectomies, 22 (15%) required 4 or more polypectomies, 17 (12%) had 5 or more polypectomies, and 11 (8%) had 6 or more polypectomies. Three of our patients had a history of 20 or more polypectomies. Therefore, nasal polyposis frequently is a recurrent problem in over 40% of the cases. Other studies *(26)* have found a recurrence rate of over 31%. Also, polyps in patients with aspirin intolerance appear to have a greater recurrence rate than aspirin-tolerant patients.

It is apparent that surgical polypectomy does not permanently eliminate this disease. However, in certain selected cases, especially in those in which corticosteroids are not effective or are contraindicated, surgical polypectomy may be considered. Steroid injection of nasal polyps has been used with some success in the hands of expert otolaryngologists *(41)*. However, injection of steroids in the nasal turbinates and polyps has resulted in 10 instances of visual loss, 5 of which were permanent as of 1981 *(42)*. Steroid emboli were demonstrated in the retinal vessels in six cases. Certainly, this type of treatment for nasal polyps should be reserved for the very skilled otolaryngologist if it is used at all.

At the present time, we believe that the treatment of choice is a 12-d course of systemic corticosteroid therapy beginning with about 60 mg of prednisone orally and decreasing by 5 mg daily. This short burst of corticosteroids should not cause a clinically significant suppression of the pituitary–adrenal axis. Occasionally, patients may need a second burst of steroids a few weeks later if they do not improve with the first course of corticosteroid treatment *(43)*.

Afterward, patients may be maintained on topical beclomethasone, Triamcinolone, or flunisolide, realizing that excessive doses of these topical medications may result in suppression of the pituitary–adrenal axis, which may be clinically significant. Newer products, such as topical budesonide and fluticasone appear to have greater topical potency with less systemic effect. Additional supportive treatment may include long-term antibiotics for sinusitis (3 wk or longer) and oral antihistamines/decongestants.

Even with systemic and topical corticosteroid therapy, nasal polyps frequently may still be a recurrent disease, and periodic bursts of systemic corticosteroids may have to be administered. When treatment with systemic corticosteroids has no effect or is contraindicated, a surgical procedure may be contemplated.

Our recent investigation *(44)* has shown that surgical polypectomy may delay the recurrence rate of polyps compared to those treated with corticosteroids, but certainly the trauma and morbidity are much worse with surgery.

Contrary to previous opinion, the surgical removal of nasal polyps does not cause or aggravate asthma. In our laboratory, 10 patients with nasal polyps and no history of asthma were studied. Results of methacholine challenge tests done before and about 5 mo after polypectomy were similar *(32)*. In a report by Miles-Lawrence et al. *(33)*, similar data were obtained. They performed methacholine challenge tests 1 mo prior to polypectomy and up to 1 yr following polypectomy. They found essentially no change in methacholine sensitivity, confirming our conclusion that polypectomy does not cause or worsen asthma. However, the reoccurrence rate for nasal polyps following polypectomy is notoriously high and may be aggravated by many nonspecific factors, such as upper respiratory infection and allergies to pollens, danders, and molds (when the chance occurrence of these diseases coexists) *(37,40)*.

To extend these laboratory findings to clinically relevant data, we evaluated pulmonary function tests just prior to polypectomy and up to 5 mo following polypectomy. There was no significant change in pulmonary function tests *(37)*.

Table 9
Effect of Polypectomy on Steroid-Dependent Asthma (6-Mo Interval)

| Patient | Age, yr | Prednisone | | Change in asthma |
		Preoperative	Postoperative, 6 mo	
M. S.	48	10 mg alt days	10 mg alt days	Same
P. B.	25	10 mg alt days	10 mg alt days[a]	Same
L. C.	66	10 mg alt days	2.5 mg daily	Better
P. M.	66	5 mg daily	10 mg alt days	Better
F. S.	42	10 mg alt days	10 mg alt days	Same
V. L.	58	10 mg daily	10 mg daily	Same
J. C.	76	10 mg alt days	10 mg alt days	Same

[a]Data collected at 9 mo.
Reprinted from ref. 37.

Table 10
Treatment of Nasal Polyps

1. Systemic corticosteroids for 6 d.
2. Topical nasal steroids: Maintenance.
3. Antibiotics for 2–3 wk.
4. Decongestants, pseudoephedrine, and antihistamines.
5. Allergy avoidance if needed.
6. Surgical polypectomy.

We also evaluated seven steroid-dependent asthmatic patients for steroid requirements before and approx 6 mo following polypectomy (Table 9). The steroid requirements were essentially unchanged in five patients and decreased in two, possibly because of less stimulation through the rhinosinobronchial reflex. Thus, our initial data with methacholine sensitivity have been confirmed with subsequent clinical information.

Patients with nasal polyps deserve an allergic evaluation despite the fact that a large percentage of them are nonatopic. If clinically relevant IgE-mediated disease is found in these patients, a course of hyposensitization may be given, especially in those with recurrent polyposis. IgE-mediated disease is not the cause of nasal polyps, but it may contribute to episodes or exacerbations (44,16).

Present-day treatment of nasal polyps is listed in Table 10. They consist of a short course of systemic corticosteroids for a period of <10d, topical nasal steroids (usually maintenance), antibiotics for 2–3 wk (45), decongestant medication, allergy avoidance and hypersensitization if needed, and surgical polypectomy. Most authorities reserve surgical intervention for medical treatment failures.

Surgical polypectomy may be used as the first means of treatment in special cases, especially those where malignancy is suspected. A combination of medical and surgical treatment at times has been used.

SUMMARY

Nasal polyps occur in many diseases. Classically, the association of asthma, chronic sinusitis, and aspirin intolerance frequently occurs as a syndrome. Other associated diseases are Young's syndrome, cystic fibrosis, Kartagener's syndrome, Churg–Strauss syndrome, and allergic fungal sinusitis. Children 16 yr or younger with nasal polyps should be evaluated for cystic fibrosis.

Nasal polyps are frequently bilateral, multiple, freely movable, pale gray in color, and arise from the middle meatus of the nose. Histologically, they classically have pseudostratified ciliated columnar epithelium, thickening of the epithelial basement membrane, high stromal eosinophil count, mucin with neutral pH, few glands, and essentially no nerve endings. Cells consist of a mixture of lymphocytes, plasma cells, and eosinophils. Polyps from patients with Young's syndrome, Kartagener's syndrome, and cystic fibrosis predominantly have neutrophils with insignificant eosinophils. Chemical mediators found in nasal polyps are as follows: histamine, serotonin, leukotrienes ([SRS-A or LTC_4, LTD_4, LTE_4], LTB_4), ECF-A, norepinephrine, kinins, TAME-esterase, and possibly PGD_2. There is more histamine in nasal polyps than in normal nasal mucosa, and norepinephrine is present in greater concentration in the base of nasal polyps than in normal nasal mucosa. The concentrations of IgA and IgE and, in some cases, IgG and IgM are greater in polyp fluid than in serum. The pathogenic mechanism of nasal polyps at this time is unknown. Recent evidence suggests that a rupture of epithelial layer and basement membrane occurs, allowing the polyp to emerge. This rupture may be associated with chronic infection *(45)* or toxic effect of the eosinophils. IgE-mediated disease is not the cause of nasal polyps, but, when present may contribute to episodes of exacerbation. Upper respiratory infections also may cause exacerbations. Despite medical or surgical management, a significant number of nasal polyps are recurrent especially in those patients with the bronchospastic form of aspirin sensitivity. For treatment, systemic corticosteroids are usually tried before surgical polypectomy. Other modes of treatment include topical nasal steroids, long-term antibiotics, decongestants, allergy avoidance and treatment. Surgical polypectomy does not increase the risk of developing asthma or making asthma worse. The association of the tetrad of nasal polyps, asthma, aspirin intolerance, and chronic rhinosinusitis has been described in detail.

REFERENCES

1. Widal MF, Abram P, Lermoyez J. Anaphylaxie et idiosyndraise. Presse Med 1922;22:191.
2. Settipane GA. Landmark commentary: history of aspirin intolerance. Allergy Proc 1990;11:251,252.
3. Davidson AE, Miller DS, Settipane RJ, Ricci AR, Klein DE, Settipane GA. Delayed nasal mucociliary clearance in patients with nonallergic rhinitis and nasal eosinophilia. Allergy Proc 1991;12(no. 6):402.
4. Wentges RTR. Edward Woakes: the history of an eponym. J Laryngol Otol 1972;86:501–512.
5. Atzelius BA. Disorders of ciliary motility. Hosp Pract 1986;21:73–80.
6. Rossman CM, Lee RM, Forrest JB, Newhouse MT. Nasal canary ultrastructure and function in patients with primary ciliary dyskinesia compared with that in normal subjects and in subjects with various respiratory diseases. Am Rev Respir Dis 1984;129:161–167.
7. Schanker HM, Rajfer J, Saxon A. Recurrent respiratory disease, azoospermia, and nasal polyposis. Arch Intern Med 1985;145:2201–2203.
8. Handelsman DJ, Conway AJ, Boylan LM, Turtle JR. Young's syndrome. Obstructive azoospermia and chronic sinopulmonary infections. N Engl J Med 1984;310:3–9.
9. Schwietz LA, Gourley DS. Allergic fungal sinusitis. Allergy Proc 1992;13:3–6.
10. Vancil ME. A historical survey of treatments for nasal polyposis. Laryngoscope 1969;79:435–445.
11. Settipane GA, Chafee FH. Nasal polyps in asthma and rhinitis: a review of 6,037 patients. J Allergy Clin Immunol 1977;59:17–21.
12. Chafee FH, Settipane GA. Aspirin intolerance: I. Frequency in an allergic population. J Allergy Clin Immunol 1974;53:193–199.
13. Settipane GA, Chafee FH, Klein DE. Aspirin Intolerance: II. A prospective study in an atopic and normal population. J Allergy Clin Immunol 1974;53:200–204.
14. Slavin RG, Linford P, Friedman WH. Sinusitis and bronchial asthma. J Allergy Clin Immunol 1982;69(part 2):102.
15. Lanoff G, Daddono A, Johnson E. Nasal polyps in children: a ten-year study. Ann Allergy 1973;31:551–554.
16. Settipane GA, ed. In: Rhinitis, 2nd ed., Providence: Oceanside Publications, 1992; pp. 175,176.
17. Ballantyne J. The nose. In: Grooves J, ed. Scott Brown's Diseases of the Ear, Nose and Throat, 3rd ed. Philadelphia: JB Lippincott, 1971; p. 179.
18. Oppenheimer EH, Rosenstein BJ. Differential pathology of nasal polyps in cystic fibrosis and atopy. Lab Invest 1979;40:445–449.
19. Wladislavosky-Wasserman P, Kern EB, Holley KE, Gleich GJ. Epithelial damage is commonly seen in nasal polyps. J Allergy Clan Immunol 1982;69(part 2):148.
20. Busuttil A. Dysplastic epithelial changes in nasal polyps. Ann Otol Rhinol Laryngol 1978;87:416–420.
21. Settipane GA, ed. Rhinitis, 1st ed., Providence: NER Allergy Proc, 1984; p. 152.
22. MacKay DN. Antibiotic treatment of rhinitis and sinusitis. Am J Rhinol 1987;1:83–85.
23. Pelletier G, Hebert J, Bedard PM, Salari H, Borgeat P. Profile of leukotrienes and histamine from human nasal polyps. J Allergy Clin Immunol 1986;77(part 2):177 (abstract).
24. Bumsted RM, El-Ackad T, Smith JM, Brody MJ. Histamine, norepinephrine and serotonin content of nasal polyps. Laryngoscope 1979;89:832–843.
25. Kaliner M, Wasserman SI, Austen KF. Immunologic release of chemical mediators from human nasal polyps. N Engl J Med 1973;289:277–281.
26. Chandra RK, Abrol BM. Immunopathology of nasal polypi. J Laryngol Otol 1974;88:1019–1024.
27. Berdal P. Serologic investigations on the edema fluid from nasal polyps. J Allergy 1952;23:11–14.
28. Mygind N, ed. Nasal polyps. In: Nasal Allergy, 2nd ed., Oxford, London: Blackwell Scientific, 1979; pp. 233–238.
29. Gray L. Deviated nasal septum. III. Its influence on the physiology and disease of the nose and ear. J Laryngol 1967;81:953–986.
30. Tos M, Mogensen C. Density of mucous glands in normal adult nasal septum. Arch Otorhinolaryngol 1977; 215:101.
31. Bernstein JM, Cropp JA, Nathanson I, Yankaskas JR. Bioelectric properties of cultured human nasal polypi and turbinate epithelial cells. Am J Rhinol 1990;4(no. 2):45–49.
31a. Tos M. The pathogenetic theories on formation of nasal polyps. Am J Rhinol 1990;4:51–56.
32. Downing ET, Braman S, Settipane GA. Bronchial reactivity in patients with nasal polyps before and after polypectomy. J Allergy Clin Immunol 1982;69(part 2):102.

33. Miles-Lawrence R, Kaplan M, Chang K. Methacholine sensitivity in nasal polyposis and the effects of polypectomy. J Allergy Clin Immunol 1982;69 (part 2):102.

34. Connell JT. Nasal disease. N Engl Soc Allergy Proc 1982;3:389–396.

35. Settipane GA. Aspirin intolerance presenting as chronic rhinitis. R I Med J 1980;63:63–65.

36. Whiteside TL, Rabin BS, Zetterberg J, Criep L. The presence of IgE on the surface of lymphocytes in nasal polyps. J Allergy Clin Immunol 1975;55:186–194.

37. Settipane GA, Klein DE, Lekas MD. Asthma and nasal polyps. In: Myers E, ed., New Dimensions in Otorhinolaryngology, Head and Neck Surgery. Amsterdam: Excerpta Medica, 1987; pp. 499,500.

38. Settipane GA, Pudupakkam RK. Aspirin intolerance. III. Subtypes, familial occurrence and cross-reactivity with tartrazine. J Allergy Clin Immunol 1975;56:215–221.

39. Simon R, Pleskow W, Kaliner M, Wasserman S. Plasma mediator studies in aspirin sensitive asthma. J Allergy Clin Immunol 1983;71(part 2):146(abstract).

40. Settipane GA. Nasal polyposis. N Engl Soc Allergy Proc 1982;3:497–504.

41. McCleve D, Gatos L, Goldstein J, Slivers S. Corticosteroid injections of the nasal turbinates: past experience and precautions. ORL J Otorhinolaryngol Related Specialties 1978;86:851–857.

42. Mabry RL. Visual loss after intranasal corticosteroid injection. Arch Otolaryngol 1981;107:484–486.

43. Settipane GA. Nasal polyps: epidemiology, pathology, immunology and treatment. Am J Rhinol 1987;1:119–126.

44. Settipane GA, Klein DE, Settipane RJ. Nasal polyps, state of the art. Rhinology 1991;11:33–36.

45. Norlander T, Fukami M, Westrin KM, Stierna P, Carlsog B. Formation of mucosal polyps in the nasal and maxillary sinus cavities by infection. Otolaryngol H, S Surg. 1993;109:522–529.

15   Sinusitis and Asthma

Associations, Influences, and Principles of Management

Georges M. Halpern, MD *and Gary A. Incaudo,* MD

CONTENTS

Chronic nocturnal cough, or worsening of asthma may be associated with sinusitis. Until proven otherwise, the treatment of sinusitis should be considered as first-line intervention.

A physiologic unity between the upper and lower airway of humans has been recognized throughout the 20th century. A number of studies have addressed and described a relationship between the inflammatory diseases occurring in the upper respiratory tract, especially sinusitis, and its consequences in the thoracic airways. At the beginning of this century, Bullen *(1)*, Gottlieb *(2)*, and Weille *(3)* found coexistent sinusitis in 20–70% of a large number of adult asthmatics. After reviewing 1074 cases of asthma, Rackemann and Tobey in 1929 wrote that "lesions in the nose and sinuses…may develop from the same fundamental cause as the asthma itself" *(4)*. More recent studies have found that 50–70% of children and adults with asthma have radiographic evidence of sinusitis *(5,6)*.

Schwartz et al. examined the sinus radiographs of 217 patients with a flare-up of asthma symptoms and found abnormal sinus radiographs in 47%, as compared with 29% of patients with rhinitis as their sole complaints *(7)*. Fuller et al. have indicated that 75% of patients admitted to Los Angeles Children's Hospital for status asthmatics had abnormal sinus radiographs *(8)*. The majority of evidence revolves around the impressive coincidence of these two entities, as well as the observations that asthma improves, sometimes dramatically, after medical or surgical management of coexisting sinusitis *(9–11)*. Despite these observations, there remains limited conclusive information whether upper respiratory tract inflammation and sinusitis specifically contribute to the pathogenesis of asthma, or whether the two problems simply "coexist" because of a common pathogenesis.

Interruption of the normal functioning of the upper airway has been shown to influence reactivity of the lower airway. The nose is our most sophisticated "air conditioner." It filters the inspired air and captures large particles by the hairs within the nostrils, whereas other noxious substances are trapped in the mucus. If nasal obstruction occurs, an increased burden of allergens and/or irritants will be delivered to the lower airways with hyperresponsiveness as a potential outcome. The nose heats and humidifies the air through the highly vascularized mucosa of the turbinates and septum. If the nose is blocked, cooler, drier air will be delivered to the lungs, which can trigger or potentiate exercise-induced asthma in the susceptible host.

Furthermore, it has been shown that chemical or mechanical irritation of the nose can induce bronchoconstriction. Exactly how and to what extent such an excitory system occurs is unknown, and a discussion of such postulates is beyond the scope of this chapter. This phenomenon appears to be more severe in patients with coexisting allergic rhinitis and asthma (12). Kaufman et al. have demonstrated a beneficial effect from trigeminal resection when reflex bronchospasm is induced by nasal and nasopharyngeal irritation (13). Observations such as these appear to confirm Sluder's original hypothesis in 1919 of the existence of a nasal-bronchial reflex in humans (14). The theory of a nasobronchial reflex contends that reflex bronchospasm occurs via stimulation of neural fibers in the nasal mucosa, which then triggers a trigeminal-afferent-vagal efferent neural arc (15).

Considerable evidence has been published demonstrating an increase in lower airway responsiveness in nasal hypersensitivity diseases. Using a ragweed bronchial inhalation challenge model, there exists considerable overlap in lower airway hyperresponsiveness between ragweed allergic patients with asthma and those with allergic rhinitis alone (16). Using increased sensitivity to methacholine or hyperventilation as a measure of more nonspecific bronchial hyperresponsiveness, a significant percentage of patients with rhinitis alone can be shown to be reactive in a range typically seen among asthmatics (17). Individuals with nasal polyps will have an estimated 25–30% risk of ultimately developing asthma (18). Attempts at demonstrating bronchial hyperreactivity with methacholine challenge in nasal polyposis have, however, been inconclusive (19,20). Nevertheless, the incidence of asthma appears to increase steadily as one progresses from nasal polyposis to associated rhinosinusitis to a history of acetylsalicylic acid (ASA) intolerance (ASA hypersensitivity tetrad). Although none of these studies illustrate a common

mechanism whereby diseases of the nose and sinus will induce asthma, they do emphasize the need to look at the upper and lower airway as systems capable of being influenced by one another.

POSTULATED MECHANISMS EXPLAINING THE RELATIONSHIP BETWEEN SINUSITIS AND ASTHMA

In 1925, Gottlieb postulated four possible mechanisms whereby inflammation of the sinuses could aggravate bronchospasm (2):

1. Mucopurulent postnasal drainage leading to continuous infection of the trachea and bronchi;
2. Absorption of toxic products from retained purulent material in the sinuses triggering an immunologically mediated asthmatic reaction;
3. Sinusitis inducing nasal obstruction, which, in turn, leads to mouth breathing of cold, dry air inducing bronchospasm; and
4. Nerve reflex bronchospasm via irritation of the nasal ganglion.

Despite our improved knowledge of the physiology and immunology of the naso-sino-bronchial system, these concepts, born almost three-quarters of a century ago, remain the fundamental postulates upon which our understanding of the relationship between sinusitis and asthma stands.

Aspiration of Infected Material

Bardin and colleagues attempted to mimic the aspiration postulate in asthmatics with sinusitis (21). They instilled a radionuclide in the maxillary sinus of four patients with maxillary sinusitis, and nine patients with sinusitis and asthma during needle puncture of the sinus. In all patients, the radionuclide could be demonstrated in the nasopharynx, sinus, and gastrointestinal tract over the next 24 h, but not in the lower airways. This negative study suggests that aspiration is not a factor in the coexistence of asthma and sinusitis.

Eosinophils

Eosinophils have unique biologic features that allow them to be major contributors to the inflammatory process: the preformed granule-associated proteins, including eosinophil peroxidase, major basic protein, cationic protein, and eosinophil-derived neurotoxin, have been identified. Major basic protein is most relevant and is capable of

Table 1
Tissue Eosinophilia in 26 Patients with Chronic Sinusitis

Group 1	Chronic sinusitis and bronchial asthma ($n = 5$)	Marked in all
Group 2	Chronic sinusitis, bronchial asthma, and allergic rhinitis ($n = 8$)	Marked in all
Group 3	Chronic sinusitis and allergic rhinitis ($n = 7$)	Marked in 6
Group 4	Chronic sinusitis ($n = 6$)	Marked in 0

Adapted from ref. 23.

contributing to mucosal injury. Activated eosinophils also generate other mediators, including leukotriene C4. In addition, eosinophils can express a release of a variety of proinflammatory cytokines, e.g., IL-1, IL-3, IL-5, and GMCSF. IL-5 has important properties in relation to the eosinophil, which may explain why airway eosinophils are phenotypically distinct from those found in circulation. Airway eosinophils are functionally upregulated and more likely to cause mucosal injury. They release more superoxide, express more activation markers and adhesion proteins, and survive longer. Eosinophils interact with a number of factors as they migrate from the circulation to the airway or sinuses. These factors include endothelial adhesion proteins, chemotactic factors, primers (such as platelet-activating factor), and cytokines (such as interleukins, granulocyte macrophage-colony stimulating factor, and tumor necrosis factor). This cellular interaction, especially with IL-5, contributes definitive changes in the eosinophils. The importance of both paracrine and autocrine interaction of eosinophils with cytokines is intriguing. Not only do eosinophils respond to cytokines generated by other cells (paracrine), but they may also produce their own cytokines (autocrine), resulting in enhanced eosinophil functions that can occur through a number of avenues.

Eosinophils have long been associated with allergic rhinitis and allergic and nonallergic forms of asthma, but the role of the eosinophil in respiratory disease in incompletely understood. Analysis of late-phase responses to nasal allergen challenge has shown a mixed inflammatory cell influx in which the eosinophil predominates (22). Analysis of nasal lavage fluids from allergens that provoked immediate and late-phase reactions revealed that the eosinophil granule major basic protein (MBP) was elevated in both phases. Significant increases in the concentrations of the eosinophil-derived neurotoxin (EDN) also occurred during the late anti-

genic response, and these correlated with the levels of MBP. The cumulative late-phase increase in MBP correlated closely with the total influx of eosinophils. The oral pretreatment with corticosteroids significantly reduced the mean of each subject's peak late-phase concentration of both MBP and EDN. In a fashion strikingly similar to the lung, this study showed that eosinophilia is present during the late-phase reaction, that eosinophil degranulation occurs during both the immediate and the late response, and that nasal eosinophilia and the release of eosinophil granule proteins are suppressed by glucocorticoid administration.

The role of eosinophil in chronic inflammatory disease of the paranasal sinuses has been investigated with sinus tissue from patients who were subjected to surgery for chronic sinusitis (23). Sinus tissue from patients with sinusitis who also had chronic asthma and/or allergic rhinitis was found to be extensively infiltrated with eosinophils. Conversely, sinus tissues from patients with chronic sinusitis alone with no evidence of allergy or asthma revealed no eosinophils (Table 1). Immunofluorescent studies demonstrated an association between the presence of extracellular deposition of MBP and damage to sinus mucosa. The histopathology of the paranasal respiratory epithelium was similar to the one described in bronchial asthma. Eosinophils seem to act as effector cells in chronic inflammatory disease in paranasal respiratory epithelium. Sinus disease in patients with asthma may well be caused by the same mechanisms that cause damage to bronchial epithelium. These authors have also described the presence of Creola bodies (clusters of exfoliated respiratory epithelial cells), Charcot-Leyden crystals (cellular eosinophil lysophospholipase), and mucous plugs in the paranasal airways. The factors that regulate the eosinophil in the sinuses affect the eosinophil in the lower airways. A number of factors, e.g., eosinophil-activating factors derived from mast cells,

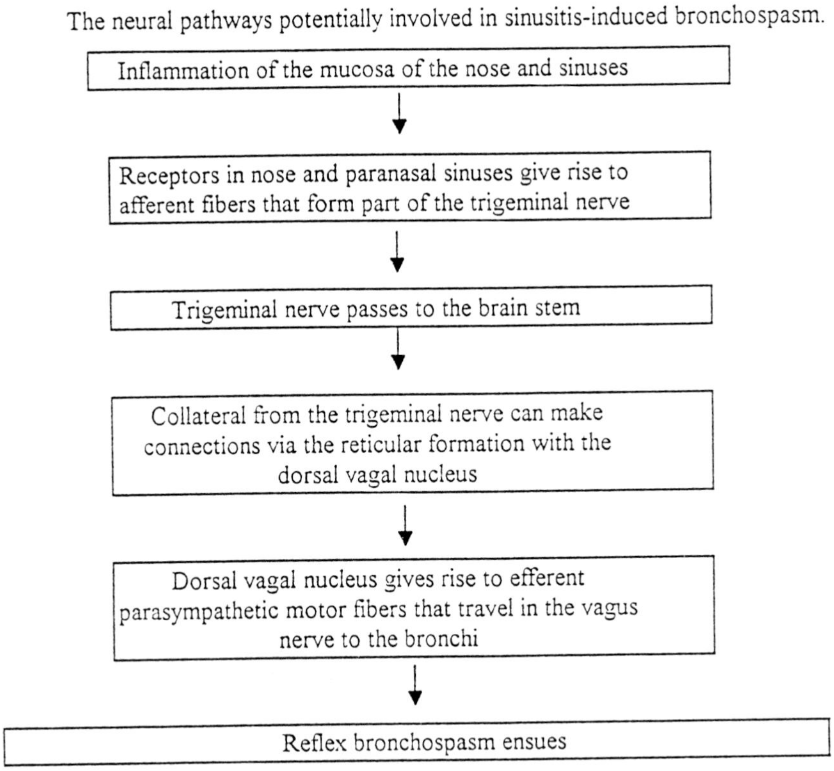

The neural pathways potentially involved in sinusitis-induced bronchospasm.

Fig. 1. The neural pathways potentially involved in sinusitis-induced bronchospasm.

monocytes, and T-lymphocytes, regulate whether this process occurs in an individual patient.

In summary, the histopathology of the paranasal respiratory epithelium in chronic sinus disease appears similar to that described in bronchial asthma. The association between eosinophilic infiltration and the release of preformed eosinophilic-derived proteins, especially MBP, onto the respiratory epithelium are dramatic and in keeping with the role for the eosinophil as an effector of damage in both the upper and lower airways.

Other Inflammatory Mediators

Stone et al. measured inflammatory mediators, leukotrienes, prostaglandin D2, and histamine in maxillary sinus lavage fluid obtained during surgery for chronic sinusitis (24). They compared the results of the these lavage to levels of mediators in nasal lavage fluid from a group of atopic rhinitis subjects. The levels of leukotrienes (mostly), histamine, and PGD2 in sinus fluid were significantly elevated over the control nasal lavage fluid, and were in the range associated with irritant receptor stimulation and local inflammation.

Nasal Sinus Bronchial Reflex

Stimulation of neural receptors in the sinuses can activate the afferent fibers that form part of the trigeminal nerve. Collaterals from the trigeminal nerve fibers enter the reticular formation where connection is made with the dorsal vagal nucleus. Parasympathetic fibers then proceed to the bronchial musculature causing bronchospasm. The surgical interruption of the vagus nerve in animals and in some patients has been demonstrated to preclude a change in airway resistance following a stimulus of the upper airway (25). This is summarized in Fig. 1.

The concepts of neurogenic inflammation and axonal reflex as proposed by Barnes may represent a scheme explaining the common association between rhinosinusitis and asthma in humans (26). In this scheme, inhaled environmental irritants or mediators of an allergenic response stimulate the sensory nonmyelinated C-fibers in the respiratory tract, causing an antidromic release of neuropeptides, such as substance P, neurokinins, and calcitonin gene-related peptide, as well as trigger cholinergic reflex-mediated effects. The neuropeptides may additionally cause further airway smooth muscle contraction, production of mucus, edema, and release of inflammatory and proinflammatory mediators from various inflammatory cells, resulting in an amplification response. The degradation of the released tachykinin neuropeptides may then be depressed owing to disruption of airway epithelium membranes to which the neutral endopeptidases are normally bound. Chronic respiratory disease may eventually result with continued stimulation. Although such theories as these may explain the common linkage between diseases of the upper and lower airways, they do not confirm or deny that eradication of inflammation in one portion of the airway will influence the expression of disease in another part of the airway.

Clinical studies have been able to verify the possible existence of an axonal reflex-mediated and/or a neurogenic inflammatory-mediated relationship between the upper and lower airways. Sluder first demonstrated in 1919 that with direct stimulation of the mucosa in the region of the sphenoid sinus, asthma can be worsened (14). Fifty years later, Kaufman and Wright placed silica particles on the nasal mucosa for 150 s and demonstrated a significant increase in measured airway resistance in human subjects without asthma (27). Parasympathetic blockade with atropine abrogated the response. Yan and Salome demonstrated a >20% fall in FEV1 in 50% of asthmatic subjects given intranasal histamine at a dosage deemed too small to have a systemic effect. The fall in FEV1 was independent of the degree of bronchial hyperreactivity demonstrated by histamine challenge (28). Using a single cold nasal stimulus, Nolte and Berger initiated an increase in lower airway resistance that could be blocked by prior intrabronchial application of a parasympatholytic agent (29).

An increase in lower airways responsiveness associated with sinusitis has also been demonstrated in a rabbit model. Brugman et al. studied sterile maxillary sinusitis in the rabbit induced by the chemotactic complement fragment C5a des arg (30). The inflammation induced a significant increase in airway responsiveness to histamine. Interestingly, when sinus inflammation was established, but the passage of fluid to the lower airways was prevented, there was no change in airway responsiveness. This observation suggests that the passage of cells or cell products to the lungs is necessary in this model for airway hyperrespon-

siveness to occur and not simply an axonal neurogenic reflex.

Other clinical studies have questioned the existence of a nasobronchial reflex in humans. Hoehne et al. and Rosenberg et al., using nasal challenges with ragweed pollen or histamine, failed to induce a drop in FEV1 in allergic subjects (31,32). Furthermore, Schumacher et al, in a placebo-controlled, double-blind study, failed to induce a nasobronchial reflex utilizing both histamine and antigen in nasal challenge with normal subjects and subjects with stable asthma and allergic rhinitis (33). The inconsistencies of clinical studies keep open the question of what role a nasobronchial reflex may have in asthma. Nevertheless, the concepts of neurogenic inflammation and axonal reflex-mediated mechanisms remain the most viable explanations of the close clinical association between rhinosinusitis and asthma.

Diminished Adrenergic Responsiveness

Szentivanyi suggested that asthmatics have an autonomic nervous system imbalance owing to an inherent adrenergic blockade (34). Evidence supports diminished adrenergic function from both in vitro and in vivo studies. Busse utilized lysosomal release from neutrophils as a model of cellular adrenergic responsiveness; responsiveness to isoproterenol from asthmatics during upper respiratory infections demonstrated decreased response, suggesting that respiratory viruses alter the inhibitory response to β-agonists, which normally prevents mediator secretion (35). This β-blockade induced by viruses results in increased release of granulocyte lysosomal products and major local inflammation. Sinusitis seems to be associated with a decrease in β-adrenergic reactivity. Data from Friedman et al. support this theory (6). Whereas prebronchodilator pulmonary function did not change significantly following antibiotic therapy in their study group, there was a significant improvement in response to bronchodilators, suggesting an enhanced β-adrenergic responsiveness with eradication of bacterial sinusitis.

THE CLINICAL ASSOCIATION BETWEEN SINUSITIS AND ASTHMA

Some investigators believe that asthma can be triggered by sinusitis, and eradication of the sinusitis will reduce or remove the need for bronchodilators. Others believe that asthma and sinusitis are both manifestations of an underlying disease, either infection in two locations within the same respiratory tract or allergic inflammation in both areas, the latter one being ultimately superinfected. Slavin should be given credit for reviving the recent interest in this subject. Phipatanakul and Slavin reported five nonatopic asthmatic patients whose asthma improved dramatically after the diagnosis and treatment of concurrent paranasal sinus diseased (39). In 1980, he and his coworkers additionally studied 15 adult patients with asthma and sinusitis; two were atopic, four were aspirin sensitive, and nine had nasal polyps (36). Of interest was the general absence of clinical signs of purulent sinus disease. There was a marked improvement of asthmatic symptoms after medical or surgical treatment of the sinus disease. A subsequent report in 1982 described subjective asthmatic improvement in 85% of 33 patients with treatment of their sinus diseased (37). Fifteen of 18 corticosteroid-dependent asthmatics were able to reduce or eliminate their steroid medication during the course of sinusitis treatment.

It has been generally unclear to what extent infections of the paranasal sinuses are involved in the observed radiographic abnormalities in asthmatics or to what extent these findings represent noninfectious inflammatory changes characteristic of asthma (38). Berman and Matheson, in a study involving nasal antral puncture, lavage, and culture of sinus fluid contents in asthmatic patients, confirmed the presence of infection in a significant number of subjects (20%), but the frequency was considerably less than the number with abnormal sinus radiographs (40%) (41a). However, organisms, such as mycoplasma or viruses, could have been missed in such studies and have been reported as causative agents in sinusitis. A more recent study evaluated the occurrence of acute sinus abnormalities during clinical exacerbations of asthma by using sinus radiographs and antral puncture analysis (39). An abnormal finding in any paranasal sinus was detected in 87% (130 of 149) of hospital admissions, and the yield of maxillary aspirate was purulent or mucopurulent in 60% (42 of 70) of aspirates. A positive bacteriological culture was obtained from 23 aspirates, and a virus was detected in 15 (7 aspirates were positive for both a virus and bacteria). Unfortunately, only those patients with clinical or radiographic evidence of sinusitis

Table 2
Disease Characteristics Before and After Treatment
for Sinusitis in 48 Children with Asthma

Characteristic	Before	After
Cough	100%	29%
Wheeze	100%	15%
Normal PFT	0	67%
Bronchodilator treatment	100%	21%

Adapted from ref. 10.

underwent antral puncture in this study, but the numbers remain impressive nevertheless.

The association between sinusitis and asthma has been noted with consistent frequency in children (40). Rachelefsky et al. have demonstrated that sinusitis and lower airway hyperreactivity can be improved, mostly in the asthmatic state, when these children receive appropriate medical treatment for their sinusitis (10). Table 2 summarizes the disease characteristics before and after treatment for sinusitis in 48 children with hyperreactivity airway disease. Seven children needed sinus lavage, whereas the rest received only appropriate medical therapy. Seventy-nine percent of these children were able to discontinue bronchodilators when their sinusitis was treated. Pulmonary function tests normalized in 67% of those with pretreatment abnormalities. The treatment included antibiotics and oral or topical decongestants. Similar results were reported by Friedman et al. (6). These authors described seven of eight patients with exacerbation of asthma and coexistent sinusitis whose asthma improved clinically after antibiotic treatment for 14–28 d. Pulmonary function tests in five of the eight patients also improved significantly. Zimmerman et al. have found, like other authors, that the incidence of sinus radiographic abnormalities is greater in children with asthma compared to controls with dental problems (31% of 138 patients with asthma vs 0 of 50 controls) (41). However, the abnormal appearance of the sinus radiograph appeared to be the same whether the asthma was mild, moderate, or severe, bringing into question the clinical relevance of the radiographic findings.

MICROBIOLOGY OF THE UPPER AND LOWER RESPIRATORY TRACT

The microbiology of sinusitis has been described in detail elsewhere in this text. The organisms most commonly seen are remarkably consistent with

Haemophilus influenzae, Streptococcus pneumoniae, and *Moraxella catarrhalis* predominating. It is interesting to note that, in community-acquired adult lower respiratory tract infections, the same spectrum of pathogens are found. Macfarlane et al. in a prospective study of adult lower respiratory tract infections in a six-partner general practice in England found that *S. pneumoniae, H. influenzae,* and *M. catarrhalis* comprised over 80% of the pathogens detected *(42).* Such a commonness of pathogens raises the possibility that antimicrobial therapy for sinusitis may also be affecting a bacterial infection of the lower respiratory tract, which could be the true exacerbating feature of a coexisting asthma.

PRINCIPLES OF DIAGNOSIS AND MANAGEMENT

Although the cause-and-effect relationship between sinusitis and asthma remains obscure, the acknowledged frequent coexistence of these two medical problems and the known physiological ties between the upper and lower airways demand that the examining physician evaluate and manage both sinusitis and asthma at the same time. The evaluation of the patient should focus on his/her general condition and history of symptoms suggestive of sinusitis and asthma. This evaluation should be comprehensive and is beyond the scope of this chapter. However, certain points are worthy of emphasis.

History

The history should focus on diseases with known associations between the upper and lower airways, such as bronchiectasis (ciliary dyskinesis or Kartagener's syndrome), cystic fibrosis, immunodeficiency disorders, and allergy. Both personal and family histories of environmentally triggered rhinitis, cough, wheeze, and/or atopic dermatitis are particularly helpful. The presence of a poor sense of smell or absence of this sense (associated with chronic sinusitis and/or nasal polyposis) or ASA intolerance should be sought. The history of nasal obstruction with or without nasal purulence should always alert the examining physician to the possibility of coexisting active sinus disease. A helpful question to ask is: "Are your asthma flare-ups commonly preceded by nasal congestion with mucous purulence?"

It is common for an asthmatic patient, particularly in childhood, to present with a persistent cough unresponsive to bronchodilator, anti-inflammatory, or brief antibiotic therapy. The cough is typically moist, present both day and night, but more common during the day, and rarely disturbing of sleep especially if asthma therapy is ongoing. There may or may not be, in such a circumstance, pulmonary function evidence of concurrent bronchospasm. However, for a patient with known asthma, the presence of a predominantly daytime rather than a nighttime cough would be unusual for asthma alone. This temporal point suggests that sinus disease may be the aggravating feature of pulmonary instability.

Physical Examination

Physical examination findings in sinus disease have been covered elsewhere in this text. However, it deserves to be emphasized that the physician should examine the upper airway of every asthmatic patient for evidence of nasal turbinate erythema, nasal polyposis, and purulent nasal or posterior pharyngeal secretions. The chest exam can also be suggestive of potential sinusitis complication. If the asthmatic patient is complaining of aggravated symptoms, but the chest exam reveals mostly rhonchi with little or no wheezing or air-flow obstruction, sinusitis should be suspected as the aggravant. This set of physical finding is particularly common in children and especially if the increasing pulmonary complaint is following an upper respiratory infection (URI). Under these circumstances, abrupt stabilization of the pulmonary complaints can often be best achieved with a 2-wk course of a broad-spectrum antibiotic rather than specifically increasing the patient's asthma therapy.

Laboratory Studies

In addition to a complete and comprehensive physical examination, some laboratory tests are occasionally useful. A complete blood count with differential, quantitative immunoglobulins, including IgG subclasses and IgE, and allergy skin tests or selected radioallergosorbent (RAST) tests should be requested in specific patients depending on the differential diagnosis derived from the history and physical findings.

The statistical studies previously discussed suggest that radiographs of the paranasal sinuses are an essential part of the evaluation of all patients with chronic asthma. As mentioned elsewhere in this text, a four-slice coronal CT scan is the most cost-effective procedure to confirm the presence of sinus disease. However, the mere presence of radiographic abnormalities of the paranasal sinuses does not establish a cause-and-effect relationship with coexisting asthma.

Principles of Management

Outcome studies of sinusitis therapy described earlier have been supportive of the concept that coexisting asthma will simultaneously improve when sinusitis is stabilized. However, there are currently no clinical criteria to predict accurately which asthmatic patient with radiographic abnormalities of the paranasal sinuses will improve with a sinusitis treatment regimen. The ultimate test in any given asthmatic patient will be to initiate sinusitis treatment when the examining physician suspects contributing sinus disease and observe the outcome. This will usually require a 14–21 d course of a broad-spectrum antibiotic accompanied by topical nasal steroids and decongestants, either orally or topically. Just as asthmatics vary with respect to their bronchodilating and anti-inflammatory needs, they will commonly vary as to the influence of sinusitis treatment on their asthma stability. It has been our experience that the aggressive treatment of purulent sinus disease is nearly universally helpful as a stabilizing factor in coexisting asthma. The more difficult decision arises when there are radiographic abnormalities of the sinuses and no signs or symptoms of purulent sinusitis. However, the studies of Slaven, Rachelefsky, Friedman, and others already discussed suggest that in the clinical setting of persistent or aggravated asthma symptoms and radiographic evidence of sinus disease, with or without clinical purulence, a medical trial of sinusitis therapy is warranted.

As has been discussed elsewhere in this text, the surgical management of sinusitis is typically undertaken when the sinusitis is severe, persistent, or refractory to medical treatment. Encouraging results have been reported. Mings et al. demonstrated a 65% improvement in asthma symptoms over 2 yr in patients surgically treated for sinus disease with bilateral intranasal sphenoethmoidectomy. Furthermore, these authors found that patients who experienced improvement over the 2-yr period commonly continued their improvement throughout a 5-yr observation period *(43)*. Friedman et al. described the surgical findings and outcomes of 50 nonatopic asthmatics who under-

went intranasal sphenoethmoidectomy for medically refractory sinus disease *(44)*. Of the 50 patients, reduction or elimination of sinusitis, relief of upper airway obstruction, and improvement in asthma occurred in 45. Twenty-six of 28 steroid-dependent patients were able to reduce or discontinue their systemic steroids following the surgical procedure. Jankowski et al. described 50 asthmatic patients with sinusitis, 30 of whom had nasal polyps and 12 were ASA-intolerant *(45)*. Ninety-one percent improved following a radical endoscopic intranasal ethmoidectomy with reference to a decrease in the frequency of attacks, decrease in respiratory difficulty subjectively, less need for asthma medications including oral corticosteroids, and a marked improvement in pulmonary function.

Not all authors have reported regularly favorable results from sinus surgery in asthmatic patients. Furthermore, the type of sinus surgery undertaken has been reported to have an influence on asthma and its evolution. Samter and Lederer; Macauley; and Moloney and Coluns observed the onset of the first attack of asthma after polypectomy in several series of patients *(18,46,47)*. Siegel et al. described a series of 61 patients with intrinsic asthma who, after limited sinus surgery, experienced no improvement or deterioration in 69% *(48)*. Of 18 patients with aspirin hypersensitivity triad, Schenck noted that six patients experienced an exacerbation of asthma following polypectomy and only five were felt to be improved *(49)*. Aspirin hypersensitivity asthmatics continued to fare poorly or experience no benefit from nasal polypectomy in studies by Brown et al. and Englisch. In over 200 asthmatics with ASA intolerance, polypectomy resulted in either no change in up to 80% or exacerbation of asthma in 5–10% *(50,51)*. The exact reason why simple polypectomy is so commonly associated with either no change or a worsening of asthma in contrast to more encouraging results from radical ethmoidectomy or sphenoethmoidectomy is unclear.

UNIQUE ASSOCIATIONS OF SINUSITIS AND ASTHMA

Cystic Fibrosis

The association of cystic fibrosis with chronic sinusitis and nasal polyposis is discussed elsewhere in this text. Chronic refractory sinusitis has been controlled in patients with cystic fibrosis by endoscopic surgery and serial microbial lavage (ESSAL) with a positive influence on pulmonary stability. Moss and King recently reported the results of the ESSAL approach in 32 patients when compared to those of conventional sinus surgery without serial antimicrobial lavage in 19 patients *(52)*. Follow-up examinations at least 1 yr following surgery were available in all but one patient. The groups were similar demographically and clinically, including presence of nasal polyposis in 34 and 42%, respectively. The ESSAL group had fewer operations per patients ($p < 0.0001$), sinus cavities entered by palpation ($p = 0.0004$), radical Caldwell-Luc procedures ($p = 0.016$), and repeat surgery ($p = 0.0001$), including in those presenting with nasal polyposis ($p = 0.0009$). Two-year repeat surgery rate was cut from 72 to 22%. Concordance between sinus and lower respiratory tract colonization was 83%, and concordance of uncommon pathogens was also found suggesting homogeneity of bacterial colonization of the respiratory tract. This ESSAL approach to treatment of sinusitis results in a dramatic reduction in recurrent sinus disease requiring surgery for at least a 2-yr follow-up period.

The Aspirin Hypersensitivity Tetrad—Nasal Polyposis–Sinusitis–Asthma–ASA Intolerance

ASA was first synthesized in 1853 by the German scientist von Gerhardt, and the clinical application of ASA in rheumatic fever was suggested in Europe in 1899. In 1911, 1 yr after ASA was released for use in the US, the first report of a serious respiratory reaction appeared in the *Journal of the American Medical Association*. G. Burton Gilbert described the case of a woman, with a history of asthma, who developed pruritis, angioedema, and dyspnea from the ingestion of 5 grains of ASA. The first description of the association between nasosinus polyposis and aspirin-induced asthma was by Widal et al. in 1922, and in most countries, this triad is called the "Fernand Widal Triad" *(53)*. Two distinct clinical syndromes of ASA intolerance had emerged. One syndrome was primarily dermatologic, involving an urticarial and angioedematous response. The other syndrome was respiratory, involving primarily the aggravation of a pre-existing asthmatic state, although some upper respiratory symptoms were a common accompaniment. As this association was recognized more fre-

quently, Samter and Beers published a typical description of ASA intolerance after personal experience of 1000 cases over a period of 10 yr, including 182 studied prospectively *(54)*. These authors expanded the definition by describing a subgroup of ASA-sensitive asthmatics who presented with a set of clinical findings consistent enough to warrant coining the term "ASA Hypersensitivity Triad" to underline the syndromic characteristics of this strange association. They were convinced they had recognized a multisymptomatic pathology that appeared to have an association of "allergic" symptoms and suggested an inflammatory origin to this "triad." The syndrome includes ASA intolerance, hyperplastic sinusitis, nasal polyposis, and asthma.

Many theories have been proposed to explain the pathogenesis of ASA intolerance. The most viable theory revolves around a disruption of the phospholipid-arachidonate metabolic pathway. Evidence in favor of an in vitro inhibition of cyclo-oxygenase and consequent "shunting" to the leukotriene pathway of asthmagenic mediators has been reviewed by Szczeklik *(55)*. Szczeklik summarized the evidence in favor of the cyclo-oxygenase inhibitory theory as follows:

1. Analgesics with anticyclo-oxygenase activity invariably precipitate bronchoconstriction in aspirin-sensitive patients;
2. Analgesics not affecting cyclo-oxygenase are devoid of bronchospastic properties in these patients;
3. There is a positive correlation between the potency of analgesics to inhibit cyclo-oxygenase in vitro and their potency to induce asthmatic attacks in the sensitive patients;
4. The degree of enzymatic inhibition that is sufficient to precipitate bronchoconstriction is an individual hallmark;
5. In vitro anticyclo-oxygenase inhibitors activate platelets to release cytotoxic mediators in aspirin-sensitive asthmatics, but not in the atopic asthmatics or healthy subjects;
6. In patients with aspirin intolerance, the inhibition of thromboxane A2(TXA_2), next to cyclo-oxygenase enzyme in the arachidonic acid cascade, neither precipitates asthmatic attacks nor alters pulmonary function; and
7. After aspirin "desensitization," crossdesensitization to other analgesics that inhibit cyclo-oxygenase also occurs.

Experimental support for the concept of a shift in arachidonic acid metabolism in favor of leukotriene production remains conflicting (56,57). The concept of arachidonic acid shunting needs an additional assumption that the airways of aspirin-sensitive patients are more sensitive to leukotrienes than those of other asthmatics. Otherwise, all asthmatics would be sensitive to nonsteroidal anti-inflammatory drugs (NSAID). Such a concept remains also inconsistently demonstrated between aspirin-intolerant asthmatics and control subjects (58,59). Nevertheless, the new generation of leukotriene inhibitors appear to have an attenuating or preventive effect on aspirin-provoked bronchospasm and rhinitis symptoms. Furthermore, during ASA desensitization, an apparent "downregulation" of cellular inflammation is seen with loss of hyperresponsiveness to the leukotriene receptors and a decrease in monocyte synthesis of arachidonate products (60,61).

ASA-sensitive respiratory syndrome usually evolves over decades with the age of onset, typically over 20 yr and observed more frequently in women (62). The clinical syndrome, usually without nasal polyposis, may be seen in children (63,64). A common first symptom is a perennial vasomotor-irritant-aggravated rhinitis, although up to one-third of these patients will have evidence of inhalant IgE-mediated disease by skin testing. Increasing nasal congestion and anosmia ensue, generally indicating the presence of hyperplastic mucosal disease with nasal polyposis. Purulent bacterial rhinosinusitis frequently complicates this stage of the syndrome, especially following an upper respiratory tract viral infection. These same infectious events often herald the onset of a chronic cough as the first symptom of evolving asthma. Treatment with corticosteroids invariably ensues, since this form of respiratory disease is highly eosinophilic and therefore steroid-responsive. A correlation between aspirin-induced asthma and HLA-DQW2 antigen has been described (65).

The clinical expression of ASA intolerance in asthmatic patients tends to be specific and unique to NSAID, but inconsistent as a function of time and ASA dosing (66). The intolerance to aspirin is usually quite acute, starting 20–180 min (average 90 min) after ingestion. The first symptom is a profuse rhinorrhea, then erythema, and possibly digestive troubles (nausea, vomiting, abdominal cramping, diarrhea), followed by the asthma attack, most often severe. Other symptoms have been observed, such as isolated nasal obstruction and rhinorrhea, urticaria, angioedema, and paradoxical bronchodilation. In a given patient, the reaction can change from time to time, in symptomatology as well as intensity. Furthermore, variations from the classic pattern of ASA idiosyncrasy have been described. For example, Lumry et al. have reported that 12% of their asthmatic patients experienced a selective nasoocular response to ASA challenge without an aggravation of bronchospasm (67).

The intolerance to aspirin includes all nonsteroid anti-inflammatory medications, which inhibit cyclo-oxygenase, but other chemical intolerances can coexist (68–71).

Metabisulfites: found in many drinks, preserves, medications;
Some azoic dyes: tartrazine, amaranth;
Some nonazoic dyes: erythrosine, indigo;
Preservatives: sodium benzoate, parahydroxy-benzoic acid, BHA, BHT; and
Acetaminophen in doses >2 g.

Cytograms show an increase of neutrophils and eosinophils that can vary according to the underlying inflammation. This secretory eosinophilia increases if asthma is associated, and even more if aspirin-induced asthma is severe. The level of eosinophil cationic protein parallels the activation of eosinophils as demonstrated by monoclonal antibodies (MAb) EG2 and Bb10, and can be correlated with the severity of the disease (72). A peripheral blood eosinophilia is commonly elevated over 500/mm^3 in this disorder (73).

The management of the ASA hypersensitivity tetrad of clinical problems involves both medical and surgical approaches. Avoidance of ASA and other NSAIDs, and the use of topical and/or systemic corticosteroids remain the typical first-line treatment approach. Antihistamines and bronchodilators may be added depending on the clinical spectrum of disease. A major difficulty in ASA-sensitive individuals with rhinosinusitis and polypoid changes is purulent sinusitis. As with other respiratory diseases where sinusitis and asthma coexist, the integrity of the sinuses appears to influence the stability of the asthma. If left untreated, rhinosinusitis in this clinical setting can dominate the course of the disease and lead to chronic systemic steroid dependency.

The hypertrophic, edematous, polypoid nature of the upper respiratory tract in the ASA hypersensitivity tetrad makes purulent sinusitis particularly difficult to treat. Broad-spectrum antibiotics, topical and systemic decongestants, and systemic steroids followed by long-term topical steroids form the backbone of therapy. At times, intractable corticosteroid-dependent asthma develops in conjunction with chronic sinusitis and nasal polyposis forcing a decision either to continue increasing the dosage of corticosteroids, despite side effects, or intervene surgically. Slavin and coworkers have demonstrated that endoscopic sinus surgery including a sphenoethmoidectomy relieved not only the sinusitis and polyposis, but also improved the asthma significantly (74). Boitout-Guillaumot has shown that after an aggressive combination of medical and surgical treatment, the blood eosinophilia may be affected, dropping significantly in more than 40% of cases (75). After 1 yr of combined treatment, all of that author's patients were either stabilized or improved, and 67% of patients considered that they were "cured." Patients had an improvement in their asthma as well as nasal polyposis: 62–72% of asthma, 72–76% of nasal/sinus polyposis. Friedman et al., McFaden et al., and Jankowski et al. have reported that up to 80% of their ASA-intolerant patients significantly reduced or eliminated their need for systemic corticosteroids with improved pulmonary function following aggressive surgical management of their hyperplastic sinusitis with nasal polyposis (44,45,76).

Initial studies using leukotriene receptor antagonists and inhibitors have confirmed a prominent role for leukotrienes as mediators of asthma (Fig. 2). This may be particularly true in the aspirin-intolerant asthmatic. Increased levels of leukotriene C4 (LCT4) have been found in the nasal lavage fluid of aspirin-intolerant asthmatics after challenge with aspirin either orally or topically (77,78). In contrast, Ferreri et al. could not verify the release of leukotrienes in nasal lavage fluid of aspirin-tolerant asthmatic patients or normal persons after they ingest aspirin. The urinary levels of leukotriene E4 (LTE4) are approximately six-fold higher in asthmatics who are aspirin-intolerant compared to levels of those who are aspirin-tolerant. Furthermore, aspirin-sensitive asthmatic patients have a four-times increase of urinary LTE4 levels 6 h after aspirin challenge, whereas no increase is observed in the aspirin-tolerant asthmatic patients (59).

Leukotriene inhibitors have emerged as potential therapeutic agents in the treatment of allergen-induced and aspirin-induced rhinitis and asthma. The 5-lipoxygenase-activating protein inhibitor MK-886 partially inhibits early- and late-phase asthma responses after allergen challenge (79). Pretreatment with the selective LTD4 antagonist SK&F 104353 was found to reduce the aspirin-induced decrease in FEV1 by a mean of 47% (80). In a similar study, the 5-lipoxygenase inhibitor zileuton significantly reduced the decrease in FEV1, angioedema, nasal congestion, and gastrointestinal symptoms that occurred after aspirin ingestion in intolerant patients (81).

Aspirin Challenge—Desensitization

As early as 1922, Widal et al. succeeded inducing tolerance by repeated administration of increasing doses of aspirin in an intolerant patient (53). This observation not only demonstrated the hypersensitivity state for the individual patient, but proved to represent a unique form of treatment in this often very-difficult-to-control disorder. The indications for ASA challenge are varied, but do not include the desire for simple verification or proof of the presence of ASA idiosyncrasy, unless it is being done for research purposes. This exclusion is based on two considerations. Although asthma induced by incremental ASA challenge can been readily controlled and no deaths have been reported in published series, the exacerbation of nasal and sinus disease that may follow can last for several weeks. In addition, there may be a variation in an individual patient's response to ASA as a function of time. For example, Matheson and Stevenson reported a patient who, on four ASA challenges over a 9-yr period, experienced a "classical" oculo-naso-asthmatic response on the first two challenges, no reaction on the third challenge, and only a nasal response following the fourth challenge (82).

The administration of ASA to an ASA-sensitive patient can also be therapeutic when administered in an incremental fashion. Lumry et al. reported that after ASA desensitization treatment of nonasthmatic ASA-sensitive patients with rhinosinusitis, 77% improved significantly as long as ASA was administered daily (67). The desensitization or tolerance is defined by the

LEUKOTRIENE FORMATION IN INFLAMMATORY CELLS[97]

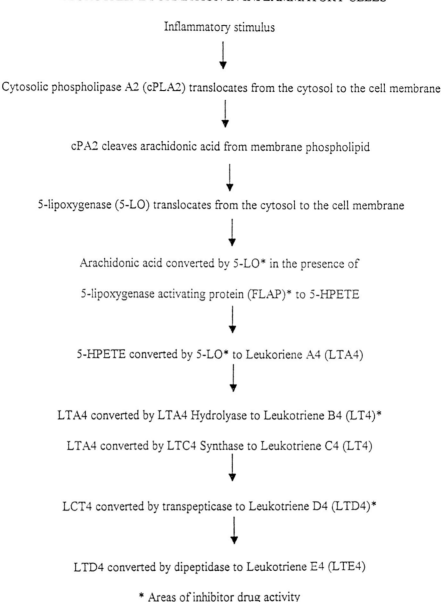

Inflammatory stimulus

Cytosolic phospholipase A2 (cPLA2) translocates from the cytosol to the cell membrane

cPA2 cleaves arachidonic acid from membrane phospholipid

5-lipoxygenase (5-LO) translocates from the cytosol to the cell membrane

Arachidonic acid converted by 5-LO* in the presence of

5-lipoxygenase activating protein (FLAP)* to 5-HPETE

5-HPETE converted by 5-LO* to Leukoriene A4 (LTA4)

LTA4 converted by LTA4 Hydrolyase to Leukotriene B4 (LT4)*

LTA4 converted by LTC4 Synthase to Leukotriene C4 (LT4)

LCT4 converted by transpepticase to Leukotriene D4 (LTD4)*

LTD4 converted by dipeptidase to Leukotriene E4 (LTE4)

* Areas of inhibitor drug activity

Fig. 2. Leukotriene formation in inflammatory cells *(86)*.

absence of any clinical reaction or deterioration of pulmonary function tests after ingestion of 650 mg of aspirin. Tolerance persists for a few days (2–5 d average), and sometimes up to 9 d once ASA is discontinued. Aspirin and other NSAIDs continue to be well tolerated during the refractory period provided continuous administration is maintained. For example, when treatment with ASA is decreased from 650 mg twice a day to 325 mg every day, nasal congestion reappears in 48–72 h within the majority of patients, but it recovers when the higher ASA dosage is reinstituted.

The induction of ASA tolerance also can have a beneficial effect on asthma in the ASA-sensitive asthmatic. Stevenson et al., in a double-blind cross-over study of 25 asthmatics with severe ASA sensitivity involving both the upper and lower respiratory tracts, demonstrated that 48% experienced a decrease in the severity of their asthma *(83)*. Sixty-seven percent also experienced significantly fewer nasal symptoms. However, the mean dose of

Table 3 *(87)*
Procedure for Oral Aspirin Challenge/Desensitization

Asthma absent clinically for several days or a FEV1 > 70% of predicted or the best previously recorded and > 1.5 L (adult)
Discontinue antihistamines, β-agonists, and cromolyn/nedocromil for a suitable time to eliminate major inhibitory activity
Administer aspirin orally every 3 h as follows:
    Day 1: 3, 30, 100 mg
    Day 2: 150, 325, 650 mg
Monitor symptom response continually and PFTs hourly during challenge
Minimum criteria for a positive challenge:
    Nasoocular: clinical evidence of nasal and ocular congestion and discharge
    Pulmonary: ≥20% fall in FEV1 from baseline of the best of two consecutive FEMs
If desensitization is required, continue 650 mg of ASA daily or change to another nonsteroidal anti-inflammatory agent
    at the desired therapeutic dosage
A refractory period of 1–5 d will ensue after desensitization

systemic corticosteroids was not reduced significantly in this study. Sweet et al. reported a retrospective review of 107 ASA-sensitive asthmatics *(84)*. Thirty-five and 32 of these patients were desensitized with ASA and treated daily thereafter for a mean duration of 3.75 yr and 2 yr, respectively. Forty-two patients avoided ASA and served as the control group. The ASA-treated groups demonstrated significant reduction in the number of emergency room visits, hospitalizations, annual sinusitis episodes, and need for sinus surgery, as well as a significant improvement in their sense of smell.

Based on clinical experience and published studies, Stevenson and Simon recommended that ASA desensitization treatment be considered for ASA-sensitive respiratory patients with the following circumstances *(85)*:

1. Patients with uncontrolled respiratory inflammation, despite the use of full topical corticosteroids and low-dose or alternate-day corticosteroids;
2. Patients who require repeated polypectomies and sinus operations; and
3. ASA-sensitive patients who require NSAID for other diseases for which there is no acceptable alternative.

It has been demonstrated that switching from one NSAID to another in the desensitized state is a safe and effective therapeutic option. Furthermore, the induction of tolerance is contraindicated if severe bronchial obstruction is present (FEV1 ≤ 1.5 L) in patients younger than 18 yr of age, in noncompliant patients, or if there are any other contraindications to aspirin or NSAIDs. Table 3 is

a representative oral aspirin challenge–desensitization protocol.

SUMMARY

There has been a century of clinical observations linking sinus disease and asthma. More importantly, evidence has been accumulating to suggest that treatment of sinus disease has a beneficial effect on any coexisting asthma. The data in children appear to be particularly strong in linking sinusitis treatment and asthma stability. Even cough presents as the most frequently encountered symptom of sinusitis of childhood, a clinical presentation commonly misdiagnosed as asthma and, therefore, treated inappropriately with bronchodilators. Nevertheless, most of the evidence for a link between sinusitis and asthma remains circumstantial.

Although multiple mechanisms have been proposed, the strongest evidence in support of a role for sinusitis in asthma stability is derived from research demonstrating a nasobronchial reflex and the influence of upper-airway mucosal-derived soluble and cellular mediators of inflammation on the lower airway. On this basis, the clinician faced with a patient suffering from chronic purulent sinusitis and asthma must exhaust all medical and/or surgical means to resolve the sinusitis state in pursuit of the greatest degree of asthma stability with the least amount of asthma medications. A more difficult decision is how to approach the asthmatic patient with radiographic evidence of sinusitis, but little or no upper respiratory symptoms. At the present time, there are no algorithms for guidance, and the clinician must use the "art" of medicine in making the correct decisions. It should be emphasized that it remains the responsibility of each physician to be aware of the relationship that exists between sinusitis and asthma and, particularly in difficult-to-control patients, to look for occult sinusitis, nasal polyposis, and/or aspirin intolerance.

REFERENCES

1. Bullen SS. Incidence of asthma in 400 cases of chronic sinusitis. J Allergy 1932;4:402–407.
2. Gottlieb MJ. Relation of intranasal disease in the production of bronchial asthma. JAMA 1925;85:105–107.
3. Weille FL. Studies in asthma: nose and throat in 500 cases of asthma. N Engl J Med 1936;215:235–239.
4. Rackemann FM, Tobey HG. Studies in asthma. IV. The nose and throat in asthma. Arch Otolaryngol 1929;9:612.
5. Rachelefsky GS, Goldberg M, Katz RM. Sinus disease in children with respiratory allergy. J Allergy Clin Immunol 1978;61:310–314.
6. Friedman R, Ackerman M, Wald E, Cassellman M, Friday G, Fireman P. Asthma and bacterial sinusitis in children. J Allergy Clin Immunol 1984;74:185–189.
7. Schwartz JH, Thompson JS, Sher TH, Ross RJ. Occult sinus abnormalities in the asthmatic patient. Arch Intern Med 1987;147:2194–2196.
8. Fuller C, Richards W, Gilsanz V, Schoettler J, Church JA. Sinusitis in status asthmaticus (abstract). J Allergy Clin Immunol 1990;85:222.
9. Phipatanakul CS, Slavin RG. Bronchial asthma produced by paranasal sinusitis. Arch Otolaryngol 1974;100:109–112.
10. Rachelefsky GS, Katz RM, Siegel SC. Chronic sinus disease with associated reactive airways disease in children. Pediatrics 1984;73:526–529.
11. Friday GA, Fireman P. Sinusitis and asthma: clinical and pathogenetic relationships. Clin Chest Med 1988;9:557–565.
12. Ogura JM, Harvey J. Nasopulmonary mechanisms—experimental evidence of the influence of the upper airway upon the lower. Acta Otolaryngol 1971;71:123–128.
13. Kaufman J, Chen J, Wright GW. The effect of trigeminal resection on reflex bronchoconstriction after nasal and nasopharyngeal irritation in man. Am Rev Respir Dis 1970;101:768,769.
14. Sluder G. Asthma as a nasal reflex. JAMA 1919;73:589–591.
15. McFadden ER Jr. Nasal-sinus-pulmonary reflexes and bronchial asthma. J Allergy Clin Immunol 1986;78:1–3.
16. Permut SM. Bronchial challenge in ragweed sensitive patients. In: Austen KF, Lichtenstein LM, eds., Asthma: Physiology, Immunopharmacology and Treatment. New York: Academic, 1977; Chapter 17.
17. Ramsdale EH, Morris MM, Roberts RS, Hargreave FE. Asymptomatic bronchial responsiveness in rhinitis. J Allergy Clin Immunol 1984;75:573–577.
18. Maloney J, Collins J. Nasal polyps and bronchial asthma. Br J Dis Chest 1977;41:1–5.
19. Downing ET, Braman S, Settipane GA. Bronchial reactivity in patients with nasal polyps before and after

polypectomy (abstract). J Allergy Clin Immunol 1982;69(part 2):102.
20. Miles-Lawrence R, Kaplan M, Chang K. Methacholine sensitivity in nasal polyposis and effects of polypectomy (abstract). J Allergy Clin Immunol 1982;69(part 2):102.
21. Bardin PG, Van Heerden BB, Joubert JR. Absence of pulmonary aspiration of sinus contents in patients with asthma and sinusitis. J Allergy Clin Immunol 1990;86:82–88.
22. Basscom R, Pipkorn U, Proud D, Dunnette S, Gleich GJ, Lichtenstein LM, Naclerio RM. Major basic protein and eosinophil-derived neurotoxin concentrations in nasal-lavage fluid after antigen challenge: effect of systemic corticosteroids and relationship to eosinophil influx. J Allergy Clin Immunol 1989;84:338–346.
23. Harlin SL, Ansel DG, Lane SR, Myers J, Kephart GM, Gleich GJ. A clinical and pathologic study of chronic sinusitis: the role of the eosinophil. J Allergy Clin Immunol 1988;81:867–875.
24. Stone BD, Georgitis JW, Matthews B. Inflammatory mediators in sinus lavage fluid (abstract). J Allergy Clin Immunol 1990;85:22.
25. Nadel JA, Widdicombe JG. Reflex effects of upper airway function on total lung resistance and blood pressure. J Appl Physiol 1962;17:861–865.
26. Barnes PJ. Asthma as an axon reflex. Lancet 1986;1:242,243.
27. Kaufman J, Wright G. The effect of nasal and nasopharyngeal irritation on airway resistance in man. Am Rev Respir Dis 1969;100:626–630.
28. Yan K, Salome C. The response of the airways to nasal stimulation in asthmatics with rhinitis. Eur J Respir Dis 1983;64(Suppl. 128):105–108.
29. Nolte D, Berger D. On vagal bronchoconstriction in asthmatic patients by nasal irritation. Eur J Respir Dis 1983;64(Suppl. 128):110–114.
30. Brugman SM, Larsen GL, Henson PM, Honor J, Irvin CG. Increased lower airways responsiveness associated with sinusitis in a rabbit model. Am Rev Respir Dis 1993;147:314–320.
31. Hoehne JH, Reed CE. Where is the allergic reaction in ragweed asthma? J Allergy Clin Immunol 1971;48:36–39.
32. Rosenberg GL, Rosenthal RR, Normal PS. Inhalational challenge with ragweed pollen and ragweed-sensitive asthmatics. J Allergy Clin Immunol 1983;71:302–310.
33. Schumacher MJ, Cota KA, Taussig L. Pulmonary response to nasal-challenge testing of atopic subjects with stable asthma. J Allergy Clin Immunol 1986;78:30–35.
34. Szentivanyi I. The beta-adrenergic theory of atopic abnormality in asthma. J Allergy 1968;42:203–232.
35. Busse WW. Decreased granulocyte response to isoproterenol in asthma during upper respiratory symptoms. Am Rev Resp Dis 1977;115:783–791.
36. Slavin RG, Cannon RE, Friedman WH, Palitons E. Sinusitis and bronchial asthma. J Allergy Clin Immunol 1980;66:250–257.
37. Slavin RG. Relationship of nasal disease and sinusitis to bronchial asthma. Ann Allergy 1982;49:76–80.
38. Adinoff AL, Cummings NP. Sinusitis and its relationship to asthma. Pediatr Ann 1989;18:785–790.
39. Rossi VJ, Pirila T, Laitinen J, Huhti E. Sinus aspirates and radiographic abnormalities in severe attacks

of asthma. Int Arch Allergy Immunol 1994;103:209–213.

40. Wald ER, Milmoe GJ, Bowen A, Ledesma-Medina J, Salamon N, Bluestone CD. Acute maxillary sinusitis in children. N Engl J Med 1981;304:749–754.

41. Zimmerman B, Stringer D, Feanny S, Reisman J, Hak H, Rashed N, et al. Prevalence of abnormalities found in sinus X-rays in childhood: lack of relation to severity of asthma. J Allergy Clin Immunol 1987;80:268–273.

41a. Berman SZ, Matheson DA, Stevenson DD, et al. Maxillary sinusitis and bronchial asthma: correlation of roentgenograms, cultures, and thermograms. J Allergy Clin Immunol 1974;53:311–317.

42. Macfarlane JT, Colville A, Guion A, Macfarlane RM, Rose DH. Prospective study of aetiology and outcome of adult lower-respiratory-tract infections in the community. Lancet 1993;341:511–514.

43. Mings R, Friedman WH, Linford P, Slaven RG. Five year follow-up of the effects of bilateral intranasal sphenoethmoidectomy in patients with sinusitis and asthma. Am J Rhinol 1988;71:123–132.

44. Friedman WH, Katsantonis GP, Slavin RG, Kannel P, Linford P. Sphenoethmoidectomy: its role in the asthmatic patient. Otolaryngol Head and Neck Surg 1982;90:171–177.

45. Jankowski R, Moneret-Vautrin DA, Goetz R, Wayoff M. Incidence of medico-surgical treatment for nasal polyps on the development of associated asthma. Rhinology 1992;30:249–258.

46. Samter M, Lederer FL. Nasal polyps: their relationship to allergy, particularly bronchial asthma. Med Clin North Am 1958;42:175–179.

47. Macauley DB. Nonspecific treatment of allergic rhinitis. Proc Roy Soc Med 1963;56:218.

48. Seigel S, Goldman JL, Arnold LM. Sinus disease, bacterial allergy and bronchial asthma. Arch Intern Med 1956;97:431–441.

49. Schenck NL. Nasal polypectomy in the aspirin sensitive asthmatic. Trans Am Acad Ophthalmol Otolaryngol 1974;78:109–119.

50. Brown BL, Harner SG, Van Dellen RG. Nasal polypectomy in patients with asthma plus sensitivity to aspirin. Arch Otolaryngol 1979; 105:413–416.

51. Englisch GM. Nasal polypectomy and sinus surgery in patients with asthma and aspirin idiosyncrasy. Laryngoscope 1986;96:374–380.

52. Moss R, King V. Long-term control of chronic refractory sinusitis and cystic fibrosis by endoscopic surgery and serial antimicrobial lavage. J Allergy Clin Immunol 1994;93:176(abstract 82).

53. Widal F, Abrami P, Lermoyez J. Anaphylaxie et idiosyncrasie. Presse Med 1922;30:189–193.

54. Samter M, Beers RF. Intolerance to aspirin: clinical studies and consideration to its pathogenesis. Ann Intern Med 1968;68:975–983.

55. Szczeklik A. Analgesics, allergy and asthma. Drugs 1986;32(Suppl. 4):148–163.

56. Szczeklik A, Virchow C, Schmitz-Schumann M. Pathophysiology and pharmacology of aspirin-induced asthma. In: Page CP, Barnes PJ, eds., Handbook of Experimental Pharmacology, vol. 98, Pharmacology of Asthma. Berlin: Springer-Verlag, 1991; pp. 291–314.

57. Sladek K, Szczeklik A. Mast cell and eosinophil activation during aspirin-provoked leukotriene release in aspirin-induced asthma. J Allergy Clin Immunol 1992;89(abstract 354):233.

58. Vaghi A, Robuschi M, Simone P, Bianco S. Bronchial response to leukotriene C4 in aspirin asthma. Abstracts SEP 4th Congress, Milano-Stresa, 1985; p. 171.

59. Christie PE, Tagari P, Ford-Hutchinson AW, Charlesson S, Chee P, Arm JP. Urinary leukotriene E4 concentration increase after aspirin challenge in aspirin sensitive asthmatic subjects. Am Rev Respir Dis 1991;143:1025–1029.

60. Arm JP, O'Hickey SP, Spur BW, et al. Airway responsiveness to histamine and leukotriene E4 in subjects with aspirin-induced asthma. Am Rev Respir Dis 1989;140:148–151.

61. Juergens UR, Christiansen SC, Stevenson DD, et al. Elevated thromboxane B2(TXB2) and leukotriene B4(LTB4) secretion from monocytes of aspirin sensitive asthmatic patients. J Allergy Clin Immunol 1991;87(abstract):221.

62. Zeitz HJ. Bronchial asthma, nasal polyps and aspirin sensitivity: Samter's Syndrome. Clin Chest Med 1988;9:567–576.

63. Rachelefsky GS, Coulson A, Siegel SC. Aspirin intolerance in chronic childhood asthma detected by oral challenge. Pediatrics 1975;56:443–448.

64. Fischer TJ, Guilfoile TD, Kesewala HH, Winant JG Jr, Kearns GL, Gartside PS, Mooman CJ. Adverse pulmonary responses to aspirin and acetaminophen in chronic childhood asthma. Pediatrics 1983;71:313–318.

65. Mullarkey MF, Thomas PS, Hansen JA, Webb DR, Nisperos B. Association of aspirin-sensitive asthma with HLa-DQW2. Ann Rev Respir Dis 1986;133:261–263.

66. Kowalski ML, Grzelewska-Rzymowska L, Szmidt M, Rozniecki J. Bronchial hyperreactivity to histamine in aspirin sensitive asthmatics: relationship to aspirin threshold and effect of aspirin desensitization. Thorax 1985; 40:598–602.

67. Lumry WR, Curd JG, Zeiger RS, et al. Aspirin sensitive rhinosinusitis: the clinical syndrome and effects of aspirin administration. J Allergy Clin Immunol 1983;71:588–593.

68. Stevenson DD, Simon RA, Lumry WA, Mathison DA. Adverse reactions to tartrazine. J Allergy Clin Immunol 1987;80:788–790.

69. Weber RW, Hoffman M, Raine DA, Nelson HS. Incidence of bronchoconstriction due to aspirin, azodyes, non-azo dyes and preservatives in a population of perennial asthmatics. J Allergy Clin Immunol 1979;64:32–37.

70. Stevenson DD, Hougham AJ, Schrank PJ, Goldlust MB, Wilson RR. Salicylate cross-reactivity in aspirin-sensitive patients with asthma. J Allergy Clin Immunol 1990;86:749–758.

71. Spector SL, Wangaard CH, Farr RS. Aspirin and concomitant idiosyncrasies in adult asthmatic patients. J Allergy Clin Immunol 1979;64:500–506.

72. Bousquet J, Chanez P, Lacoste JY, Enander I, Venge P, Peterson C, Ahlstedt S, Michel FB, Godard P. Indirect evidence of bronchial inflammation assessed by titration of inflammatory mediators in BAL fluid of patients with asthma. J Allergy Clin Immunol 1991;88:649–660.

73. Moneret Vautrin DA, Wayoff M, Bonne CI. Les mechanismes de l'intolerance a l'aspirine. Ann Otolaryngol Chis Cervicofac 1985;23:357–363.

74. Slavin RG, Linford PA, Friedman WH. Sphenoethmoidectomy in the treatment of nasal polyps, sinusitis and bronchial asthma. J Allergy Clin Immunol 1983;71:156.

75. Boitout-Guillaumot A. La triade de Fernand Widal. Thesis Medicine, Nancy, France, 1993; p. 203.

76. McFadden EA, Kanny RJ, Fink JN, Toohill RJ. Surgery for sinusitis and aspirin triad. Laryngoscope 1990; 100:1043–1046.

77. Ferreri NR, Howland WC, Stevenson DD, Spiegelberg HL. Release of leukotrienes, prostaglandins, and histamine into nasal secretions of aspirin-sensitive asthmatics during reaction to aspirin. Am Rev Respir Dis 1988; 137:847–854.

78. Picado C, Ramis I, Rosello J, Prat J, Bulbena B, Plaza V, et al. Release of peptide leukotriene into nasal secretions after local instillation of aspirin in aspirin-sensitive asthmatic patients. Am Rev Respir Dis 1992;145:65–69.

79. Friedman BS, Bel EH, Buntinx A, Tanaka W, Han YH, Shingo S, et al. Oral leukotriene inhibitor (MK-886) blocks allergen-induced airway responses. Am Rev Respir Dis 1993;147:839–844.

80. Christie PE, Smith CM, Lee TH. The potent and selective sulfidopeptide leukotriene antagonist SK&F 104353, inhibits aspirin-induced asthma. Am Rev Respir Dis 1991;144:957,958.

81. Israel E, Fischer AR, Rosenberg MA, Lilly CM, Callery J, Shapiro J, et al. The pivotal role of 5-lipoxygenase products in the reaction of aspirin-sensitive asthmatics to aspirin. Am Rev Respir Dis 1993;148:1447–1451.

82. Matheson DA, Stevenson DD. Hypersensitivity to non-steroidal anti-inflammatory drugs: indications and methods for oral challenges. J Allergy Clin Immunol 1979;64:569–576.

83. Stevenson DD, Pleskow WW, Simon RA, et al. Aspirin-sensitive rhinosinusitis asthma: a double blind cross-over study of treatment with aspirin. J Allergy Clin Immunol 1984;85:59–66.

84. Sweet JM, Stevenson DD, Mathison DA, et al. Long term effects of aspirin (ASA) desensitization treatment for ASA sensitive patients with asthma. J Allergy Clin Immunol 1990;85:59–65.

85. Stevenson DD, Simon RA. Sensitivity to aspirin and non-steroidal antiinflammatory drugs. In: Middleton E, Reed CE, et al., eds., Allergy: Principles and Practice, vol. II. St. Louis: Mosby, 1993; pp. 1747–1765.

86. Henderson WR. The role of leukotrienes in inflammation. Ann Intern Med 1994;121:684–697.

87. Incaudo GA, Gershwin ME. Aspirin and related nonsteroidal anti-inflammatory agents, sulfites and other food additives as precipitating factors in asthma. In: Gershwin ME, ed., Bronchial Asthma, 2nd ed. Orlando: Grune & Stratton, 1986; pp. 213–232.

16 Fungal Sinusitis

Pathogenesis and Treatment

Harold S. Novey, MD

CONTENTS

INTRODUCTION, HISTORICAL PERSPECTIVE, AND PREVALENCE

Fungi resemble cave dwellers. They inhabit dark, warm, moist enclosed spaces. Fungi may enter and occupy any human body orifice, and given sufficient nutrients, will proliferate usually in concentric rings until the space is completely occupied. Fungal otitis, rhinitis, vaginitis, pharyngitis, proctitis, enteritis, bronchitis, and paranasal sinusitis have all been described.

In 1791, a 22-yr-old soldier with maxillary pain was described as cured of a fungus tumor by cautery *(1)*. The organism was not otherwise identified. A hundred years later, specific diagnoses were made of noninvasive and invasive paranasal sinus disease by *Aspergillus* species *(1)*. Until 1980, fungal sinusitis was rarely reported with the exception of an endemic area in the Sudan, Africa. Only 103 cases of *Aspergillus*-related sinusitis outside of Sudan had been documented *(2)*. However, during the recent decade and a half, the prevalence of fungal sinusitis has apparently risen dramatically. Although the exact incidence is still unknown, over this brief span, there have been reports, for example, of 85 cases from a single ear, nose, and throat (ENT) center in Nantes, France *(3)*; 79 cases from a clinic in Lausanne, Switzerland *(4)*; and another 22 from clinics at the Johns Hopkins University and the University of Pittsburgh *(1)*, as well as dozens of smaller multiple case reports *(5–9)*. The increased prevalence has been ascribed to improved diagnoses, widespread antibacterial therapy, and higher rates of acquired immunodeficiency.

Of the more than 12,000 genera of fungi *(10)*, only about 18 genera have been associated with paranasal sinusitis (Table 1), and of these, fully 90% of the cases have been attributed to *Aspergilli*, most notably *fumigatus* and *flavus* species *(11)*. It is noteworthy from the list that most of the fungi are ubiquitous and not usually considered human pathogens. Fungi responsible for such diseases as coccidiomycosis, histoplasmosis, and blastomycosis have rarely if ever been incriminated in isolated sinusitis.

From: *Diseases of the Sinuses* (M. E. Gershwin and G. A. Incaudo, eds.), ©1996 Humana Press Inc., Totowa, NJ.

Table 1
Fungal Genera Incriminated in Fungal Sinusitis

Aspergillus, ~90%
Mucor and *Candida*, ~5%
The remaining 5%:
  Penicillium
  Fusarium
  Bipolaris (Drechslera)
  Curvularia
  Alternaria
  Exserohilum
  Paecilomyces
  Pseudoallescheria
  Rhizopus
  Schizophyllum
  Cunninghamilla
  Conidiobolus
  Basidiobolus
  Absidia
  Rhinosporidium

Table 2
A Clinicopathological Classification of Fungal Sinusitis

Noninvasive
  Acute—rare, and not recently reported
  Chronic or indolent
  Mycetoma
  Allergic
Invasive
  Acute or chronic

CLASSIFICATION AND CLINICAL PRESENTATIONS

Based on criteria of clinical severity, fungal sinusitis can be classified into just two categories: noninvasive and invasive forms (Table 2). The invasive type has the poorer prognosis, is subject to more serious complications, and requires more extensive treatment. Invasion and dissemination are abetted by immunodeficiency states, but fungal invasion has also occurred in otherwise healthy individuals.

Noninvasive Fungal Sinusitis

This category can be subdivided into three syndromes based on clinical findings. Acute noninvasive fungal sinusitis has been reported in the older literature, but appears to be rare presently, and thus will not be discussed here.

CHRONIC OR INDOLENT FORM

Signs and symptoms of sinusitis persist over a 3-mo duration. Usually bacterial sinusitis is suspected, but remission does not occur despite extensive antibiotic therapy. The patients are characteristically otherwise healthy. They are most likely to experience unilateral headaches and unilateral nasal obstruction. Nasal secretions may be purulent, caseous, or pseudomembranous. Radiography usually reveals abnormalities, often unilateral and involving a single sinus.

MYCETOMA

This form is rarer than the chronic type of sinusitis, may be asymptomatic, and usually occurs following bacterial sinus disease or sinus injury. Symptomatic patients resemble those with the chronic type and invariably have single sinus involvement. The distinction is mainly based on the histological description of minimal if any inflammatory reaction of sinus mucosa to the mycelial mass or fungal ball. Its counterpart is found in the mycetoma of the pulmonary cavity.

ALLERGIC FUNGAL SINUSITIS

The clinical presentation is similar to the chronic or indolent form. However, the patients usually have pre-existing asthma or other allergic diseases, nasal polyposes, occasionally peripheral eosinophilia, and on sinus irrigation, a characteristic secretion termed allergic mucin. Associated immunological responses resemble those found in its lower respiratory tract counterpart, allergic bronchopulmonary (aspergillosis) mycosis.

Invasive Form

Fungal invasion into the sinus mucosa is its hallmark. Multiple sinuses are usually involved, and such complications as orbital proptosis, epiphora, diplopia, and facial edema are common. An immunocompromised state arising from hematological cancers, irradiation, cytotoxic drugs, HIV, and other causes is usually, but not invariably, present. The two most common types or noninvasive fungal sinusitis are discussed in more detail, as follows.

CHRONIC NONINVASIVE FUNGAL SINUSITIS

A fairly typical example of the chronic noninvasive, nonallergic type of fungal sinusitis is illustrated in this previously unreported case history. A 39-yr-old female in prior good health developed decay under the crown of a right upper molar tooth in 1980 and chronic dental pain. Eventually two right upper molars had root canal treatment and finally three right upper molars were extracted, but cheek pain persisted. A cyst filling 2/3 of the right maxillary sinus was seen on a paranasal sinus radiograph, and led to a Caldwell-Luc procedure with antrostomy. Under the serous cyst, an area of vascular necrotic bone over the alveolar ridge was found and debrided with the cyst. However, the maxillary area stabbing pain persisted, and only seemed to ameliorate after prolonged antibacterial regimens, which were frequently administered.

Three years later, a right maxillary sequestrectomy was performed with removal of inflamed maxillary bone. A palatal transpositional greater palatine artery flap was required to close the communication between the maxillary sinus and dental alveolus. The pathology examination found a granulomatous foreign body-type reaction within masses of brown granular debris. Postoperative cephalosporin therapy was riven for 3 mo. Finally, the patient's facial neuralgia ceased and she has remained pain free to date. However, a year later, in 1984, after a nonspecific upper respiratory infection, foul-smelling purulent discharge presented from the right nasal passage. The drainage did not clear after courses of cefaclor, doxycycline, and erythromycin. Cultures had shown evidence of micrococci sensitive to the antibiotics used. Another Caldwell-Luc surgical procedure this time found the right maxillary sinus virtually filled with thick granulation tissue, which sealed the antral window. The material was excised and clusters of branching septate hyphae among chronic inflammatory tissue were seen on pathology examination. *Aspergillus fumigatus* was readily cultured and was the only organism grown in several media.

There was no history of exposure to birds or moldy hay. Allergy skin tests were negative to extracts of *Aspergillus* species, and no *Aspergillus* precipitins were present in the patient's serum. Her total serum IgE was normal, 23 U/mL, and total eosinophil count was only 141 cells/mm³. The patient has remained asymptomatic during the past 10 yr. Repeat paranasal radiographs and antral washings have been essentially negative.

This patient developed fungal sinusitis limited to one maxillary sinus following dental treatment and extensive antibiotic administration. Whether the fungal organism entered during the dental surgery or subsequently after the sinus surgeries

cannot be determined. Antibacterial drugs likely removed competing organisms to fungal occupation of the sinus. Neither the pathological specimens nor the immunological studies indicated an allergic component. Tissue invasion by hyphae was not present. This case should be classified as the chronic or indolent type of noninvasive fungal sinusitis, the most common form in healthy persons.

ALLERGIC FUNGAL SINUSITIS

In 1983, Katzenstein, a pathologist, in collaboration with allergists, reported on a review of 119 surgically excised specimens from paranasal sinuses *(12,13)*. Katzenstein, who had earlier first described the condition called bronchocentric granulomatosis and its association in some cases with aspergillosis, noted the similarity in seven specimens with mucoid impactions found in allergic bronchopulmonary aspergillosis (ABPA). The material consisted of necrotic eosinophils amid other cellular debris within a background of pale eosinophilic-to-basophilic, amorphous mucin (Figs. 1 and 2). Charcot-Leyden crystals were plentiful (Fig. 3). Gomori methenamine silver stains uncovered thin, septate hyphae resembling *Aspergilli* within the mucin (Fig. 4). Additionally, the patients had immunologic features comparable to ABPA patients. Peripheral eosinophilia, increased serum IgE levels, serum precipitins to *Aspergillus* antigens, specific serum IgE and IgG antibodies, and skin tests reactions to fungal extracts were found (Table 3). Since her report, there have been, according to Goldstein *(14)*, a total of 70 well-documented cases of allergic fungal sinusitis. Forty-two of these have been associated with *Aspergilli* and the remainder to a variety of genera, most commonly *Bipolaris, Curvularia,* and *Alternaria.* The prevalence of this condition, as with ABPA, is unknown, but a 6–6.5% rate postoperatively is suggested by two retrospective reviews of surgical specimens totaling 333 cases *(14)*.

The immunological responses are usually more muted than those in ABPA. The serum total IgE levels, though elevated, rarely reach 1000 U. Additionally, peripheral eosinophilia may not be present and when present have usually been <1000 cells/mL. Thus, systemic responses to the fungal sinus antigens generally are less than to antigens in bronchi. Allergic *Aspergillus* sinusitis and allergic bronchopulmonary aspergillosis can coexist, and six such cases have been reported *(15)*.

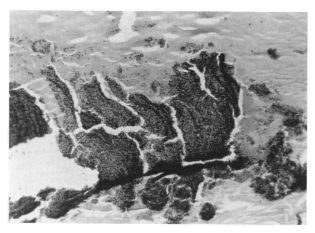

Fig. 1. "Allergic mucin" composed of mucin and abundant degenerated cellular debris obtained from resected maxillary sinus material, a hallmark of allergic fungal sinusitis (×100). (Reprinted from ref. *31* with permission.)

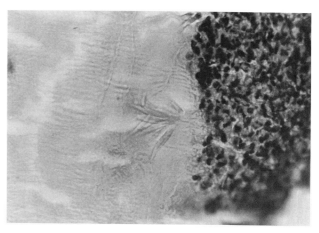

Fig. 3. Charcot-Leyden crystals in the exudate from the maxillary sinus, similar to the characteristic finding in secretions from asthmatic bronchi (×250). (Reprinted from ref. *31* with permission.)

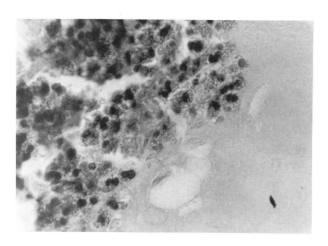

Fig. 2. Much of cellular debris in allergic mucin consisted of eosinophils (×395). (Reprinted from ref. *31* with permission.)

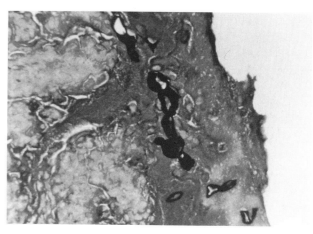

Fig. 4. The diagnosis of allergic fungal sinusitis was confirmed by the finding of noninvasive septate hyphae in the paranasal sinus exudate (methenamine silver stain, ×250). (Reprinted from ref. *31* with permission.)

PATHOGENESIS

The fungi associated with sinusitis are incidentally saprophytic and not inherently pathogenic to humans. The ability of inhaled conidia to germinate in the sinuses probably depends on local factors, such as nutrients in the mucus, and impaired mucociliary activity, drainage, and aeration. Studies in birds and mammals revealed that inhaled conidia in bronchoalveolar spaces germinate rapidly and produce hyphal branching, but further proliferation may be halted by a dense leukocytic response by the host. This reaction may result in the formation of fibrous capsules and eventually lead to the destruction of the hyphae. In natural

infection in mammals, resistance to *Aspergilli* is manifested by the development of eosinophilic "asteroid" sheaths around hyphae. The sheath is composed of a layer of hard refractive material 0.5–1.0 μ thick surrounded by macrophages and eosinophils *(16)*.

The appearance of straight or spirally unbranched hyphae signal release from resistance by the host. Branches may become so close that a compact mass or fungus ball is formed with a clearly delimited leading edge. Clinical findings may result from pressure of the mass on soft tissue or bone, blockage of drainage from osteomeatal obstruction, and

Table 3
Immunological Responses in Allergic Fungal Sinusitis

Positive immediate and delayed skin test reactions to
  specific fungal antigens
Elevated total serum IgE
Specific serum IgE and IgG fungal antibodies
Precipitating IgG antibodies to specific fungal antibody
Generally immunocompetent

Table 4
Predisposing Factors for Fungal Sinusitis

Precedent bacterial (or viral) sinusitis
Multiple sinus surgeries
Multiple courses of antibacterials for sinusitis
Dental fillings of maxillary teeth
Nasotracheal and nasogastric intubations >5 d
Immunocompromised states
  Diabetic ketoacidosis
  Hematological malignancy
  Bone marrow transplantation
  Prolonged neutropenia
  Primary and acquired immunodeficiency
Residence in northern Sudan, Africa

local inflammatory reactions. Tissue invasion for the most part requires a breach of normal defense barriers. Neutrophils or macrophages prevent fungal spread in murine models. There is a direct correlation between dissemination and degree of neutropenia in hematological disorders, and evidence of cessation of spread if the neutropenia is reversed. High-dose corticosteroids allows conidia to germinate and proliferate within macrophages with subsequent invasion of adjacent tissues. Mice exposed to the inhalation of *Aspergillus flavus* spores and subjected to either irradiation, cyclophosphamide, corticosteroids, or bone marrow transplantation had a much higher death rate than untreated mice. Combinations of the above treatments were more lethal than any single one. Human counterparts are suggested by untreated leukemia patients who have less opportunistic fungal infections than leukemics treated with steroids, antibiotics, or cytotoxic drugs (17).

Of 1331 cancer patients treated at the University of Maryland during a 5-yr period, 52 developed sinusitis of which 21 were diagnosed as fungal, mostly from *Aspergillus* species (18). Predisposing factors for fungal sinusitis were granulocyte counts <500/μL (mean duration 42 vs 14 d for nonfungal sinusitis), and prolonged antibiotic therapy (mean duration 22 vs 9 d). A similar incidence of invasive fungal sinusitis, 2.6%, occurred among 423 consecutive bone marrow transplant recipients from 1986 to 1992 at the Hadassah University Hospital, Jerusalem (19). Again there was a direct correlation with duration of neutropenia. In both series, the most prevalent underlying disease was acute myelogenous leukemia (Table 4).

An exception to an immunodeficiency basis for invasive fungal sinusitis is the special situation in the Sudan. In the northern hot and arid areas, fungal, mostly *A. flavus,* invasive sinusitis is relatively common. Spores are plentiful in the ambient air, bedding, straw roofs, timbers, and earth floors of

the dwellings, and in nasal swabs from asymptomatic individuals (2). Veress et al. (20) believe three factors play a role in the Sudanese pathogenicity: recurrent nasal inflammation from the hot, dry, sandy environment; dissemination of spores in sandstorms; and an unspecified immune process once fungal invasion has begun. The Sudan experience may be widening based on a recent report from Saudi Arabia of rhinocerebral *Aspergillus* sinusitis in otherwise healthy individuals (21). Washburn et al. at the NIH and at Johns Hopkins (1) described seven cases of chronic invasive fungal sinusitis without evidence of immune disorders. One of the seven patients was a native of Sudan. Among their immunological studies were:

1. Phagocytic and fungicidal activity of peripheral blood mononuclear cells against *A. fumigatus* conidia;
2. Superoxide generation, reduction of nitroblue tetrazolium, and chemotaxis;
3. Esterase and myeloperoxidase staining of monocytes;
4. Natural killer cell functional activity;
5. Lymphocyte subpopulations;
6. Serum immunoglobulin levels;
7. Delayed-type hypersensitivity skin tests; and
8. HIV testing, including Western blot.

No immunological abnormalities were found in the patients studied.

Another factor predisposing to fungal sinusitis is immune hyperreactivity to fungal antigens resulting in inflammatory reactions. Models for this mechanism exist in pulmonary fungal allergic reactions, such as ABPA mycosis and hypersensitivity pneumonitis to *Aspergillus clavatus* in malt worker's lung. Based on these premises, allergic fungal sinusitis is believed to be mediated by the combination of IgE (Type I) and immune complex (Type III) reactions. Mast cell degranulation induced by IgE antibodies on membrane receptors binding with fungal antigens leads to release of vasoactive agents. These, in turn, promote extravascular deposition of complexes of circulating fungal non-IgE antibodies and antigen. Phagocytic cells, in the process of clearing the complexes, release various proteolytic enzymes that are proinflammatory. Specific T-cell activity may also contribute to inflammatory and granulomatous pathology.

The sinus aspergillomas have immunological responses similar to pulmonary aspergillomas. In both cases, serum-precipitating antibodies (IgG, IgM, and IgA classes) to *Aspergillus* antigens have been found *(22)*, but brisker precipitin reactions result from the pulmonary lesions. Unlike allergic fungal sinusitis and ABPA, the precipitins arising from mycetomas appear to be secondary and not contributory to the local pathology.

In addition to opportunistic infections, colonization, and antigenic activity, fungi can exert pathogenicity by toxic metabolites. Although fungal toxicosis has been found among plants, domesticated animals, and birds, there have apparently been no documented reports involving human sinuses *(23)*.

DIAGNOSIS

There are two broad historical clues that suggest that a patient's sinusitis might be of fungal origin. One is sinusitis that is chronic, recurrent, and seemingly unaffected by several courses of antibiotics or even by surgical attempts to improve drainage. The other is either acute or chronic sinusitis in immunodeficient patients.

Predisposing factors include prolonged antibiotic therapy, dental fillings or extractions abutting the maxillary sinuses, and prolonged oro-nasal intubations (Table 4). In one series, there was a 26% rate of sinusitis proved by CT scan in patients whose tracheas were intubated by the nasal route longer than 5 d *(24)*. A critical care unit reported a 5% rate of acute sinusitis over a 2-yr period in patients on nasotracheal intubation. Specific etiological diagnoses were not made in many cases, but there is a report of *Candida* pan-sinusitis in a patient requiring oro-tracheal and nasogastric intubation

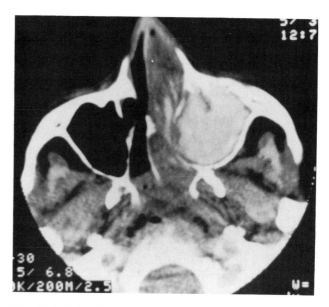

Fig. 5. Axial CT scan, without contrast media, reveals a hyperdense expanded left maxillary antrum with thinning of the medial wall. A low-attenuation mass is present in the left nasal cavity, extending from the choanal area into the nasopharynx. Diagnosis: allergic fungal sinusitis. (Reprinted from ref. *31* with permission.)

following multiple traumas from an auto accident *(24)*. In another study, 85 cases of *Aspergillus* paranasal sinusitis were diagnosed over a 15-yr period in an ENT clinic in Nantes, France *(3)*. The diagnosis was made by pathological examination, and all patients who were immunodeficient were excluded. A common factor in these otherwise healthy patients was indications of dental pathology. Eighty of the 85 showed on imaging a dense opacity within the affected maxillary sinus caused by a foreign body. In 72 cases, the density was associated with a dental filling. The intrasinus foreign body was identified as dental paste. The authors concluded that overfilling of maxillary teeth with dental paste gave rise to the foreign bodies, and colonization by *Aspergilli* was aided by zinc in the paste. Low concentrations of zinc accelerated fungi growth when added to culture media *(3)*.

Signs and symptoms of fungal sinusitis are similar to sinusitis of nonfungal origin. However, unilateral disease as indicated by symptoms, physical signs, or imaging is more common in fungal sinusitis, especially in the noninvasive category (Figs. 5 and 6). The maxillary sinus is most likely to be involved initially, but unilateral, isolated fungal disease has been reported for each of the sinuses. Nasal secretions may be mucopurulent, occasion-

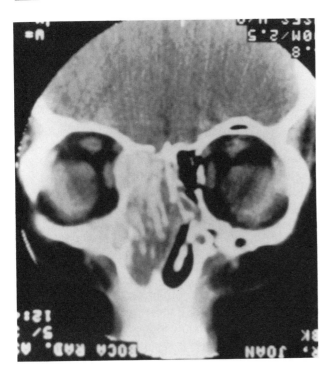

Fig. 6. Coronal CT image, without contrast material, the hyperdense mass filling the left ethmoid sinus and bulging into the left orbit. This 62-yr-old woman complained of obstruction of the left nasal cavity, anosmia, and tearing from the left eye. Same subject as in other figures. (Reprinted from ref. *31* with permission.)

ally blood-flecked, or containing caseous or pseudomembranous material, but cannot be considered specific for fungal infection.

Imaging can confirm sinus disease, but not an etiological diagnosis in most cases. However, in a series of 293 patients who underwent computed tomography (CT) for sinusitis, 25 were subsequently diagnosed as fungal following surgery and pathological examination. Most of them had foci of increased attenuation on scans. When magnetic resonance imaging (MRI) was performed on seven patients, a characteristic area of decreased signaling within a soft tissue mass was found on T2-weighted images *(25)*. In an effort to determine the basis of the CT and MRI images, the pathological specimens were subjected to special stains and chemical analysis for calcium, and furnace atomic absorption spectrometry for metals. The CT findings were attributed to calcium phosphate and sulfate deposits within necrotic debris, and the hypodense signal was attributed to interference by magnetic elements produced by fungal metabolites. The fungal sinusitis specimens contained higher

Table 5
Diagnostic Features of Fungal Sinusitis

History of chronic sinusitis resistant to antibacterials
Unilateral symptoms and signs
Purulent nasosinus drainage
Expulsion of caseous, membranous, hemorrhagic exudates
Sinus imaging abnormalities—MRI may be most specific
Confirmation by stains and cultures of sinus secretions

concentrations of manganese and iron than specimens from nonfungal sinusitis. Som and Curtin *(26)* caution that these findings can also be mimicked by desiccated secretions and hemorrhage, and thus cannot be definitive of fungal involvement (Table 5).

Definitive diagnosis requires identification of fungi within the sinus contents or, in the case of invasive disease, within sinus and adjacent tissue. Fungal elements may be revealed on H and E mounts, if plentiful, but special stains, such as Gomori methenamine silver, Fontana-Masson melanin, or periodic acid-Schiff stains may he required. Confirmation and speciation of the organism can be obtained by cultures of specimens from surgery and sinus irrigation using media designed for fungal growth. Nasal secretions *per se* do nor serve as suitable material, since even a positive culture may result from airborne or local contaminants *(1)*.

Differential diagnosis of unilateral sinus disease must consider neoplasm, such as an inverting papilloma, squamous cell carcinoma, lymphoma, and other, rarer tumors. More benign conditions to be differentiated include mucoceles, polyps, inclusion cysts, mucin impactions, and Pindborg tumors. Destructive lesions may be the results of nonfungal granulomas, especially Wegener's granulomatosis. A thorough history, physical examination and radiography may suffice to differentiate among the benign presentations, but surgical intervention will usually be needed to diagnose seriously ill patients.

TREATMENT

A diagnosis of fungal sinusitis usually means surgical intervention is the treatment of choice *(1,11)*. Medical treatments alone have proven unsuccessful. These have included use of systemic and topical antifungicides, desensitization attempts with fungal extracts, radiation therapy, and systemic iodides *(27)*. The key to successful surgery is removal of the fungal material and diseased mucosa (if present), maintenance of drainage, and aeration of the involved sinuses.

Diagnosis based on the classification of noninvasive or invasive type will dictate the degree of surgical intervention and whether ancillary medical treatments will be tried. The invasive category is the most serious, the noninvasive chronic and mycetoma forms more benign, and the allergic category is usually in between. Fungal invasion into the sinus mucosa can lead to unrestricted spread. *Mucor* species have a predilection for invading blood vessels and hematogenous dissemination *(28)*. Involvement of the lungs, spleen, and liver has occurred with some frequency. *Aspergilli* can also invade blood vessels, as well as dura and bone. Proptosis, diplopia, chemosis, and ophthalmoplegia signify orbital involvement, and intracranial extension via the dura may also have occurred. Hyphae may enter the internal carotid artery intracranially causing thrombi, emboli, or rupture with fatal hemorrhage *(2)*. If the fungus spreads to the orbit or intracranially, a life-threatening situation has arisen. Without prompt and sufficient surgical debridement, the mortality rate is high. Most surgeons advise wide excision of involved bone and tissue, while preserving the natural brain barriers—dura and orbital periosteum—even when locally involved *(1)*. Combinations of surgery with antifungal agents have been used. Intravenous and topical amphotericin, and oral imidazole derivatives (conazole agents) administered singly or in combination, have met with success, but not in all cases.

Improvement in invasive sinusitis, at least temporarily, will occur if the underlying immunocompromised conditions are also improved. Reversal of diabetic ketoacidosis has aided in the control of mucormycosis *(28)*. Correction of neutropenia with granulocyte transfusions and remission of leukemia under treatment have slowed fungal invasion *(18,19)*.

Visual impairment has occurred in patients diagnosed with allergic fungal sinusitis. In a series of five cases, the mycotic mass produced bony erosions into the orbital fossae, presumably from pressure expansion *(29)*. Patients treated with surgical excision and corticosteroids seemed to have fared better and had less recurrence than patients on surgery alone. Corey *(30)* recommends a postoperative prednisone dose of 80–100 mg daily over several weeks before tapering to lower mainte-

nance doses until a disease-free state can be confirmed by monitoring with sinus endoscopy and radiographic or MRI imaging.

In those noninvasive cases without extrasinus pathology, surgical procedures and maintenance of aeration usually suffice, although some authors have added antifungal therapy *(1,14)*.

In summary, surgical excision of the mycotic masses is the treatment of choice. Steroid treatment, similar to the experience with ABPA, has been added for some patients with the allergic sinusitis form of fungal disease. Antifungal regimens have been tried in some cases of chronic, noninvasive, and mycetoma types of fungal sinusitis, and in the majority of cases of invasive fungal sinusitis in recent years. Efforts should be made to correct or improve any immunodeficient states. It must be realized that the treatment modalities discussed above are anecdotal and empiric. Controlled studies of even a small series of cases have not been reported.

SYNOPSIS

Fungal-caused sinusitis has long been established, but there has been evidence during the past 15 yr of an increasing prevalence globally. Among reasons cited are improved diagnoses, heavy antibiotic use, and more acquired immunodeficiencies. Although about 18 different genera of fungi have been associated with sinusitis, most cases are caused by *Aspergilli*. Pathogenic mechanisms involve:

1. Colonization of damaged sinuses to produce localized mucosal inflammation;
2. A space-occupying noninflammatory fungal mass causing pressure symptoms;
3. Allergic inflammation mediated by Type I and III reactions; or
4. Opportunistic invasion usually in immunocompromised hosts.

These four mechanisms have their clinical correlates in the respective syndromes: chronic or indolent noninvasive, mycetoma, allergic fungal sinusitis, and acute and chronic invasive sinusitis. Mortality is highest in the invasive type, but morbidity is significant in the noninvasive forms, especially in allergic fungal sinusitis.

Surgical debridement, drainage, and aeration are the treatments of choice. Antifungicides have been added to the treatment of some cases of noninvasive forms, and most cases of mycotic invasion. Systemic corticosteroid therapy has supplemented surgical treatment for the allergic form, but the effectiveness of these approaches has not been subjected to definitive studies. Awareness of and earlier diagnosis of the fungal forms of sinusitis should lead to decreased morbidity and mortality.

REFERENCES

1. Washburn RG, Kennedy DW, Begley MG, Henderson DK, Bennett JE. Chronic fungal sinusitis in apparently normal hosts. Medicine 1988;67:231–247.

2. Jahrsdoerfer RA, Ejercito VS, Johns MME, Cantrell RW, Sydnor JB. Aspergillosis of the nose and paranasal sinuses. Am J Otolaryngol 1979;1:6–14.

3. Legent F, Billet J, Beauvillain C, Bonnet J, Miegeville M. The role of dental canal fillings in the development of Aspergillus sinusitis. Arch Otorhinolaryngol 1989;246:318–320.

4. Grigoriu D, Bambule J, Delacretaz J. Aspergillus sinusitis. Postgrad Med J 1979;55:619–621.

5. Petersen JM, Baldone SC, Sresthadatta T. Paranasal sinus aspergillosis: a report of two cases and review of the literature. J Am Osteopath Assoc 1982;81:549–553.

6. von Haacke N. Aspergillosis of the paranasal sinuses. J Laryngol Otol 1984;98:193–197.

7. Pingree TF, Holt GR, Otto RA, Rinaldi MG. Bipolaris-caused fungal sinusitis. Otolaryngol Head and Neck Surg 1992;106:302–305.

8. Watters GWR, Milford CA. Isolated sphenoid sinusitis due to Pseudallescheria boydii. J Laryngol Otol 1993;107:344–346.

9. Morrison VA, Weisdorf DJ. Alternaria: a sinonasal pathogen of immunocompromised hosts. Clin Infect Dis 1993;16:265–270.

10. James PW, Hawsworth DL. Dictionary of the Fungi. Kew, Surrey: Commonwealth Mycological Institute, 1971.

11. Lin WS, Hung HY. Transnasal endoscopic surgery of sphenoid sinus aspergillosis. J Laryngol Otol 1993;107:837–839.

12. Katzenstein A-LA, Sale SR, Greenberger P. Allergic Aspergillus sinusitis: a newly recognized form of sinusitis. J Allergy Clin Immunol 1983;72:89–93.

13. Katzenstein A-LA, Sale SR, Greenberger PA. Pathologic findings in allergic aspergillus sinusitis: a newly recognized form of sinusitis. Am J Surg Pathol 1983;7:439–443.

14. Goldstein MF. Allergic fungal sinusitis: an underdiagnosed problem. Hosp Pract 1992;27:73–92.

15. Shah A, Bhagat R, Panchal N, Jaggi OP, Khan ZU. Allergic bronchopulmonary aspergillosis with middle lobe syndrome and allergic Aspergillus sinusitis. Eur Respir J 1993;6:917,918.

16. Austwick PKC. Pathogenicity. In: Raper KB, Fennell DI, eds., The Genus Aspergillus. Huntington, NY: Robert E. Krieger, 1977; pp. 90, 91.

17. Lemos LB, Jensen AB. Pathology of aspergillosis. In: Al-Doory Y, Wagner GE, eds., Aspergillosis. Springfield, IL: Charles C. Thomas, 1985, p. 172.

18. Viollier A-F, Peterson DE, De Jongh CA, et al. Aspergillus sinusitis in cancer patients. Cancer 1986;58:366–371.

19. Drakos PE, Nagler A, Or R, et al. Invasive fungal sinusitis in patients undergoing bone marrow transplantation. Bone Marrow Transplantation 1993;12:203–208.

20. Veress B, Malik OA, El Tayeb AA, El Daoud S, El Mahgoub S, El Hassan AM. Further observations on the primary paranasal Aspergillus granuloma in the Sudan. Am J Trop Med Hyg 1973;22:765–772.

21. Kameswaran M, Al-Wadei A, Khurana P, Okafor BC. Rhinocerebral aspergillosis. J Laryngol Otol 1992;106:981–985.

22. Mahgoub EL. Mycological and serological studies on Aspergillus flavus isolated from paranasal aspergilloma in Sudan. J Trop Med Hyg 1971;74:162–165.

23. Austwick PKC. Pathogenicity. In: Raper KB, Fennell DI, eds., The Genus Aspergillus, Huntington, NY: Robert E. Krieger, 1977; p. 83.

24. Wolf M, Zillinsky I, Lieberman P. Acute mycotic sinusitis with bacterial sepsis in orotracheal intubation and nasogastric tubing: a case report and review of the literature. Otolaryngol Head Neck Surg 1988;98:615–617.

25. Zinreich SJ, Kennedy DW, Malat J, et al. Fungal sinusitis: diagnosis with CT and MR imaging. Radiology 1988;169:439–444.

26. Som PM, Curtin HD. Chronic inflammatory sinonasal diseases including fungal infections: the role of imaging. Radiol Clin North Am 1993;31:33–44.

27. McGuirt WF, Harrill JA. Paranasal sinus aspergillosis. Laryngoscope 1979;89:1563–1568.

28. Kohn R, Hepler R. Management of limited rhino-orbital mucormycosis without exenteration. Ophthalmology 1985;92:1440–1444.

29. Daghistani KJ, Jamal TS, Zaher S, Nassif OI. Allergic Aspergillus sinusitis with proptosis. J Laryngol Otol 1992;106:759–803.

30. Corey JP. Allergic fungal sinusitis. Otolaryng Clin North Am 1992;25:225–230.

31. Case Records of the Massachusetts General Hospital. Weekly clinicopathological exercises. Case 20—1991. A 62-year-old woman with obstruction of the left nasal cavity and paranasal sinuses by a mass. N Eng J Med 1991;324:1423–1429.

17   Rhinocerebral Mucormycosis

Katherine A. Kendall, MD *and Craig W. Senders,* MD

CONTENTS

INTRODUCTION

Rhinocerebral mucormycosis is an uncommon, but rapidly progressive, fungal infection of the nose and sinuses that plagues diabetics and other immunocompromised patients. Its invasion results in fulminating disease that often runs its course within days. The organisms are inhaled and deposited in the nasal and pharyngeal mucosa. In the appropriate host, invasion occurs rapidly, leading to involvement of the paranasal sinuses with subsequent spread into the orbit and cranial cavity. Mucormycosis is the most acutely fatal fungal infection known *(1)*. Survival depends on prompt diagnosis and the aggressive institution of appropriate therapies *(1,2)*. A diagnosis of mucormycosis must be suspected in immunocompromised patients presenting with sinusitis, especially if there has been a slow or minimal clinical response to antibiotics.

From: *Diseases of the Sinuses* (M. E. Gershwin and G. A. Incaudo, eds.), ©1996 Humana Press Inc., Totowa, NJ.

The term mucormycosis encompasses a group of invasive infections caused by fungi within the taxonomic order mucorales, usually *Rhizopus, Absidia,* and *Mucor (1,3)*. These fungi are ubiquitous in nature, subsisting on decaying vegetation and organic material. The spores are airborne and can be easily inhaled *(4–6)*. Mucorales are cultured from nasal swabs in healthy people where no pathologic abnormality owing to the noninvasive presence of the fungi can be found *(1,4)*. When these fungi become invasive, the clinical course of infection by the various species is indistinguishable, and the identification of the species involved is not required to make a diagnosis of mucormycosis and institute therapy *(1,3)*. *Rhizopus* is the species most frequently associated with rhinocerebral mucormycosis *(4)*. The noninvasive presence of fungi on nasal examination must be distinguished from the invasive and often lethal mucormycosis.

Opportunistic infections with mucormycoses occur in patients who are exposed to cytotoxic and immunosuppressive treatments, as well as in patients with poorly controlled diabetes mellitus. Some underlying debilitating disease is identified in over 95% of mucormycosis cases *(5)*. Diabetes, particularly when accompanied by ketoacidosis, is the most common underlying disease. There has been, however, an increase in mucormycosis reported in patients with leukemia or lymphoma, burns, renal failure with or without acidosis, and prolonged postoperative courses. Other associated conditions include multiple myeloma, carcinoma, sepsis, cirrhosis, severe diarrhea, malnutrition, and congestive heart failure *(2,4–8)*.

PATHOPHYSIOLOGY

The reason for the tendency of these infections to occur in immunosuppressed or ketoacidotic patients is speculative. Ketosis and acid pH may enhance the invasion and growth of the fungi *(5,9)*. Certain mucorales species are known to have an active ketone-reductase system, and this allows them to thrive in an acid environment *(1,10,11)*. They are also capable of growing in tissues with a low oxygen tension.

Animal models have been used to study host resistance in an attempt to explain why diabetic and immunocompromised patients fail to contain a mucor infection adequately. When large numbers of spores are instilled in the nares of normal mice or rabbits, only a local mild inflammatory reaction develops. The spores fail to germinate and are killed during a period of several weeks. In contrast, when spores are introduced into ketoacedotic rabbits, fulminant infection is induced. Normal rabbits made hyperglycemic by a constant glucose infusion (but not ketoacidotic) did not develop vascular invasion or tissue infarction when spores were introduced intranasally, suggesting that hyperglycemia alone is not responsible for the immunologic defect *(1)*. Acidosis and decreased tissue oxygen tension appear to be major components in allowing the fungus to proliferate *(12)*. The inflammatory response in ketoacidotic animals also differs from controls. There is a neutrophil-rich exudate surrounding hyphael elements in control animals that is attenuated in the ketoacidotic animals *(2)*.

Human diabetics have decreased phagocytic and chemotactic activity of neutrophils resulting in a depressed local inflammatory response. It is postulated that this is a major factor in the ability of the fungi to invade *(1,2,5,10–13)*. Humoral factors may also play a role in host defenses. Normal human serum can prevent the growth of rhizopus spores on a nutrient medium. The serum of hyperketotic patients appears actually to enhance growth of the rhizopus spores. This property disappears when the ketoacidotic state is controlled.

Patients undergoing hemodialysis and treatment with deferoxamine for iron and aluminum overload have recently been reported to be susceptible to infections with mucorales. This drug is known to chelate iron, and it is postulated that iron thus becomes more available to the fungus, enhancing its growth *(3,10)*.

Mucormycosis infections are classified into rhinocerebral, pulmonary, widely disseminated, gastrointestinal, and cutaneous *(3)*. Rhinocerebral infection is the most common form of the disease *(4,5)*.

SPREAD OF INFECTION

Rhinocerebral mucormycosis usually begins in the nasal passages or palate and extends to the adjacent paranasal sinuses. The first cellular form of these fungi infecting humans is probably the airborne spore, and only the immunocompromised person fails to respond to this invasion by phagocytic containment. The spores are metabolically inert, but spore germination is initiated in a water-containing environment, such as the nares. A healthy person probably produces compounds that inhibit some aspect of spore germination, but once germinated, the fungus evolves into its hyphael form, which has the necessary features for invasiveness *(2)*.

The propensity of the fungus for invasion of the internal elastic lamina of blood vessels is the hallmark of mucormycosis *(5,11)*. Hyphael invasion of blood vessels leads to thrombosis and subsequent tissue infarction, which produces pale ischemic tissues and black necrotic purulence. The fungus proceeds to invade the adjacent hypoxic and acidotic tissue directly, thus propagating the infection *(4,12,13)*. Initially, fungi invade arteries, and later, fungi invade veins and lymphatics *(1,6)*. The infection tends to progress through the ethmoid sinuses and spreads to the retro-orbital region via extension of thrombosis along the vasculature that connects these structures or by direct extension through the soft tissues *(1)*. Ocular and optic nerve ischemia from fungal infiltration is responsible for the frequent loss of vision seen in these patients *(8)*.

Mucormycosis tends to extend through the orbital apex into the brain. Some investigators feel that the most common route of central nervous system infection is by direct extension of the infection from the paranasal sinuses *(3)*. Not only can the infection reach the cranial cavity through the cribriform plate and orbital apex, but also through invasion of the vascular system, such as the carotid artery *(1,4–6)*. Embolization of septic thrombi is also a potential route of spread to the brain *(2,9)*. In our experience, orbital involvement with mucormycosis is tantamount to the development of intracranial infection, and we recommend that these patients be treated as if intracranial infection already existed *(14)*.

CLINICAL PRESENTATION

Patients may present initially with orbital and facial pain out of proportion to physical signs. A black eschar or pale area on the palate or nasal mucosa is a diagnostic clue to the presence of mucormycosis. A characteristic brick-red discoloration of the nasal mucosa occurs, followed by the development of the eschar *(5,6)*. Many patients may complain of epistaxis, and the intranasal eschar of mucormycosis can be mistaken for dried blood *(1)*. Other common initial findings of rhinocerebral mucormycosis include lethargy and headache. Patients with mucormycosis appear to be systemically ill.

Loss of ocular movement, ptosis, proptosis, periorbital paresthesias, and cellulitis occur as a result of orbital invasion by the fungus *(1,9)*. As orbital involvement progresses, pupillary dilatation and loss of vision occur. Abedi et al. report in a review of 179 cases that the most common presenting signs of mucormycosis are cranial nerve defects, facial swelling, proptosis, palatal ulcer, and decreased mental status *(15)*. The fifth and seventh cranial nerves may become involved later. Palatal and facial skin necrosis may also occur *(1)*.

The early visual loss with retinal artery occlusion seen in mucormycosis helps to distinguish it from cavernous sinus thrombosis although cavernous sinus thrombosis, and internal carotid artery thrombosis may complicate mucormycosis *(4)*. Bacterial cavernous sinus thrombosis usually presents with a prodrome of deep retro-orbital pain, and severe orbital congestion and cellulitis, lacrimation, lid edema, and ptosis. Exophthalmos and decreased visual acuity are late findings in bacte-

rial cavernous sinus thrombosis, but occur early in the course of mucormycosis owing to the involvement of the orbital apex with central retinal artery thrombosis *(1,2,13)*. *See* Chapter 11 for additional details regarding bacterial sinusitis.

Brain involvement commonly arises from infarction due to direct vascular invasion by the fungi *(4)*. The intracranial lesions that result from mucormycosis infection can be categorized into three types:

1. Those that result from direct tissue invasion and necrosis, such as meningitis, brain abscess, and cranial nerve palsies;
2. Those secondary to vascular injuries, such as cavernous sinus thrombosis, internal carotid thrombosis or aneurysm, and ischemic infarcts; and
3. Those resulting from space-occupying lesions manifested as hydrocephalus and behavioral changes *(10)*.

DIAGNOSIS

A high index of suspicion is key to making an early diagnosis. Particular mention should be made of the clinical syndrome of the diabetic patient presenting in ketoacidosis with obtundation. If the obtundation does not respond to correction of the metabolic abnormalities, a diagnosis of mucormycosis should be entertained and a work-up initiated *(2)*.

A biopsy specimen of the involved tissues is required to make a diagnosis of mucormycosis. Within the tissues are found the broad, thick-walled nonseptate hyphae with right angle branching that are characteristic of mucormycosis *(5,7,9)* (Fig. 1). Ante mortem cultures are frequently negative. Thus, biopsy of suspicious lesions for histopathologic examination must be done. Swabs of the infected regions may be negative. Thus, the procurement of tissue is a requirement *(9)*. Microscopic examination of involved tissues should be done by mixing a small portion of the material with two to three drops of 10–20% potassium hydroxide on a glass slide or by frozen section. The organisms can be easily visualized with hematoxylin and eosin stains, silver nitrate stains, and PAS stains *(1,3,9)*. The initiation of treatment is based on the histopathology found on frozen section. Culture of biopsy material can be used to confirm the diagnosis, but to delay treatment while waiting for culture results would likely be lethal in cases of invasive

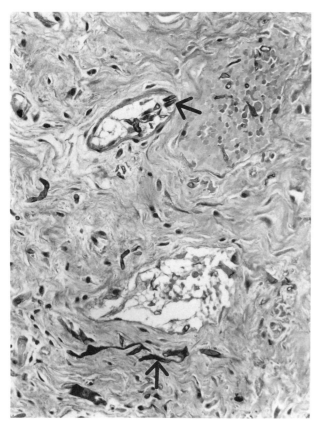

Fig. 1. Histological section of infected tissue demonstrating the broad septate hyphae of mucormycosis.

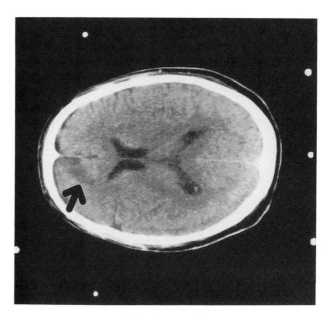

Fig. 2. CT scan of patient with intracranial mucormycosis demonstrating cerebritis.

mucormycosis. The organisms are aerobic and grow well on many media in 2–5 d at 37° *(3)*. Pathological evaluation of involved tissues reveals vasculitis with thrombosis, hemorrhage, and infarction *(3,5,6)*.

Radiographic findings in mucormycosis are nonspecific. Multiple sinuses may be involved, and there is typically an absence of air–fluid levels *(6)*. Spotty destruction of the bony walls of the sinuses is often seen on CT scans and nodular thickening of the sinus mucosa may be present *(1,2,9,13,16,17)*. The fungus can extend beyond bony partitions without evidence of bone destruction, because it travels along the vascular channels that penetrate the bone, such as the anterior and posterior ethmoid arteries *(2)*.

CT scans can be particularly helpful in identifying the presence of orbital and intracranial disease *(2,3,6,7,9)*. CT signs specific for orbital involvement with mucormycosis include no contrast enhancement of the superior ophthalmic vein and the ophthalmic artery *(2)*. Cerebritis, or the early

stages of brain abscess formation, is represented on CT by hypodense regions within the cerebral tissues *(15)*. These lesions may also be the result of infarct *(2)* (Fig. 2). Invasion of the cerebrum with frank abscess formation usually occurs in the frontal or temporal lobes, and, after the infusion of iv contrast, the typical well-defined ring enhancement seen on CT scans with bacterial abscesses is not always seen with mucormycosis *(2,7)*. T2-weighted MR images may be more sensitive than CT in detecting intracranial spread, and allow the early detection of meningeal irritation, intracranial vascular occlusion, and parenchymal involvement before clinical signs develop *(7,10)*. Fungal infiltration of fat planes of the face and orbit can also be seen on MRI *(7,17)*. High concentrations of calcium, iron, and manganese may be found in the fungal-infected tissue. These elements have the ability to disturb the magnetic field and will create a hypointense signal on MRI *(4)*.

Cerebral spinal fluid (CSF) findings in intracranial mucormycosis infections are also nonspecific. The CSF may be normal, or contain increased cell numbers and mild protein elevation *(2,8)*. CSF and blood cultures are rarely positive *(2)*.

DIFFERENTIAL DIAGNOSIS

The differential diagnosis of invasive mucormycosis infection includes invasive infection with

Aspergillus species. The clinical picture of the two conditions is similar, and biopsy is required to differentiate the two *(3,13)*. Mucormycosis appears as broad, thick-walled hyphae that branch at right angles compared to *Aspergillus,* which is segmented *(7)* (Fig. 1). Bacterial cavernous sinus thrombosis must also be delineated from mucormycosis. Malignancy should always be included in the differential diagnosis *(9,13)*.

TREATMENT

Invasive mucormycosis infection is fatal without therapy. Successful treatment relies on early diagnosis, systemic antifungal therapy, aggressive surgical debridement, and control of the underlying disease. Early recognition and aggressive treatment are considered to be responsible for the growing number of survivors of infectious mucormycosis *(2)*.

SURGICAL THERAPY

The surgical removal of all necrotic tissue is the mainstay of therapy. Debridement of the paranasal sinuses, orbital exenteration, and craniotomy may be required *(11,15)*. Survival is markedly improved in patients with intracranial extension of disease who undergo aggressive debridement. Anand et al. reviewed 123 cases of intracerebral mucormycosis and found a survival rate of 70% in patients who underwent craniotomy for eradication of intracranial disease compared to a 25% survival rate in patients who did not have a craniotomy *(10)*.

AMPHOTERICIN B THERAPY

Despite aggressive surgical therapy, the prognosis for rhinocerebral mucormycosis remained poor until the introduction of the antifungal agent, Amphotericin B, in 1958 *(7,9)*. Amphotericin B remains the most reliable single agent against mucormycosis *(2)*. Gass reported the first survivor of rhinocerebral mucormycosis who was treated with amphotericin B *(19)*. Since that time, results have been variable in part owing to the fact that minimal inhibitory concentrations (MICs) for mucormycosis have not been established. The in vivo form of mucormycosis seems to be more sensitive to amphotericin B than the spore used in in vitro studies. As a result, in vitro sensitivities do not have much value as a guide to clinical effective-

ness of the drug *(2)*. The rate of amphotericin B administration varies with the patient's overall condition and the severity of infection. Traditionally, a 1-mg test dose is recommended followed by a progressive daily escalation of the dose. In seriously ill patients with rapidly progressing disease, valuable time is lost while patients remain on suboptimal doses by this schedule. Patients should be brought to the maximum dose as soon as they are clinically able to tolerate it. An increase of the dose by 0.25 mg/kg/d until a dose of 1 mg/kg/d is reached is often recommended *(7)*. Each iv dose is given over 4–6 h. A premedication of acetaminophen, benadryl, and demerol may be administered to help counteract the fevers and chills that are commonly experienced during the infusion. These signs may be confused with further extension of the disease *(11)*. The daily dose is continued until the patient's condition improves to the point where no further spread of infection has been noted for at least 7 d, at which time an every-other-day regimen can be established. A total of 2–6 g of amphotericin B may be required to clear the infection, although the regimen must be tailored for individual patients *(7,12)*. Some authors recommend treatment for at least 2 mo *(2,5)*.

In cases of intracranial mucormycosis, there is a need to improve the delivery of the amphotericin B to the brain tissues since its passage through the blood–brain barrier is poor. We have successfully treated patients with proven intracerebral mucormycosis by instilling the amphotericin B directly into the ventricles via a surgically placed Ommaya reservoir. Patients who require orbital exenteration for debridement of involved tissues should be considered to have intracranial spread of infection despite no evidence of cerebritis on a CT scan, since experience shows that the vast majority of these patients go on to develop frank intracranial disease. We recommend that these patients undergo placement of an Ommaya reservoir and are started on intrathecal amphotericin B *(18)*.

Therapy with amphotericin B may be limited by its nephrotoxity and bone marrow suppression, particularly in an already immunocompromised patient population. The renal toxicity is directly related to the serum concentration and the total dose of the drug given *(11)*. Some authors recommend allowing the serum creatinine to reach 3.0 before holding a dose of amphotericin B in order to stabilize a patient's kidney function. Hypermagnesemia and hypocalcemia are also side effects of the therapy *(5,11)*.

There have been reports in the literature of successful mucormycosis treatment using a liposomal form of amphotericin B that is less toxic, and may have an improved therapeutic effect because of better CSF penetration and enhancement of the therapeutic index over 20-fold. Reported dosages are 1 mg/kg for up to 28 d, followed by the use of regular amphotericin B for a total dose of only 2 g. The liposomal preparation of amphotericin B improves the intracellular delivery of the drug to phagocytes *(5)*. These reports are preliminary and the number of patients treated is small, but this form of the drug holds promise *(5,7)*.

Despite therapy with amphotericin B, early and repeated surgical resection of all infected tissues is required for successful treatment of mucormycosis. All necrotic tissue must be removed. Amphotericin B is fungistatic only and cannot reach tissues infected secondary to thrombosed vasculature *(11)*. This drug is thus often unable to eradicate the primary focus of infection, but is effective in controlling micrometastasis and preventing further progression of the primary focus *(15)*. Some institutions irrigate wounds with amphotericin B or apply it to dressings in an attempt to saturate infected tissues directly with the drug *(7)*.

METABOLIC MANAGEMENT

Correction of diabetic ketoacidosis is an integral part of any therapeutic attempt at controlling the mucormycosis. There have been reports linking mucormycosis in well-controlled diabetics with disease that is more localized and more responsive to therapy. Those patients in whom control of the underlying debilitating disease is not possible have a uniformly dismal outcome *(11,15,17)*.

HYPERBARIC OXYGEN THERAPY

Hyperbaric oxygen therapy has been used as an adjunct in the treatment of invasive mucormycosis with success *(14)*. The mechanism of action of the hyperbaric oxygen is not clear. It is believed that the increased oxygen tension within the tissues improves migration of polymorphonuclear leukocytes (PMNs) and macrophages, allows fibroblasts to lay down collagen (which provides a framework for new vessel formation) and may alleviate acidosis and hypoxia in marginal tissues, thus preventing fungal proliferation. Hyperoxia inhibits fungal growth in vitro *(6,9,12)*. Current treatment regimens consist of 2-h exposures to 100% oxygen at 2 atm every 12 h for up to 30 treatments. Contraindications to the use of hyperbaric oxygen treatments include the presence of intracranial air and medical instability of the patient. Possible complications include hyperoxic seizures and pneumothorax. It is recommended that patients undergo the placement of pressure equalization tubes in the tympanic membranes prior to treatment. The tubes enable rapid middle ear pressure equalization during therapy *(2,6)*.

OUTCOME

Accurate data on the effectiveness of treatment for mucormycosis are difficult to find. Patients treated successfully generally have less extensive mucormycosis than those treated unsuccessfully. This finding confirms the notion that early diagnosis leads to a more favorable outcome *(2)*. Survival rates range from 35 to 70% *(8)*. Poor prognosis is clearly related to the severity of the underlying disease and the ability to correct it *(10)*. Diabetic patients have a better prognosis than patients presenting with leukemia in whom the induction of a remission is unlikely *(11,15,17)*. Patients presenting with facial necrosis, nasal deformity, internal carotid artery occlusion, cavernous sinus thrombosis, and intracerebral mucormycosis have an extremely poor prognosis *(1,9,10,12)*. There are several reports in the literature where none of the patients presenting with orbital or intracranial extension of disease survive despite amphotericin B and surgical debridement *(7,8)*.

At least 70% of survivors are left with residual defects. Cranial nerve palsies and blindness are the most commonly reported sequelae *(11)*.

REFERENCES

1. Eisenberg L, Wood T, Boles R. Mucormycosis. Laryngoscope 1977;87:347–356.
2. Lehrer RI, Howard DH, Sypherd PS, Edwards JE, Segal GP, Winston DJ. Mucormycosis. Ann Int Med 1980;93(1):93–108.
3. Sugar AM. Mucormycosis. Clin Infectious Diseases 1992;14(Suppl. 1):S126–S129.
4. Terk MR, Underwood DJ, Zee CS, Colletti PM. MR imaging in rhinocerebral and intracranial mucormycosis with CT and pathologic correlation. Magn Reson Imaging 1992;10:81–87.

5. Fisher EW, Toma A, Fisher PH, Cheesman AD. Rhinocerebral mucormycosis: use of liposomal amphotericin B. J Laryngol Otol 1991;105:575–577.

6. Ferguson BJ, Mitchell TG, Moon R, Camporesi EM, Farmer J. Adjunctive hyperbaric oxygen for treatment of rhinocerebral mucormycosis. Rev Infectious Diseases 1988;10(3):551–559.

7. Nussbaum ES, Hall WA. Rhinocerebral mucormycosis: changing patterns of disease. Surg Neurol 1994;1:152–156.

8. Sponsler TA, Sassani JW, Johnson LN, Towfighi J. Ocular invasion in mucormycosis: survey of ophthalmology. 1992;36(5):345–350.

9. Kemper J, Kuijper EJ, Mirck PGB, Balm AJM. Recovery from rhinocerebral mucormycosis in a ketoacidotic diabetic patient: a case report. J Laryngol Otol 1993; 107:233–235.

10. Anand VK, Alemar G, Griswold JA. Intracranial complications of mucormycosis: an experimental model and clinical review. Laryngoscope 1992;102:656–662.

11. Blitzer A, Lawson W, Meyers BR, Biller HF. Patient survival factors in paranasal sinus mucormycosis. Laryngoscope 1980;90:635–648.

12. Couch L, Theilen F, Mader JT. Rhinocerebral mucormycosis with cerebral extension successfully treated with adjunctive hyperbaric oxygen therapy. Arch Otolaryngol Head and Neck Surg 1988;114:791–794.

13. Ziegler EI. Cerebral mucormycosis; neurologic infections. In: Braude AJ, ed., Medical Microbiology and Infectious Diseases. Philadelphia, PA: W. B. Saunders, 1985, pp. 1085–1088.

14. De La Paz MA, Patrinely JR, Marines HM, Appling WD. Adjunctive hyperbaric oxygen in the treatment of bilateral cerebro-rhino-orbital mucormycosis. Am J Ophthalmology 1992;114:208–211.

15. Abedi E, Sismanis A, Choi K, Pastore P. Twenty-five years' experience treating cerebro-rhino-orbital mucormycosis. Laryngoscope 1984;94:1060–1062.

16. Estrem SA, Tully R, Davis WE. Rhinocerebral mucormycosis: computed tomographic imaging of cavernous sinus thrombosis. Ann Otol Rhinol Laryngol 1990; 99:160,161.

17. Gamba JL, Woodruff WW, Djang WT, Yeates AE. Craniofacial mucormycosis: assessment with CT. Radiology 1986;160(1):207–212.

18. LePage E. Using a ventricular reservoir to instill amphotericin B. J Neurosci Nursing 1993;25(4):212–217.

19. Gass JDM. Acute orbital mucormycosis. Report of two cases. Arch Ophthal 1961;65:214–221.

18 Sinus Disease in Cystic Fibrosis

Michael J. Light, MD, Richard B. Moss, MD,
and Terence M. Davidson, MD

CONTENTS

INTRODUCTION
CYSTIC FIBROSIS
CF SINUS DISEASE
ACUTE AND CHRONIC SINUSITIS
MEDICAL MANAGEMENT
SURGICAL TREATMENT
REFERENCES

INTRODUCTION

The current understanding of pathophysiology, diagnosis, and management of sinus disease has resulted in a more aggressive approach that appears to benefit children and adults with cystic fibrosis (CF). Chronic sinusitis, with and without nasal polyps, is problematic in the majority of CF patients, and previous treatment strategies have been associated with disappointing results. The new approaches for management of chronic sinus disease are clearly associated with improved outcome. The otolaryngologist has become an integral member of the team caring for CF patients.

CYSTIC FIBROSIS

The CF gene is carried by about 5% (1 in 20) of the Caucasian population. The incidence of CF is approx 1:2500 live births of the Caucasian population and 1:10,000 African-American live births. The incidence in the Hispanic population is unknown, but has been suggested to be about

1:11,500 live births (1). CF is rare in Polynesians and extremely rare in Asians. It is estimated that there are 25,000–30,000 patients with CF in the US. Median survival approaches 30 yr of age, and there is optimism that major breakthroughs in care will result in further improvement in life expectancy. The major problem with CF is chronic inflammatory pulmonary disease, which results in destructive lung changes.

In 1989, it was announced that the CF gene and its gene product had been identified. The protein that results from the CF gene is CFTR, which is the cystic fibrosis transmembrane conductance regulator. The defect that comprises approx 70% of the alleles of individuals with CF is a deletion of 3 bp that code for the amino acid phenylalanine at position 508 of chromosome seven. There are more than 400 other defects that have been found to account for the remaining 30% of CF alleles. The definitive diagnostic test remains the sweat chloride test, performed by pilocarpine iontophoresis. Sodium or chloride concentration >60 mmol/L is necessary to confirm the diagnosis.

The chloride defect that appears to be key to the resultant thick mucus that is characteristic of CF

From: *Diseases of the Sinuses* (M. E. Gershwin and G. A. Incaudo, eds.),
©1996 Humana Press Inc., Totowa, NJ.

357

was first recognized in the early 1980s. Quinton *(2)* demonstrated that the high sweat chloride was related to very low chloride permeability in the sweat duct, so that salt could not be absorbed. Knowles et al. *(3)* demonstrated that there is defective regulation of the secretory chloride channel of the apical membrane of the respiratory mucosal cell. In the respiratory tract, there is production of mucus that has reduced water content, leading to impaired mucociliary transport and stasis of mucus and infection. The resultant thick mucus in the gastrointestinal tract leads to meconium ileus in the newborn. In the pancreas, the thick secretions prevent sodium bicarbonate and digestive enzymes from passage through the pancreatic duct, resulting in pancreatic malabsorption in about 90% of CF patients.

Antibiotics and airway clearance techniques are employed to reduce pulmonary morbidity. Newer modalities to thin the mucus of airway secretions include recombinant human DNase (alpha dornase) and amiloride. RhDNase has been approved recently by the FDA and is marketed as Pulmozyme (R, Genentech Inc., San Francisco, CA). Pulmozyme functions to reduce the viscosity of CF sputum by depolymerizing the DNA, which is abundant in infected CF sputum. Pulmozyme has been shown to improve pulmonary function and reduce respiratory tract infection *(4)*. The sodium channel blocker amiloride inhibits transepithelial sodium transport in the human airway *(5)*. Aerosol administration of amiloride slows accelerated sodium transport rates in the CF airway epithelium and appears to normalize the viscoelastic property of CF airway secretions.

Various techniques are being employed to transfer a functional CFTR gene into the airway cells of patients with CF. The CFTR gene has been transferred using an attenuated adenovirus into the nasal epithelium with normalization of electrophysiologic properties. Initial studies have delivered adenovirus-mediated gene into the lung, and liposomes have delivered the gene into the sinuses *(6–8)*.

CF SINUS DISEASE

CF patients have normal ciliary beat frequency *(9),* but mucociliary transport is frequently impaired, and ultrastructural abnormalities are frequently found. It is not clear whether the findings are related to the chronic infection or if there is an inherent defect of the cilia. Evaluation of the structure and function of cilia of CF patients by Jorissen *(10)* has shown no difference in ciliary activity in vitro, suggesting that the abnormal mucociliary function is the result of *in situ* effects of the mucus, infection, or both.

Moss and coworkers *(11)* collected maxillary antral secretions at the time of endoscopic sinus surgery from 11 patients with CF. They analyzed histopathology and microbiology, as well as biochemical and rheologic properties of these secretions. Macroscopically, CF sinus secretions were grossly inspissated and tenaciously adherent to the underlying mucosa. All samples analyzed were colonized by *Pseudomonas aeruginosa*; one sample also contained *Aspergillus fumigatus* with a surrounding granulocytic infiltrate (Fig. 1A,B). Unlike sputum, where there is usually a massive polymorphonuclear cell infiltrate, sinus secretions from CF patients were primarily acellular masses of mucinous material (Fig. 2) with islands of desquamative epithelium (Fig. 3).

Purulence was assessed by measuring DNA concentration. CF sinus secretions exhibited DNA concentrations of 34–1776 µg/mL (mean ± SE, 524 ± 190) (Table 1). This is about 1 log lower than that seen in CF sputum, where mean DNA concentration is 7900 ± 1200 µg/mL. Compactibility, a measure of viscoelastic properties, of CF sinus secretions was also sharply reduced compared to CF sputum; only about 25% of samples showed a positive response to the in vitro action of rhDNase with a ≥25% increase in compaction after exposure to 16 µg/mL rhDNase (Table 1). Thus, sinus secretions in CF appear to be severely inspissated and infected mucin collections with a lesser acute inflammatory cellular response than that seen in the lower respiratory tract.

Rulon et al. *(12)* suggested that viscid mucus causes cystic dilatation of the nasal mucosal glands, which results in compression and obstruction of terminal capillaries. Resulting edema then leads to polypoid prolapse. Polyps associated with CF are similar to those related to allergy with mucous gland hyperplasia, mucous cysts, and epithelial dysplasia. The difference between CF and allergy polyps has been defined by Oppenheimer *(13)*. The CF polyps have a fine basement membrane and few eosinophils, and the mucous glands contain acid mucins. Polyps from atopic patients have thick basement membranes, high eosinophil counts, and

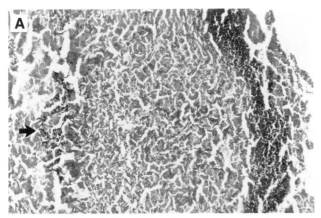

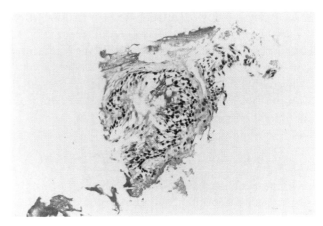

Fig. 2. Low-power view of desquamated epithelial cluster and adherent mucus in sample from another patient.

Fig. 1. Histochemistry of sinus secretions from CF patients. Sections were obtained at surgery, frozen, sectioned, and stained with PAS-Diastase to show mucin while degrading glycogen. **(A)** Low-power view from a patient with sample DNA content of 650 µg/mL but no compaction to recombinant DNase, showing concretized mucus glycoprotein (stained pink, in middle), inflammatory cell infiltrate (stained violet, right), and fungal colonization (arrow) within inspissated mucous mass. **(B)** High-power view of sample shows hyphae of *A. fumigatus* (arrow).

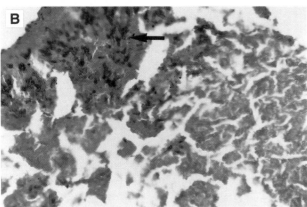

Fig. 3. Low-power view of pauci-cellular mass of mucous glycoprotein comprising sinus secretory concretion in sample from a third CF patient.

neutral mucins. The pathogenesis of polyps in CF remains unclear. It is likely that the mucous glands, which have thickened mucus, become dilated and inflamed.

Nasal polyps are found in 6–48% of CF patients *(14–19),* and the relationship between polyps and sinus disease is unclear. Polyps have been noted as young as 2 yr of age. They are multiple and usually bilateral, presenting during childhood and becoming less frequent in adolescence. Polyps are unusual before 5 and are initially seen before 20 yr of age. The onset of nasal polyps may precede the diagnosis of CF and so should be considered an indication to perform the sweat test *(20).* One study concerning polyps in adults described the highest incidence

Table 1
DNA and Compaction Results of CF Sinus Secretions

Patient	DNA g/mL	Compaction saline	Compaction rhDNase
1	159	66	44
2	1776	18	10
3	147	TC	TC
4	620	TC	TC
5	40	TC	TC
6	34	TC	TC
7	650	3	2
8	46	TC	TC
9	44	TC	TC

TC = too concretized to perform compaction assay.

CF sputum samples exhibited a mean DNA concentration of 7900 ± 1200 µg/mL and a mean % change in compaction compared to saline of 13 ± 4%; mean ± SE, n = 18.

(15), but overall there appears to be a decline after 14 yr of age. Kerrebijn et al. *(21)* reported that 44% of their adult CF patients had nasal polyps, half of whom had nasal obstruction. Earlier studies evaluating incidence of polyps often utilized visualization by looking through nasal speculum. The true incidence of nasal polyps is not known.

ACUTE AND CHRONIC SINUSITIS

It has been suggested that 5–10% *(22)* of upper respiratory infections (URIs) of younger children are accompanied by acute sinusitis. Most viral URIs tend to last 5–7 d and improve by 10 d. More intense symptoms than usual or persistence beyond this time may suggest that acute sinusitis is complicating the URI. The use of long-term antibiotics in children with CF may reduce the frequency of acute sinusitis. Perhaps two-thirds of CF children are prescribed oral antibiotics on multiple occasions either for treatment of URIs or as prophylaxis for *Staphylococcus aureus* or *Haemophilus influenzae.*

The relationship between sinus disease and lower airway disease continues to be conjectural. Sinus disease is thought to contribute to the pathogenesis of asthma *(23)*. The incidence of allergic upper airway disease in CF patients appears to be similar to that of the general population *(16,17)*.

If there is a reduction in pulmonary symptoms after sinus surgery, it is tempting to relate the two events, but there are not good scientific data to recommend surgery unless there are significant nasosinus symptoms. Chronic pulmonary disease dominates the clinical picture in CF. The sinuses may contribute to some of the respiratory symptoms, but how much can be attributed directly to the sinuses has not been quantitated. Umetsu and colleagues *(24)* reported four patients with CF who underwent aggressive treatment of sinus disease, and they suggested that there was potential to improve lower respiratory disease.

Symptoms related to sinus disease in CF include nasal congestion, nasal obstruction, postnasal drip, cough, facial pain, and persistent headache. Nasal congestion and stuffiness tend to be worse at night. Cough in CF tends to be worst first thing in the morning, whereas cough related to sinus disease tends to occur earlier in the night. There may be hyposmia or anosmia, and halitosis is common.

Sinus pain tends to be maxillary and/or periorbital. It is often made worse by coughing. The pain can be differentiated from the headache associated with hypoxia, which tends to be temporal or parietal. The headache caused by hypoxia or carbon dioxide retention tends to be worst first thing in the morning.

Examination may reveal tenderness over the maxillary sinuses or the bridge of the nose. Speculum examination of the nose may show mucosal hyperemia or turbinate hypertrophy with purulent nasal discharge. Polyps may be visible and tend to be bilateral.

The most common organisms causing sinusitis in normal children are *Pneumococcus,* nontypeable *H. influenzae,* and *Moraxella (Branhamella) catarrhalis. S. aureus, Streptococcus viridans,* and anaerobes are seen with chronic sinusitis. In patients with CF, the most common organisms associated with sinusitis include *S. aureus,* nontypeable *H. influenza, Pseudomonas aeruginosa,* streptococci, and anaerobes *(25)*. It is noteworthy that *Streptococcus pneumoniae* and *M. catarrhalis* are rarely cultured from the CF patient.

Shapiro et al. *(25)* showed that 19 of 20 patients had organisms in the sinus cavities, and the one patient who did not was the only one to have radiographically normal sinuses. They compared routine (nonquantitative) cultures from the nasopharynx, throat, or sputum to quantitative cultures from sinus aspirates. If the "predominant" and "present" colonization categories of these routine cultures are combined, there is an 84% concordance of organisms with sinus aspirates. Wong and colleagues *(26)* have shown that nonquantitative cultures cannot be correlated with quantitative cultures. Moss and King *(27)* have confirmed a high concordance of nonquantitative cultures from sinuses with cultures from sputum, suggesting common colonization throughout the respiratory tract. Gonzalez et al. *(28)* have demonstrated this definitively by performing DNA fingerprinting on multiple isolates of *P. aeruginosa* isolated from sinuses and sputum of six patients with CF. They found that all patients had at least one strain of common genetic origin cocolonizing the sinuses and lower respiratory tract (Fig. 4). Three patients also had additional cocolonizing strains identified. Phenotypic identification methods, such as antibiogram and morphology, were unreliable.

Opacification of the sinuses on radiologic examination is the rule. The opacification is the result of mucosal hypertrophy, with thick mucoid

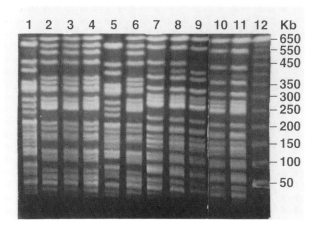

Fig. 4. Isolates of *P. aeruginosa* collected from sputum and sinuses from two CF patients, and analyzed by pulsed-field gel electrophoresis after digestion with the restriction enzyme *Spe*I. Isolates from patient GJ are shown in lanes 1–6 and patient TR in lanes 7–11; with phage standard in lane 12. The sputum isolate from GJ in lane 1 (strain A) is identical to the sinus isolate in lane 5, whereas a cocolonizing sinus strain B is seen in lanes 2–4 and 6. The sputum isolate from TR in lane 7 (strain A) is identical to the sinus isolates in lanes 8 and 11, and nearly identical (strain variant) to sinus isolates in lanes 9 and 10. No unrelated cocolonizing *P. aeruginosa* is identified in this patient.

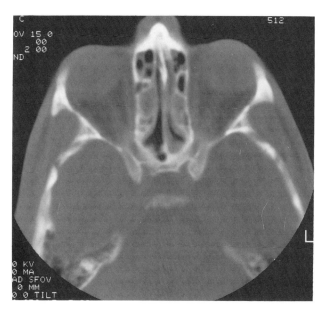

Fig. 5. CT scan—axial view showing ethmoid sinus disease.

secretions. Air–fluid levels tend not to be seen in CF patients. The frontal sinuses usually do not develop, presumably because of early inflammation. Plain film evaluation of the CF sinuses has included the Water's view, Caldwell, basal and lateral views, and almost always shows opacification so that clear or air-filled sinuses should cast doubt on the diagnosis of CF *(29)*. Plain films tend to be inaccurate for diagnosing sinus disease, and computed tomography (CT) is the preferred imaging method for all sinus disease, including the CF patient. This is particularly necessary to guide the surgeon performing endoscopic sinus surgery.

Maxillary mucoceles tend to be seen in patients with CF as an incidental finding *(30)*. Sharma et al. *(31)* have reported three cases of mucopyocele of the frontal sinus with erosion of one or more of the walls of the sinus. In each case, there was operative obliteration of the sinus with autologous adipose tissue, after removal of the mucopyocele, but all three recurred. Severe frontal headache may be caused by frontal mucopyocele, and the diagnosis can be confirmed by CT scan.

CT examination is used to confirm clinical impression of sinusitis. Coronal CT sections are

obtained of the maxillofacial area *(32)*, which allows visualization of the sinuses and their connections. April et al. *(33)* have shown that the degree of involvement of the sinuses of children with CF was more severe than in other chronic sinus disease. The CF patients demonstrated bilateral uncinate process demineralization with medial displacement of the lateral nasal wall in the middle meatus. In addition, 75% of maxillary sinuses showed increased attenuation on the soft-tissue window, presumably from long-standing chronic infection and viscid mucus.

Axial CT scan may be useful to delineate ethmoid sinus disease, as shown in Fig. 5. Figure 6 is a coronal CT scan showing extensive pan-sinusitis with nasal polyps, and Fig. 7 shows a postoperative scan with recurrence in the maxillary and ethmoid sinuses after surgery. Figure 8 shows a postoperative scan of a good result with minimal maxillary thickening.

MEDICAL MANAGEMENT

Even though the incidence of chronic sinus disease is almost universal in CF patients, the proportion of patients with symptomatic sinusitis is much less. Acute sinusitis with maxillary or frontal pain or tenderness, with fever and nasal discharge has been reported by Cepero et al. *(14)* to be 11%.

Acute sinusitis may be bacterial or viral. Antibiotic treatment may be indicated, and should be directed at the results of cultures if available. Small

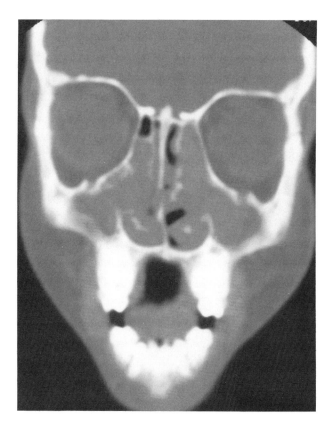

Fig. 6. Preoperative coronal CT scan. Extensive disease of paranasal sinuses and turbinates. The medial wall of maxillary sinuses has been eroded bilaterally, and there is almost complete opacification. Frontal sinuses not developed. Bilateral nasal polyps.

children may require longer-term antibiotics to improve the sinusitis. It is possible that chronic antibiotic therapy that is commonly utilized for CF patients may reduce the incidence of acute sinusitis and prevent complications, such as orbital cellulitis.

Topical steroids have been shown to produce variable response in CF patients with nasal polyps. It has been recommended to use preoperative steroids in a dose of 2 mg/kg/d for 10–14 d to shrink nasal polyps, and this does not appear to worsen bleeding during surgery. There is also a suggestion that postoperative topical steroids may reduce the potential for recurrence. These recommendations are not universally followed, nor is there good evidence that they are indicated *(34)*. Donaldson and Gillespie *(35)* treated a series of patients with and without polyps, and both groups had subjective improvement with less nasal obstruction. They recommended intranasal steroids prior to resorting to surgery.

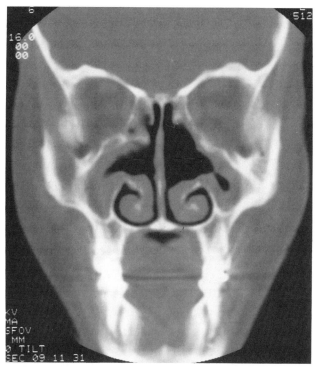

Fig. 7. Postoperative coronal CT scan. Poor result showing thickening of mucosa of maxillary and ethmoid sinuses. The inferior turbinates are swollen.

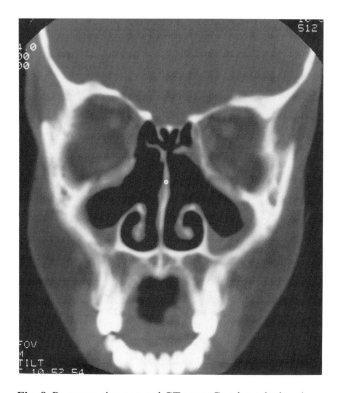

Fig. 8. Postoperative coronal CT scan. Good result showing aeration of nasal passages, ethmoid, and maxillary sinuses. Minor residual thickening of base of maxillary sinuses.

SURGICAL TREATMENT

Consideration for surgery is based on symptoms and signs discussed above and radiologic evidence confirming chronic sinusitis. There should be a reasonable trial of medical treatment prior to selection for surgery. The presence of nasal polyps is an indication for surgery if there are obstructive symptoms or if there is discomforting sinus disease. Removal of polyps may be justified even though there is potential for recurrence because of the improvement that can be achieved, even if only temporary *(36)*. It is usual for sinuses to be opacified without significant clinical symptoms so that the radiographic appearance does not constitute an indication for surgery. It has been suggested that 20% of CF patients will require surgical treatment for sinus disease *(37)*.

If there is significant pulmonary disease, it is recommended to consider admission for iv antibiotics and aggressive pulmonary care a few days prior to surgery to optimize pulmonary status. It is also important to be aware that problems with clotting may be the result of liver disease or from malabsorption of fat-soluble vitamins. Hematologic work-up may be indicated prior to surgery, including platelet count, PT, PTT, and perhaps bleeding time.

Findings at surgery are variable. In the nose, polyps are seen most commonly in the middle meatus, and the septum may be deviated. In the maxillary sinuses, the mucosa is thickened and polypoid. The secretions are viscous varying from putty-like consistency to hard concretions as previously noted. There may be destruction of the medial wall of the antrum. The ethmoids tend to be thickened with polypoid mucosa and mucopus. There may be destruction of the lamina papyracea and widening of the ethmoid cells.

Until the late 1980s, conventional surgery for sinonasal disease included polypectomy, Caldwell-Luc, ethmoidectomy, and intranasal antrostomy. The introduction of endoscopic sinus surgery (ESS) by Messerklinger *(38)* and Stammberger *(39)* has only recently been applied to pediatric patients. The results for treatment of CF children and adults have been associated with considerable benefit. The results compare well with previous treatment in terms of operative time and blood loss, and are much improved with regard to recurrence rates *(40)*.

There are reports of high incidence of recurrence. Cuyler *(41)* reported follow-up of 10 children with CF who had endoscopic sinus surgery for pansinusitis. The Messerklinger technique was used, and all 10 had recurrence or persistence of disease when followed with CT scan 2 yr after surgery. All patients believed there was improvement following surgery despite the CT findings. The comment was that "elimination of sinus disease with cystic fibrosis currently does not seem possible with medical or surgical therapy." David *(42)* reported that of 106 children with CF, 19 had between them 49 operations for removal of nasal polyps with a range between 1 and 6 operations, and the mean number of operations was 2.6. There were 29 children who had 80 operations on their sinuses, with a mean of 2.8.

Until the late 1980s, it was thought to be unnecessary to perform sinus surgery at the same time as nasal polypectomy in CF patients, because there seemed to be no additional benefit. It has now been shown that the risk of recurrence of nasal polyps is significantly less if sinus surgery is performed. Cepero et al. *(14)* noted that the extent of intranasal surgery for polypectomy was inversely proportional to the recurrence rate. Simple polypectomy was ineffective treatment, and when performed with a Caldwell-Luc and either an intranasal or extranasal ethmoidectomy, the recurrence rate of polyps was <13%.

As has been noted, the results of ESS have been sufficiently encouraging that many CF centers are now more aggressive in surgical management *(14,15,27,40)*. The major disadvantage is that many patients who are being treated have significant compromise of pulmonary function that increases the risk of performing surgery. This is particularly the case in programs that recommend sinus surgery prior to lung transplantation.

There are different philosophies about the advantage of performing ESS prior to lung transplantation. One view is that there has been no demonstrated advantage to performing sinus surgery prior to lung transplantation. Flume and colleagues reviewed the airway pathogens prior to surgery and after, comparing this to lung transplantation for other indications. They found no suggestion that the presence of untreated chronic sinus disease increased the risk of postoperative infection *(43)*. The opposing view is that leaving a sump of infection, which is usually *P. aeruginosa,* increases the chance of seeding the donor lungs with infectious material from the sinuses *(44)*.

In addition to an aggressive surgical approach for the CF patient, it is possible that recurrence rates are in part dependent on persistent infection following surgery. For this reason, some CF centers are employing antral lavage with antibiotics as a necessary function of the postoperative management. The protocol suggested by Moss and King *(27)* uses implanted irrigation cannulae into the maxillary antrum. The cannulae used are 19-gage butterfly iv catheters with the needle and plastic butterfly cut off leaving the external Luer-lock connection. The catheters are passed into the maxillary antra and sutured in place. Antimicrobial lavage is started immediately following surgery with tobramycin 40 mg (1 cc) being instilled three times daily and left in place for 2–3 min. The head is then turned to allow the fluid to drain out. Following 7–10 d of treatment, the catheters are removed. Monthly examinations under local anesthesia with instillation of antibiotics are performed with more frequent lavage if indicated.

The recurrence rate with ESS followed by antral lavage has been shown to reduce the recurrence rate compared to conventional surgery from 72 to 22% at 2 yr follow-up *(27)*.

A similar approach has been used at the University of California, San Diego where flushing of the sinuses starting a few days after surgery is performed using a Waterpik and Ethicore nasal adaptor, and mixing the tobramycin (20 mg, 0.5 cc) with the final 30–50 cc of hypotonic saline.

Although experience performing more extensive surgery for chronic sinus disease for CF patients is only recent, preliminary results suggest that recurrence is less. The addition of antibiotic antral lavage also may reduce recurrence. It is hoped that aggressive management of CF sinus disease will result in improvement in overall pulmonary status.

REFERENCES

1. FitzSimmons SC. The changing epidemiology of cystic fibrosis. J Pediatr 1993;122:1–9.
2. Quinton P. Chloride impermeability in cystic fibrosis. Nature 1983;301:421,422.
3. Knowles MR, Stutts MJ, Spock A, et al. Abnormal ion permeation through cystic fibrosis respiratory epithelium. Science 1983;221:1067–1070.
4. Ramsey BW, Astley SJ, Aitken ML, et al. Efficacy and safety of short-term administration of aerosolized recombinant human deoxyribonuclease in patients with cystic fibrosis. Am Rev Respir Dis 1993;148:145–151.
5. Knowles MR, Church NL, Waltner WE, et al. A pilot study of aerosolized amiloride for the treatment of lung disease in cystic fibrosis. N Engl J Med 1990;322:1189–1194.
6. Collins FS. Cystic fibrosis: molecular biology and therapeutic implications. Science 1992;256:774–779.
7. Wilson JM. Cystic fibrosis. Vehicles for gene therapy. Nature 1993;365:691,692.
8. Zabner J, Couture LA, Gregory RJ, Graham SM, Smith AE, Welsh MJ. Adenovirus-mediated gene transfer transiently corrects the chloride transport defect in nasal epithelia of patients with cystic fibrosis. Cell 199;75:207–216.
9. Rutland J, Cole PJ. Nasal mucociliary clearance and ciliary beat frequency in cystic fibrosis compared with sinusitis and bronchiectasis. Thorax 1981;36:654–658.
10. Jorissen M, Van der Schueren B, Van den Berghe H, Cassiman J-J. In vitro ciliogenesis in respiratory epithelium of cystic fibrosis patients. Ann Otol Rhinol Laryngol 1991;100:366–371.
11. Moss R., Desch J, King V, Toy KJ, Sinicropi D, Shak S. Biochemical and biophysical characterization of sinus secretions in CF (abstract). Pediatr Pulmonol 1993;9(Suppl.):266.
12. Rulon JT, Brown HA, Logan GB. Nasal polyps and cystic fibrosis of the pancreas. Arch Otolaryngol 1963;78:192–199.
13. Oppenheimer EH, Rosenstein BJ. Differential pathology of nasal polyps in cystic fibrosis atopy. Lab Invest 1979;40:455–459.
14. Cepero R, Smith RJH, Catlin FI, Bressler KL, Furuta GT, Shandera KC. Cystic fibrosis—an otolaryngologic perspective. Otolaryngol Head Neck Surg 1987;97:356–360.
15. Crockett DM, Mcgill TJ, Healy GB, Friedman EM, Silkeld LJ. Nasal and paranasal sinus surgery in children with cystic fibrosis. Ann Otol Rhinol Laryngol 1987;97:367–372.
16. Cuyler JP, Monaghan AJ. Cystic fibrosis and sinusitis. J Otolaryngol 1989;18:173–175.
17. Drake-Lee AB, Morgan DW. Nasal polyps and sinusitis in children with cystic fibrosis. J Laryngol Otol 1989;103:753–755.
18. Reilly JS, Kenna MA, Stool SE, Bluestone CD. Nasal surgery in children with cystic fibrosis: complications and risk management. Laryngoscope 1985;95:1491–1493.
19. Stern RC, Boat TF, Wood RE, Matthews LW, Doershuk CF. Treatment of nasal polyps in cystic fibrosis. Am J Dis Child 1982;136:1067–1072.
20. Wiatrak BJ, Myer CM, Cotton RB. Cystic fibrosis with sinus disease in children (letter). Am J Dis Child 1993;147:258–260.
21. Kerrebijn JDF, Poublon RML, Overbeek SE. Nasal and paranasal disease in adult cystic fibrosis patients. Eur Respir J 1992;5:1239–1242.
22. Wald ER. Current concepts—sinusitis in children. N Engl J Med 1992;326:319–323.
23. Slavin RG. Asthma and sinusitis. J Allergy Clin Immun 1992;90:534–537.
24. Umetsu DT, Moss RB, King VV, Lewiston NJ. Sinus disease in patients with severe cystic fibrosis and relation to pulmonary exacerbation. Lancet 1990;335:1077,1078.
25. Shapiro ED, Milmoe GJ, Wald ER, Rodnan JB, Bowen A'D. Bacteriology of the maxillary sinuses in patients with cystic fibrosis. J Infectious Dis 1982;146:589–593.

26. Wong K, Roberts MC, Owens L, Fife M, Smith AL. Selective media for the quantitation of bacteria in cystic fibrosis sputum. J Med Microbiol 1984;17:113–119.

27. Moss RB, King VV. Management of sinusitis in cystic fibrosis by endoscopic surgery and serial antimicrobial lavage. Arch Otolaryngol 1995;121:566–572.

28. Gonzalez A, Troup N, Mickelson P, Moss R. Pseudomonas aeruginosa in sinuses and airways of CF patients: genomic fingerprinting by pulsed field gel electrophoresis (abstract). Pediatr Pulmonol 1994;10(Suppl.):252.

29. Amodio JB, Berdon WE, Abramson S, Baker D. Cystic fibrosis in childhood: pulmonary, paranasal sinus, and skeletal manifestations. Semin Roentgenol 1987;22:125–135.

30. Wagenmann M, Naclerio RM. Complications of sinusitis. J Allergy Clin Immunol 1992;90:552–554.

31. Sharma GD, Doershuk CF, Stern RC. Erosion of the posterior or inferior wall of the frontal sinus due to mucopyocele in three patients with cystic fibrosis (abstract). Pediatr Pulmonol 1993;9(Suppl.):266.

32. Zinreich SJ, Kennedy DW, Rosenbaum AE, Gayler BW, Kumar AJ, Stammberger H. Paranasal sinuses: CT imaging requirements for endoscopic surgery. Radiology 1987;163:769–775.

33. April MM, Zinreich SJ, Baroody FM, Naclerio RM. Coronal CT scan abnormalities in children with chronic sinusitis. Laryngoscope 1993;103:985–990.

34. Parsons DS, Phillips SE. Functional endoscopic surgery in children: a retrospective analysis of results. Laryngoscope 1993;103:899–903.

35. Donaldson JD, Gillespie CT. Observations on the efficacy of intranasal beclomethasone dipropionate in cystic fibrosis patients. J Otolaryngol 1988;17:43–45.

36. Lanza DC, Kennedy DW. Current concepts in the surgical management of nasal polyposis. J Allergy Clin Immunol 1992;90:543–546.

37. Ramsey B, Richardson MA. Impact of sinusitis in cystic fibrosis. J Allergy Clin Immunol 1990;90:547–552.

38. Messerklinger W. Endoscopy of the Nose. Baltimore, MD: Urban and Schwarzenberg, 1978.

39. Stammberger H. Functional Endoscopic Sinus Surgery. Philadelphia, PA: B. C. Decker, 1991.

40. Duplechain JK, White JA, Miller RH. Pediatric sinusitis. Arch Otolaryngol Head Neck Surg 1991;117:422–426.

41. Cuyler JP. Follow-up of endoscopic sinus surgery on children with cystic fibrosis. Arch Otolaryngol Head Neck Surg 1992;118:505,506.

42. David TJ. Nasal polyposis, opaque paranasal sinuses and usually normal hearing: the otorhinolaryngological features of cystic fibrosis. J Royal Soc Med 1986;79(Suppl. 12):23–26.

43. Flume PA, Egan TM, Paradowski LJ, Detterbeck FC, Thompson JT, Yankaskas JR. Infectious complications of lung transplantation. Impact of cystic fibrosis. Am J Respir Crit Care Med 1994;149:1601–1607.

44. Lewiston N, King V, Umetsu D, et al. Cystic fibrosis patients who have undergone heart-lung transplantation benefit from maxillary sinus antrostomy and repeated sinus lavage. Transplant Proc 1991;23:1207,1208.

19 Immunity, Infection, and Nasal Disease

Steven H. Yoshida, PHD *and M. Eric Gershwin,* MD

CONTENTS

INTRODUCTION

Mucosal surfaces provide interfaces between the external and internal environments through which gases, nutrients, waste products, and other materials move. The properties of host mucosal surfaces that allow for these functions also provide ideal sites for the entry of microbial pathogens. Probably for this reason, the immune system developed defensive components with functions specialized for mucosal areas. These include mucus and its constituents, secretory immunoglobulins, and unique subsets of leukocytes that localize to or maturate in mucosal regions. They function to prevent attachment of microbes to host tissues and thereby prevent entry, and to signal and mobilize other immune components if entry has been achieved.

The nose is an important component of respiration in that it is the first mucosal site normally exposed to inspired air. Since the nose functions as a filter to trap airborne impurities and as a sensory tissue for monitoring the host's environment, it is under constant infectious, allergen, and chemical challenges. As a primary site of environmental

contact, the nose should be included in any discussion of mucosal immunology. This chapter summarizes current information on nasal immunity, including its components, functions, and regulation. In addition, nasal manifestations related to immunodeficiencies are also reviewed. Although the above comments allude to the importance of the nose in the overall context of mucosal immunity, there appears to be little information on nasal immune mechanisms relative to other regions of the mucosa, such as the gut.

INTERNAL NASAL ANATOMY

The general internal anatomy of the nose has been reviewed *(1,2)* and is described briefly here (Table 1). The nasal septum divides the nasal cavity into two fossae. At the extreme anterior end, the nasal vestibule is lined by skin containing hair and sebaceous and sweat glands. More posteriorly, the septal cartilage joins the perpendicular plate of the ethmoid bone and the vomer. Three turbinates or conchae, the inferior, middle, and superior, project from the walls as scrolls or baffles. The superior and middle turbinates are formed from the ethmoid bone, whereas the inferior is formed from a separate bone. Each turbinate protects its corresponding

From: *Diseases of the Sinuses* (M. E. Gershwin and G. A. Incaudo, eds.), ©1996 Humana Press Inc., Totowa, NJ.

Table 1
Gross Structure of the Nasal Mucosa

Turbinates	Scrolls or baffles that project from the walls of the nasal septum and function to increase the surface area of the nasal mucosa; the inferior, middle, and superior turbinates are normally found in all people; occasionally, a fourth, superior turbinate is present
Blood supply	External carotid artery → sphenopalantine artery → posterior portions of the nasal septum and lateral walls; the internal carotid artery → lateral wall and the anterosuperior septa; venous blood → anterior facial vein → sphenopalantine vein → ethmoid veins; lymphatic drainage follows venous drainage
Nerve supply	Sensory function Fifth cranial nerve → first (ophthalmic) division → anterior ethmoid nerve → superior and anterior parts of the septa and lateral walls Fifth cranial nerve → second (maxillary) division → sphenopalantine → posterior sections of nose Motor function Sympathetic and parasympathetic neurons

meatuses into which drain the paranasal sinuses. Although the nasolacrimal ducts drain into the anterior portion of the inferior meatus, the posterior end is close to the orifice of the Eustachian tube in the nasopharynx. Near the central portion of the middle meatus is the ethmoid infindibulum, which is a channel for the drainage of three sinuses, the maxillary, frontal, and anterior ethmoids. The superior meatus is a collection site for the posterior ethmoid cells. Slightly above and posterior to the superior turbinate is the sphenoethmoidal recess, which contains the ostium of the sphenoid sinus.

The blood supply to the nose is provided by both the external and internal carotid systems (1,2). The external carotid artery conducts blood primarily through the internal maxillary artery and its terminal branch, the sphenopalantine. The sphenopalantine artery then supplies most of the posterior portions of the nasal septum and the lateral wall of the nose. The internal carotid artery also distributes blood to the lateral wall as well as the anterosuperior parts of the septum via the anterior and posterior ethmoidal arteries. Venous blood is retrieved by the anterior facial vein, the sphenopalantine vein via the pteryogid plexus, and the ethmoidal veins. Lymphatic drainage of the nose generally parallels the venous drainage.

Innervation is also important for the sensory and motor functions of the nose. The sensory nerve supply of the internal nose is derived primarily from the fifth cranial nerve (1,2). The ophthalmic (first) division then branches into the nasociliary or anterior ethmoidal nerve. This neural segment serves the superior and anterior parts of the septum and lateral wall of the nose. The sphenopalantine of the maxillary (second) division innervates the posterior sections of the nose. Olfaction is mediated by sensory epithelial cells, which send fibers through the cribriform plate to the olfactory bulb. The autonomic nerve supply provides both vasomotor and secretomotor functions to the mucosa of the nasal cavities, and contains both sympathetic and parasympathetic components. These latter neural functions are partly responsible for the regulation of secretion and mucus flow, which then contributes to the inflammatory and immune components of the nose.

There are four air-filled sinuses on each side of the nasal cavity that are designated the ethmoid, maxillary, frontal, and sphenoid paranasal sinuses (1,3,4). Although the functions of these sinuses are controversial, various purposes for their presence have been suggested. These include resonance, weight reduction, conditioning of inspired air, regulation of intranasal pressure, facial architecture, and protection of intracranial structures from trauma.

THE PHYSIOLOGY OF THE NOSE

The functions of the nose are primarily related to respiration, and are generally categorized as olfaction, air humidification, air temperature control, and air cleansing (Table 2). Antimicrobial and immunological activities of the nose are discussed in later sections.

The olfactory area is located in a narrow niche bordered by the superior turbinate, the upper septum, and the cribriform plate (1,4). The olfactory mucosa consists of four cell types:

1. The olfactory receptor;
2. The sustentacular or supporting cells;

Table 2
General Nasal Functions

Functions	*Components*
Olfaction	Olfactory receptor cells are located near superior turbinate; high lipid content of these cells accumulates lipophilic substances
Air humidification, temperature control, and cleansing	Turbinates increase surface area for efficient temperature and humidity regulation; turbinate size can be altered by changing blood flow; hair, cilia, and mucus remove particulate matter from inspired air
Antimicrobial activity and immunology	Mucociliary action acts as a physical barrier to the accumulation of xenobiotics; immunoglobulins and other antimicrobial proteins are released into the nasal lumen; leukocytes are found in the nasal mucosal and participate in inflammation
Xenobiotic metabolism	Human nasal cells contain enzymatic activities, such as P-450, 15-lipoxygenase, and glutathione-S-transferase; functions are not understood

3. Basal cells, which rest on the basement membrane; and
4. Microvillar cells.

The microvillar cells are located near the epithelial surface and project tufts of microvilli into the mucus layer. There are 10–20 million bipolar olfactory receptor cells scattered among the sustentacular cells. The high lipid content of olfactory cells allows for the intracellular accumulation of lipid-soluble fragrances. The axons of the olfactory cells pass through the basement membrane and the cribriform plate. They then travel to the olfactory area of the cortex through the first cranial nerves. In addition to the sense of smell, the taste of food is recognized through simultaneous stimulation of the taste buds on the tongue and the olfactory cells. Thus, when odors cannot reach the olfactory area, food tastes are initially diminished. However, if olfaction is absent for an extended period, a compensatory increase in the sensitivity of taste can develop.

Air conditioning is a principal function of the nose. The temperature of inspired air is adjusted to approximate body temperature during its passage through the nose *(1,4)*. Turbinate structure increases the surface area of the internal nose, and capillaries associated with erectile tissues enable blood spaces to enlarge or contract. Thus, as cold air flows across these turbinates, the nasal turbinates respond by swelling, which then allows for an increased transfer of heat from the blood to the air. The efficiency of this system is witnessed by a change of less than 1°C in the air reaching the laryngeal inlet despite variations in external air temperature from 25 to

0°C. When the air entering the nose is higher than body temperature, the direction of heat exchange is generally reversed. If the air outside the body is lower than body temperature, conservation of heat during exhalation is also partly a turbinate function. Inevitably, some heat is lost. This loss, which may range from 10–50%, depends on the degree of dilation of mucosal arterioles and degree of engorgement of blood spaces.

Humidification of inspired air is also an important air-conditioning function of the nose *(1,4)*. When the outside air is dry, water must be transferred to the inspired air during its passage through the nose. This water is provided by the blanket of mucus that covers the surface of the nasal mucosa. It is estimated that as much as a liter of water can be evaporated from the nose in 24 h in order to maintain a 75–90% saturation humidity. As the air absorbs water from the mucosa, the submucosal glands replenish the water supply. The nasal mucosa rarely becomes dry unless the epithelial layer of the nose is damaged.

The entire lining of the nose is covered by this secretory mucus blanket *(5)* consisting of two layers, the surface gel/mucus layer and the lower aqueous/serous layer. Because the mucous membrane is not keratinized, mucus must provide many of the protective functions usually reserved for the outermost skin layer. Mucous glycoproteins act as a replaceable, flexible, continuous extracellular surface that protects the mucous membranes. Its multiple functions include insulating and waterproofing the epithelium by enclosing the aqueous layer beneath, lubrication, humidification of the inspired air, and facilitation of heat transfer between the nose and air. In order to restrict oxygen-induced injuries to the mucous membranes, nasal secretions also contain antioxidants. These include lactoferrin, transferrin, ceruloplasmin, glutathione, and ascorbate. However, the major antioxidant found in nasal secretions is uric acid. Resting concentrations of 5 μM are known to rise to 16 μM following submucosal gland stimulation. Evidence suggests that although uric acid is stored by serous cells, it is probably derived from plasma *(6)*.

Air contains particulate matter that the nose attempts to remove to prevent their reaching the pharynx and lungs *(4,7)*. Particles are trapped in the surface layer and transported by mucociliary action to the posterior pharynx at a rate of approx 1 cm/min, where it is eventually swallowed or expelled. Under resting conditions, this mucus layer is replaced every 10–20 min. Each surface respiratory epithelial cell has 25–30 cilia of 5–7 μm in length, and most cilia beat 10–40 times/s. Via this barrier function, microbes and particulate matter are trapped in the mucus and removed. The serous layer does not turn over as rapidly, and its greater stability may provide additional protective functions for host defense since secretory constituents become concentrated there.

Human nasal cells also have a variety of enzymatic capabilities that are able to metabolize xenobiotics. Glutathione-*S*-transferase, 15-lipoxygenase, P-450, epoxide hydrolase, and other enzymatic activities have been described *(8)*. Although the functions of these processes are not known, they may contribute to the toxic effects of inhalants, such as formaldehyde, dimethylnitrosamine, and benzo-a-pyrene.

THE NASAL MUCOSA

Cellular Components

The respiratory mucosa contains a variety of cell types that form an epithelium on a basement membrane that is itself over a lamina propria *(9)* (Table 3). Cells in the nasal vestibule and anterior fossa are characterized as a squamous epithelium with hair follicles. Posteriorly, cells become hair-free and convert to a transitional, pseudostratified epithelial type. All epithelial cells are in contact with the basement membrane, but not all reach the surface and none directly contact the lamina propria. Basal cells lie between the columnar cells, are attached to the basement membrane and are the precursors of columnar and goblet cells *(4,9)*.

Table 3
Cells of the Nasal Mucosa

Cells	Functions
Columnar epithelial cells	Secretion of mucus
Goblet cells	Secretion of mucus containing primarily acidic glycoproteins and sulfated mucopolysaccharides
Basal cells	Precursors of columnar and goblet cells
Leukocytes	Effectors of inflammation and antibody production

Constituents of the mucus and serous layers are secreted by seromucinous and intraepithelial glands that are found throughout the mucosa *(4,9)*. The seromucinous glands, which secrete acid mucopolysaccharides and mucoproteins, are compound alveolar in type and may contain both mucous and serous glands within an individual alveolus. The intraepithelial glands are aggregations of tall columnar cells that secrete sulfated mucosal elements. The surface of each columnar cell is covered with microvilli, which aid in maintaining fluid on the epithelial surface and in chemical exchange. Goblet cells are a specialized type of apocrine gland with mucinogen granules containing primarily acidic glycoproteins and sulfated mucopolysaccharides. The surfaces of goblet cells are covered with microvilli with small openings through which granules are discharged. Their distribution in the nasal mucosa is irregular and are often seen with eosinophils and mast cells, and they may increase in number with allergies. Normally, the ratio of columnar to goblet cells is approx 5:1.

Leukocytes are often found scattered throughout the nasal mucosa *(9)*. Under the appropriate stimuli, they leave the venous circulation, enter the connective tissues of the lamina propria, and travel to the epithelium using ameboid movement. Resident granulocytes are common cellular constituents of the nasal mucosa. Eosinophils and mast cells, although rare in the epithelium, are frequently observed in the lamina propria and secretions of normal individuals. Also, approximately one-third of mucosal mast cells were shown to stain for surface IgE in normal human turbinates *(10)*. However, cellular characteristics do change in clinical situations. Inhalant allergies and nonallergic eosinophilic rhinitis are associated with increases in eosinophil counts. Food allergies and allergic pollen extracts also increase mast cell numbers in nasal secretions *(9,11)*. Polymorphonuclear leukocytes (PMNs) are often present concurrently with eosinophils in nasal secretions. Although some PMNs are always observed in a healthy nose, increased numbers are usually associated with bacterial infections. Lymphocytes are also found in the nasal mucosa. Among T-lymphocytes, both CD4 and CD8 T-cells are represented, and approx 80–90% of T-cells express the αβ receptor *(10,12,13)*. Macrophages and B-lymphocytes are also found in the mucosa, but in fewer numbers than T-cells *(9,11)*. Antibody-producing plasma cells in normal human turbinates are found in close proximity to the submucosal glands and are primarily IgA$^+$ *(10)*. Intraepithelial dendritic cells have also been described in the nasal turbinate *(13)*. These cells express surface markers CD14 and KiM1P, which identify them as of the mononuclear phagocyte lineage. Despite the presence of leukocytes in the nasal mucosa, organized subepithelial lymphoid tissues have not been found in nasal turbinates *(13)*.

Immunological and Inflammatory Components of Mucus

IgA and IgG are the primary immunoglobulins found in nasal secretions *(5)* (Table 4). IgG is mainly derived from the plasma, and its distribution in the nasal mucosa is a function of vascular permeability. There is also some IgG production by plasma cells present within the mucosa. Regardless of their source, IgG, although present throughout the mucosa, is most concentrated in the lamina propria. This suggests that its primary function is to limit invasions by microorganisms that pass the surface fluid layers and reach the epithelium. IgA, on the other hand, is produced by plasma cells located near submucous glands. Dimeric IgA released by B-lymphocytes binds to secretory components produced by nearby serous cells to form secretory IgA. This secretory IgA is then transported through the serous cells to become part of their glandular secretions. IgA acts primarily by neutralizing microorganisms in the surface fluid layer to prevent their attachment to the underlying mucosa. IgG and IgA constitute approx 2–4 and 15%, respectively, of total resting secretory proteins.

There are also nonspecific antimicrobial proteins released by the nasal mucosa *(5,14)*. Lactoferrin is an iron-binding protein that has bactericidal and

Table 4
Components of Normal Mucus

Constituents	Characteristics[a]
Mucus glycoproteins	(10–15%) provides structural gel-like qualities to mucus
Lipids	Structural molecules in mucus
Albumin	(15%) Nonspecific binder of particulates
Antioxidants	Uric acid, lactoferrin, glutathione, transferrin, ceruloplasmin, ascorbate; minimize oxygen-induced injury
Immunoglobulins	(2–4%) IgG, (15%) secretory IgA, (<1%) IgM
Lactoferrin	(2–4%) Iron binder
Lysozyme	(15–30%) Antimicrobial enzyme
Secretory leukoprotease inhibitor	(10%) Regulates inflammatory proteases

[a]Numbers in parentheses represent fraction of total protein.

bacteriostatic effects on both gram-positive and gram-negative bacteria. Lysozyme is bactericidal and bacteriostatic for some gram-positive bacteria. These compounds may work in conjunction with other immune components. For example, the activity of lactoferrin may be enhanced by IgA, and lysozyme may contribute to the lytic activity of complement. Both lactoferrin and lysozyme are components of serous cell secretions and comprise approx 2–4 and 15–30%, respectively, of resting secreted proteins.

Regulation of Nasal Secretion

Processes that lead to increase vascular permeability and glandular secretion rates also contribute to the antimicrobial activity of the nasal mucosa. The increased volume of secretions leads to better clearance of particulate matter as well as the availability of IgG and other plasma proteins. The regulation of secretion is governed by several signaling mechanisms, including soluble inflammatory molecules as well as neuronal controls.

Arterial blood flow and, consequently, plasma extravasation are subject to nervous control owing to the innervation of arterial vessels by sensory, parasympathetic, and sympathetic nerves. Additionally, binding sites for various neuropeptides have been discovered in vessel walls. Therefore, of interest is the manner by which neuropeptide-containing nerves contribute to the control of arterial

Table 5
Regulation of Nasal Secretion

Stimuli	Effects	
	Vascular permeability	Glandular secretion
Parasympathetic neurons	Increase	Increase
Cholinergic receptors		Increase
α-Adrenergic receptors		Increase
Muscarinic receptors		Increase
Trigeminal sensory neurons	Increase	
Tachykinins	Increase	Increase
Bradykinin	Increase	Increase
Histamine	Increase	Increase
Endothelin-1	Decrease	

and arteriovenous anastomosis dilation, plasma extravasation, myoepithelial cell contraction, and epithelial permeability.

Innervation of the nose includes parasympathetic and sensory connections with the glands and vascular beds (12) (Table 5). In general, stimulation of parasympathetic nerves leads to increased secretion of glandular material and, to a lesser extent, plasma proteins. Also, cholinergic stimulation increases glandular release of lysozyme, lactoferrin, and IgA levels without altering the baseline levels of plasma proteins, such as IgG and albumin. Finally, β-adrenergic stimulation has no effect on secretions, whereas α-adrenergic stimuli have mild effects on glandular secretions (15).

Neuropeptides contained in parasympathetic neurons include acetylcholine, vasoactive intestinal peptide (VIP), and peptide histidine methionine (PHM). The characterization of these neuropeptides is not fully developed. However, what is known is that VIP receptors in the nasal mucosa are primarily found on the epithelium, vessels, and glands. Also, the putative functions of VIP are vessel dilation, glandular secretion, and increasing plasma flux (16). The effects of PHM are considered similar to those of VIP.

Neuropeptide Y (NPY) coexists with norepinephrine in sympathetic neurons (16), and like norepinephrine, NPY acts as a vasoconstrictor. The localization of NPY binding sites on the smooth muscles of arterioles and arteriovenous anastomoses provides additional data suggesting that NPY regulates human nasal blood flow.

Additional evidence for neuronal influences on nasal mucosal function is provided by studies on

muscarinic receptors. The muscarinic agonist, methacholine (MCh), is able to induce glandular secretions both in vivo and in vitro, confirming direct stimulation (15). Nasal challenge with MCh also induces hypersecretion, indicating that glandular secretion is mediated by muscarinic receptors. Recently, muscarinic receptors were identified in the nasal mucosa (17); M_1 and M_3 receptor subtypes were found in submucosal glands, and M_3 receptors were noted in vessels. Both M_1 and M_3 receptors appeared to be involved in glycoconjugate and lactoferrin release. M_2 receptors were not detected.

Trigeminal sensory nerves contain neuropeptides that affect secretory cell activity when released. These neurons are known to be stimulated by a variety of substances, including capsaicin, nicotine, cigaret smoke, histamine, serotonin, bradykinin, acetylcholine, and prostaglandins (16). When these nerve fibers are depolarized, neuropeptides are released and diffuse to adjacent structures. Since epithelial injury or mast cell degranulation can lead to the release of various inflammatory mediators that depolarize sensory nerves, neuropeptides can be present over a relatively widespread area near submucosal vessels and glands. Therefore, a small-scale injury can be amplified to generate a large-scale reaction.

Several other neuropeptides that regulate nasal secretion have been described (16). Trigeminal sensory neurons are known to contain calcitonin gene-related peptide (CGRP), substance P (SP), neurokinin A (NKA), and gastrin-releasing peptide (GRP). CGRP receptors are concentrated primarily on arterioles, to a lesser extent on venous vessels, and are not present on glandular cells. This distribution is consistent with the physiologic role of CGRP as a potent arterial vasodilator. Thus, CGRP probably contributes to nasal secretion by arterial vasodilation, increasing nasal blood flow, and increasing plasma flux across fenestrated capillaries. Tachykinins are a family of small peptides that include SP, NKA, and neurokinin B (NKB). SP binding sites are widely distributed on the epithelium, glands, and vessels of the human nasal mucosa. In accord with its binding characteristics, SP stimulates epithelial cell secretion, mucoglycoconjugate secretion of human nasal explants, and vasodilation, as well as chemoattracting inflammatory cells. Binding sites for NKA are located on the arterial walls of human nasal mucosa, and the functions of NKA include mucoglycoconjugate release and bronchoconstriction. GRP may act as a secretogogue for both serous and mucosal cells, and as a growth factor. GRP receptors have been identified on the epithelium and submucosal glands of the human nasal mucosa.

Bioactive molecules of nonneuronal origin also possess vasoactive properties or alter nasal secretion characteristics. Bradykinin (BK) is generated by the action of plasma or tissue kallikrein on the substrate, kininogen. BK receptors are found on blood vessels, and topical application of BK increase secretion and nasal blood flow *(5)*. Although increases in vascular permeability induced by BK are probably a result of direct binding to BK-specific receptors, the mechanism of glandular secretion is less well understood. The absence of BK receptors on glandular cells suggests that BK stimulates glandular secretion indirectly, perhaps through the involvement of platelet-activating factor or arachidonic acid metabolites *(18)*.

As an inflammatory mediator, histamine is capable of increasing the vascular permeability of the nasal mucosa. In fact, histamine receptors have been detected on the endothelium of vessels in human nasal turbinates *(19)*. However, the ability of histamine to activate secretion may be indirect, either through the activation of chemical intermediates, such as prostaglandins, or through the stimulation of sensory nerves *(15,20)*. Relatedly, it has been suggested that IL-4 may alter the affects of histamine on the vascular bed *(21)*. Since nasal congestion is a side effect of IL-4 treatment, the effects of IL-4 on nasal provocation tests were studied. Pretreatment with IL-4 decreases the secretion of histamine-related products, such as plasma proteins, but does not alter the outcome of methacholine challenge, which stimulates glandular secretion. The means by which IL-4 is able to induce nasal congestion, increase histamine in nasal lavages, and downregulate vascular responsiveness to histamine are not known.

Endothelin-1 (ET-1) is a vaso- and bronchoconstrictor that is synthesized by endothelial and epithelial cells *(22,23)*. Studies with cultured human nasal mucosal explants show that ET-1 induces the release of PGE2, PGD2, PGF2α, TXB2, and 15-HETE; ET-1 appears to be an inducer of arachidonic acid metabolism. ET also acts on glandular receptors to induce both serous and mucous cell secretions. In the nasal mucosa, ET is present in the vascular endothelium and the serous cells of submucosal glands. *In situ* hybridization of nasal turbinate tissues with ET-1 mRNA suggests that ET may be synthesized by endothelial cells, smooth muscle cells of the venous sinusoids, small veins, small muscular arteries, and possibly macrophages and mast cells. Thus, ET affects vasomotor tone as well as regulates secretions.

The activities of these secretogogues and proinflammatory agents are also regulated by various enzymes. SP, endothelin, SIP, and NKA are metabolized by peptidases found in nasal secretions *(15)*. Angiotensin-converting enzyme (ACE) may be involved in the regulation of BK *(24)*, since BK is a known substrate of ACE in vitro. Although ACE is measurable in the human nasal mucosa, methacholine does not augment ACE release. Studies on the distribution of ACE suggest that its origins include the plasma and possibly mononuclear cells, such as macrophages and lymphocytes. Thus, ACE in the interstitial and epithelial lining fluids may regulate the actions of inflammatory peptides, such as BK. Another potential regulator of inflammatory mediators is secretory leukoprotease inhibitor (SLPI; *25*). SLPI is found in serous cells in the nasal mucosa. It constitutes a large portion of the total proteins in nasal secretions, which increases on nasal challenge. Since SLPI is thought to regulate elastase activity as well as inhibit mast cell chymase activity and histamine release, it may function to minimize mucosal injury by regulating inflammatory proteases.

NASAL MANIFESTATIONS OF IMMUNODEFICIENCY

The prominence of the nose as an initial site of contact with foreign materials underscores the importance of immune components in minimizing particulate and microbial contact with the mucosa. Therefore, the nasal mucosa may be particularly susceptible to microbial invasion during states of immunodeficiency. It is known that some patients with chronic or recurrent sinusitis suffer from immunodeficiency diseases. However, the diagnosis of immunodeficiency as a primary cause of nasal problems may be difficult because of the similarities of symptoms with those of allergic or immunologically normal individuals. Chronic sinusitis or the recurrence of sinusitis after the termination of antibiotic therapy may often be the most overt

Table 6
Nasal Manifestations of Immunodeficiencies

Deficiencies	Characteristics
CVID	Chronic rhinosinusitis, decreased numbers of ciliated and goblet cells, impaired mucociliary transport, increases in abnormal cilia, infections
SIAD	Increases in goblet cells, impaired mucociliary transport, chronic infections
IgG$_3$ deficiency	Sinusitis, infections, asthma
AIDS	Sinusitis, infections, dermatitis lymphoma, Kaposi's sarcoma, atopy

indication that immunodeficiency is a contributing factor to disease *(26)*. Therefore, followup immunological tests may be helpful in correctly diagnosing any potential immunodeficiencies related to nasal infections. It should be noted that although AIDS is a form of acquired immunodeficiency associated with nasal infections, many immunodeficiency diseases are genetic and often involve humoral immune deficiencies.

The characteristics and genetics of selective IgA deficiency (SIAD), common variable immunodeficiency (CVID), and IgG$_3$ deficiency were recently reviewed by Smith et al. *(27)* (Table 6). The frequency of SIAD among Caucasians is approx 1:500 and is the most prevalent of human immunodeficiencies. The genetics of SIAD probably involves multiple loci and may be associated with HLA haplotypes A1, B8, and DR3, but not complement. This deficiency can be transferred by bone marrow cells, thus implicating a defect in hematopoietic cells as an etiologic factor. Although decreases of both IgA$_1$ and IgA$_2$ are found in both sera and secretions, only about one-third of people with SIAD are prone to infections. This suggests that the presence of other antibody isotypes are able to provide sufficient immunoglobulin functions for normal health. The prevalence of CVID is reported as 1:20,000, and this immunodeficiency may also be associated with the same HLA haplotypes as SIAD. People with CVID often have abnormally low levels of IgG as well as IgA and are highly prone to recurrent infections. The B-lymphocyte abnormalities responsible for these deficiencies in humans are not known. There is the possibility that a developmental block may occur involving I (interven-

ing) regions upstream of switch sequences. This was suggested by data on peripheral blood mononuclear cells from IgA-immunodeficient patients, which showed a lack of I-region transcripts. However, the ability of TGF-β to induce in vitro transcription of the I region of IgA suggests that perhaps a regulatory or signaling pathway, and not a primary genetic defect within the Ig loci, is involved. Smith et al. *(27)* hypothesized that some patients may be unable to convert IgA$^+$ B-lymphocytes to IgA-secreting plasma cells. Since SIAD and CVID may be manifestations of a common abnormality, similar molecular and cellular events may lead to CVID.

Karlsson et al. *(28,29)* compared the sinusitis characteristics of CVID and SIAD patients. Overall, chronic rhinosinusitis was more prominent in patients with CVID, and upper respiratory tract infections preceded the appearance of lower respiratory tract infections by several years. Surface morphology of the nasal mucosa differed between individuals of the two groups. Frequencies of decreases in ciliated cells and increases in abnormal cilia were higher in CVID patients when compared to SIAD patients. Patients with CVID also tended to show lower numbers of goblet cells, whereas people with SIAD had increased numbers of goblet cells. Although mucociliary transport was impaired in both patient groups when compared to normal controls, it was more severe in the CVID individuals. Patients with CVID had the highest frequency of isolatable pathogenic bacteria from the nose and/or nasopharynx and had the most purulent infections. The authors suggested that epithelial and ciliary damage are caused by granulocyte enzymes released during infections and that the intensity of damage is related to the severity of infection. This was supported by the observation that SIAD patients as well as CVID patients who underwent immunoglobulin transfusion therapy had less mucosal damage and less severe infections. These data also emphasized the importance of antibodies in host defense within the nasal mucosa.

Ciliary defects attributable to primary ciliary dyskinesia (PCD) also lead to sinusitis and recurrent pulmonary infections. This is an autosomal recessive disorder that affects 1 in 15,000–30,000 people *(30)*. The physical abnormality is owing to a lack of one or both dynein arms among microtubule doublets. Radial spoke defects result in biphasic rotations about a vertical axis to give a

Table 7
IGG Subclasses

IgG subclasses	Characteristics
IgG_1 and/or IgG_3	Linkage disequilibrium between G_1 and G_3 genes Concurrent deficiencies observed 50% of adult levels reached by 1 yr of age Deficiencies primarily in adults, especially women Primarily responsive to protein antigens, viral antigens IgG_3 associated with atopy
IgG_2 and/or IgG_4	Close proximity of G_1 and G_4 genes on chromosome 14 Concurrent deficiencies observed 50% of adult levels reached by 4 yr of age Deficiencies primarily in male children Primarily responsive to carbohydrate antigens of bacteria

"washing machine" effect. The loss of both arms causes cilia to vibrate or rotate. These abnormalities decrease mucociliary clearance rates, and the ability to remove particulates and pathogens from the respiratory tracts. Chronic sinusitis, bronchitis, and otitis media then result from this dysfunction in natural immunity. If untreated, these problems will progress to bronchiectasis, pulmonary hypertension, and corpulmonale.

IgG subclass deficiencies are also associated with nasal diseases (Table 7). Among adult patients and, in particular, females, the most common abnormality is of IgG_3 *(31,32)*. Immunoglobulin allotypes, HLA haplotypes, and defects in isotype switching are associated with IgG_3 deficiency *(31)*. It has been reported that the concurrence of IgG_1 and IgG_3 deficiencies is the result of a linkage disequilibrium between the G1m(a) and G3m(g) gene allotypes *(33)*. As with IgG_1 and IgG_3, IgG_2 and IgG_4 deficiencies are coupled owing to the physical proximity of their genes. These linkages are also noted during normal development; IgG_1 and IgG_3 reach 50% of adult levels at 1 yr of age, whereas the same is said for IgG_2 and IgG_4 at 4 yr *(32)*.

Reviews of IgG subclass deficiencies and their associations with recurrent infections suggest that IgG_2 defects may be more common than previously thought *(32–34)*, particularly among male children.

Although immunoglobulins of the subclasses IgG_1 and IgG_3 primarily react with protein antigens, especially viral antigens, IgG_2 and IgG_4 are preferentially produced in response to carbohydrate antigens. In agreement, IgG_2 subclass deficits are associated with respiratory infections caused by bacteria with polysaccharide capsules, such as *Haemophilus influenzae* and *Streptococcus pneumoniae*. Children with IgG_2 deficiencies also show deficits in responses to a variety of immunizations, such as tetanus toxoid, *H. influenzae* capsular antigens, measles, and polio.

Rhinosinusitis and rhinopharyngitis are observed with IgG_3 deficiency *(35,36)*. Barlan et al. *(31)* noted high frequencies of asthma (55%) and recurrent sinus infections (95%) in patients with IgG_3 subclass deficiency. Armenaka et al. *(37)* reported that serum IgG_3 levels were depressed in people with chronic sinusitis, but not chronic rhinitis or normals. They also observed that atopic patients with chronic sinusitis had a greater frequency of IgG_3 deficiency than nonatopics. One reason for the association of atopy, sinusitis, and IgG_3 deficiency may be owing to sinus inflammation and asthma provoked by recurrent infections, which are in turn the result of the antibody defect. IgG_3 consumption as a result of chronic infection was also considered a possibility. Further insights into the relationships among atopy, infections, and immunodeficiencies provided by data from intravenous immunoglobulin (IVIG) administration are discussed on the next page.

Other immunodeficiency states, including those involving cellular immune components, are associated with sinusitis *(38)*, necrosis of the nose *(39)*, and lymphadenopathy *(40)*. Cellular immune defects with chronic purulent rhinosinusitis have been related to the presence of a retroviral-like protein in patient sera *(41,42)*. This factor, p15E, shows structural similarity to the envelope protein of murine and feline leukemia virus. Treatment with the bovine thymic extract, TP-1, results in improved immune status, and decreases in both nasal infections and serum p15E levels. Although the therapeutic mechanism of TP-1 is not known, an effect on T-cell maturation and/or function is possible. Sinusitis may also be a result of abnormal neural control of nasal secretions. Recurrent sinusitis is partly owing to decreased responsiveness to cholinergic stimulation, and correspondingly lower releases of immunoglobulins and lysozyme *(43)*.

Table 8
Infectious Organisms of the Nose and Sinus in AIDS

Acanthamoeba castellani
Aspergillus fumigatus
Alternaria alternata
Cryptococcus neoformans
Cytomegalovirus
Haemophilus influenzae
Legionella pneumophilia
Pseudallescheria boydii
Pseudomonas aeruginosa
Rochalimaea henselae
Staphylococcus aureus
Streptococcus pneumoniae

Table 9
Mechanism of Action of Intravenous Immunoglobulins

Antisera against certain infectious microbes can replace host antigen-specific antibodies

IVIG contains components that regulate the function of inflammatory cytokines; natural autoantibodies specific for IL-1 and TNF neutralize these cytokines; autoantibodies also inhibit the release of IL-1 and TNF from leukocytes; IVIG also inhibit the release of T-cell cytokines and downregulate IL-2 receptor expression

Natural autoantibodies found in IVIG may function to correct irregularities in immune networks via interactions with lymphocyte surface molecules, immunoglobulins, plasma proteins, and other cellular constituents

Infection with the human immunodeficiency virus (HIV) is accompanied by nasal manifestations (Table 8). According to a review by Rubin and Honigberg (44), sinusitis incidences of 10–68% have been reported among HIV-infected individuals. A predisposition for elevated IgE levels and other symptoms of atopy was also noted. Meiteles and Lucente (45) presented an overview of organisms recovered from sinonasal infections of AIDS patients, and concluded that these people are susceptible to a variety of common as well as rare infectious agents. Nasal dermatitis, lymphoid proliferation, lymphoma, and Kaposi's sarcoma are also characteristic of AIDS. More recently, HIV and nasal problems were associated with cryptococcal (46), rickettsial (47), *Pseudomonas* (48,49), and fungal (50) infections. Sinusitis and HIV are also found concurrently with gross mucosal abnormalities (51) and atopy (52).

The use of immunoglobulin prophylaxis has achieved some success in relieving the severity of sinusitis associated with immunodeficiencies. In the previously mentioned paper by Karlsson et al. (28), mucociliary function was reported to be impaired in patients with CVID. However, patients who received adequate immunoglobulin therapy had better mucociliary activity than those that did not. Hanson et al. (33) also demonstrated a positive effect of IVIG on respiratory infections and asthma. The dose and timing of IVIG administration is of critical importance in the success of treatment. The experience of Williams et al. (53) suggests that early intervention in primary hypogammaglobulinemia increases the effectiveness of IVIG in preventing sinusitis. Established infections are

more resistant to immunoglobulin treatments. Respiratory infections associated with IgG$_3$ deficiencies (31) and alcohol-related liver disease (54) are also alleviated through IVIG. Three HIV-infected children who received IVIG were also seen to have fewer respiratory infections following treatment (55). These data show that passive immunoglobulin therapy has the potential to re-establish immunocompetence in immunodeficient patients.

Although gammaglobulins have protective effects against infections during immunodeficient states, their modes of action are controversial (Table 9). Barlan et al. (31) reported that the positive effects of IVIG on IgG$_3$-deficient patients could not be owing to IgG$_3$ replacement, since the IVIG preparation did not contain IgG$_3$. Also, the selection of batches of normal gammaglobulins used are probably not based on their antigen specificities. If so, then IVIG targeting of specific microbial antigens is probably not the principal mechanism involved. Although there is some evidence that IVIG may neutralize effector molecules, such as complement (56) and microbial toxins (57), it appears that much of the beneficial functions of IVIG are the result of other mechanisms. Indeed, papers cited in this chapter implicate allergies in the pathogenesis of sinusitis and rhinitis. Spector (58) suggested that granulocytes recruited by the inflammatory response contribute to nasal mucosal damage, which then increases the host's susceptibility to infection. It has also been reported that among HIV-infected patients, atopy and not hypogammaglobulinemia is important in the development of sinusitis (52). Therefore, it is possible that sinus infections are products of defects in immune regulation that are clinically manifested by both immuno-deficiencies and allergies. This implies that the benefits of IVIG treatments rely primarily on the ability of humoral components to reinstate immuno-regulatory networks.

Pooled human immunoglobulins have well-documented effects on endogenous cytokine levels. In particular, attention has focused on interleukin-1 (IL-1) and tumor necrosis factor (TNF). As reviewed by Abe et al. *(59)*, both cytokines are proinflammatory and mediate productive responses to infectious microbes. They can also generate undesirable side effects, such as septic shock. Since natural autoantibodies found in normal human sera contain specificities for cytokines, including IL-1 and TNF, IVIG is thought to replace some of the regulatory constraints of inflammatory cytokines. Natural IgG can also inhibit the release of IL-1 and TNF from peripheral blood mononuclear cells. In addition, exogenous IgG has the potential to modulate IL-1 activity by influencing the expression of the IL-1 receptor antagonist (IL-1ra). This receptor antagonist is structurally related to IL-1 and will bind to the IL-1 receptor, but does not appear to stimulate a cellular response. Early in vitro studies demonstrated the ability of IgG to induce IL-1ra release by monocytes probably by signaling through Fc receptors *(60)*. For now, however, there is little evidence to support the idea that IVIG therapy in humans is able to generate sufficient IL-1ra to affect IL-1 activity *(61)*. Cytokines other than IL-1 and TNF are also affected by IVIG therapy. Andersson et al. *(62)* used an in vitro system to demonstrate the ability of IVIG to inhibit the production and release of TH_1 and TH_2 cytokines that normally occur following PMA/ionomycin stimulation. The lower activation state of responder cells to mitogens was also noted by a decrease in IL-2 receptor expression.

The incorporation of exogenous immunoglobulins into a host's natural autoantibody network and the consequences of this integration were reviewed by Kazatchkine et al. *(63)*. A characteristic of natural autoreactive antibodies is high connectivity at their variable regions. That is, these antibodies tend to recognize self-molecules, including each other. These interactions contribute to the maintenance of immunological homeostasis as it relates to the expression of autoreactive antibody repertoires. Since IVIG contains antibody reactivities against a wide range of self-molecules, this exogenous source of highly connected antibodies probably operates through network interactions. These interactions include:

1. The neutralization of circulating autoantibodies;
2. The recognition of lymphocyte surface structures, such as antigen receptors, major histocompatibility molecules, CD4, CD5, and Fc receptors; and
3. Reactivity with intracellular components and plasma proteins.

A major product of this autoreactive antibody network is the V-region-dependent selection of B-cell repertoires. Sundblad et al. *(64)* showed that connectivity between the existing antibody repertoire and the emerging repertoire, as represented by bone marrow B-lymphopoiesis, results in continuous adjustments in the autoreactive antibody specificities. Such interactions allow the immune system to absorb information about self without the generation of highly aggressive autoreactivity. These authors suggested that autoimmune disease is a manifestation of defects in connectivity that result in abnormalities in both peripheral repertoires and the selection of emergent B-cell clones. The purpose of administrating IVIG as a treatment for autoimmune diseases and allergies is then to re-establish connectivity and normalize immunological homeostasis. Such discussions of the mechanisms of action of IVIG support the proposal that abnormalities in the regulation of inflammation are primary factors contributing to the development of sinusitis.

CONCLUSION

The nasal mucosa conditions and cleans inspired air before it enters deeper regions of the body. However, this filtering capacity results in the accumulation of foreign substances in the nose. Since these impurities include both particulate and infectious materials, mechanisms for washing the nasal interior and immune resistance are well developed. The increase in chronic sinusitis that accompanies host immunodeficiency states confirms the importance of immune responses in maintaining the health of the nasal mucosa and perhaps overall health.

This overview does reveal limitations in knowledge on nasal immune mechanisms. For example, there is a lack of information on antigen presentation and other leukocyte functions in the nose. Interactions between nasal immune/inflammatory manifestations and systemic immunity are also not clear. However, such information is hopefully forthcoming, particularly because of interest in immunization via mucosal vaccinations *(65)*. General concepts on mucosal immunity probably apply to the nose. For instance, IgA is an important component of nasal as well as overall local immunity. However, comparisons between specific mucosal sites show that differences do exist. As an example, although serum IgG_3 deficiency may be reflected by a decrease in IgG_3^+ cells in the rectal mucosa, a similar serum deficiency appears to correlate with an increase in IgG_3^+ cells in the nasal mucosa *(36)*. Therefore, further information on nasal immunity will contribute to an appreciation of the nose and define its place among mucosal immune defenses.

REFERENCES

1. Hollinshead WH, Rosse C. The ear, orbit, and nose. In: Textbook of Anatomy, 4th ed. Philadelphia: Harper and Row, 1985; pp. 943–986.
2. Walike JW, Larrabee, WF Jr. Anatomy of the nose and nasopharynx. In: English GM, ed., Otolaryngology, Vol. 2: Diseases of the Nose and Sinuses. Philadelphia: JB Lippincott, 1994; pp. 1–19.
3. Wagenmann M, Naclerio RM. Anatomic and physiologic considerations of sinusitis. J Allergy Clin Immunol 1992;490:419–423.
4. Taylor M. Physiology of the nose, paranasal sinuses, and nasopharynx. In: English GM, ed., Otolaryngology, Vol. 2: Diseases of the Nose and Sinuses. Philadelphia: JB Lippincott, 1994; pp. 1–75.
5. Kaliner MA. Human nasal respiratory secretions and host defense. Am Rev Respir Dis 1991;144:S52–S56.
6. Peden DB, Swiersz M, Ohkubo K, et al. Nasal secretion of the ozone scavenger uric acid. Am Rev Respir Dis 1993;148:455–461.
7. Kaliner MA. Human nasal host defense and sinusitis. J Allergy Clin Immunol 1992;90:424–430.
8. Dahl AR, Hadley WM. Nasal cavity enzymes involved in xenobiotic metabolism: effects on the toxicity of inhalants. CRC Crit Rev Toxicol 1991;21:345–372.
9. Krause HE. Nasal cytology in clinical allergy. In: Krause HF, ed., Otolaryngic Allergy and Immunology. Philadelphia: WB Saunders, 1989; pp. 112–122.
10. Igarashi Y, Kaliner MA, Hausfeld JN, et al. Quantification of resident inflammatory cells in the human nasal mucosa. J Allergy Clin Immunol 1993;91:1082–1093.
11. Borres MP, Irander K, Björkstén B. Metachromatic cells in nasal mucosa after allergen challenge. Allergy 1990;45: 98–103.
12. Fokkens WJ, Holm AF, Rijntjes E, et al. Characterization and quantification of cellular infiltrates in nasal mucosa of patients with grass pollen allergy, non-allergic patients with nasal polyps and controls. Int Arch Allergy Appl Immunol 1990;93:66–72.
13. Graeme-Cook F, Bhan AK, Harris NL. Immunohistochemical characterization of intraepithelial and sub-

14. epithelial mononuclear cells of the upper airways. Am J Pathol 1993; 143:1416–1422.
14. Bernstein JM. Mucosal immunology of the upper respiratory tract. Respiration 1992;59(suppl 3):3–13.
15. Mullol J, Raphael GD, Lundgren ID, et al. Comparison of human nasal mucosal secretion in vivo and in vitro. J Allergy Clin Immunol 1992;89:584–592.
16. Braniuk JN, Kaliner MA. Neuropeptides and nasal secretion. J Allergy Clin Immunol 1990;86:620–627.
17. Okayama M, Mullol J, Baraniuk JN, et al. Muscarinic receptor subtypes in human nasal mucosa; characterization, autoradiographic localization, and function in vitro. Am J Respir Cell Mol Biol 1993;8:176–187.
18. Baraniuk JN, Silver PB, Kaliner MA, et al. Ibuprofen augments bradykinin-induced glycoconjugate secretion by human nasal mucosa in vivo. J Allergy Clin Immunol 1992;89:1032–1039.
19. Okayama M, Baraniiuk JN, Haausfeld JN, et al. Characterization and autoradiographic localization of histamine H1 receptors in human nasal turbinates. J Allergy Clin Immunol 1992;89:1144–1150.
20. Raphael GD, Igarashi Y, White MV, et al. The pathophysiology of rhinitis. V. Sources of protein in allergen-induced nasal secretions. J Allergy Clin Immunol 1991; 88:33–42.
21. Emery BE, White MV, Igarashi Y, et al. The effect of L-4 on human nasal mucosal responses. J Allergy Clin Immunol 1992;90:772–781.
22. Wu T, Mullol J, Rieves RD, et al. Endothelin-1 stimulates eicosanoid production in cultured human nasal mucosa. Am J Respir Cell Mol Biol 1992;6:168–174.
23. Mullol J, Chowdhury BA, White MV, et al. Endothelin in human nasal mucosa. Am J Respir Cell Mol Biol 1993; 8:393–402.
24. Ohkubo K, Lee CH, Baraniuk JN, et al. Angiotensin-converting enzyme in the human nasal mucosa. Am J Respir Cell Mol Biol 1994;11:173–180.
25. Lee CH, Igarashi Y, Hohman RJ, et al. Distribution of secretory leukoprotease inhibitor in the human nasal airway. Am Rev Respir Dis 1993;147:710–716.
26. Polmar SH. The role of the immunologist in sinus disease. J Allergy Clin Immunol 1992;90:511–555.
27. Smith CIE, Islam KB, Vorechovsky OO, et al. X-linked agammaglobulinemia and other immunoglobulin deficiencies. Immunol Rev 1994;138:159–183.
28. Karlsson G, Petruson B, Björkander J, et al. Infections of the nose and paranasal sinuses in adult patients with immunodeficiency. Arch Otolaryngol 1985;111:290–293.
29. Karlsson G, Hansson H-A, Petruson B, et al. The nasal mucosa in immunodeficiency. Surface morphology, mucociliary function and bacteriological findings in adult patients with common variable immunodeficiency or selective IgA deficiency. Acta Otolaryngol 1985;100: 456–469.
30. Le Mauviel L. Primary ciliary dyskinesia. West J Med 1991 Sep;155:280–283.
31. Barlan IB, Geha RS, Schneider LC. Therapy for patients with recurrent infections and low serum IgG3 levels. J Allergy Clin Immunol 1993;92:353–355.
32. Fadal RG. Chronic sinusitis, steroid-dependent asthma, and IgG subclass and selective antibody deficiencies. Otolaryngol Head Neck Surg 1993;109:606–610.

33. Hanson LA, Söderström R, Avanzini A, Bengtsson U, Björkander J, Söderström T. Immunoglobulin subclass deficiency. Pediatr Infect Dis J 1988;7:S17–S20.

34. Shackelford PG, Polmar SH, Mayus JL, Johnson WL, Corry JM, Nahm MH. Spectrum of IgG2 subclass deficiency in children with recurrent infections: prospective study. J Pediatr 1986;108:647–653.

35. Hanson LA, Söderström R, Nilssen DE, et al. IgG subclass deficiency with or without IgA deficiency. Clin Immunol Immunopathol 1991;61:S70–S77.

36. Nilssen DE, Söderström R, Brandtzaeg P, et al. Isotype distribution of mucosal IgG-producing cells in patients with various IgG subclass deficiencies. Clin Exp Immunol 1991;82:17–24.

37. Armenaka M, Grizzanti J, Rosenstreich DL. Serum immunoglobulins and IgG subclass levels in adults with chronic sinusitis: evidence for decreased IgG3 levels. Ann Allergy 1994;72:507–514.

38. Braegger C, Bottani A, Hallé F, et al. Unknown syndrome: ischiadic hypoplasia, renal dysfunction, immunodeficiency, and a pattern of minor congenital anomalies. Med Genet 1991;28:56–59.

39. Koch C, Pedersen FK, Bendtzen K, et al. Necrotic ulceration of the nose in a patient with primary immunodeficiency syndrome characterized by severe defects in the production of cytokines. Immunodeficiency 1993;4: 141–144.

40. Maennle DL, Grierson HL, Gnarra DG, et al. Sinus histiocytosis with massive lymphadenopathy: a spectrum of disease associated with immune dysfunction. Pediatr Pathol 1991;11:399–412.

41. Tas M, Leezenberg JA, Drexhage HA. Beneficial effects of the thymic hormone preparation thymoxtimulin in patients with defects in cell-mediated immunity and chronic purulent rhinosinusitis. A double-blind crossover trial on improvements in monocyte polarization and clinical effects. Clin Exp Immunol 1990;80:304–313.

42. Scheeren RA, Keehnen RMJ, Meijer CJLM, et al. Defects in cellular immunity in chronic upper airway infections are associated with immunosuppressive retroviral p15E-like proteins. Arch Otolaryngol Head Neck Surg 1993; 119:439–443.

43. Jeney EVM, Raphael GD, Meredith SD, et al. Abnormal nasal glandular secretion in recurrent sinusitis. J Allergy Clin Immunol 1990;86:10–18.

44. Rubin JS, Honigberg R. Sinusitis in patients with the acquired immunodeficiency syndrome. Ear Nose Throat J 1990;69:460–463.

45. Meiteles LZ, Lucente FE. Sinus and nasal manifestations of the acquired immunodeficiency syndrome. Ear Nose Throat J 1990;69:454–459.

46. Mares M, Sartori MT, Carretta M, et al. Rhinophyma-like cryptococcal infection as an early manifestation of AIDS in a hemophilia B patient. Acta Haematol 1990;84:101–103.

47. Hnatuk LAP, Brown DH, Snell GED. Bacillary angiomatosis: a new entity in acquired immunodeficiency syndrome. J Otolaryngol 1994;23:216–220.

48. O'Donnell JG, Sorbello AF, Condoluci DV, Barnish MJ. Sinusitis due to Pseudomonas aeruginosa in patients with

human immunodeficiency virus infection. Clin Infectious Dis 1993;16:404–406.

49. Grant A, von Schoenberg M, Grant HR, Miller RF. Paranasal sinus disease in HIV antibody positive patients. Genitourin Med 1993;69:208–212.

50. Meyer RD, Gaultier CR, Yamashita JT, et al. Fungal sinusitis in patients with AIDS: report of 4 cases and review of the literature. Medicine 1994;73:69–78.

51. Chong WK, Hall-Craggs MA, Wilkinson ID, et al. The prevalence of paranasal sinus disease in HIV infection and AIDS on cranial MR imaging. Clin Radiol 1993;47: 166–169.

52. Small CB, Kaufman A, Armenaka M, et al. Sinusitis and atopy in human immunodeficiency virus infection. J Infect Dis 1993;167:283–290.

53. Williams P, While A, Wilson JA, et al. Penetration of administered IgG into the maxillary sinus and long-term clinical effects of intravenous immunoglobulin replacement therapy on sinusitis in primary hypogammaglobulinaemia. Acta Otolaryngol 1991;111:550–555.

54. Spinozzi F, Cimignoli E, Gerli R, et al. IgG subclass deficiency and sinopulmonary bacterial infections in patients with alcoholic liver disease. Arch Intern Med 1992;152:99–104.

55. Hague RA, Burns SE, Hargreaves FD, et al. Virus infections of the respiratory tract in HIV-infected children. J Infect 1992;24:31–36.

56. Rosen FS. Putative mechanisms of the effect of intravenous g-globulin. Clin Immunol Immunopathol 1993;67: S41–S43.

57. Meissner HC, Schlievert PM, Leung DYM. Mechanisms of immunoglobulin action: observations on Kawasaki Syndrome and RSV prophylaxis. Immunol Rev 1994; 139:109–123.

58. Spector SL. The role of allergy in sinusitis in adults. J Allergy Clin Immunol 1992;90:518–520.

59. Abe Y, Horiuchi A, Miyake M, et al. Anti-cytokine nature of natural human immunoglobulin: one possible mechanism of the clinical effect of intravenous immunoglobulin therapy. Immunol Rev 1994;139:5–19.

60. Arend WP, Leung DYM. IgG induction of IL-1 receptor antagonist production by human monocytes. Immunol Rev 1994;139:71–78.

61. Dinarello CA. Is there a role for interleukin-1 blockade in intravenous immunoglobulin therapy? Immunol Rev 1994;139:173–188.

62. Andersson U, Björk L, Skansén-Saphir U, et al. Pooled human IgG modulates cytokine production in lymphocytes and monocytes. Immunol Rev 1994;139:22–42.

63. Kazatchkine ME, Dietrich G, Hurez V, et al. V region-mediated selection of autoreactive repertoires by intravenous immunoglobulin (i.v.Ig). Immunol Rev 1994;139: 79–107.

64. Sundblad A, Marcos M-AR, Malanchere E, et al. Observations on the mode of action of normal immunoglobulin at high doses. Immunol Rev 1994;139:125–158.

65. Walker RI. New strategies for using mucosal vaccination to achieve more effective immunization. Vaccine 1994; 12:387–400.

20   Autoimmune-Mediated Sinus and Midfacial Diseases

Thomas Cupps, MD

CONTENTS

INTRODUCTION

Relative to other pathologic processes, autoimmune-mediated diseases rarely involve sinus and midfacial structures. In the setting of an established systemic autoimmune disease, clinically significant involvement of the sinuses and midfacial structures is not common. When present, autoimmune-mediated diseases of these structures are most commonly seen in the setting of a systemic disease process. Autoimmune mediated involvement of these facial structures may be seen as the initial clinical manifestation or early in the course of several systemic diseases. An appreciation of the pattern of autoimmune disease involvement of midfacial structures may prove useful in directing a timely diagnostic evaluation looking for a systemic autoimmune process.

DISEASE MECHANISMS

Based on available clinical, laboratory, and research findings, autoimmune-mediated mecha-

From: *Diseases of the Sinuses* (M. E. Gershwin and G. A. Incaudo, eds.), ©1996 Humana Press Inc., Totowa, NJ.

nisms are felt to be important in the pathogenesis of these autoimmune-mediated sinus and midfacial syndromes. In all likelihood, different immunoregulatory mechanisms will be important in the pathogenesis of these syndromes. Our current understanding of the pathogenesis of autoimmune-mediated clinical syndromes is limited. A complete understanding of pathogenesis would require detailed knowledge of the following phases of disease expression:

1. The initial or "triggering" event;
2. The host's immunoregulatory response that leads to a sustained immune response directed at apparently normal tissue; and
3. The mechanisms of immune-mediated damage of normal structures leading to the clinically recognized pattern of disease involvement.

Because the first two phases may be completed prior to the clinical expression of disease, more detailed information characterizing the third phase is available for review.

There is little direct information defining the triggering events for any of the autoimmune-mediated syndromes involving the sinuses and midfa-

Table 1
Reactivity to Self-Antigens

Syndrome	Self-antigen	T-cell	B-cell
Wegener's granulomatosis	Proteinase 3 (PR3)	+	+
Churg-Strauss syndrome	Myeloperoxidase	?	+
Behçet's syndrome	Heat shock protein	+	−
Relapsing polychondritis	Cartilage antigen (type II collagen?)	+	+
McCabe's Syndrome	Cochlear antigen	?	+
Sarcoidosis	Kveim reagent?	+	−

cial structures. Because of the involvement of the upper respiratory tract and, in some syndromes, the lower respiratory tract in these diseases, respiratory pathogens and/or inhaled antigens have been postulated as potential triggering agents. Since the initial clinical description of Wegener's granulomatosis, for example, attempts to identify an infectious agent in both lung and sinus tissue have been uniformly unsuccessful. However, the failure to identify a pathogen does not exclude an infectious agent as a triggering event. An active infection could resolve with complete clearance of the infectious agent prior to the onset of clinically apparent autoimmune disease. The frequent history of a viral-like prodrome and epidemiologic data demonstrating a seasonal variation in the frequency of presentation provide indirect evidence for an infectious agent as the initial event in the pathogenesis of Wegener's granulomatosis. An inhaled antigen has been implicated as a cause of disease in a case of Churg-Strauss syndrome (1).

A detailed understanding of how a triggering event leads to a breakdown in host tolerance and progresses to an autoimmune disease is not currently available for any of these clinical syndromes. If respiratory tract pathogens or inhaled antigens are initial triggering events, a pattern of "molecular mimicry" may be a potential mechanism of lost self-tolerance. An infectious agent or inhaled antigen stimulates a physiologic host immune response that then crossreacts with a host protein with a similar amino acid sequence or epitope. The role for the immune response to the host antigens (Table 1) in the autoimmune-mediated syndromes of the sinus and midfacial structures has not been fully defined.

Of these syndromes, the mechanism of immune-mediated damage in Wegener's granulomatosis has been studied in greatest detail (2–4). A variety

Table 2
Levels of Serum Mediators
in Active Wegener's Granulomatosis

Elevated	Unchanged
C-ANCA (antibody to PR3)	Interleukin-1 (IL-1)
Interleukin-2 (IL-2)	Interferon-γ
IL-2 receptor (IL-2R)	Soluble CD4 (sCD4)
Interleukin-6 (IL-6)	Soluble CD8 (sCD8)
Interferon-α	
Tumor necrosis factor (TNF)	
Soluble intercellular adhesion molecule (sICAM)	
Soluble vascular adhesion molecule (sVCAM)	
Soluble E-selectin	

of soluble immunoregulatory molecules can be detected in increased concentrations in the serum of patients with active disease (Table 2). Clinical recurrence of Wegener's granulomatosis is often preceded by increasing titers of antineutrophil cytoplasmic antibodies (ANCA) with a course granular cytoplasmic pattern (C-ANCA) and/or IL-2R. In situ studies done on renal biopsies from patients with Wegener's granulomatosis demonstrate the local production of IL-1β and TNF-α and upregulation of IL-2R (5). Clearly these soluble mediators are important in the expression of the inflammatory lesions in Wegener's granulomatosis. The regulatory mechanisms that control the upregulation of these mediators are less well defined.

The potential role of C-ANCA and proteinase 3 (PR3) in the pathogenesis of Wegener's granulomatosis has been investigated in considerable detail (2–4). PR3, a neutral serine protease, is present in the cytoplasm of PMNs, monocytes, and endothelial cells. Following activation with a variety of

Table 3
Activities of C-ANCA

Binds to proteinase 3 (PR3)
Decrease enzymatic activity of PR3
Decrease PR3 binding to α_1-antitrypsin
Binds to (regulated by) anti-idiotype antibody
Binds to activated PMNs
    Enhances oxidative burst
        Fc-dependent mechanisms
        Fc-independent mechanisms
    Enhances degranulation
    Enhances chemotaxis
Binds to activated endothelial cells
    Complement-mediated lysis of endothelial cells
    Enhanced cytotoxic responses toward endothelial cells

stimulants, including TNF-α, PR3 can be detected on the surfaces of these cells. With the translocation to the cell surface, the PR3 is available for binding to C-ANCA. A variety of functional activities has been defined for C-ANCA (Table 3). The role of any of these functional activities in the clinical expression of Wegener's granulomatosis remains undefined. The mechanisms of the failure of both T-cell and B-cell tolerance leading to the production of C-ANCA have not been defined.

OVERVIEW OF CLINICAL SYNDROMES

Wegener's Granulomatosis

DEFINITION

Although a precise, generally accepted classification scheme for the vasculitides remains elusive, efforts to develop diagnostic criteria (6) and establish standard nomenclature (7) do allow for a more precise definition of the systemic vasculitic syndromes, including Wegener's granulomatosis. The American College of Rheumatology 1990 criteria (traditional format for classification) identified four major criteria that are useful in the classification of Wegener's granulomatosis:

1. Abnormal urinary sediment (red cell casts or >5 red blood cells/high-power field);
2. Abnormal findings on chest radiograph (nodules, cavities, or fixed infiltrates);
3. Oral ulcers or nasal discharge; and
4. Granulomatous inflammation on biopsy (6).

The presence of two or more of these major criteria is associated with a sensitivity of 88.2% and a specificity of 92.0%. The potential limitations of these classification criteria should be emphasized. They are designed to distinguish Wegener's granulomatosis from other major vasculitic syndromes, but have no validity in the exclusion of other clinical entities. The criteria are developed from patient populations with fully developed disease; consequently, the utility of this classification scheme to establish the diagnosis of Wegener's granulomatosis at the initial presentation of the disease is limited.

Because the precise pathogenesis remains undefined, the clinical definition of Wegener's granulomatosis is based on characteristic patterns of clinical, laboratory, and pathologic findings (7,8). Wegener's granulomatosis is a systemic syndrome characterized by necrotizing granulomatous vasculitis and inflammation with a predilection for the upper and lower respiratory tracts. Renal involvement with a necrotizing glomerulonephritis is present in the majority of patients. C-ANCA is present in over 90% of patients with active systemic Wegener's granulomatosis (8,9).

CLINICAL OVERVIEW

Symptoms related to the head and neck are the most common presenting complaints in Wegener's granulomatosis and are present in approx 75% of patients. Symptoms related to the lungs are present in less than half of the patients. Renal involvement is generally asymptomatic, but evidence of renal disease may be seen in approx 25% of patients at the time of initial diagnosis. When fully manifest, Wegener's granulomatosis affects the paranasal sinuses, oropharynx, lungs, and kidneys. Involvement of joints, skin, eyes, and nervous system is identified in less than half of the patients.

SINUS AND MIDFACIAL DISEASE

Because the majority of presenting signs and symptoms of Wegener's granulomatosis are related to the head and neck, knowledge of the pattern of disease activity in the sinus and midfacial structures frequently provides clinical clues that will facilitate an appropriate diagnostic evaluation.

Nose and Paranasal Sinuses. Wegener's granulomatosis most commonly presents with a pattern of chronic recurrent episodes of sinusitis manifest by nasal congestion, facial pain, or rhinitis for a variable period of time before the correct diagnosis is established. During the initial presentation, patients are treated with repeated courses of antibiotics, topical nasal glucocorticoids, and surgical drainage of the sinuses. Clinical improvement is commonly noted, but the problems recur. The nasal mucosa, particularly over the nasal turbinates and medial wall of the maxillary sinuses, may become friable with the appearance of granulation tissue. Mucosal ulceration with crusting is commonly present. The rhinitis may be serous or muco-purulent. Epistaxis has been reported, but is not common. The maxillary sinuses are most commonly involved followed by the ethmoid sinuses. Less commonly, the sphenoid and frontal sinuses are affected. Erosion through the bone of the medial wall of the maxillary sinuses has been described. Overall symptoms related to the head and neck region are present in 85% of patients at some point during the course of the disease.

Chronic dysfunction of the sinuses is seen in 50% of patients. Atrophic rhinitis with mucosal gland atrophy may be a long-term sequela of the initial sinusitis. Impaired mucosal host-defense function is frequently manifest by chronic recurrent episodes of sinusitis caused by *Staphylococcus aureus*. The chronic nasal carriage of *S. aureus* defines a subset of patients with Wegener's granulomatosis at increased risk of disease relapse *(10)*.

In addition to the nasal mucosa, the cartilaginous portion of the nasal septum may be involved. The clinical findings include nasal septal perforation as well as multiple small perforations. More diffuse involvement with destruction of the cartilaginous portion of the nasal septum results in collapse of the anterior portion of the nose producing the so-called saddle nose deformity. Rarely, a pattern of nasal chondritis similar to the pattern described in relapsing polychondritis has been described. Clinical involvement of the nose is present in 5% of patients at presentation. Long-term cosmetic and/or functional impairment of the nose is present in 30% of patients.

Oropharyngeal and Laryngotracheal Involvement. Symptoms related to the mouth and throat, including sore throat, laryngitis, shortness of breath, and stridor, are present in 10% of patients at presentation. Shallow ulcers up to a centimeter in diameter can be seen in the oral mucosa. Of note, the mucosal ulcers involving the roof of the mouth do not characteristically erode into or perforate the bone of the hard palate. Gingivitis, secondary to a characteristic pattern of friable gingival hyperplasia, is present in 5% of patients at presentation. In the absence of appropriate therapeutic intervention, the gingivitis may produce

alveolar bone resorption with secondary loosening of the teeth.

Laryngotracheal inflammation may produce laryngitis with altered voice tonal quality. Although not common, inflammation of the subglottic region may compromise air flow, producing stridor and shortness of breath. Rarely, urgent intervention is required to protect the integrity of the airway. Chronic problems with tracheal stenosis are seen in 13% of patients with Wegener's granulomatosis and may require therapeutic intervention as well *(8)*.

Eye and Associated Structures. Approximately 20% of patients with Wegener's granulomatosis have eye involvement at presentation. Both proptosis and corneoscleral ulceration have been reported as the initial manifestation of disease *(11)*. Ultimately, between 40 and 50% of patients will develop some form of eye disease. Virtually any structure related to the eye may be involved. Proptosis secondary to retro-orbital inflammation with progression to fibrosis is the single most common manifestation. Inflammation of the anterior structures, including conjunctivitis, episcleritis, scleritis, and corneoscleral ulceration, is present in 15% of patients. Less common manifestations of disease include uveitis, dacryocystitis, and vasculitis of retinal, choroidal, or optic nerve vessels. Visual loss as a result of the retro-orbital disease is present in 8% of patients *(8)*.

Ear. At presentation, 15% of patients will have symptoms related to the ears, including pain and decreased auditory acuity. Ultimately, 35% of patients will have some hearing impairment, although complete hearing loss is rare, affecting 1% of individuals. Suppurative otitis media is the most common manifestation. The problem may follow a chronic recurrent course. Inflammation with residual scarring of the Eustachian tube is a contributory factor in some patients. Damage to the structures of the inner ear is the most common cause of partial auditory impairment. Although less common, sensorineural impairment presumably secondary to vasculitis-induced ischemia may result in the acute onset of severe audiovestibular dysfunction *(12)*. A full functional recovery has been reported with the rapid initiation of appropriate therapy in the setting of acute onset of sensorineural impairment *(13)*. Rarely, a pattern of auricular chondritis has been reported in association with Wegener's granulomatosis.

LABORATORY AND PATHOLOGY

Routine Laboratory. Abnormal laboratory studies including leukocytosis, thrombocytosis, elevated erythrocyte sedimentation rate and c-reactive protein, positive rheumatoid factor and polyclonal increases in IgG and IgA are consistent with active systemic inflammatory process, but are not specific for Wegener's granulomatosis. The presence of hematuria, RBC casts, and proteinuria on routine urinalysis is useful to identify renal involvement.

Serology. As previously noted, the C-ANCA directed toward PR3 is a specific marker for Wegener's granulomatosis. The sensitivity of the C-ANCA varies with both extent and activity of disease *(9)*. The sensitivity of the C-ANCA exceeds 90% in patients with generalized active disease, but is in the range of 60% for more localized active disease. Following successful therapy in patients with both generalized and localized disease, the sensitivity drops to the 40% range. Although not currently included, the C-ANCA will undoubtedly be part of future disease criteria for Wegener's granulomatosis.

In general, there is an association between the titer of C-ANCA and disease activity. In some patients, a rising titer of C-ANCA may precede clinical exacerbations of disease. However, a rising titer is variably associated with clinically apparent disease activity. At present, committing a patient to the potential morbidity of immunosuppressive therapy based on a rising C-ANCA titer may be premature *(8)*. Close clinical follow-up in this setting looking for subtle manifestations of disease activity would be prudent.

Imaging Studies. Routine sinus radiographs generally demonstrate a pattern of both acute and chronic sinusitis. CT studies of the sinuses may be useful for identifying possible bony involvement. Both CT and MRI studies are useful to identify retro-orbital disease (Fig. 1). A wide variety of parenchymal lesions can be seen on chest radiographs, including infiltrates and nodules with or without cavitation. The lesions may be unilateral or bilateral. Of particular note, pleural effusions and hilar adenopathy are very rare findings in Wegener's granulomatosis. Pulmonary CT studies are more sensitive than routine chest radiographs and may be useful in identifying the more subtle parenchymal lesions for possible biopsy.

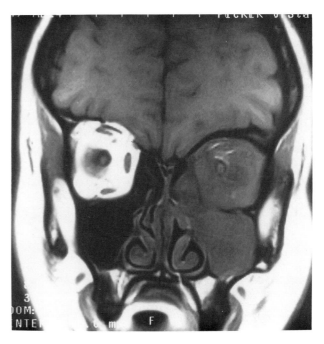

Fig. 1. MRI of the retro-orbital space. The patient developed recurrent retro-orbital Wegener's granulomatosis of the left eye following a prolonged disease-free period of time. The MRI (TR = 783, TE = 16, TI = 0, RF = 90) demonstrates the loss of the retro-orbital adipose signal and loss of definition of the extraocular muscles when compared to the normal right eye.

Pathology. The histopathologic findings in Wegener's granulomatosis have been studied in detail *(14,15)*. An open-lung biopsy provides the highest diagnostic yield for the definitive tissue diagnosis of this disease. The major diagnostic findings include:

1. Parenchymal necrosis;
2. Vasculitis of small and medium-sized vessels, including arteries, arterioles, capillaries, venules, and veins; and
3. Granulomatous inflammation accompanied by an inflammatory infiltrate composed of neutrophils, lymphocytes, plasma cells, histiocytes, and eosinophils.

Capillaritis is present in 30% of biopsy specimens. A wide variety of other pathologic patterns can be seen as a minor component of the biopsy as well *(14)*. The characteristic findings can be identified in 20% of biopsies from the head and neck region (Fig. 2) *(15)*. The finding of granulomatous inflammation in the absence of vasculitis may provide supportive evidence for the diagnosis (Fig. 3).

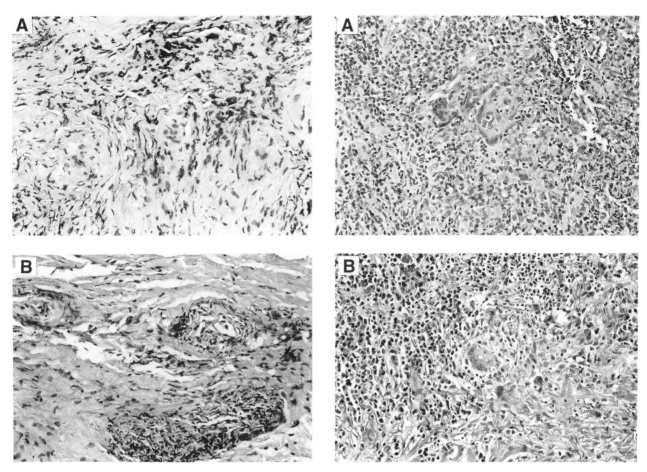

Fig. 2. Biopsy of retro-orbital lesion in a patient with Wegener's granulomatosis. **(A)** A pattern of chronic inflammation with granuloma formation is present. Hematoxylin and eosin stain (original magnification ×200). **(B)** Vasculitic lesion with a predominately mononuclear cell infiltration of the blood vessel wall. Hematoxylin and eosin stain (original magnification ×200).

Fig. 3. Biopsies from a patient chronic sinusitis, diabetes insipidus, and a low-titter positive C-ANCA without lung or renal disease. **(A)** Biopsy of sinus tissue showing granuloma, multinucleated giant cells, and acute and chronic inflammation. Hematoxylin and eosin stain (original magnification ×200). **(B)** Trans-sphenoidal biopsy of the pituitary fossa lesion showing granulomas, multinucleated giant cells, and chronic inflammation. Hematoxylin and eosin stain (original magnification ×200).

The most common pattern on renal biopsy is a focal segmental glomerulonephritis. A pattern of diffuse proliferative glomerulonephritis with crescent formation may be seen in the cases with rapidly progressive renal dysfunction. Vasculitis with granuloma formation is not commonly seen.

THERAPY AND PROGNOSIS

General Treatment. Initial treatment with low-dose oral daily cyclophosphamide (2 mg/kg body wt) and prednisone (1 mg/kg body wt) followed by a taper of the prednisone to an alternate-day regimen over 3 mo is effective in inducing remission in the majority of patients *(8)*. Over 90% of patients will improve on this regimen with 75% of patients going into complete remission. However, over 50%

of patients who enter a remission will have at least one relapse. Because of significant drug-associated morbidity with this therapeutic approach, alternative treatment protocols have been studied. Intermittent high-dose iv cyclophosphamide does not appear to be as effective in inducing durable remissions *(16)*. Preliminary experience with the combination of glucocorticoids and weekly low-dose methotrexate suggests that this regimen may be an effective treatment alternative in at least a subset of patients with Wegener's granulomatosis *(17)*.

Sinus and Midfacial Treatment Concerns. Because of the damage to the mucosa, chronic sinus problems are a common sequelae. Recurrent episodes of bacterial sinusitis, most commonly secondary to *S. aureus,* require repeat courses of antibiotic therapy. Distinguishing episodes of bacterial sinusitis from reactivation of Wegener's granulomatosis may be problematic. Surgical intervention to enhance sinus drainage may benefit some patients. Patients with more severe sinus mucosal involvement may benefit from the regular use of saline nasal sprays.

Chronic or recurrent tracheal stenosis can be a long-term management problem as well. Therapeutic alternatives include mechanical dilatation and/or laser therapy. Surgical options include open reconstructive surgery or chronic tracheostomy. When feasible, surgery should not be performed during periods of active disease. Experience with reconstructive surgery to repair the nasal deformities is limited. There has been a general reluctance to proceed with cosmetic reconstructive surgery because of concerns about reactivation of the disease.

Churg-Strauss Syndrome

DEFINITION

The American College of Rheumatology 1990 criteria (traditional format) identified six major criteria for the classification of the Churg-Strauss syndrome (allergic angiitis and granulomatosis):

1. Asthma;
2. Eosinophilia >10%;
3. Neuropathy, including both mono- and polyneuropathy;
4. Nonfixed, migratory pulmonary infiltrates;
5. Paranasal sinus abnormality; and
6. Extravascular eosinophils *(18).*

The presence of any four or more of the six criteria yields a sensitivity of 85% and a specificity of 99.7% in relationship to other major vasculitic syndromes. The same potential limitations in the classification scheme noted for Wegener's granulomatosis apply to the Churg-Strauss syndrome classification criteria.

Given the limitations of our understanding of the pathogenesis, the clinical definition of the Churg-Strauss syndrome is also based on characteristic patterns of clinical, laboratory, and pathologic findings *(7,19–22).* Although it is generally accepted that the Churg-Strauss syndrome is a distinct clinical entity, a consensus on a precise clinical definition is currently lacking. Because incomplete or

"limited" forms of this disease exist, establishing a uniformly accepted clinical definition is problematic *(21).* However, the Churg-Strauss syndrome is a distinct clinical entity characterized by the following elements:

1. History of allergic rhinitis and asthma;
2. Peripheral blood eosinophilia generally >1.5×10^9/L;
3. Noninfectious, migratory pulmonary infiltrates;
4. Systemic vasculitis; and
5. Extravascular necrotizing granuloma generally with an eosinophilic infiltrate.

It should be emphasized that, in an individual patient, not all elements will present at a given time during the course of the disease and that "limited" forms of the syndrome exist. Although the ANCA with a perinuclear staining pattern (P-ANCA) with specificity for myeloperoxidase is present in the majority of patients with Churg-Strauss syndrome *(23),* the test lacks diagnostic specificity because this autoantibody is also present in patients with Wegener's granulomatosis, polyarteritis nodosa, and idiopathic crescentic glomerulonephritis *(24).*

CLINICAL OVERVIEW

Several distinct phases in the clinical expression of the Churg-Strauss syndrome are recognized. In the majority of patients, there is a prodromal phase characterized by allergic rhinitis and asthma. The mean time from the onset of asthma to the development of systemic vasculitis is 8 yr (range 0–30 yr) *(20).* A shorter time interval is associated with more severe disease with a mean time interval of just over 3 yr in patients who died of disease. Initially, the asthma is readily treated in the majority of patients. Over time, management becomes more problematic. Many patients have received at least abbreviated courses of systemic glucocorticoid therapy prior to the diagnosis of the systemic vasculitis. Because of problems in the treatment of bronchospasm, chest radiographs are obtained that demonstrate a pattern of migratory infiltrates. During the transition to the vasculitic phase, systemic involvement becomes apparent. The majority of patients will develop problems with the skin (purpura and nodules), peripheral nervous system (mononeuritis multiplex), and hypertension. Involvement of the gastrointestinal tract, heart, and kidneys is also commonly seen. During the transition to the systemic phase of the Churg-Strauss syndrome, the marked changes in the degree of bronchospasm may be noted. Both marked exacerbation with glucocorticoid-resistant status asthmaticus and significant improvement of the bronchospasm have been observed.

SINUS AND MIDFACIAL DISEASE

Nose and Paranasal Sinuses. In approx 70% of patients, allergic rhinitis represents the initial manifestation of the Churg-Strauss syndrome, and leads to nasal obstruction, recurrent sinusitis, and nasal polyposis. The allergic rhinitis generally predates clinically apparent asthma. Although less common than allergic rhinitis, a necrotizing process of the upper respiratory tract similar to the pattern seen in Wegener's granulomatosis can be identified and is clinically manifest by nasal pain, and purulent and/or hemorrhagic discharge. The nasal mucosa is friable with crusting and may have a granular appearance. Nasal septal perforation is rare and progression to a saddle nose deformity is not characteristically seen.

Oropharyngeal and Laryngotracheal Involvement. Primary involvement of these structures is not common. Symptoms in the oropharynx are generally secondary to the sinusitis.

Eye, Ear, and Associated Structures. Involvement of these structures in Churg-Strauss syndrome is rare. When present, the eye involvement is the result of ischemic optic neuropathy secondary to vasculitis of the short posterior ciliary arteries. Retro-orbital disease is not seen.

LABORATORY AND PATHOLOGY

Routine Laboratory. The findings on routine laboratory studies during the vasculitic phase of the Churg-Strauss syndrome reflect a nonspecific pattern of systemic inflammation. Leukocytosis, an elevated erythrocyte sedimentation rate, and a polyclonal increase in Ig commonly occur. Although mild eosinophilia consistent with allergic rhinitis characterizes the initial phase of the disease, increasing levels of eosinophilia occur as the pattern of asthma evolves into the systemic vasculitic phase of the disease. The mean peak eosinophil count in 85 patients reported by Lanham et al. *(21)* was 12.9×10^9. Elevated serum levels of IgE are reported in the majority of patients as well.

Serology. As previously noted, the majority of patients with Churg-Strauss syndrome will have serum P-ANCA to myeloperoxidase. However, this test lacks diagnostic specificity, and the rela-

tionship between the P-ANCA titer and disease activity is undefined.

Imaging Studies. Routine films or CT studies of sinuses frequently show a pattern of pan-sinusitis, including both acute and chronic changes. Retro-orbital involvement and destruction of bony elements are not typically present. The pattern of chest radiographs in Churg-Strauss syndrome is variable. Most commonly, radiographs demonstrate transient, patchy infiltrates without a particular distribution. Less common findings include hilar lymphadenopathy, diffuse interstitial infiltrates, and a miliary pattern. Massive bilateral nodular infiltrates that progress to a confluent pattern have been described, but progression to cavitary lesions is unusual. Pleural effusions have been reported in 30% of cases.

Pathology. A variety of pathologic lesions can be seen in Churg-Strauss vasculitis. The essential diagnostic lesions are vasculitis and extravascular necrotizing granulomas usually with eosinophilic infiltrates *(22)*. Transmural inflammation of small muscular arteries is the most common vasculitic lesion. Intermediate-sized arteries, veins, and venules may be involved to a lesser degree. Early lesions may have a predominant eosinophilic infiltrate. As the lesion matures, a mixed cellular infiltrate with eosinophils is common. Vasculitic lesions in varying stages of maturation may be seen in a given biopsy site. Renal biopsy may show focal segmental necrotizing glomerulonephritis, crescents, vasculitis, or eosinophilic interstitial infiltrates.

THERAPY AND PROGNOSIS

General Treatment. Glucocorticoid therapy (i.e., prednisone 1 mg/kg) is generally effective in suppressing signs and symptoms of active disease. Lanham et al. *(21)* have recommended continued treatment with high-dose glucocorticoids until improvement of the mononeuritis multiplex and/or glomerulonephritis is noted. After the initial response, the glucocorticoids are tapered based on clinical response. Treatment of 1 yr appears to be adequate to induce long-term remissions in the majority of cases. A subset of patients may require cytotoxic therapy in addition to the glucocorticoid treatment. Both azathioprine and cyclophosphamide have been used successfully in such glucocorticoid-refractory cases.

During aggressive therapy for the systemic vasculitis, the symptoms of allergic rhinitis and asthma tend to abate. Because the systemic gluco-corticoids are tapered and discontinued, clinical recurrence of the rhinitis and bronchospasm may require additional therapy. The return of these symptoms is not necessarily indicative of recurrence of the systemic vasculitis. Prognosis for the majority of patients with treated Churg-Strauss syndrome is good. In a 16-patient series reported by Lanham et al. *(21)*, only a single patient died from the disease. Relapse of the disease was seen in six patients, and the majority of these relapses occurred during the initial treatment period following a reduction in the glucocorticoid dose. Late recurrence or a chronic relapsing disease course is not common. Long-term sequelae, including chronic neuropathy, impaired renal function, and hypertension, occur in 20% of patients. Aggressive management of the hypertension in the setting of mild renal failure is important to prevent progression to chronic renal failure. Angiotensin enzyme inhibitors are frequently very effective in controlling hypertension in the setting of systemic vasculitis.

Sinus and Midfacial Treatment Concerns. After successful therapy of the systemic vasculitis and withdrawal of the immunosuppressive therapy, treatment for recurrent allergic rhinitis is commonly required. In the small subset of patients who develop necrotizing sinusitis, chronic sinusitis similar to the pattern described in patients with Wegener's granulomatosis may also develop.

Behçet's Syndrome

DEFINITION

Several different sets of classification criteria have been proposed for the diagnosis of Behçet's syndrome (reviewed in *[24]*). These classification criteria emanate from different countries and emphasize that the clinical expression of Behçet's syndrome may vary by geographic location. The classification criteria proposed by The International Study Group for Behçet's Disease *(25)* have been validated on an international patient cohort *(26)* and are summarized as follows: Recurrent oral ulceration is an absolute diagnostic criterion. Minor aphthous, major aphthous, or herpetiform ulceration observed by a physician or reported reliably by a patient with recurrence at least three times in one 12-mo period is required. In addition, any two

of the following four criteria must be identified during the course of the disease:

1. Recurrent genital ulceration: recurrent genital aphthous ulceration or scarring, especially in males, observed by a physician or reliably reported by the patient;
2. Eye lesions: anterior uveitis, posterior uveitis, cells in the vitreous on slip lamp examination, or retinal vasculitis observed by a qualified physician (ophthalmologist);
3. Skin lesions: erythema nodosum-like lesions observed by a physician or reliably reported by the patient, pseudofolliculitis, papulopustular lesions, or acneiform nodules consistent with Behçet's syndrome—observed by a physician in postadolescent patients not receiving glucocorticoids; and
4. Positive pathergy test: to be read by a physician 24–48 h after oblique insertion of a 20-gage or smaller needle under sterile conditions. A positive test is characterized by the development of a 3–10-mm nodule or pustule at the site of the needle insertion.

Of note, the incidence of the pathergic responses appears to vary by geographic region with a particularly low incidence in North American patients with Behçet's syndrome *(27)*. The International Study Group classification criteria have a sensitivity of 90% and a specificity of 95% when applied prospectively to an international patient cohort *(26)*.

With only a limited understanding of the pathogenesis of this disease, the clinical definition of Behçet's syndrome is also based on the characteristic patterns of clinical, laboratory, and pathologic findings *(27–32)*. Behçet's syndrome is a systemic disease characterized by a chronic relapsing inflammatory process, including recurrent aphthous stomatitis, aphthous genital ulceration, a variety of other skin lesions (cutaneous nodules, pustules, and erythema nodosum), inflammatory eye disease, thrombophlebitis, synovitis, neurologic dysfunction, ulcerative gastrointestinal tract disease, and vasculitis. No histopathologic pattern is diagnostic of this disease, although vasculitis is a frequent finding.

CLINICAL OVERVIEW

The full clinical expression of Behçet's syndrome generally evolves over several years. Although the course of individual patients varies greatly, a pattern of disease expression is apparent. In over 70% of cases, the initial manifestation of Behçet's syndrome is a pattern of recurrent crops of aphthous ulcers. Less common presenting signs include eye lesions and joint involvement. The presenting complaints bringing the patient to medical attention follow a different pattern with eye and oral symptoms accounting for 25% of the patients each. Presenting complaints related to joint symptoms, neuropsychiatric concerns, and thrombophlebitis each account for another 10%. After the initial presentation with recurrent episodes of oral ulcers, and skin and eye involvement, the development of genital ulcers follows. Given the sequential pattern of disease expression, it is not surprising that a mean time of 6 yr has been reported from the initial clinical presentation to the diagnosis of Behçet's syndrome (28). Late manifestations of Behçet's syndrome include central nervous system disease and vascular compromise. Vascular lesions include both large artery vasculitis and veno-occlusive disease. Less common manifestations of Behçet's syndrome include ulcerative bowel disease with a predilection for the terminal ileum and colon, immune complex-mediated glomerulonephritis, myositis, and amyloidosis.

SINUS AND MIDFACIAL DISEASE

Nose and Paranasal Sinuses. Involvement of the nose and paranasal sinuses is not a prominent feature of Behçet's syndrome. A rare association between relapsing polychondritis and Behçet's syndrome has been reported, however (32).

Oropharyngeal and Laryngotracheal Involvement. Recurrent crops of aphthous ulcers are the most common initial manifestation and are required for the definitive diagnosis of Behçet's syndrome. The oral lesions of Behçet's syndrome tend to be round or oval in shape. The lesions vary in size from 3 to 15 mm in diameter. When adjacent ulcers become confluent, larger lesions up to 30 mm may be seen. The lesions are shallow with an erythematous rim and a yellow necrotic base. The majority of lesions heal within 7–14 d without scarring. Less commonly, herpetiform lesions can occur. The oral lesions seen in Behçet's syndrome and the oral lesions seen in idiopathic recurrent oral ulceration are similar in appearance. However, certain patterns of involvement are more common in Behçet's syndrome. Patients with Behçet's syndrome have an increased number of concurrent ulcers and more frequent involvement of the soft palate and oropharynx (33). The oral ulcers tend to be symptomatic. With severe involvement of the oropharynx, oral intake may be decreased because of pain.

Rarely, clinical signs, such as dilation of sublingual veins or facial swelling, may be seen in the setting of a superior vena cava syndrome. Neuro-Behçet's with brainstem involvement may produce a pattern of pseudobulbar palsy.

Eye, Ear, and Associated Structures. Eye involvement is seen in 75% of patients at some point during the course of the disease. Although any structure of the eye can be affected, inflammation of the elements of the anterior segment of the eye is the most common pattern of involvement. Relapsing iridocyclitis and/or anterior uveitis with hypopyon is the most common pattern of eye disease in Behçet's. Conjunctivitis and corneal ulceration are seen less commonly. Disease of the posterior segment is seen in >50% of patients with a pattern of choroiditis, retinal vessel involvement (arteritis, phlebitis, and thrombosis), and optic neuritis. Vitreous involvement with inflammation and/or hemorrhage is seen less commonly. Chronic sequelae include cataracts, glaucoma, optic nerve atrophy, and impaired vision. Rarely, papilledema secondary to intracranial hypertension can be seen with dural sinus thrombosis.

Ear disease is distinctly uncommon in Behçet's syndrome. Sensorineural hearing loss is rarely seen. The acute onset of hearing loss suggests a vasculitic process. Vestibular dysfunction is highly suggestive of neuro-Behçet's with involvement of the brainstem.

LABORATORY AND PATHOLOGY

Routine Laboratory and Serology. The findings on routine laboratory studies during active flares of the disease reflect a nonspecific pattern of systemic inflammation. Leukocytosis, elevated erythrocyte sedimentation rate, and increased levels of acute phase reactants, including c-reactive protein, may be seen during periods of active disease. In the subset of patients with glomerulonephritis, the urinalysis will reflect an active urinary sediment. Serologic studies are characteristically negative. Anticardiolipin antibodies can be seen in 30% of patients, but do not correlate with thrombotic events.

Imaging Studies. Chest radiographs may be entirely normal. In the rare patient with pulmonary hemorrhage secondary to Behçet's syndrome, pulmonary infiltrates are described. Evidence of vascular disease, such as superior vena cava syndrome or aortitis, may be seen on routine chest radiographs. Radiographic evidence of sinusitis or retro-orbital disease is characteristically not seen. Contrast studies of the gastrointestinal tract may show a pattern of mucosal ulceration with bowel wall involvement. MRI studies of the central nervous system provide important diagnostic information in neuro-Behçet's. Focal small areas of increased signal intensity can be seen in the white matter. Gray matter lesions are less commonly seen. Frequent and severe involvement of the brainstem and posterior fossa has been described.

Pathology. Although the precise pattern of pathology may vary according to the organ system involved, vasculitis is a key feature of the histopathology in Behçet's syndrome. The earliest feature of the ulcerative lesions is a mononuclear cell infiltrate of the dermis and basal layers of the epidermis, which leads to the epidermal slough. A small vessel vasculitis may or may not be seen below the ulcerative lesion. Virtually any size blood vessel, from large elastic arteries (including the vasa vasorum) to arterioles and large veins to venules, can be involved. Lymphocytes and plasma cells are the dominant cells in the inflammatory lesions. Giant cells and granuloma formation are not characteristic. Disruption of the internal elastic lamina may result in pseudoaneurysm formation. Superimposed thrombosis can be seen in both arterial and venous lesions. Vasculitic lesions in various stages of evolution are commonly seen together. Necrosis is not a dominant feature of the vasculitis seen in Behçet's syndrome.

TREATMENT AND PROGNOSIS

General Treatment. Optimal management of patients with Behçet's syndrome remains problematic. Because of the wide spectrum of disease expression, the pattern of clinical involvement will dictate the level of therapeutic intervention. A wide variety of therapeutic measures have been tried with limited success in Behçet's syndrome, including NSAIDs, colchicine, dapsone, levamisole, and thalidomide. Glucocorticoids, administered both topically and systemically, will suppress symptoms of disease activity, but do not appear to alter the course of the underlying disease, particularly eye involvement. Positive therapeutic responses have been reported with several different immunosuppressive agents. Both azathioprine *(31)* and cyclosporin *(34)* reportedly have a positive therapeutic effect on the ocular manifestations of Behçet's disease. Chlorambucil is reported to have a positive therapeutic effect on both uveitis and meningoencephalitis *(35)*. A major source of disease-associated morbidity is eye involvement with approx 30% of patients with ocular disease progressing to blindness. Although the disease-associated mortality is <5%, the principal source of mortality is central nervous system (CNS) involvement. Based on these observations, immunosuppressive therapy is warranted in patients with Behçet's syndrome who have progressive eye and CNS disease. The duration and level of therapeutic intervention are dictated by the course and level of disease activity.

Sinus and Midfacial Treatment Concerns. Topical analgesics can be used to provide symptomatic relief of the oral lesions. Topical glucocorticoids may provide symptomatic relief as well.

Relapsing Polychondritis

DEFINITION

Several different classification criteria have been proposed for relapsing polychondritis *(36,37)*. The classification criteria are empirical and can be summarized as follows: (1) proven inflammatory episodes involving at least two of three sites—auricular, nasal, or laryngotracheal cartilage, or (2) one of those sites and two other manifestations, including ocular inflammation (conjunctivitis, keratitis, episcleritis, uveitis), hearing loss, vestibular dysfunction, or seronegative inflammatory arthritis. A detailed analysis of the sensitivity and specificity of these classification criteria is not currently available.

Given the limited understanding of pathogenesis, the clinical definition of this syndrome is based on the characteristic patterns of clinical and pathologic findings. Relapsing polychondritis is a rare clinical syndrome characterized by episodic and generally progressive inflammation of cartilaginous structures throughout the body, including ears, nose, eyes, and joints. Laryngeal, bronchial, and costal cartilage is also affected. The pattern and sequence of involvement tend to vary. The clinical manifestation of relapsing polychondritis may be associated with a variety of other autoimmune diseases. Biopsies of actively involved cartilage demonstrate a characteristic perichondral inflammation composed of mononuclear cells.

CLINICAL OVERVIEW

The most common clinical manifestations of relapsing polychondritis in descending order of frequency are auricular chondritis (39%), arthritis (36%), laryngotracheal symptoms (26%), and nasal chondritis (25%). Ocular, auditory, and vestibular dysfunction more commonly evolve later during the course of the disease. Vascular abnormalities, such as aortitis, cardiac valvular insufficiency, and aneurysm formation, may also develop as late complications of the disease. Evidence of renal involvement, most commonly glomerulonephritis, is seen in 25% of patients. Systemic vasculitis is present in approx 10% of patients. In addition to the aortitis, vasculitis of muscular arteries can occur, particularly in the CNS. Other diseases seen in association with relapsing polychondritis include rheumatoid arthritis, systemic lupus erythematosus, undifferentiated connective tissue disease, myeloproliferative syndromes, and others.

SINUS AND MIDFACIAL DISEASE

Nose and Paranasal Sinuses. Over half the patients with relapsing polychondritis will have an episode of nasal chondritis during the course of the disease. The saddle nose deformity is present in 18% of patients at disease presentation and will ultimately develop in 29% of patients. Disease involvement of the paranasal sinuses and the bony portion of the nasal septum is typically absent.

Oropharyngeal and Laryngotracheal Involvement. The oropharynx is spared in this disease. In contrast, laryngotracheal involvement is present in a quarter of patients at presentation and ultimately will develop in half of the patients. Pain of the involved structure is the characteristic clinical manifestation of this disease feature. Hoarseness, stridor, wheezing, and shortness of breath have been reported as well. Life-threatening obstruction of the airway is rarely reported at disease presentation. Strictures of these structures are identified in 15% of patients at presentation and develop in 23% of patients during the course of the disease. Although present in a minority of patients, tracheal and bronchial strictures are a significant source of both morbidity and mortality.

Eye, Ear, and Associated Structures. Eye involvement is present in 20% of patients at presentation and will be identified in 50–65% of patients during the course of the disease. Inflammation of the anterior structures of the eye, including conjunctivitis, episcleritis, scleritis, and rarely keratitis, can be seen. Although involvement of the posterior structures is less common, iridocyclitis, chorioretinitis, retinal hemorrhage, and retinal vasculitis have been reported. Miscellaneous abnormalities include cataract formation, optic neuritis, and extraocular muscle palsies. Involvement of the retro-orbital structures is exceedingly rare, but may be seen in overlap syndromes with elements of both relapsing polychondritis and Wegener's granulomatosis.

Auricular chondritis is the most common presenting manifestation of relapsing polychondritis and ultimately develops in 85% of patients. During an acute flare of auricular chondritis, the pinna becomes erythematous, painful, and swollen. Characteristically, the inflammation is limited to the cartilaginous portion of the pinna and external auditory canal. With recurrent episodes, the cartilage is replaced by fibrous tissue, and the structural integrity of the pinna is compromised. Otitis media is seen in 5% of patients.

Although only 10% of patients have evidence of audiovestibular dysfunction at presentation, changes in auditory acuity and/or vestibular function develop in 45% of patients as the disease progresses. Sensorineural impairment is the predominant cause of audiovestibular dysfunction.

LABORATORY AND PATHOLOGY

Routine Laboratory. Anemia is reported in over half the patients with relapsing polychondritis. An elevated erythrocyte sedimentation rate is common during an acute flare of the disease. Evidence of renal disease identified by an elevated serum creatinine or an abnormal urinalysis is present in a quarter of patients.

Serology. Serologic studies in patients with relapsing polychondritis alone are generally negative. The presence of an elevated rheumatoid factor or a positive ANA would suggest the presence of an associated autoimmune disease, such as rheumatoid arthritis or systemic lupus erythematosus. Studies of the relationship of relapsing polychondritis to ANCA are currently unavailable.

Imaging Studies. Routine radiographs of the chest have a low diagnostic yield. Abnormalities of the aortic contour may be seen in patients with aortitis and aneurysm formation. CT studies of the neck and chest are useful to characterize the tracheal and bronchial lesions *(38)*. Several patterns of involvement are seen on the CT studies. Diffuse thickening of the tracheobronchial wall with loss of the normal smooth contour is seen at sites of disease activity. Strictures are manifest by further narrowing of the lumen.

Generally, radiographs of the hands do not show evidence of erosive disease, unless the patient has concurrent rheumatoid arthritis. The radiographic abnormalities of patients with the seronegative arthritis of relapsing polychondritis include juxta-articular osteopenia followed by narrowing of the joint spaces secondary to cartilage loss.

Other Studies. Pulmonary function studies are useful to define the functional impact of the relapsing polychondritis on the tracheobronchial tree. The flow-volume loop studies are useful to identify the dynamic lesions that may develop following the destruction of the tracheobronchial rings.

Pathology. The characteristic histopathology is chondritis secondary to infiltration by lymphocytes and plasma cells. The changes on light microscopy can be summarized as a loss of basophilic staining of the cartilage matrix, perichondral inflammation, and eventual cartilage destruction with replacement by fibrous tissue. The renal biopsies show mild mesangial proliferation and segmental necrotizing glomerulonephritis with or without crescent formation. The vasculitic lesions show a pattern of panarteritis.

THERAPY AND PROGNOSIS

General Treatment. The optimal approach to the management of patients with relapsing polychondritis has not been defined. There is a wide spectrum in the pattern of disease involvement and clinical progression; consequently, the level of therapeutic intervention is dictated by the clinical course of the disease. A variety of therapeutic agents, including NSAIDs, dapsone, colchicine, glucocorticoids, azathioprine, cyclophosphamide, chlorambucil, and cyclosporin, have been tried in relapsing polychondritis with varying degrees of efficacy. In a subset of individuals, approx 25% of patients, the use of NSAID alone provides adequate suppression of the inflammation. Glucocorticoid therapy is sufficient treatment in another 25% of patients. Of note, however, progressive organ system damage can proceed despite suppression of the signs and symptoms of inflammation. Although no

firm guidelines have been established, consideration for the use of cytotoxic agents is appropriate in the following situations:

1. Progressive renal disease despite glucocorticoid therapy;
2. Progressive damage to the respiratory tree; or
3. The presence of systemic vasculitis.

Because relapsing polychondritis tends to follow a prolonged course, extended treatment with maintenance doses of glucocorticoids may be required in a significant subset of patients.

There is a well-defined disease-associated mortality. The 5-yr survival in one series was 74% *(37)*. In the presence of systemic vasculitis, the 5-yr survival rate dropped to 45%. The major reported causes of death include infection, sequelae of systemic vasculitis, respiratory failure, and renal failure.

Sinus and Midfacial Treatment Concerns. Sinus problems are not a significant management problem in relapsing polychondritis. Damage to the trachea from recurrent episodes of chondritis can produce significant long-term management problems. Both anatomic obstruction in the form of strictures and dynamic obstruction in the form of tracheomalacia may require surgical intervention. If possible, surgery should not be performed during an episode of active inflammation. Cyclosporin has been used successfully in some patients with progressive eye disease.

Cogan's Syndrome

DEFINITION

Although specific diagnostic criteria have not been established for Cogan's syndrome, the clinical syndrome is defined by a characteristic pattern of clinical and pathologic findings *(39,40)*. Cogan's syndrome is an uncommon disease characterized by an unusual noninfectious interstitial keratitis and recurrent Meniere-like episodes of audiovestibular symptoms progressing to irreversible hearing loss. A systemic form of Cogan's syndrome with disseminated vasculitis and CNS findings is recognized *(39)*.

CLINICAL OVERVIEW

Cogan's syndrome is a disease of young adults with a mean age at onset of 25 yr. Generally, the eye and audiovestibular symptoms are temporally linked at presentation. The symptoms tend to be acute in onset with a Meniere-like pattern. Associated findings seen only in a subset of patients include headache, diarrhea, arthralgia, and myalgia. Approximately 10–15% of patients will develop isolated aortitis or a systemic vasculitis of the aorta, aortic arch, and muscular arteries. The vasculitis is the principle cause of mortality in Cogan's syndrome.

SINUS AND MIDFACIAL DISEASE

Nose and Paranasal Sinuses. The nose and paranasal sinuses are not characteristically involved in Cogan's syndrome. A pattern of polychondritis has been reported in approx 2% of patients with Cogan's syndrome.

Oropharyngeal and Laryngotracheal Involvement. Except for the rare patients with associated polychondritis, these structures are not affected in Cogan's syndrome.

Eye, Ear, and Associated Structures. The characteristic interstitial keratitis is the most common manifestation of eye disease in Cogan's syndrome. Clinically, the interstitial keratitis presents with the acute onset of blurred vision, photophobia, tearing, and eye pain. On physical examination, the pupil may appear cloudy. Early on, the most frequent ocular lesion is bilateral peripheral subepithelial keratitis consisting of faint, nummular lesions (41). Later in the course of Cogan's syndrome, the pattern of interstitial keratitis changes. In patients with established disease, slit-lamp examination reveals a pattern of discrete areas of oval or round patches of inflammation that have a granular consistency and appear yellow, gray, or white in color. Generally, the posterior half to third of the cornea is most severely involved with relative sparing of the anterior portion. Corneal vascularization can be seen in the more severe cases. In the typical Cogan's syndrome, approx 5% of patients will have an associated conjunctivitis and/or iritis. However, in the so-called atypical Cogan's syndrome (39), involvement of any ocular structure can be seen. In addition to the findings seen in classical Cogan's syndrome, episcleritis, scleritis, retinal vascular disease, uveitis, papilledema, and exophthalmus have been reported. Involvement of the posterior segment of the eye is generally associated with the systemic disease pattern.

Episodes of audiovestibular dysfunction are typically acute in onset, with varying degrees of hearing impairment. Partial recovery may be seen, particularly with timely therapeutic intervention. However, progressive loss of hearing frequently develops with recurrent episodes of acute impairment. Vestibular dysfunction is characterized by acute onset of nausea, vomiting, and vertigo.

LABORATORY AND PATHOLOGY

Routine Laboratory Studies. Routine laboratory studies demonstrate a nonspecific pattern of systemic inflammation. During acute flares of the disease, leukocytosis, anemia, and an elevated erythrocyte sedimentation rate are typical. Less than a quarter of patients will have cryoglobulins.

Serology. Although the ANA is generally negative, approx 8% of patients will have a low-titer positive rheumatoid factor. The results of ANCA testing have not been reported in large series of patients with Cogan's syndrome.

Imaging Studies. Routine chest radiographs are generally negative, unless aortic disease is identified. Angiography is useful to identify the patients with systemic vasculitis.

Pathology. The interstitial keratitis is caused by an infiltration of lymphocytes and plasma cells. A similar pattern of chronic inflammation occurs in the cochlea and labyrinth. The aortitis and systemic vasculitis lesions have a mixed pattern of inflammation with polymorphonuclear leukocytes, monocytes, lymphocytes, plasma cells, and, in some cases, granuloma formation.

THERAPY AND PROGNOSIS

Topically glucocorticoids are effective in suppressing the acute flares of interstitial keratitis. Failure to use topical glucocorticoids was associated with neo-vascularization of the cornea in one patient. When the disease is limited to the anterior segment of the eye, the prognosis for normal vision is excellent.

Systemic glucocorticoid therapy (i.e., prednisone 1 mg/kg) is recommended for audiovestibular involvement (39). The need for rapid initiation of therapy has been emphasized, since the prognosis for recovery of hearing is improved when therapy is started within 2 wk of the onset of symptoms. The role for more prolonged therapy with glucocorticoids remains undefined. Later in the course of the disease, fluctuation of hearing may be secondary to cochlear hydrops rather than recurrent episodes of inflammation. The outcome for auditory acuity is quite variable. Acuity in the lower frequency range is generally more severely affected. Progression to deafness ultimately occurs in a significant number of patients. Systemic manifestations of Cogan's syndrome, particularly inflammation of the posterior segment of the eye, aortitis, and systemic vasculitis, may progress despite systemic glucocorticoid therapy. Treatment with the immunosuppressive drugs, such as cyclophosphamide or cyclosporin, appears to be effective in patients with glucocorticoid-refractory disease (40). Aortic valve replacement may be required in some patients with severe aortitis.

McCabe's Syndrome
(Autoimmune Inner Ear Disease)

DEFINITION

McCabe's syndrome or autoimmune inner ear disease is a relatively uncommon disease characterized by progressive bilateral sensorineural hearing impairment that responds to immunosuppressive therapy (42). The assumption that the syndrome is an autoimmune diathesis is based on the observation that immunosuppressive therapy is an effective form of treatment.

CLINICAL OVERVIEW

The auditory dysfunction presents in a subacute pattern and progresses over weeks to months. The process is bilateral, but may be asymmetric in the degree of hearing impairment early in the course of the disease. The decreased auditory acuity is secondary to a sensorineural impairment with localization to the cochlea. Vestibular compartment involvement is common and presents with "storms" of vertigo marked by many spells in a day. The patients also have low-grade symptoms of vertigo between the spells.

SINUS AND MIDFACIAL DISEASE

By definition, the pathology in McCabe's syndrome is limited to the cochlea, labyrinth, and adjacent structures. Facial nerve involvement has been reported in some cases of McCabe's syndrome.

LABORATORY AND PATHOLOGY

Laboratory. Routine laboratory studies are generally unremarkable. Anticochlear antibodies reacting with a 62–68 kDa inner ear antigen have been reported in approximately one-third of patients with progressive disease. Experience with imaging studies in McCabe's is limited. In a single patient, a gadolinium-enhanced MRI demonstrated increased uptake in the cochlea. Following therapy, the MRI returned to a normal pattern.

Pathology. Histopathologic studies in this disease are limited (12) and the findings can be summarized as follows:

1. Destruction of inner ear tissues, including the sense organs, supporting structures, and the membranous labyrinth;
2. Scattered infiltrates and free-floating aggregates of lymphocytes, plasma cells, and macrophages;
3. Focal or diffuse areas of fibrosis; and
4. In some, but not all cases, a pattern of endolymphatic hydrops is seen.

THERAPY AND PROGNOSIS

Dr. McCabe advocates early aggressive therapy with glucocorticoids and cyclophosphamide (42). In his experience, the use of glucocorticoids alone is ineffective with progression to deafness. The duration of therapy is determined by serial audiometry (42). Long-term remissions with stable auditory acuity following a course of immunosuppressive therapy have been reported.

Sarcoidosis

DEFINITION

Well-defined diagnostic criteria for sarcoidosis have not been established. Sarcoidosis, a systemic granulomatous disease of undetermined etiology and pathogenesis, most often involves lymph nodes, lungs, liver, spleen, skin, eyes, phalangeal bones, and parotid glands.

CLINICAL OVERVIEW

There is a wide spectrum of clinical disease expression in sarcoidosis ranging from incidental findings on a chest radiograph to progressive, potentially life-threatening disease. Constitutional symptoms, including fatigue, weakness, weight loss, anorexia, fever, and sweats, are the most common initial manifestations of the disease. The specific pattern of clinical expression varies based on organ system involvement. Cardiac, CNS, and advanced pulmonary disease mark a more severe spectrum of sarcoidosis. In contrast to other systemic autoimmune diseases, glomerular pathology is typically absent.

SINUS AND MIDFACIAL DISEASE

Sarcoidosis involves structures of the head and neck in approx 10% of cases (43,44). In the more chronic cases of sarcoidosis lasting >5 yr, the frequency of head and neck disease approaches 30% (45). In both the acute and chronic series, anterior uveitis is the most common head and neck manifestation of disease. Of note, involvement of structures of the head and neck may be the initial manifestation of disease.

Nose and Paranasal Sinuses. Involvement of these structures can be seen in 1% of patients with sarcoidosis *(43)*. Lupus pernio, a distinctive, chronic, persistent, violaceous, plaque-like skin lesion with a predilection for the nose, cheeks, and ears, is frequently associated with upper respiratory tract sarcoidosis *(46)*. Granulomatous sinusitis presents most commonly with symptoms of nasal obstruction (82%) and epistaxis (23%). Less frequent manifestations include dyspnea, nasal pain, anosmia, and epiphora. The mucosa of the nasal septum and inferior turbinates are commonly involved. Extensive granulomatous inflammation may result in drying and crusting of the mucosa as normal mucosal structures are compromised. Sarcoidosis can also be manifest as single or multiple submucosal nodules, 1–7 mm in diameter. Although unusual, sarcoidosis involving the nasal septum may produce septal perforation and collapse. On several occasions, the damage to the septum evolved after some form of surgical intervention. Rarely, the disease affects the bony structures of the nose and paranasal sinuses, producing lytic-like lesions.

Oropharyngeal and Laryngotracheal Involvement. Rarely parotid gland swelling (bilateral or unilateral) can occur in patients with sarcoidosis. Despite recurrent episodes of parotid swelling, clinically significant xerostomia is a very rare sequela. Less commonly, granulomatous inflammation of the laryngotracheal structures may produce hoarseness and very rarely may threaten airway patency. A mass effect from marked cervical lymphadenopathy may produce laryngotracheal symptoms. Very rarely, sarcoid involvement of the bone may produce lesions of the hard palate.

Eye, Ear, and Associated Structures. Involvement of the eye and associated structures is an important manifestation of sarcoidosis. Eye disease is present in 20% of patients at the time of initial evaluation, and a total of 30% will have evidence of eye involvement during the course of the disease. The most common manifestation of sarcoidosis in the eye, anterior uveitis, occurs in 70% of patients with ocular involvement. Posterior uveitis occurs in approx 25% of the patients and is manifest in descending order of frequency by

periphlebitis, vitritis, choroiditis, and choroidal nodules. With rare exception, involvement of the posterior segment is associated with anterior uveitis. Optic neuropathy is a very unusual complication of ocular sarcoidosis. Conjunctival involvement is seen in 10–15% of patients with ocular sarcoidosis. Scleral and corneal inflammation is characteristically absent. Glaucoma and less commonly retinal detachment may be late complications of ocular sarcoidosis.

Sarcoidosis may affect extraocular structures as well. Lacrimal gland involvement occurs in up to 30% of patients with ocular sarcoidosis and is generally present early in the course of the disease. Inflammatory masses in the retro-orbital space and myositis of the extraocular muscles are less common manifestations of the disease. Inflammation of the retro-orbital structures may produce diplopia and/or ptosis. Neuropathies of cranial nerves III, IV, or VI, as well as sarcoidosis of the brainstem, may produce ophthalmoplegia. Nodular lesions of the eyelids have been reported in 10% of patients with ocular sarcoidosis.

Direct involvement of the ear in sarcoidosis is rare. As previously noted, the pinna may be involved as part of lupus pernio. Nerve or brainstem involvement may produce vestibular symptoms.

LABORATORY AND PATHOLOGY

Routine Laboratory and Serology. Routine laboratory studies are nonspecific. Acute-phase reactants may be elevated in the setting of active disease. With hepatic involvement, liver function studies may be abnormal. Elevated serum and/or urinary calcium may be present in a subset of patients. The angiotensin-converting enzyme (ACE) level may be elevated as well. Unfortunately, the ACE determination lacks diagnostic specificity.

Imaging Studies. Sinus films may show evidence of acute and/or chronic sinusitis. Chest radiographs are useful to stage the pulmonary disease based on the pattern of hilar and parenchymal involvement. Gallium 67 scanning may show increased uptake in the lung if an active alveolitis is present. Uptake in both parotid and lacrimal glands can be seen as well. MRI of the retro-orbital space may help define the pattern of disease involvement in patients presenting with diplopia *(47)*.

Pathology. The characteristic histopathologic pattern of sarcoidosis is noncaseating epithelioid-cell granulomas with multinucleated giant-cell formation and an associated mononuclear cell infiltrate. This pattern is not diagnostic of sarcoidosis, and infectious agents, including mycobacteria, fungus, and parasites, should be excluded.

TREATMENT AND PROGNOSIS

General Considerations. Given the wide clinical spectrum of sarcoidosis, the level and duration of therapy are determined by the pattern of disease activity. In many patients, the pulmonary involvement runs a self-limited course, and treatment is not required. Patients with active pulmonary alveolitis, CNS, and cardiac involvement generally respond to systemic glucocorticoid therapy. A subset of patients may follow a prolonged course requiring more long-term therapy. A variety of glucocorticoid-sparing agents, including azathioprine, hydroxychloroquine, and methotrexate, have been used with reported efficacy. Although the overall prognosis in unselected patient populations with sarcoidosis is excellent *(44)*, progressive lung disease and cardiac involvement are associated with an increased risk of diseased associated mortality.

Sinus and Midfacial Treatment Concerns. The anterior uveitis is responsive to both topical and/or systemic glucocorticoid therapy with an excellent prognosis. Progression to chronic uveitis particularly with disease of the posterior segment and the development of glaucoma increases the risk of a poor visual outcome. Disease of the retro-orbital structures requires systemic glucocorticoid therapy. Both topical and systemic glucocorticoids provide symptomatic improvement of the granulomatous sinusitis. Atrophic rhinitis may be a long-term outcome of the sinus disease, however.

Systemic Lupus Erythematosus (SLE)

DEFINITION

SLE is a systemic autoimmune disease characterized by the production of antibodies to components of the cell nucleus in association with a diverse array of clinical manifestations. The classification criteria for SLE are well established. The present review will focus on the sinus and midfacial manifestation of SLE.

SINUS AND MIDFACIAL DISEASE

Nose and Paranasal Sinuses. Autoimmune-mediated sinusitis is not characteristically seen in SLE. Because of the host-defense abnormalities, chronic bacterial sinusitis may occur with increased frequency in patients with SLE. Except for the malar rash and less commonly the discoid lesion, nasal involvement with SLE is uncommon. Shallow ulcers, which are similar in appearance to the oral lesions, can appear in the nasal mucosa, particularly in the anterior portion of the nasal septum. Nasal septal perforation is very infrequent. As previously noted, relapsing polychondritis can be seen rarely in a patient with SLE.

Oropharyngeal and Laryngotracheal Involvement. The complaint of a sore throat is common in SLE. Oral ulcerations occur in approx 30% of patients during the course of SLE. The characteristic oral lesion is an erythematous papule that progresses to a small painless shallow ulcer, most commonly located on the soft or hard palate. Less commonly, the ulcer may enlarge to >1 cm and become increasingly symptomatic. Oral ulcers may herald a systemic flare of SLE. Gingival hypertrophy and gingivitis are other uncommon manifestations. Parotid gland swelling (unilateral or bilateral) is seen in 8% of SLE patients. The frequent association of Sjogren's syndrome with SLE is well recognized. Laryngotracheal involvement is less common. Rarely, inflammation and edema of the epiglottis, glottis, and/or subglottic regions may produce symptoms. Very rarely, such inflammation may necessitate acute surgical intervention to protect airway integrity. Subglottic stenosis has been reported as a long-term complication. Although uncommon, paralysis of the recurrent laryngeal nerve or cricoarytenoid arthritis may produce symptoms.

Eye, Ear, and Associated Structures. Eye disease occurs in approximately one-third of patients. Periorbital edema, lacrimal gland enlargement, and discoid lesions of the skin around the eye can occur in a subset of patients. Although the posterior segment of the eye is most frequently involved, conjunctivitis and episcleritis (both infectious and autoimmune) are present in 15% of patients. Scleritis is not a characteristic complication of SLE. Corneal involvement is also rare in SLE. Abnormal corneal staining with fluorescein is reported and partly may reflect the keratoconjunctivitis sicca seen in association with Sjogren's syndrome. Keratitis or keratopathy caused by SLE is very rare. Iritis or anterior uveitis occasionally occurs. A variety of pathologic processes may affect the posterior elements of the eye. The cytoid bodies or white patches are the most common retinal lesions in SLE. Other lesions include flame hemorrhages, retinal vasculitis, choroiditis, vaso-occlusive lesions, neo-vascularization, and vitreous hemorrhage. Retinal disease is associated with an increased incidence of both anticardiolipin antibody and CNS involvement. Although retro-orbital structures are not involved, ophthalmoplegia secondary to cranial neuropathy can occur.

Ear involvement in SLE is limited. Discoid lesions may involve the pinna of the ear. Tinnitus is a common symptomatic complaint, but is most often related to drug-associated toxicity. Reversible hearing loss presumably mediated by autoimmune mechanisms has been reported in several patients. Rarely, otitis media has been seen in SLE.

Sjogren's Syndrome

DEFINITION

Sjogren's syndrome is a chronic progressive lymphocyte-mediated autoimmune disease affecting predominately the exocrine glands. The principal clinical manifestations result from mucosal dryness. Sjogren's syndrome can present as a primary disease process or in association with other autoimmune diseases, such as rheumatoid arthritis or SLE. Autoantibodies to Ro(SS-A) and La(SS-B) are seen in the majority of patients. The present review will focus on the sinus and midfacial manifestations of Sjogren's syndrome.

SINUS AND MIDFACIAL DISEASE

Nose and Paranasal Sinuses. Nasal crusting can occur secondary to dryness of the mucosa. Chronic sinusitis secondary to compromised host-defense responses represents an additional complication.

Oropharyngeal and Laryngotracheal Involvement. Xerostomia is one of the hallmarks of Sjogren's syndrome, and is manifest by sore throat, oral burning, hoarseness or change in tonal quality, problems with mastication of dry foods, and dental caries. On examination, dry lips with cheilosis and a decrease in the saliva pool in the sublingual vestibule are frequently seen. Xerotrachea is generally manifest by a nonproductive cough. Problems with airway obstruction are not seen. Parotid or submental gland swelling is seen in 50% of patients.

Eye, Ear, and Associated Structures. The keratoconjunctivitis sicca from the decreased tear film is clinically manifest by a sandy/scratchy sensation under the lid. The decreased tear film leads to damage of both corneal and bulbar conjunctival epithelium. Damage to the cornea can be demonstrated by Rose Bengal staining. Except for optic neuritis, which is frequently associated with CNS manifestations of Sjogren's syndrome, other structures of the eye are not involved. With the exception of lacrimal gland swelling, retro-orbital structures are not affected.

Vogt-Koyanagi-Harada Syndrome

The Vogt-Koyanagi-Harada syndrome (uveo-meningoencephalitis syndrome) is a rare clinical entity that classically presents in distinct phases *(48)*. The initial manifestation is an acute onset meningoencephalitic prodrome with headache, nausea, vomiting, and meningeal signs. Neurologic dysfunction follows, resulting in papilledema, cranial neuropathies, nystagmus, hemiparesis, and mental status changes. Although the neurologic symptoms may fluctuate during this initial phase of the disease, permanent sequelae are uncommon. A severe, protracted bilateral granulomatous uveitis involving both the anterior and posterior segments of the eye develops during or following the meningeal phase. An associated hearing loss and/or tinnitus commonly is present. Morbidity from the granulomatous uveitis can occur, including retinal detachment, glaucoma, and cataracts. After 3 mo or more, patients may enter a final phase characterized by symmetric pigment loss involving the face, eyebrows, and eyelashes along with circumscribed alopecia.

Idiopathic Midline Destructive Disease (IMDD)

DEFINITION

IMDD (idiopathic midline granuloma) is a rare clinical syndrome marked by a localized relentlessly progressive destructive disease of the upper respiratory tract *(49,50)*. Other causes of the midline granuloma syndrome (Table 4) must be excluded before the diagnosis of IMDD can be established. In a review of 11 patients, the following clinicopathologic features were identified:

1. Presence of locally destructive lesions always restricted to the upper respiratory tract;
2. Absence of a systemic disease during a follow-up period;
3. Biopsies that show a pattern of acute and chronic inflammation with variable amounts of necrosis in the absence of atypical or neoplastic cells; and
4. Inability to demonstrate an infectious etiology *(50).*

Table 4
Diseases that May Present
with the "Midline Granuloma" Syndrome

Bacterial
   Actinomycosis
   Brucellosis
   Klebsiella rhinoscleromatis
   Leprosy
   Tuberculosis
   Syphilis
   Yaws
Fungal
   Blastomycosis
   Candida
   Coccidiomycosis
   Histoplasmosis
   Rhinosporidiosis
   Phycomycosis
Parasitic
   Leishmaniasis
   Myiasis
Inflammatory/autoimmune
   IMDD
   Wegener's granulomatosis
Neoplastic
   Carcinoma
   Sarcoma
   Conventional lymphoma
   Angiocentric lymphoma
   Lymphomatoid granulomatosis

CLINICAL OVERVIEW

By definition, manifestations of a systemic disease process are absent. In particular, direct involvement of the eye, CNS, lower respiratory tract, and kidneys is absent.

SINUS AND MIDFACIAL DISEASE

The initial presentation of IMDD is a pattern of pan-sinusitis with progression to destructive lesions of the nasal septum, hard, and soft palate.

Nose and Paranasal Sinuses. In the setting of chronic pan-sinusitis, ulcerative lesions of the nasal septum develop. The ulcers are nonhealing, and slowly progress with destruction of both the cartilaginous and bony nasal septum. In some patients, the inflammatory process will erode into the paranasal sinuses. Secondary infections are common. Breakdown of the skin on the face occurs in a third of patients.

Oropharyngeal and Laryngotracheal Involvement. The ulcerative, destructive lesions of IMDD

may involve both the hard and soft palate. The lesions may progress, producing holes in the affected structures. Tracheal involvement is reported in 10% of patients.

Eye, Ear, and Associated Structures. Direct involvement of the eye is not seen. The eye may be secondarily involved as the inflammatory process erodes in the bony orbit. Extension into the orbit was reported in 30% of patients. Extension into the ear is rare. Symptoms of otitis media secondary to Eustachian tube damage can occur.

LABORATORY AND PATHOLOGY

In the absence of a secondary infection, routine laboratory studies are negative. Serologic studies are also characteristically negative, although the results of ANCA serologies have not been reported in IMDD. Imaging studies, including sinus series and CT studies, are useful to document the site and extent of sinusitis and bony involvement.

The histopathologic pattern seen in IMDD is acute and chronic inflammation with varying degrees of necrosis. Granulocytes, lymphocytes, histiocytes, monocytes, and plasma cells can be seen. Eosinophils are sparse, if present at all. Although inflammatory cell infiltration of the outer portion arterioles was identified in almost half of the patients, a pattern of fibrinoid necrosis, hyalinization of the vascular wall, thrombosis, or granulomatous vasculitis was not seen. Granuloma formation and giant cells are identified in <25% of patients. Malignant and atypical cells are characteristically absent. As previously noted, infectious agents should be excluded by appropriate cultures and special stains.

TREATMENT AND PROGNOSIS

A variety of therapies have been tried without success in IMDD, including glucocorticoids, cytotoxic agents, and low-dose irradiation protocols. High-dose irradiation therapy (tissue dose of 4000–5000 rad in daily fractions of 200 rad) is reported to be effective in arresting the progressive tissue destruction in IMDD *(49,50)*. Morbidity from therapy, including death from irradiation-induced necrosis of the brainstem and secondary neoplasms, is significant.

APPROACH TO THE DIFFERENTIAL DIAGNOSIS

Given the clinical diversity of the autoimmune diseases that may affect the sinus and midfacial

Table 5
Pattern of Direct Eye Involvement

Disease	Conjunct/episcler	Scleritis	Cornea	Anterior uveitis	Posterior uveitis	Retinal vessels	Optic nerve	Retro-orbital Lacrimal	Other	Ophthalmoplegia	Visual loss
WG	++	+++	+	++	++	++	++	++	+++	++	++
CSS	+	–	–	–	–	±	+	–	–	±	–
Behçet's	+	+	±	+++	++	++	++	–	–	±	+++
RPC	±	±	±	±	±	–	–	–	–	–	–
Cogan's	±	–	+++[a]	±	–	–	–	–	–	–	–
McCabe's	–	–	–	–	–	–	–	–	–	–	–
Sarcoid	–	–	–	+++	++	–	±	++	+	++	–
SLE	+	+	±	+	++	++	+	+	–	+	+
Sjogren's	++	–	sicca	–	–	–	+	++	–	–	–
VKH	–	–	–	+++[b]	+++[b]	–	–	–	–	–	–
IMDD	–	–	–	–	–	–	–	(Indirect)		–	++

Abbreviations: WG, Wegener's granulomatosis; CSS, Churg–Strauss syndrome; RPC, relapsing polychondritis; SLE, systemic lupus erythematosus; VKH, Vogt–Koyanagi–Harada syndrome; IMDD, idiopathic midline destructive disease.
[a]Interstial keratitis.
[b]Granulomatous inflammation.

structures, no single approach to the differential diagnosis of these syndromes is feasible. It should be emphasized that the initial symptoms of these autoimmune diseases may be indistinguishable from other more common clinical syndromes that affect the oropharynx and sinuses. With the exception of McCabe's syndrome and IMDD, the autoimmune diseases affecting the sinuses and midfacial structures are systemic syndromes; consequently, the pattern of disease activity at other sites is useful in narrowing the differential diagnosis. A detailed history and physical examination looking for disease activity of the eyes, central and/or peripheral nervous system, lymph nodes, lungs, or kidneys may direct subsequent diagnostic studies.

The presence of a malar or discoid rash would suggest the diagnosis of SLE. Although rare, the nodular or plaque-like lesions of the lupus pernio rash are suggestive of sarcoidosis. Swelling of the cartilaginous portion of the nose or the pinna suggests the diagnosis of relapsing polychondritis. With the exception of the submucosal nodular lesions seen in sarcoidosis, the pattern of nasal mucosal involvement is nondiagnostic. Perforation of the cartilaginous portion of the nasal septum can be seen in Wegener's granulomatosis, relapsing polychondritis, IMDD, sarcoidosis, and rarely the Churg-Strauss syndrome. Except for IMDD and other diseases of the midline granuloma syndrome, perforating lesions of the hard or soft palate are exceedingly rare. Although there is considerable overlap,

the pattern of eye involvement may prove useful in the differential diagnosis (Table 5). A detailed ophthalmologic evaluation will help define the precise pattern of disease involvement. With the exception of the lacrimal glands, disease of retro-orbital structures is unusual, except in Wegener's granulomatosis and sarcoidosis.

Although routine laboratory studies may demonstrate a pattern consistent with systemic inflammation, the pattern lacks diagnostic specificity. An active urinary sediment with RBC casts reflecting a glomerular lesion may be seen in Wegener's granulomatosis, Churg-Strauss syndrome, Behçet's syndrome, relapsing polychondritis, or SLE. Serologic studies including ANCA and ANA may provide important diagnostic information in the appropriate clinical setting. The PR3-specific ANCA has high sensitivity and specificity for active systemic Wegener's granulomatosis. The myeloperoxidase-specific ANCA can be seen in the Churg-Strauss syndrome and less commonly in Wegener's granulomatosis, as well as other diseases. The diagnostic utility of the ANA in the setting of SLE and associated syndromes is well defined.

In selected clinical settings, imaging studies will provide clinically useful information. The pattern of acute and/or chronic sinusitis seen on routine sinus films lacks diagnostic specificity. CT studies of the sinuses are useful to identify involvement of bony structures. Perforation of the bones of the maxillary sinuses is seen rarely in Wegener's granulomatosis. Sarcoidosis involvement of the facial bones can be seen as well. Bony involvement of the hard palate suggests the diagnosis of IMDD or one of the other diseases of the midline granuloma syndrome. Retro-orbital disease identified on CT or MRI would suggest the diagnosis of Wegener's granulomatosis or sarcoidosis. Chest radiographs may provide useful diagnostic information in patients with Wegener's granulomatosis, Churg-Strauss syndrome, and sarcoidosis.

Biopsies of sinus and midfacial structures may also provide important diagnostic information. A histopathologic pattern of acute and chronic inflammation lacks diagnostic specificity. Granulomas or giant cells may be seen in sinus biopsies in patients with Wegener's granulomatosis, Churg-Strauss syndrome, sarcoidosis, and less commonly IMDD. The failure to find granulomas or giant cells, however, does not exclude these syndromes. In the setting of destructive midfacial lesions, appropriate studies to exclude neoplastic and infectious etiologies should be performed on the biopsy specimens. In some clinical settings, biopsies from sites of disease activity other than midfacial structures may be more productive in establishing a definitive diagnosis.

ACKNOWLEDGMENTS

The expert review of the manuscript by Dana Ascherman, Witold Turkiewicz, and Ethan Gamound is greatly appreciated.

REFERENCES

1. Guillevin L, Amouroux J, Arbeille B, Boura R. Arguments favoring the responsibility of inhaled antigens. Chest 1991;100:1472,1473.
2. Jennette JC, Ewert BH, Falk RJ. Do antineutrophil cytoplasmic autoantibodies cause Wegener's granulomatosis and other forms of necrotizing vasculitis? Rheum Dis Clin North Am 1993;19:1–14.
3. Hagen EC, Ballieux EPB, van Es LA, Daha MR, van der Woude FJ. Antineutrophil cytoplasmic autoantibodies: a review of the antigens involved, the assays, and the clinical and possible pathogenetic consequences. Blood 1993;81:1996–2002.
4. Mayet WJ, Csernok E, Szymkowiak C, Gross WL, zum Büschenfelde KHM. Human endothelial cells express Proteinase 3, the target antigen of anticytoplasmic antibodies in Wegener's granulomatosis. Blood 1993; 82:1221–1229.
5. Noronha IL, Krüger C, Andrassy K, Ritz E, Waldherr R. In situ production of TNF-alpha, IL-1Beta and IL-2R in ANCA-positive glomerulonephritis. Kidney Intern 1993; 43:682–692.
6. Leavitt RY, Fauci AS, Bloch DA, et al. The American College of Rheumatology 1990 Criteria for the classification of Wegener's granulomatosis. Arthritis Rheum 1990;33:1101–1107.
7. Jennette JC, Falk RJ, Andrassy K, et al. Nomenclature of systemic vasculitides, proposal of an international consensus conference. Arthritis Rheum 1994;37:187–192.
8. Hoffman GS, Kerr GS, Leavitt RY, et al. Wegener granulomatosis: an analysis of 158 patients. Ann Intern Med 1992;116:488–498.
9. Nölle B, Specks U, Lüdemann J, Rohrbach MS, DeRemee RA, Gross WL. Anticytoplasmic autoantibodies: their immunodiagnostic value in Wegener granulomatosis. Ann Intern Med 1989;111:28–40.
10. Stegeman CA, Tervaert JWC, Sluiter WJ, Manson WL, de Jong PE, Kallenburg CGM. Association of chronic nasal carriage of *Staphylococcus aureus* and higher relapse rates in Wegener granulomatosis. Ann Intern Med 1994;120:12–17.
11. Haynes BF, Fishman ML, Fauci AS, Wolff SM. The ocular manifestations of Wegener's granulomatosis. Am J Med 1977;63:131–140.
12. Schuknecht HF. Ear pathology in autoimmune disease. Adv Otorhinolaryngol 1991;46:50–70.
13. Clements MR, Mistry CD, Keith AO, Ramsden RT. Recovery from sensorineural deafness in Wegener's granulomatosis. J Laryngol Otol 1989;103:515–518.
14. Travis WD, Hoffman GS, Leavitt RY, Pass HI, Fauci AS. Surgical pathology of the lung in Wegener's granulomatosis. Am J Surg Pathol 1991;15:315–333.
15. Devaney KO, Travis WD, Hoffman G, Leavitt R, Lebovics R, Fauci AS. Interpretation of head and neck biopsies in Wegener's granulomatosis: a pathologic study of 126 biopsies in 70 patients. Am J Surg Pathol 1990; 14:555–564.
16. Hoffman GS, Leavitt RY, Fleischer TA, Minor JR, Fauci AS. Treatment of Wegener's granulomatosis with intermittent high-dose intravenous cyclophosphamide. Am J Med 1990;89:403–410.
17. Hoffman GS, Leavitt RY, Kerr GS, Fauci AS. The treatment of Wegener's granulomatosis with glucocorticoids and methotrexate. Arthritis Rheum 1992;35:1322–1329.
18. Masi AT, Hunder GG, Lie JT, et al. The American College of Rheumatology 1990 Criteria for the classification of Churg-Strauss syndrome (allergic granulomatosis and angiitis). Arthritis Rheum 1990;33:1094–1100.
19. Churg J, Strauss L. Allergic granulomatosis, allergic angiitis, and periarteritis nodosa. Am J Pathol 1951; 27:277–301.
20. Chumbley LC, Harrison EG Jr, DeRemee RA. Allergic granulomatosis and angiitis (Churg-Strauss Syndrome): report and analysis of 30 cases. Mayo Clin Proc 1977; 52:477–484.
21. Lanham JG, Elkon KB, Pusey CD, Hughes GR. Systemic vasculitis with asthma and eosinophilia: a clinical approach to the Churg-Strauss syndrome. Medicine 1984;63:65–81.
22. Lie JT and members and consultants of the American College of Rheumatology subcommittee on classification of vasculitis. Illustrated histopathologic classification criteria for selected vasculitis syndromes. Arthritis Rheum 1990;33:1074–1087.

23. Tervaert JWC, Limburg PC, Elema JD, et al. Detection of autoantibodies against myeloid lysosomal enzymes: a useful adjunct to classification of patients with biopsy-proven necrotizing arteritis. Am J Med 1991;91:59–66.

24. Tervaert JWC, Goldschmeding R, Elema JD, et al. Association of autoantibodies to myeloperoxidase with different forms of vasculitis. Arthritis Rheum 1990; 33:1264–1272.

25. The International Study Group for Behçet's Disease. Evaluation of diagnostic (classification) criteria in Behçet's disease—towards internationally agreed criteria. Br J Rheum 1992;31:299–308.

26. O'Neill TW, Rigby AS, Silman AJ, Barnes C. Validation of the international study group criteria for Behçet's disease. Br J Rheum 1994;33:115–117.

27. O'Duffy JD. Vasculitis in Behçet's disease. Rheum Dis Clin North Am 1990;16:423–431.

28. O'Duffy JD, Carney JA, Deodhar S. Behçet's disease: report of 10 cases, 3 with new manifestations. Ann Intern Med 1971;75:561–570.

29. Chajek T, Fainaru M. Behçet's disease. Report of 41 cases and a review of the literature. Medicine 1975;54:179–196.

30. Shimizu T, Ehrlich GE, Inaba G, Hayashi K. Behçet disease (Behçet syndrome). Semin Arthritis Rheum 1979;8: 223–260.

31. Yazici H, Pazarli H, Barnes CG, et al. A controlled trial of azathioprine in Behçet's syndrome. N Engl J Med 1990;322:281–285.

32. Firestein GS, Gruber HE, Weisman MH, Zvaifler NJ, Barger J, O'Duffy JD. Mouth and genital ulcers with inflamed cartilage: MAGIC Syndrome, five patients with features of relapsing polychondritis and Behçet's disease. Am J Med 1985;79:65–72.

33. Main DMG, Chamberlain MA. Clinical practice: clinical differentiation of oral ulceration in Behçet's disease. Br J Rheum 1992;31:767–770.

34. Nussenblatt RB, Palestine AG, Chan C, Mochizuki M, Yancey K. Effectiveness of cyclosporin therapy for Behçet's disease. Arthritis Rheum 1985;28:671–679.

35. O'Duffy JD, Robertson DM, Goldstein NP. Chlorambucil in the treatment of uveitis and meningoencephalitis of Behçet's disease. Am J Med 1984;76:75–84.

36. McAdam LP, O'Hanlan MA, Bluestone R, Pearson CM. Relapsing polychondritis: prospective study of 23 patients and a review of the literature. Medicine 1976; 55:193–215.

37. Michet CJ Jr, McKenna CH, Luthra HS, O'Fallon WM. Relapsing polychondritis: survival and predictive role of early disease manifestations. Ann Intern Med 1986; 104:74–78.

38. Booth A, Dieppe PA, Goddard PL, Watt I. The radiological manifestations of relapsing polychondritis. Clin Radiol 1989;40:147–149.

39. Haynes BF, Kaiser-Kupfer MI, Mason P, Fauci AS. Cogan syndrome: studies in 13 patients, long-term follow-up, and a review of the literature. Medicine 1980; 59:426–441.

40. Allen NB, Cox CC, Cobo M, et al. Use of immunosuppressive agents in the treatment of severe ocular manifestations of Cogan's syndrome. Am J Med 1990;88: 296–301.

41. Cobo LM, Haynes BF. Early corneal findings in Cogan's syndrome. Ophthalmology 1984;91:903–907.

42. McCabe BF. Autoimmune inner ear disease: therapy. Am J Otol 1989;10:196,197.

43. McCaffrey TV, McDonald TJ. Sarcoidosis of the nose and paranasal sinuses. Laryngoscope 1983;93:1281–1284.

44. Reich JM, Johnson RE. Course and prognosis of sarcoidosis in a nonreferral setting. Am J Med 1985; 78:61–67.

45. Jabs DA, Johns CJ. Ocular involvement in chronic sarcoidosis. Am J Ophthal 1986;102:297–301.

46. Neville E, Mills RGS, Jash DK, MacKinnon DM, Carstairs LS, James DG. Sarcoidosis of the upper respiratory tract and its association with lupus pernio. Thorax 1976;31:660–664.

47. Hoogland YT, Kattah JC, Cupps T. Ophthalmoplegia: differential diagnostic considerations in sarcoidosis. J Rheum 1993;20:1262,1263.

48. Ellner JJ, Bennett JE. Chronic meningitis. Medicine 1976;55:341–369.

49. Fauci AS, Johnson RE, Wolff SM. Radiation therapy of midline granuloma. Ann Intern Med 1976;84: 140–147.

50. Tsokos M, Fauci AS, Costa J. Idiopathic midline destructive disease (IMDD), a subgroup of patients with the "midline granuloma" syndrome. Am J Clin Pathol 1982;77:162–168.

21 Rhinopathic Headaches

Referred Pain of Nasal and Sinus Origin

Dean M. Clerico, MD

CONTENTS

INTRODUCTION

Headache is universal in the human experience. Despite the familiarity most of us have with the symptom, the cause of most headaches remains a mystery. Much of modern research has focused on headache mechanisms (such as spreading cerebral electrical depression, serotonin receptor properties, and vasodilatory mechanisms) rather than headache causation. Pain referred from the sinonasal tract is one preventable cause of headache. The anatomical basis for the relationship between headache and the sinonasal tract is the trigeminal nerve (CN V). The fifth cranial nerve not only provides sensory fibers to the nasal cavity and paranasal sinuses, but innervates pain-sensitive structures in the cranial cavity, such as dura and intracranial blood vessels, thus providing the basis for referred headache. The headache and facial pain that accompany acute sinusitis are fairly well recognized, chiefly owing to the obvious nasal symptoms, such as purulent rhinorrhea, nasal congestion and obstruction, post-nasal drip, and cough. The concept of headache referred from the sinonasal cavity with-

out overt nasal symptoms or gross mucosal disease is rapidly gaining acceptance, largely owing to the enhanced diagnostic capabilities afforded by rigid nasal endoscopy and coronal computed tomography (CT). This chapter will focus on headache as a symptom of various sinonasal pathophysiologic processes, which may or may not be accompanied by nasal symptoms or inflammatory sinus disease. The term "primary headache" will be used in this chapter to denote the vascular- or tension-type headaches (migraine, cluster, chronic daily headache, tension headache, and so on) traditionally thought to be unrelated to any underlying organic pathology.

NEURORHINOLOGY

The nasal cavity is richly innervated by a variety of neural inputs, including special sensory (olfaction associated with cranial nerve 1), general sensory (via the ophthalmic [V1] and maxillary [V2] divisions of the trigeminal nerve), autonomic sympathetic (via the cervical sympathetic chain), and parasympathetic (from the superior salivatory nucleus in the midbrain), as well as the largely unknown functions of the nervus terminalis and vomeronasal organ.

From: *Diseases of the Sinuses* (M. E. Gershwin and G. A. Incaudo, eds.),
©1996 Humana Press Inc., Totowa, NJ.

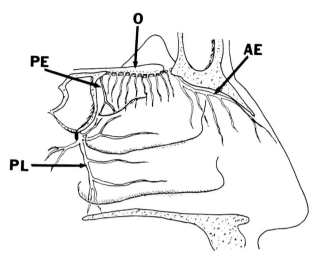

Fig. 1. Innervation of the lateral nasal wall seen in sagittal view. AE, anterior ethmoidal nerve; O, olfactory bulb; PE, posterior ethmoidal nerve; PL, posterolateral branch of V2.

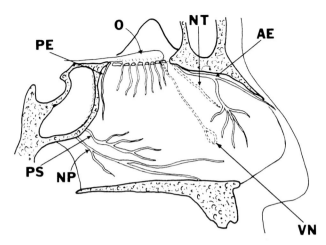

Fig. 2. Innervation of the nasal septum in the sagittal view. AE, anterior ethmoidal nerve; NT, nervus terminalis; O, olfactory bulb; PE, posterior ethmoidal nerve; PS, posterosuperior medial nasal nerve; NP, nasopalatine nerve; VN, vomeronasal nerve and organ.

Gross Anatomy

The trigeminal nerve houses sensory ganglionic cell bodies in the semilunar (or Gasserian) ganglion, located within the middle cranial fossa. The nerve trifurcates upon emerging from this ganglion; the ophthalmic and maxillary divisions supply the nasal cavity while the mandibular division supplies the oral cavity and will not be discussed further. The ophthalmic division traverses the cavernous sinus and enters the posterior orbit through the superior orbital fissure, thereafter giving rise to the nasociliary nerve. The nasociliary nerve then subdivides into posterior and anterior ethmoid branches. Along with their respective arteries, the anterior and posterior ethmoid nerves emerge from within the orbit to cross the skull base and roof of the ethmoid sinus from lateral to medial, then enter the cribriform plate. The anterior ethmoid nerve divides into internal and external branches, the internal branch supplying the anterosuperior aspect of the lateral nasal wall and septum while the external branch supplies the skin over the dorsum of the nose. The posterior ethmoid nerve innervates the posterosuperior regions of the lateral nasal wall and septum (Figs. 1 and 2).

The maxillary division exits the cranial cavity through the foramen rotundum, traverses the pterygopalatine (or sphenopalatine) fossa, and runs along the roof of the maxillary sinus within the infraorbital canal to terminate as the infraorbital nerve (supplying sensation to the middle third of

the face). Branches of V2 (the major one being the nasopalatine nerve) divide within the pterygopalatine fossa, emerge from the sphenopalatine foramen, and supply the posteroinferior regions of the nasal cavity (Figs. 1 and 2).

Trigeminal Physiology and Microanatomy

The mucosa of the sinonasal tract contains a rich network of sensory nerve endings carrying various neuropeptides such as substance P (SP), calcitonin gene related peptide (CGRP), and neurokinin A. The sensory nerves and their terminals, which provide information about noxious stimuli, are generally termed nociceptors. The majority of sensory fibers in the nasal cavity are so-called C-fiber polymodal nociceptive afferents, indicating that they are small unmyelinated fibers that respond to a variety of noxious stimuli (mechanical, thermal, inflammatory, and chemical irritant stimuli). Cutaneous polymodal nociceptive afferents display several properties which may eventually be demonstrated in nasal models, such as sensitization (lowered thresholds for stimulation) after repeated applications of low-intensity stimuli *(1)*. The sensitivity of nociceptors increases following mild injury *(2)*, analogous to the increased sensitivity of skin after sunburn. A condition known as hyperalgesia results, in which a stimulus of lower-than-normal intensity elicits pain.

Sensory nerve endings traverse the basement membrane and extend into the epithelium, some of

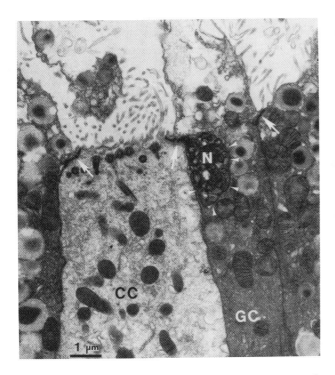

Fig. 3. Electron micrograph showing the closest approach of a free trigeminal nerve ending to the surface of the nasal mucosa of a rat. The nerve process (N) shown lies between a goblet cell (GC) and a ciliated cell (CC), just below the level of the tight junctions (arrows). The plasma membrane of the nerve terminal is outlined by the arrowheads. (Reprinted from ref. *2a*. Courtesy of Marcel Dekker, Inc.)

which extend to within just a few microns of the epithelial surface. These free nerve endings are situated just below intercellular tight junctions (Fig. 3). Activation of these terminals by chemical stimuli may result from direct contact of the chemical with the nerve after diffusion through mucus and lipid barriers or indirectly through inflammatory mediators like bradykinin, which is released as a consequence of epithelial cell damage. A mechanical pressure stimulus may initiate a nerve stimulus directly via contact of the stimulus to the nerve ending, or indirectly as a result of mediators released during localized trauma and cell damage.

Polymodal nociceptors, such as those found in the sinonasal cavity, can be activated by a variety of mechanical, chemical, inflammatory, and thermal stimuli. These nociceptors have small-diameter unmyelinated C fibers which are slow-conducting nerves (in the order of 0.5–2 m/s). A noxious stimulus activates the nociceptor by depolarizing the membrane of the sensory ending. Mucosal contact points may represent areas of localized tissue dam-age, and hyperalgesia may result as the area or duration of mucosal contact increases. Hyperalgesia can occur both at the site of tissue damage and in the surrounding undamaged areas (Fig. 4).

Animal studies have shed considerable light on the properties of the two main nasal sensory nerves: the ethmoidal and nasopalatine nerves. Ethmoidal nerve afferents can be divided into two classes *(3)*: low threshold mechanoreceptors (LTM) responsive to light tactile input but unresponsive to noxious chemical or mechanical stimuli, and wide dynamic range (WDR) neurons responsive to both noxious and nonnoxious chemical or mechanical stimuli applied to the nasal cavity. Ethmoidal afferents project mainly to subnuclei interpolaris and caudalis of the spinal trigeminal nucleus (sp. V) *(4)*. The caudalis nucleus, which receives the bulk of ethmoidal nerve projections, contains a higher percentage of WDR neurons. These brain stem neurons also receive input from a number of other oral-facial regions *(3)*, providing a neuroanatomical basis for referred pain and headache of nasal and sinus origin (discussed below).

All airway epithelia contain enzymes such as neutral endopeptidase (NEP), which degrades sensory neuropeptides such as SP. NEP is found in the epithelial cells and submucosal glands. One possible mechanism of hyperalgesia is the decreased production of NEP from epithelial cells, such as may occur from the mild trauma caused by mucosa-to-mucosa contact, or as a result of inflammatory changes within the nasal epithelium. NEP represents one possible peripheral nonneurologic mechanism by which the response of the nasal epithelium to noxious stimuli may be modified, with subsequent modulation of referred pain.

The effects of SP can be blocked with topical application of capsaicin, the pungent extract of red pepper. Initial application of capsaicin causes SP release with associated irritative symptoms, but repeated application depletes SP stores in sensory terminals and leads to the selective destruction of C-fiber afferents. Intranasal application of capsaicin evokes an immediate burning pain in the ipsilateral nasal, ocular, and temporal areas, as well as lacrimation and rhinorrhea *(5)*. Repeated applications of capsaicin in the nasal cavity have been found helpful in patients with cluster headaches (*see* section on Literature Review later in chapter).

A dense network of SP-containing nerve endings exists around the parasympathetic neurons of

A

B

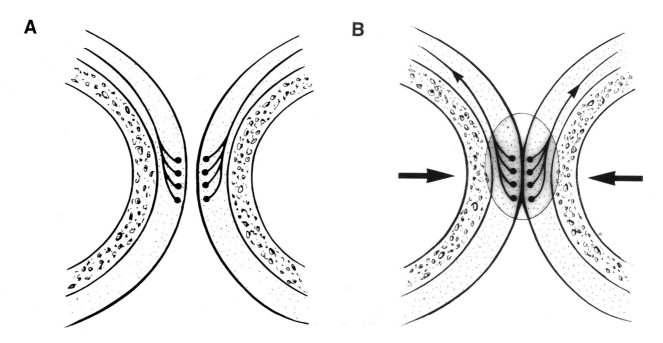

Fig. 4. Schematic demonstrating the phenomenon of mucosal contact causing a pain reflex with hyperalgesia. **(A)** depicts two mucosa-covered structures with intact sensory supply in close approximation but not contacting each other. **(B)** demonstrates that with mucosal contact, such as by the continued pneumatization of a concha bullosa or the continued growth of a septal spur (arrows), sensory stimulation results in the transmission of an electrical signal back to the CNS (arrow heads), as well as the release of neuropeptides (such as SP) at the site of stimulation and the surrounding mucosa (shaded area). This local release of SP excites other free nerve endings and induces inflammatory changes in the mucosa.

the sphenopalatine ganglion *(6)*. Sensory stimulation in the nasal cavity may therefore initiate such autonomic symptoms as rhinorrhea, nasal congestion, and lacrimation; these parasympathetic symptoms are prominent components of the cluster headache syndrome.

The trigeminally-derived sensory innervation of the nose was once thought to represent a so-called "common chemical sense" distinct from the special chemical sense of olfaction. Nasal trigeminal chemoreceptors, usually associated with painful or irritating chemical stimuli, are now thought to be simply a class of pain receptors (i.e., polymodal nociceptors containing SP) rather than a separate chemical sense *(7)*.

Referred Pain

The phenomenom of referred pain is well known in other parts of the body, such as the radiating left arm and shoulder pain that can accompany myocardial infarction. Two mechanisms have been proposed to account for referred pain. One is the convergence theory. According to this hypothesis, afferent fibers from nociceptors in the viscera (in

this case, the sinonasal tract) and afferents from specific areas of the periphery (such as the scalp, dura, or cranial vessels) converge on the same projection neurons in the trigeminal nucleus. The thalamus receives input from the trigeminal nucleus, and relays information to the cortex. These higher cortical centers do not distinguish the actual source of the noxious stimulus and mistakenly identify the sensation with the more peripheral structure. The variable nature of pain responses suggests the possible existence of modulatory systems within the central nervous system (CNS) that regulate pain. The gate control theory proposed by Melzack and Wall in 1965 *(8)* states that central messages reflecting an individual's attentional, cognitive, and emotional state descend from the brain through the brain stem and spinal cord to influence nociceptive impulses coming from the periphery, either inhibiting or facilitating this sensory input.

The other theory of referred pain involves an axon reflex (Fig. 5). An axon reflex involves both an affecter and effector function. In addition to serving as affectors mediating sensation and nociception, the intraepithelial sensory neurons also

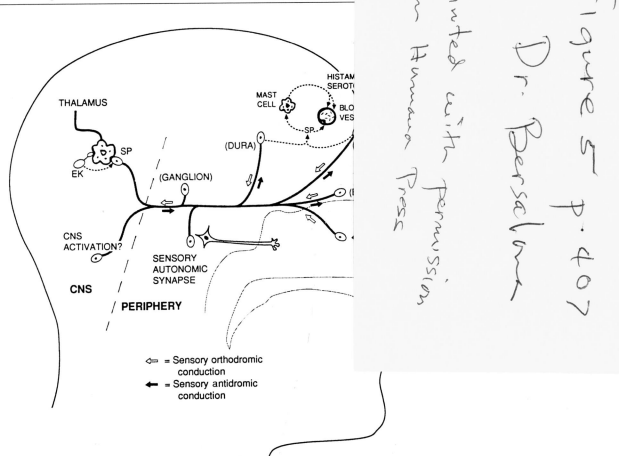

Fig. 5. Diagram depicting how an intranasal irritant stimulus (mechanical, thermal, chemical, or inflammatory) can induce referred reflex pain in other areas in the distribution of the trigeminal nervous system, as well as autonomic phenomena. The intranasal stimulus initiates an orthodromic sensory impulse back to the CNS. However, the signal may also get rerouted along other branches of the stimulated nerve (antidromic conduction). These branches innervate pain-sensitive structures such as the dura, eye, and skin of the scalp. The release of substance P (SP) as a result of antidromic conduction at these other peripheral terminals leads to inflammatory events pictured. Since SP-immunoreactive nerves have been found in high concentration around the sphenopalatine ganglion, reflex parasympathetic stimulation may also ensue. The CNS probably modulates incoming impulses through a variety of mechanisms, including the influence of enkephalins (EK). (Reprinted with permission from ref. *8a*.)

serve an effector function. Stimulation of these neurons causes the release of their neuropeptides, such as SP and CGRP, from four categorically different sites *(9)*: the site of stimulation, terminals more peripheral than the area of stimulation, collateral terminals, and central terminals. The affector limb of this reflex occurs when various stimuli (mechanical, chemical, inflammatory, or thermal) initiate an orthodromic impulse along afferent C fibers, resulting in the release of SP in the CNS. This intracranial release of SP, which is a potent vasodilator and inflammatory mediator, may account for the phenomena directly involved in headache causation (such as spreading electrical depression, intracranial vasodilation, and so on).

The nociceptive stimulus can also initiate an antidromic (away from the CNS) impulse, conducting electrical messages to nerve endings peripheral or collateral to the area stimulated. The effector limb of the reflex occurs with the release of neuropeptide mediators at these peripheral or collateral terminals *(10)*, which consist of trigeminal nerve endings innervating other cephalic structures. After their release, these neuropeptides can exert a wide variety of effects collectively referred to as "neurogenic inflammation." These effects include vasodilation, increasing venular permeability and plasma extravasation, promoting histamine release from mast cells, and others. Therefore, the mechanisms exist whereby mechanical stimulation in the nose

Table 1
Summary of Wolff's Intranasal Stimulation Studies on Human Volunteers[a]

Site stimulated	Pain intensity	Pain quality	Pain distribution
Nasopharynx	1+ to 2+	Aching	Throat
Septum	1+ to 2+	—	Local
Middle part			Zygoma, preauricular
Ethmoid part			Outer, inner canthus
Inferior turbinate	4+ to 6+	Dull, aching	
Anterior			Upper teeth
Middle			Under eye, zygoma, ear
Posterior			Same as above
Middle turbinate	4+ to 6+	—	Zygoma, ear, temple
Superior turbinate		—	Medial canthus, forehead, lateral nose
Natural maxillary os	6+ to 9+	Sharp, burning	Local, nasopharynx, molars, zygoma, temple
Nasofrontal duct	5+ to 7+	—	Medial canthus, under eye, zygoma, temple
Frontal sinus	1/2+	—	Forehead
Ethmoid sinus	5+ to 6+	—	
Anterior			Over eye, medial canthus, upper jaw, deep in eye
Posterior		Aching	Upper teeth, lateral canthus, lateral nose
Sphenoid sinus			
Anterior wall	5+ to 6+	—	"Deep in head," over eye, upper teeth
Interior	1+ to 2+		Vertex of skull
Maxillary sinus	Mild	—	
Roof			Eye
Lower lateral wall			Jaw, molars

[a]Adapted with permission from ref. 12a.

(such as by mucosal contact) triggers an axon reflex resulting in inflammatory events elsewhere in the distribution of the trigeminal nerve (such as the dura, intracranial vasculature, the eye, and so on), and causing the sensation of pain perceived as coming from these other structures. These structures are either more pain sensitive than the nasal cavity or central mechanisms result in misinterpreting the neural input. Referred pain results. Thus headache may represent, in many cases, a "nasocranial reflex" analogous to other nasal reflexes with systemic responses (11,12).

Wolff's Experiments

Despite a rather rich neural supply, the nose has a limited ability to localize mechanical and other noxious stimuli, as demonstrated by Wolff's studies. Harold Wolff, in his classic experiments performed in the 1940s, determined patterns of referred pain from stimulation of various points in the nasal cavity. He studied both pain distribution and intensity referred from stimulating nasal and sinus structures with a blunt probe, faradic electric current, and epinephrine-soaked cotton pledgets (see Table 1). Wolff performed these studies on volunteers consisting of five normal subjects, ten subjects who had undergone complete excision of a left acoustic neuroma with facial nerve resection, five with chronic sinusitis, four with acute sinusitis, and one subject with an oroantral fistula. Wolff also noted that some patients with migraines report accompanying ipsilateral nasal obstruction and rhinorrhea with headache (13). His theory was that general vasodilatory mechanisms produced simultaneous nasal congestion and distention of cranial arteries, the latter being the true source of pain.

Wolff's findings can be summarized as follows:

1. The mucosa covering the sinus ostia are the most pain-sensitive areas in the sinonasal cavity, followed by the turbinates, then the septum and mucosa within the sinuses (more recent studies with a pressure probe have confirmed that the middle turbinate is more pain sensitive than the inferior turbinate or septum [14]);

2. Stimulation within the sinonasal cavity produced referred pain rather than pain at the site of stimulation; and

3. If a headache was not associated with inflammation and engorgement of the turbinates, it was in all probability not referred from nasal and sinus structures.

Careful inspection of Wolff's experiments will leave the rhinologist with several questions. How was he able (presumably with a head mirror and nasal speculum) to identify and stimulate areas such as the frontal ostium, superior turbinate, and inside the sphenoid sinus in normal subjects? These areas are frequently inaccessible in normal noses even to the modern endoscopist. And how, while attempting to stimulate deeper structures, could he avoid simultaneously stimulating proximal structures (such as the septum and the middle and inferior turbinates) and therefore confuse the issue of where pain is actually referred from? So while some neurologists (15) have taken Wolff's studies as the final word in nasally referred headache and used his data to discount the occurrence of referred headache emanating from intranasal structures such as the septum, modern means of examining the nasal cavity utilizing the nasal telescope have exposed flaws in Wolff's method.

CLINICAL ENTITIES

Headache associated with sinus inflammatory disease may take one of two forms. In most cases, headache is reported as one of a constellation of symptoms among others well recognized as sinus in origin. Less frequently, patients presenting with chronic headache alone in the absence of nasal or sinus symptoms are found to have occult sinusitis or sinonasal anatomical variations or abnormalities. Occasional reports have surfaced in the literature, describing patients with sinusitis masquerading as primary vascular-type headaches (16,17). Therefore, while certain pain characteris-

tics and referral patterns typify sinus-related headaches, the reader should therefore keep in mind the high degree of variability associated with headache referred from the sinonasal tract.

Acute Sinusitis

Headache associated with acute sinusitis has been reviewed by several authors (18–20). The diagnosis is usually obvious because of the associated nasal symptoms, such as congestion, obstruction, and purulent discharge. An antecedent viral upper respiratory infection is the cause in most cases. Fever is often present, and the associated pain is usually well localized and located over the involved sinus. Certain headache features are prominent in acute sinusitis regardless of the sinus involved. The pain is typically worsened by bending over, coughing, or straining. Headache, along with postnasal drainage, is usually worse in the morning upon awakening, and can be relieved somewhat by maintaining an upright position. The pain of acute sinusitis is typically more severe than that associated with chronic sinus disease, probably because chronic inflammation appears to be associated with a lower density of sensory nerve endings in the sinonasal mucosa. In acute sinusitis, the mucosal nerve density is relatively normal. Patients occasionally report vascular features in acute sinusitis, such as dizziness, nausea, photophobia, and a pulsatile quality to the pain. Anterior rhinoscopy and plain sinus radiographs are more helpful in diagnosing acute sinusitis than in chronic sinusitis, a condition in which nasal endoscopy and CT scanning are the diagnostic procedures of choice. Although patients commonly present with more than one sinus involved in the acute infection, each sinus will be discussed separately.

ACUTE ETHMOID SINUSITIS

Acute ethmoiditis typically presents as symptoms of nasal obstruction, purulent rhinorrhea, and headache or pain located in the medial canthal area (Fig. 6). Symptoms may be unilateral or bilateral, depending on whether the ethmoid involvement is unilateral or bilateral. Physical examination may demonstrate tenderness to palpation over the medial canthus, lacrimal fossa, and/or bridge of nose. Because the ethmoid sinus is the crossroad for drainage from the other dependent sinuses, spread of infection to these other sinuses is common. Orbital symptoms, such as pain and burning

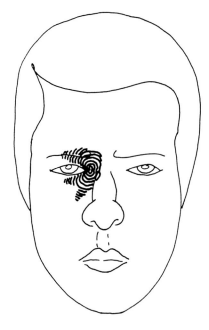

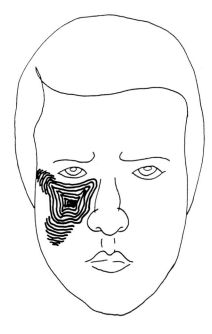

Fig. 6. Area of referred pain in acute ethmoid sinusitis. (Reproduced with permission from ref. *20a.*)

Fig. 7. Area of pain in acute maxillary sinusitis. (Reproduced with permission from ref. *20a.*)

in the eye, are common with acute ethmoiditis, but the presence of orbital signs on physical exam, such as periorbital edema or proptosis, should alert the physician to the possible spread of infection from the ethmoid sinus into the neighboring orbit. Orbital spread of acute ethmoiditis is much more common in children than in adults. Plain films may show clouding or loss of definition to the bony partitions of the ethmoid sinus, but these changes are often subtle. CT evaluation is reserved for the patient with signs of orbital involvement or the patient with refractory or recurrent disease.

ACUTE MAXILLARY SINUSITIS

Acute maxillary sinusitis typically presents as pain and pressure over the involved sinus(es) along with nasal congestion and purulent nasal discharge. The pain often radiates to the teeth, zygoma, periorbital or temporal areas (Fig. 7). Occasionally, patients may present only with dental pain, especially if the maxillary sinusitis is of dental rather than rhinologic origin. Tenderness to palpation over the involved sinus can usually be elicited. Intranasal examination may reveal mucosal edema and erythema, and pus will be seen often in the middle meatus if that area can be visualized. Plain films are diagnostic more often in acute maxillary sinusitis than in acute ethmoiditis, demonstrating either an air-fluid level or total opacification of the

infected sinus. If appropriate antibiotics and vaso-constricting agents are not successful in alleviating symptoms, antral puncture and irrigation may be necessary.

ACUTE FRONTAL SINUSITIS

The pain of acute frontal sinusitis is often severe, located over the forehead, and associated with tenderness on percussion of the involved sinus (Fig. 8). The pain becomes intolerable with bending over or straining. Because of the potential for intracranial spread via the valveless diploic veins, acute frontal sinusitis should be considered a medical emergency. Children and adolescent males in particular seem more prone to intracranial spread of frontal infection. Hospitalization and intravenous antibiotics are recommended after the diagnosis is confirmed with radiographic studies. If clinical improvement does not occur early in the course of medical therapy, surgical intervention is indicated.

ACUTE SPHENOID SINUSITIS

Acute sphenoid sinusitis is a diagnostic challenge owing to the location of the sphenoid sinus and the variable presentation of symptoms that accompany sphenoiditis. Pain may be unilateral or bilateral, even when only one side of the sphenoid is involved. The headache is usually poorly localized, but patients complain most commonly of

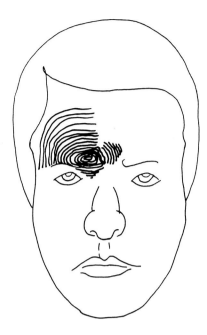

Fig. 8. Areas of referred pain seen in acute frontal sinusitis. (Reproduced with permission from ref. *20a*.)

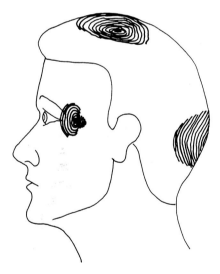

Fig. 9. Patterns or referred pain in acute sphenoid sinusitis. (Reproduced with permission from ref. *20a*.)

retro-orbital or vertex pain (Fig. 9). The sphenoid is the most difficult sinus both to examine and to image with plain films. Because of the sphenoid's close proximity to the cavernous sinus and the vital structures it contains, acute sphenoiditis is also considered a medical emergency. In-patient observation and intravenous antibiotics are indicated, and surgical drainage should be considered if a clinical response to medical therapy does not rapidly ensue.

Chronic Sinusitis

Chronic sinus disease can masquerade as a variety of conditions, including chronic primary headache. While acute sinusitis can be diagnosed with relative ease, diagnosing headache and facial pain secondary to chronic sinus disease can be a challenging endeavor. Chronic sinusitis often presents without obvious nasal symptoms, such as congestion, obstruction, or postnasal drip. In the absence of classic sinus symptoms, it is not surprising that clinicians overlook the sinonasal tract as the site of pathology in patients presenting with headaches. Traditional methods of examining the area tend to confirm this lack of suspicion, since anterior rhinoscopy and plain sinus films are frequently normal in these patients. Plain films provide very little detail about the ethmoid sinus, which is the seat of pathology in most cases of chronic sinus disease. Nasal symptoms, no matter how seemingly insignificant, should not be taken lightly in the patient presenting with chronic headaches, but should alert the clinician to the possibility of underlying chronic sinus disease.

While tenderness over the involved sinus(es) is a reliable sign in acute sinusitis, it may or may not be present in chronic sinusitis. The severity of pain is also variable, with some patients complaining of debilitating pain and others of minor discomfort. The severity of pain bears little relation to the extent of sinus disease, but pain and other sinus symptoms are exacerbated by a viral upper respiratory infection, which may precipitate episodes of acute sinusitis. Headache associated with chronic sinus disease may be located over the involved sinus or may be referred elsewhere in the distribution of the branch of the trigeminal nerve innervating the involved sinus (*see* section on Referred Pain earlier in chapter). Patients describe the character of the pain most frequently as a pressure sensation, but the pain can take on almost any quality, including sharp and lancing (resembling trigeminal neuralgia), throbbing and pulsating (resembling a vascular headache), or tight and drawing (resembling tension-type headache). The pain may be constant or variable, and often most intense in the morning on awakening. Changes in barometric pressure, such as those encountered during changes in weather or air travel, typically trigger headache or facial pain. Patients with allergy may experience seasonal variation in headache, suggesting a nasal or sinus causation.

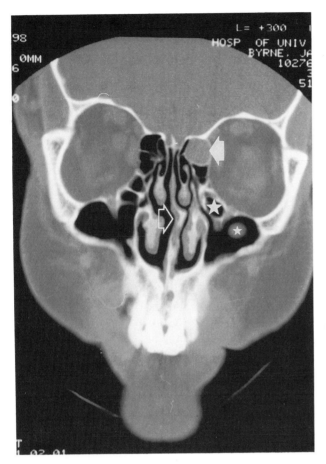

Fig. 10. Coronal CT of a patient with a 14-yr history of cluster headaches resulting in narcotic addiction and hospitalization for pain management. Patient had unilateral pain in the forehead and eye with ipsilateral lacrimation and clear rhinorrhea. CT demonstrates septal deviation (open arrow), an opacified ethmoid cell in the neighborhood of the anterior ethmoidal nerve (arrow), a Haller cell (large star), and a pedunculated polyp (small star); all of these findings were ipsilateral to the side of pain. Surgical correction of these abnormalities relieved the patient's headaches. (Reprinted with permission from ref. *8a.*)

Headache or facial pain secondary to chronic inflammatory sinus disease typically responds at least in part to antibiotics, and to topical and systemic corticosteroids. However, symptoms commonly recur at some point after discontinuation of medical therapy. If symptoms recur frequently, or if symptoms are debilitating when they do occur, CT evaluation of the sinuses is indicated (Fig. 10). The clinician should also inquire as to possible underlying conditions which may predispose to the development of sinus disease, such as allergy, immunodeficiency, mucociliary disorders, cystic fibrosis, autoimmune disease, and chemical inhalation (e.g., cigaret smoke exposure, occupational chemical exposure, building-related exposure, and so on).

The accurate diagnosis of headache owing to chronic sinus disease requires taking a thorough history, a careful nasal endoscopic examination, and, in many cases, CT evaluation. Diagnostic nasal endoscopy is indispensible in the evaluation of chronic sinus disease. The technique has been described elsewhere in this volume (Chapter 29). Patients are selected for CT evaluation based on history, nasal endoscopic exam, and their response to medical therapy. Coronal CT remains the imaging modality of choice for evaluating sinus disease. Using the same CT parameters as those for intracranial examination is inappropriate and may fail to reveal significant ostiomeatal complex pathology *(21)*. So-called "bone windows" should be used in CT evaluation of the sinuses. The presence of sinus opacification, anatomical abnormalities, or mucosal thickening on CT does not mean necessarily that these findings are the cause of symptoms. CT findings must be interpreted with reference to the patient's symptoms, including the location of pain, as incidental abnormalities are fairly common on CT exam of asymptomatic subjects *(22,23)*.

Referred Headache from Sinonasal Mucosal Contact Areas

HISTORICAL PERSPECTIVE

The concept of intranasal anatomical variations and/or abnormalities causing referred headache, without concomitant inflammatory, degenerative, or neoplastic disease, dates back at least to the last century. Anatomical variations or abnormalities, such as septal spurs and deviations or a pneumatized middle turbinate (concha bullosa), have been identified as causes of headaches in some patients from this early time. The earliest known association between headache and nasal obstruction was by John Jacob Wepfer in 1728 (cited in ref. *24*). In the following century, John Roe, an otorhinolaryngologist from Rochester, New York, recorded these remarkable insights:

"There is perhaps no single affection that causes so large an amount of human suffering, and which is regarded so lightly, as that known by the generic term, headache. . . . Headaches caused by chronic abnormal conditions of the nasal passages, in which the nasal derangement played a

less conspicuous part, were sometimes attributed to other causes, and the nasal disease was entirely overlooked or unsuspected. In case of entire failure to detect a cause, the headache was often termed 'nervous' or 'congestive,' or by that most comforting of terms, 'idiopathic.' Headaches that have their exciting cause in the nose are reflex in character. This is a self-evident fact, for the reason that the manifestation of pain is at a point more or less remote from its exciting cause in the nose. . . . The exciting cause of nasal headache is an irritation of the terminal nerve-filaments in the nasal chambers, which excites an undue activity in the communication ganglion, and from which an irritation is reflected to the terminal filaments of other communication nerves. . . . In the nose, the irritation is occasioned by some abnormal condition which brings together parts that normally should be separate, and produces more or less pressure between them. . . . It is not uncommon that a sensation of fulness is felt at the base of the nose and about its bridge, associated with more or less head pain, due to an enlarged middle turbinated body wedged in tightly against the septum...when there is constant pain there is a correspondingly constant pressure, and in temporary attacks of pain the pressure is correspondingly temporary. . . . Certain atmospheric conditions will excite headache. It is usually when there is a low temperature and low barometer, with the air surcharged with moisture—a condition that causes these diseased nasal tissues to become engorged and also distended by the absorption of water from the atmosphere. . . . The location of the pains in the head has no constant relation to the disease nor to its seat in the nose, and it has no such relation to the distribution of the nerves or blood vessels. Notwithstanding the fact that the location of the pain in the head bears no constant relation to the location of the disease in the nose, it is observed that from certain portions of the nasal chamber pain is more often reflected to certain regions of the head than to other regions. The pain reflected from the region of the middle turbinated bone is commonly referred to the temple, sometimes invading the whole region from the nose to the parietal eminence, and extending to the vertex; while pain reflected from the region of the superior turbinated bone is commonly felt in the frontal and supraorbital region. Sometimes the pain will completely surround the eye, or be centered in the back of the eyeball. . . . In all cases where there is not an unquestionable relation of cause and effect between some other local or general disease and the headache, the nasal passages should be interrogated, even in the absence of urgent or distinctive symptoms of nasal disease. . . . It is too frequently the case that a well-pronounced nasal trouble is looked upon as nothing more nor less than an ordinary 'nasal catarrh;' while the headache that results from the disease in the nose is considered to be chronic neuralgia, . . . In case the headache is associated with pronounced nasal irritation, and there is an absence of any other pronounced cause, . . . we have presumptive evidence that the headache originates in the nose. . . . Further evidence we should seek for, by careful examining the nasal passages" (25).

Other attempts to explain headache causation with nasal involvement followed during the turn of the century. Sphenopalatine neuralgia (Sluder's syndrome) was first described by Sluder in the early part of this century. The syndrome is characterized by unilateral pain in the lower half of the head and face, mainly in the distribution of the maxillary division of the trigeminal nerve (V2). The pain is episodic and recurrent, lasting from minutes to days. Common locations for pain include the periorbital area, base of the nose, and the mastoid process (26). Eagle (27) found a high incidence of septal deformities in a series of patients with this disorder, and advocated submucus resection of the septum when spurs and deviations were present. Others like Vail (28) suggested that the vidian nerve, rather than the sphenopalatine ganglion, was the site of pathology. Vail's description of vidian neuralgia is essentially identical to Sluder's syndrome. Vail supposed either occult of frank sphenoid sinusitis as the cause of such headaches. Later work by Stewart and Lambert (29), Cushing (30), and others shed doubt on both theories. Wolff was of the opinion that since various interventions (such as septal surgery [according to Eagle], sphenoid-otomy [according to Vail], or cocainization of the sphenopalatine ganglion [according to Sluder]) have a similar therapeutic effect, there must not be any specific etiologic relationship between intranasal structures and the pain encountered in this syndrome. Wolff concluded that sphenopalatine or vidian neuralgia was actually a vascular syndrome (in keeping with his general theory of vascular headaches) involving the internal maxillary artery *(31)*. Most investigators now consider Sluder's syndrome to be equivalent to cluster headache *(32)*.

Reports in the literature describing "vacuum headaches" have appeared since at least 1891 (according to ref. *33*). The theory is that narrow ostia may close off and create negative pressure within the affected sinus. Rapid changes in barometric pressure, such as experienced by aviators, may cause recurrent headaches secondary to sinus ostial obstruction *(34,35)*. Many rhinologists suspect this happens in nonaviators as well, as many patients with known sinus disease experience worsening of symptoms with weather-related barometric pressure changes. A significant percentage of migraine sufferers also experience weather-related exacerbations of their headaches *(36)*, suggesting possible rhinologic involvement in these patients.

The term "rhinogenic headache" has been employed, but since it means "headache which generates a nose," the term is misapplied *(37)*. "Cephalgiagenic rhinopathy" more accurately describes the process of a nasal problem causing headache, but the term is awkward and unwieldy. "Septal contact headache," "mucosal contact headache," and "middle turbinate headache syndrome" *(38)* are terms that allude to a particular mechanism of or structure involved in referred headache. These terms suggest that whenever two apposing mucosal surfaces come into contact with each other (such as between a deviated septum and a turbinate), headache ensues. "Headache of sinus and nasal origin," a term proposed by several investigators, is general enough to include both the entity of mucosal contact, as well as that of occult sinus inflammatory disease. Table 2 lists some of the names that have been used to describe this entity.

LITERATURE REVIEW

Rhinogenic headache *(39)* described in recent texts is thought to be caused by septal impaction or contact (with the lateral nasal wall), allergic and vasomotor rhinitis and nasal polyps, trauma, posttraumatic conditions, intranasal tumors, and septal hematoma. Various anatomical structures within the nasal cavity have been implicated as a cause of mucosal contact—induced headache in the absence of sinusitis, including the nasal septum *(40,41)*

Table 2
Some Terms that Have Been Used
to Describe Headache Referred from the Sinonasal
Tract in the Absence of Sinus Inflammatory Disease

Nasal headache	Rhinogenic headache
Sinus headache	Rhinologic headache
Headache of nasal origin	Sinugenic headache
Headache of sinus origin	Septal contact headache
Headache of nasal and sinus origin	Mucosal contact headache
Congestive headache	Barosinusitis/barosinus headache
Vasomotor headache	Middle turbinate headache
Vacuum headache	Nasal contact headache

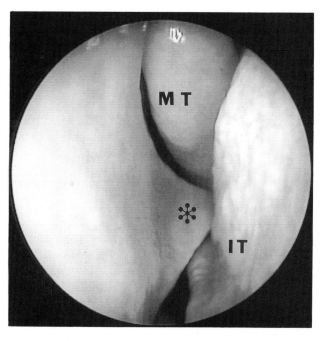

Fig. 11. Left-sided septal spur (asterisk) impacting the inferior turbinate (IT) as seen with a 0° nasal telescope. Injection of the spur with local anesthesia abolished the patient's pain, suggesting that the septum, rather than the inferior turbinate, was the cause of pain. MT, middle turbinate.

(Fig. 11), the middle turbinate *(39,42)* (Fig. 12), and the inferior turbinate *(43,44)*.

Schønsted-Madsen et al. *(45)* reported on a series of 157 patients with headache and nasal obstruction secondary to septal deviation. Surgical correction of the septal deviation was successful in alleviating chronic headache complaints in the majority of cases. Saunte and Soyka concede that septal deformity (such as a spur) can cause headache even without nasal symptoms *(39)*.

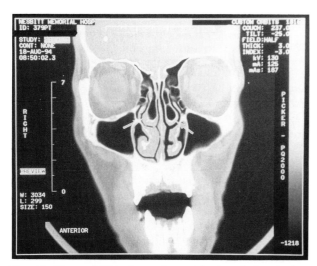

Fig. 12. Coronal CT of a patient with chronic headaches revealing bilateral concha bullosa (arrows) in the absence of mucosal disease. Limited endoscopic surgery succeeded in resolving symptoms.

Chow *(46)* reported his experience with 18 patients with headache referred from the sinonasal tract. He does not give details on the headache features, such as location, chronicity, character of pain, and so on. None of the patients reported headache as their chief complaint, and none had inflammatory disease of the sinuses. The cause of headaches was determined to be septal spurs in 12, mucus retention cysts in three, a mucosal contact point between the middle turbinate and the lateral nasal wall in two, and a dehiscent infraorbital nerve in one. Fifteen of eighteen (83%) reported significant improvement after medical or surgical therapy, but the mean length of follow-up and the specific therapies employed are not described.

Castellanos and Axelrod *(47)* studied 246 patients with a major complaint of headache whose previous neurologic evaluations were unrevealing. Flexible fiberoptic rhinoscopy and routine sinus radiographic examinations were performed on each subject. Twenty-six percent had neither rhinoscopic nor radiographic evidence of infection. Sixty percent demonstrated only rhinoscopic evidence of infection (purulent material emanating from a sinus drainage area), while 34% had both rhinoscopic and radiographic evidence of infection. A high percentage of patients with identifiable disease reported either seasonal or perennial rhinitis, while few without disease reported nasal symptoms. Headache characteristics were not described in this study, so it is unclear whether any of these patients suffered from primary headaches. Patients with identifiable sinus disease responded well to oral antibiotic therapy, with resolution of headaches and nasal symptoms in the great majority of cases. The response rates for patients with radiographic disease were slightly lower than that for patients with rhinoscopic disease only, suggesting the early stages of sinusitis are more antibiotic-responsive than later stages. In this study, the chronicity and responsiveness of headache to medical therapy depended on the radiographic presence of disease. The group without any evidence of disease was also treated with antibiotic therapy, and responded poorly.

Cook et al. *(48)* recently reviewed their experience with 18 patients with a chief symptom of recurrent sinusitis and headache, but who had normal CT studies of the sinuses. Seven of these patients were referred for neurology evaluation, of which three were diagnosed with migraine and one with depression. The surgical procedure was limited to uncinectomy and middle meatal antrostomy with partial middle turbinectomy. They report no benefit to the four patients with a diagnosis of migraine or depression after surgery.

Stammberger and Wolf *(49)* recognize three different groups of headache patients:

1. Those with headaches clearly connected to some sinus problem, such as inflammatory disease, neoplasm, barotrauma, and so on;
2. Those with headaches clearly traceable to nonsinus causes such as migraine, neuralgias, vascular disorders, and so on; and
3. Those whose problems are not clear and in whom there seems to be no overt indication of sinus disease.

These authors report a variety of sinonasal anatomical variations and/or abnormalities with patients in the third category (Tables 3 and 4).

Bonaccorsi, in his experience with 1000 patients, reports 89% improvement in headache symptoms employing sphenoethmoidectomy *(50)*. He reports that even minor abnormalities, such as contact between the septum and middle or superior turbinates, can have pathological significance in patients with a "lowered pain threshold and elevated central integrative capability." Bonaccorsi *(51)* and several other investigators *(52,53)* have noted an association between migraine headaches and sinonasal disorders. Clerico has also reported on a series of

Table 3
Frequent Anatomic Variations Predisposing to Headaches and Recurrent Sinusitis[a]

Septal deviations/spurs
Agger nasi cells
Uncinate process
    Medially bent
    Laterally bent
    Curved anteriorly
    Fractures
    Contacting turbinate
    Pneumatized
Middle turbinate
    Concha bullosa
    Paradoxically bent
    Bulging into lateral nasal wall
Ethmoid bulla
    Large, filling middle meatus
    Contact areas
    Anterior growth
    Protruding from middle meatus
Combination of all of the above

[a]Adapted with permission from ref. 48.

Table 4
Frequent Endoscopic and/or CT Findings in Patients with Sinugenic Headaches[a]

Septal deviation/spurs[b]
Diseased agger nasi cells[c]
Diseased frontal recess[c]
Uncinate process
    Medially bent, contacting middle turbinate[c]
    Laterally bent[b]
    Curved anteriorly ("doubled middle turbinate")[c]
    Fractures (trauma, iatrogenic)[b]
Abnormalities of the middle turbinate
    Concha bullosa (pneumatized middle turbinate)[c]
    Paradoxically bent[b]
    Bulging into lateral nasal wall
Ethmoidal bulla
    Large, filling middle meatus[d]
    Contact areas (especially polyps from turbinate sinus)[c]
    Anterior growth, overlapping hiatus semilunaris[b]
    Protruding from middle meatus[c]
Combination of all of the above, resulting in an obstruction of the frontal recess or of other parts of the middle meatus
Isolated sphenoid disease[b]

[a]Adapted with permission from ref. 49a. [b]Rare finding; [c]more frequent finding; [d]very frequent finding.

patients with sinonasal anatomical variations and abnormalities and occult sinus inflammatory disease masquerading as refractory primary headache syndromes *(8a)*. Other evidence for a sinonasal causation in primary vascular-typed headaches is that capsaicin has been found helpful when applied intranasally in relieving pain in patients with cluster headaches *(54,55)*. These recent reports challenge the traditional theory that headache owing to paranasal sinus disease is not accompanied by migrainous or vascular features *(38)*. As stated in a recent comprehensive textbook on headache, "hypertrophic turbinates and…chronic sinusitis [are] not validated as a cause of headache or facial pain." *(38)*. Migraine and tension-type headaches are often confused with sinus-related headaches owing to the similarity of pain location. The question remains whether primary headaches coexist with referred headaches of sinonasal origin, and whether sinonasal disorders represent just one of many potential triggers of head and face pain, or is there a cause-and-effect relationship between sinonasal disorders and so-called primary headaches? Little research has been done to answer this question. Regardless of the exact mechanism, the reports cited above suggest that the diagnosis of primary headache (such as migraine, tension-type,

or cluster headache) does not necessarily preclude a sinonasal causation.

MECHANISMS

Stammberger and Wolf *(48)* point out that ostiomeatal complex disease can cause headaches by several mechanisms: constant intense mucosal contact according to the referred pain concept, malventilation of nonventilation of the sinuses with resulting hypoxia, or pressure from proliferation polyps. The authors go on to say that all of the above conditions, even when very small and circumscribed, may have one dominating clinical symptom: headache.

Tables 3 and 4 list the various anatomical structures and pathophysiologic processes that may be involved in rhinopathic headache. Stammberger points out that not all of these conditions should be considered diseases, but all can give rise to mucosal contact, and all these conditions, even when small and circumscribed, may present with headache as the dominant clinical symptom. The inferior turbinate is not a common cause of referred headache in the author's experience.

Stammberger also stresses the importance of the ethmoid bulla as a cause of headaches, even when

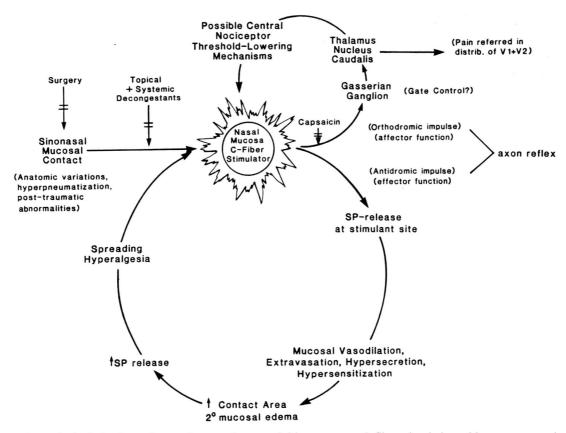

Fig. 13. Schematic depicting how sinonasal mucosal contact initiates sensory C-fiber stimulation with consequent release of SP, and the triggering of both orthodromic and antidromic impulses. Central processes may work to modulate pain; peripheral processes may be self-perpetuating, with resultant hyperalgesia. The pathway may be interrupted at its origin (i.e., relieving the contact with surgery), or further downstream with various medical interventions (topical agents, capsaicin).

it is uninvolved with inflammatory disease. In his experience, a large or overly-pneumatized ethmoid bulla is the most common cause of referred headache of sinus origin in the absence of sinusitis (*see* Table 4). The mechanism of pain is presumed to result from contact between the bulla and the middle turbinate located medial to it.

Stammberger and Wolf *(48)* found SP present in 17 of 23 samples from normal controls in concentrations averaging 2.0 ng/g of tissue. In five of nine samples from patients with chronic sinusitis, SP was present in 0.75 ng/g quantities, and SP was not detected at all in polyp tissue. This interesting biochemical finding correlates with the clinical spectrum of pain from sinus disease. The pain of acute sinusitis is typically more severe than that of chronic sinusitis. Patients with sinonasal polyps are comparatively pain free, oftentimes despite massive polyposis.

The presence of higher levels of SP in normal mucosa also explains how mucosal contact in the absence of inflammatory sinus disease can cause pain. Mucosal contact serves as the mechanical stimulus that releases SP, found in relatively higher amounts in this normal noninflamed tissue, and initiates an axon reflex (Fig. 13).

Many patients exhibit mucosal contact on intranasal or CT examination who are headache-free, just as many asymptomatic subjects display mucosal changes in the paranasal sinuses on CT. Obviously mucosal contact alone is not sufficient cause for referred pain. It may be that the extent or duration of mucosal contact is a significant determinant of headache. Other factors altering pain threshold, such as CNS modulation (secondary to endogenous opiod release or brainstem modulatory nuclei activation), the presence of inflammation at the site of peripheral stimulation, integrity of mucosal defense mechanisms (including the activity of neutral endopeptidase [NEP]), hormonal influences, autonomic responses, and psychological factors may act in concert with mucosal contact to create the subjective sense of pain.

Chemical-Induced Rhinopathic Headaches

Airborne chemical irritants and pollutants can affect both the olfactory and trigeminal systems when inhaled intranasally. One manifestation of this exposure is headaches. Inhaled pollutants and irritants can act centrally via trigeminal reflex pathways or by direct transport into the CNS via olfactory pathways. The trigeminal nerve also modulates olfactory afferent inputs into the CNSs (56). Inhaled irritants stimulate trigeminal afferents in the nasal mucosa (57), which then can result in central reflexes. Since trigeminal-derived fibers are localized to intracranial blood vessels, reflex vasodilation can occur as a result of intranasal stimuli that cause the release of SP (58).

Lewis et al. (59) have coined the term "nose–brain barrier" to describe the protective functions of the nasal cavity in limiting access of inhaled environmental toxic substances to the CNS. Because olfactory neuroepithelium is unique in that it is the only area of the body in direct contact with both the CNS and the external environment, the nasal cavity possesses various defenses against inhaled toxins. Components of this nose–brain barrier include a high concentration of xenobiotic (foreign substance)-metabolizing enzymes, tight junctions between epithelial cells lining the nasal cavity, mucosal immune defenses, and sinonasal mucus secretions. Experimental studies have detected olfactory bulb accumulation of substances introduced into the nasal cavity. Information gained by these transport studies indicates that CNS penetration of many substances takes place through both intraneuronal and extraneuronal routes. Efferent projections from the olfactory bulbs are diffuse, extending to limbic areas, the hypothalamus and the hippocampus. Intranasal inhalation of certain chemical substances can therefore have a broad impact on the CNS. Inhaled pollutants may directly cause headache through CNS penetration, or indirectly by promoting inflammatory changes in the nasal mucosa (60), thus initiating trigeminal reflex pain.

The ethmoidal nerve contains many mechanoreceptor fibers as well as fibers responding only to chemical stimulation (61). Some chemical pollutants, such as ozone, increase the responsiveness of the ethmoidal and nasopalatine nerves to odors (60), perhaps providing a basis for the hypersensitivity to odors perceived by many individuals with multiple chemical sensitivity syndrome (MCS).

Table 5
Pertinent Headache Characteristics to Elicit
from Patient During History Taking

Location	Severity	Chronicity
Duration (each episode)	Frequency	Character of pain
Associated symptoms	Triggering factors	Daily variation
Neurological workup?	Seasonal variation	Previous trauma?
Treatments and response to treatments		

Headache is also a prominent complaint in MCS patients.

Several investigators have reported that odors can precipitate a migraine attack in susceptible individuals (62,63). Hirsch (64) reported that 18% of migraine sufferers were found to be hyposmic or anosmia compared to a 1% rate in the general population. Others have reported that patients with migraine have a heightened sensitivity to odors, particularly during headache attacks (65,66). Whether chemical sensitivity is a causative factor or simply an epiphenomenon in these subjects is not known.

Concurrent Disorders

The clinician should keep in mind that primary headaches and sinonasal disease can coexist independent of each other. The mere presence of headache and sinus symptoms simultaneously does not necessarily infer cause and effect. Appropriate diagnostic and therapeutic measures must be taken (see next section).

DIAGNOSIS AND TREATMENT

The rhinologist must rely heavily on the patient's history (see Table 5) as well as diagnostic nasal endoscopy and coronal CT scanning, to diagnose rhinopathic headache. Other more obvious environmental causes of headache (such as response to ingested food, drink, or medication, occupational exposure to vasoactive chemicals, and so on) should be excluded. Historical clues that suggest a rhinopathic origin include the presence of nasal symptoms no matter how seemingly insignificant, weather-related exacerbations of headache (particularly with low barometric pressure or rapid changes in barometric pressure), onset or worsening of headache with viral upper respiratory infections, or nasal allergy. The absence of nasal symptoms does not rule out the diagnosis of rhinopathic headache; conversely, the presence of nasal symptoms in a headache patient does not necessarily implicate the sinonasal tract in headache causation. The location of the headache may give clues to the site of pathology, as Wolff's mapping of referred pain suggests. In acute sinusitis, pain is mostly felt in the skin or bones overlying the involved sinus(es). Pain associated with acute sinusitis typically is more severe than that associated with chronic sinusitis, presumably because normal mucosa has a greater density of sensory nerve fibers and is therefore more pain sensitive than chronically hypertrophic or hyperplastic mucosa *(20)*. This characteristic of normal mucosa also provides the rationale behind how mucosal contact can elicit a pain reflex. In situations of chronic sinusitis or referred headache secondary to mucosal contact, the location of pain less reliably indicates the site of pathology *(53,67)*.

Inflammatory sinus disease may be suspected from the history, and should be confirmed with diagnostic nasal endoscopy or CT scanning. Office endoscopic examination is indispensible for viewing the nasal cavity in great detail. Musosal abnormalities, anatomical variations and abnormalities, and sinus disease, which has extended into the nasal cavity, are all appreciable through nasal endoscopy. Rigid telescopes are preferred over flexible fiberoptic scopes because of the superior optics and the ability to use a free hand for instrumentation within the nasal cavity alongside the scope. In most cases, direct visualization of the ostiomeatal complex is possible with adequate topical anesthesia.

Nasal endoscopy can only indirectly evaluate the paranasal sinuses. Coronal CT scanning with window width/length ratios that highlight bony detail remains the modality of choice for imaging the sinuses. Mucosal changes and structural/anatomical variations within the sinus complex can be identified in this way. The information gathered from nasal endoscopy and CT scanning should be considered complementary rather than mutually exclusive.

In the absence of inflammatory disease, areas of mucosal contact should become the focus of attention. Such areas include septal spurs and deviations, paradoxical curvature of the middle turbinate, pneumatized middle and/or superior turbi-

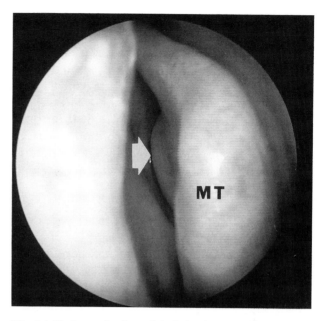

Fig. 14. Endoscopic view of the left middle turbinate (MT) with a paradoxical curvature, and the superior turbinate contacting the nasal septum (arrow). Topical anesthesia applied directly to the superior turbinate markedly reduced the patient's headache. CT later confirmed pneumatization of the superior turbinate, and endoscopic ethmoidectomy provided complete relief of headaches.

nates (Fig. 14), and ethmoid asymmetry (where ipsilateral enlargement or hypertrophy of the ethmoid/middle turbinate complex is associated with contralateral septal deflection). If the patient has a headache at the time of initial examination, areas of mucosal contact should be topically anesthetized under direct endoscopic visualization. The author's procedure is to first apply decongestant (1% ephedrine) and anesthetic (2% Pontocaine®) sprays; if there is no pain relief after 5–10 min, a cotton-tipped applicator soaked in 4% cocaine solution (other topical anesthetics may be substituted) is inserted between areas of mucosal contact under visualization with either the 0° or 30° rigid telescope. The applicator is left in place for 5–10 min, then removed. The patient should then be allowed time for the effect of the mechanical stimulation from the applicator to subside. After another 5–10 min, the patient is then questioned about headache pain. A significant reduction in pain severity score (>50%) should be achieved to suspect rhinopathic headache. If pain is not present at the time of initial examination, the patient is encouraged to return to the office on a day when headache is present and significant. The above procedure is then repeated if necessary. Occasionally, injection of local anesthetic (1% lidocaine with epinephrine 1:100,000) into an area of mucosal contact may be necessary to relieve pain and therefore make the diagnosis. In pediatric patients who cannot cooperate with office nasal endoscopic examination, administration of topical intranasal decongestant and corticosteroid sprays offers both diagnostic and therapeutic potential. If headaches resolve or improve with this therapy, sinonasal causation is likely.

The clinician must be ever mindful of a placebo effect with this office diagnostic procedure and the possibility of false positive responses. The effect of cocaine applied intranasally for headache relief was questioned as early as 1900 (68). The author has personal experience with one such case. Pain relief after topical application of anesthetic is not a foolproof diagnostic test; objective evidence of mucosal disease or contact should accompany such a response. Good clinical judgment is required, and several office sessions with the patient may be needed before both patient and physician are convinced of any relationship between sinonasal findings and headache.

As Stammberger and Wolf point out, negative findings with anterior and posterior rhinoscopy and conventional radiographs do not necessarily rule out a sinus-related headache. They state that only the combination of diagnostic nasal endoscopy with CT provides sufficient information to make such a diagnosis. However, pathology suspected via these modalities may not be confirmed by provocative testing (such as with topical anesthesia to the site) as the source of pain. In other words, the simple presence of an intranasal deformity or abnormality does not predict its role in headache causation. Topically anesthetizing the area with the aid of an endoscope is more reliable than simple visualization in identifying the source of pain.

Treatment of rhinopathic headaches should start with the most conservative measures first and proceed to endoscopic surgery only in refractory cases when the patient's quality of life is significantly affected by symptomatology. In the case of chemical-induced headaches, both patient and physician should energetically attempt to identify the offending substance(s). Avoidance is the key to headache prevention in such cases. In suspected cases of mucosal contact head-

aches, attempts to decongest and shrink nasal mucosa should be instituted. Home remedies to shrink nasal mucosa such as steam inhalation and saline irrigation have a mild decongestant effect and will lessen mucosal contact and encourage sinus drainage. These measures may provide symptomatic relief in the mildest of cases. Topical decongestants work rapidly and often represent the most effective medical therapy for rhinopathic headaches, but should be limited to short courses of therapy interspersed with drug holiday periods to avoid rebound (rhinitis medicamentosa). Systemic decongestants can also be quite effective but many patients either develop tolerance to the medication or experience unpleasant side-effects (insomnia, nervousness, the "jitters"). Topical corticosteroid sprays are safe for long-term use but somewhat less effective than topical decongestant therapy. Systemic steroids also represent a short-term therapy owing to the relatively high risk of complications with long-term use. Experimental therapies with capsaicin, SP-antagonists, and NEP-like substances may hold promise for the future treatment of mucosal contact phenomena. In any patient with sinusitis, antibiotic therapy should be instituted. The principles of antimicrobial therapy for inflammatory sinus disease are presented elsewhere in this volume. The patient should also undergo appropriate allergy workup and treatment when indicated.

Surgical therapy is indicated if the diagnosis of rhinopathic headache is well established and if more conservative measures fail. Endoscopic sinonasal surgery is preferred since this approach offers optimal visualization and the opportunity for maximal preservation or normal mucosa. Endoscopic surgery for rhinopathic headaches may not be truly "functional" in the sense that some "normal" structures may need to be sacrificed if they are involved in mucosal contact phenomena. Preservation of healthy mucosa is a priority after mucosal contact areas have been addressed. The surgery should tailor the patient's needs and, at least ideally, be limited to those areas confirmed as the cause of referred pain by office diagnostic procedures. Concha bullosae and septal spurs represent common causes of referred headache and are managed best by endoscopic surgery. Figure 15 shows an algorithm for the management of rhinopathic headaches.

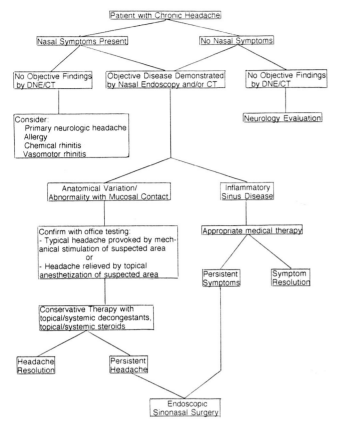

Fig. 15. An algorithm for the diagnosis and management of rhinopathic headaches. DNE, diagnostic nasal endoscopy.

SUMMARY

Various sinonasal abnormalities have been identified as etiologic factors in chronic headaches since the last century. The prevailing opinion within the field of neurology, that sinus abnormalities other than acute purulent sinusitis are rarely if ever a cause of headache *(69)*, is based on antiquated methods of rhinologic diagnosis and treatment. Modern modalities such as diagnostic nasal endoscopy and coronal sinus CT scanning have yet to be employed widely in the workup of headache patients. A subset of patients with primary headaches have sinonasal anatomical variations/abnormalities or occult inflammatory disease that either cause or exacerbate their headaches. The presence or absence of nasal symptoms is often unreliable as an indication of underlying pathology. Based on preliminary reports, endoscopic sinonasal surgery addressing areas of sinonasal pathology holds promise as an effective treatment modality for these patients.

ACKNOWLEDGMENT

I would like to thank David I. Barras for his valuable suggestions in reviewing the manuscript.

REFERENCES

1. Mayer DJ, Frenk H. The role of neuropeptides in pain. In: Nemeroff CB, ed., Neuropeptides in Psychiatric and Neurological Disorders. Baltimore: Johns Hopkins University Press. 1988; p. 201.
2. Sessle BJ. Neural mechanisms of oral and facial pain. Otolaryngol Clin North Amer 1989;21:1059–1072.
2a. Finger TE, et al. Affector and effector functions of peptidergic innervation of the nasal cavity. In: Green BG, Mason JR, Kare MR, eds., Chemical Senses, Vol. 2: Irritation. New York: Marcel Dekker, 1990; pp. 1–17.
3. Lucier GE, Egizii R. Characterization of cat nasal afferents and brain stem neurones receiving ethmoidal input. Exp Neurol 1989;103:83–89.
4. Lucier GE, Egizii R. Central projections of the ethmoidal nerve of the cat as determined by the horseradish peroxidase tracer technique. J Comp Neurol 1986; 247:123-132.
5. Sicuteri F, Fanciullacci M, Nicolodi M, Geppetti P, Fusco BM, Marabini S, Alessandri M, Campagnolo V. Substance P theory: a unique focus on the painful and painless phenomena of cluster headache. Headache 1990;30:69–79.
6. Lundblad L, Lundberg JM, Brodin E, Änggård A. Origin and distribution of capsaicin-sensitive substance P-immunoreactive nerves in the nasal mucosa. Acta Otolaryngol 1983;96:485–493.
7. Silver WL, Farley LG, Finger TE. The effects of neonatal capsaicin administration on trigeminal nerve chemoreceptors in the rat nasal cavity. Brain Res 1991;561: 212–216.
8. Melzack R, Wall PD. Pain and mechanisms: a new theory. Science 1965;150:971–979.
8a. Clerico DM. Sinus headaches reconsidered: referred cephalgia of rhinologic origin masquerading as refractory primary headaches. Headache 1995;35:185–192.
9. Maggi CA, Meli A. The sensory-efferent function of capsaicin-sensitive neurons. Gen Pharmacol 1988;19: 1–43.
10. Silver WL, Finger TE. The trigeminal system. In: Getchell TV, Doty RL, Bartoshuk LM, Snow JB Jr, eds., Smell and Taste in Health and Disease. New York: Raven, 1991; p. 105.
11. Eccles R. Neurological and pharmacological considerations. In: Proctor DF, Andersen I, eds., The Nose: Upper Airway Physiology and the Atmospheric Environment. Amsterdam: Elsevier, 1982; pp. 191–214 (198–202).
12. Raphael GD, Meredith SD, Baraniuk JN, Kaliner MA. Nasal reflexes. In: Settipane GA, ed., Rhinitis, 2nd ed. Providence, RI: OceanSide, 1991; pp. 135–142.
12a. In: Dalessio DJ, Silberstein SD, eds., Wolff's Headache and Other Head Pain, 6th ed. New York: Oxford University Press, 1993; pp. 297–305.
13. Wolff HG. Headache and Other Head Pain. Oxford University Press, New York, 1948; p. 548.

14. Fairley JW, Yardley MPJ, Durham LH. Pressure applied to middle turbinate causes pain at lower threshold than inferior turbinate or nasal septum (Abstract). Abstract book—14th Congress European Rhinologic Society, Rome, Oct. 6–10, 1992;96.

15. Pearce JMS. Chronic headache: the role of deformity of the nasal septum (letter to the editor). Br Med J 1984; 288:1005.

16. Takeshima T, Nishikawa S, Takahashi K. Cluster headache like symptoms due to sinusitis: evidence for neuronal pathogenesis of cluster headache syndrome. Headache 1988;28:207,208.

17. Faleck H, Rothner AD, Erenberg G, Cruse RP. Headache and subacute sinusitis in children and adolescents. Headache 1988;28:96–98.

18. Levine HL. Headache associated with sinus disease. In: Tollison CD, Kunkel RS, eds., Headache: Diagnosis and Treatment. Baltimore: Williams & Wilkins, 1993; pp. 247–256.

19. Rosenblum BN, Friedman WH. Paranasal sinus etiologies of headache and facial pain. In: Jacobson AL, Donlon WC, eds., Headache and Facial Pain. New York: Raven, 1990; pp. 233–244.

20. Friedman WH, Rosenblum BN. Paranasal sinus etiology of headaches and facial pain. Otolaryngol Clin North Amer 1989;22:1217–1228.

20a. Kennedy DW, ed., Sinus Disease: Guide to First-Line Management. Darien, CT: Health Communications, 1994; pp. 22–26.

21. Kennedy DW, Loury MC. Nasal and sinus pain: current diagnosis and treatment. Sem Neurol 1988;8:303–314.

22. Calhoun KH, Waggenspack GA, Simpson CB, Hokanson JA, Bailey BJ. CT evaluation of the paranasal sinuses in symptomatic and asymptomatic populations. Otolaryngol Head Neck Surg 1991;104: 480–483.

23. Havas TE, Motbey JA, Gullane PJ. Prevalence of incidental abnormalities on computed tomographic scans of the paranasal sinuses. Arch Otolaryngol Head Neck Surg 1988;114:856–859.

24. Wells WA. Some nervous and mental manifestations occurring in connection with nasal disease. Am J Med Sci 1898;116:677–692.

25. Roe JO. The frequent dependence of persistent and so-called congestive headaches upon abnormal conditions of the nasal passages. Med Record 1888;34:200–204.

26. Wolff HG. Headache and other head pain. Oxford University Press, New York, 1948; p. 499.

27. Eagle WW. Sphenopalatine ganglion neuralgia. Arch Otolaryngol 1942;35:66.

28. Vail HH. Vidian neuralgia. Ann Otol 1932;41:837–846.

29. Stewart D, Lambert V. The sphenopalatine ganglion. J Laryngol 1930;45:753–758.

30. Cushing H. The major trigeminal neuralgias and their surgical treatment, based on experiences with 332 Gasserian operations. The varieties of facial neuralgia. Am J Med Sci 1920;160:157–163.

31. Wolff HG. Headache and other head pains. Oxford University Press, New York, 1948; p. 502.

32. Manzoni GC, Prusinski A. Cluster headache. In: Olesen J, Tfelt-Hansen P, Welch KMA, eds., The Headaches. New York: Raven, 1993; p. 544.

33. Pratt FJ, Pratt JA. Intranasal Surgery. FA Davis, Philadelphia, 1924.

34. Bolger WE, Parsons DS, Matson RE. Functional endoscopic sinus surgery in aviators with recurrent sinus barotrauma. Aviat Space Environ Med 1990;61:148–156.

35. Bolger WE, Parsons DS. Treatment of recurrent sinus barotrauma in aviators: comparison of functional endoscopic and "classic" sinus surgery techniques. Am J Rhinol 1990;4:75–81.

36. Robbins L. Precipitating factors in migraine: a retrospective review of 494 patients. Headache 1994;34: 214–216.

37. Fairley JW. Personal communication.

38. Goldsmith AJ, Zahtz GD, Stegnjajic A, Shikowitz M. Middle turbinate headache syndrome. Am J Rhinol 1993;7:17–23.

39. Saunte C, Soyka D. Headache related to ear, nose, and sinus disorders. In: Olesen J, Tfelt-Hansen P, Welch KMA, eds., The Headaches. New York: Raven, 1993; pp. 753–757.

40. Ryan RE Sr, Ryan RE Jr. Headache of nasal origin. Headache 1979;19:170–173.

41. Koch-Henriksen N, Gammelgaard N, Hvidegaard T, Stoksted P. Chronic headache: the role of deformity of the nasal septum. Br Med J 1984;288:434,435.

42. Clerico DM, Fieldman RF. Referred headache of rhinogenic origin in the absence of sinusitis. Headache 1994;34:226–229.

43. Greenfield HJ. Headache and facial pain associated with nasal and sinus disorders: a diagnostic and therapeutic challenge. Part I. Insights in Otolaryngol 1990;5:2–8.

44. Greenfield HJ. Headache and facial pain associated with nasal and sinus disorders: a diagnostic and therapeutic challenge. Part II: Clinical application. Insights in Otolaryngol 1991;6:2–8.

45. Schønsted-Madsen U, Stoksted P, Christensen PH, Koch-Henriksen N. Chronic headache related to nasal obstruction. J Laryngol Otol 1986;100:165–170.

46. Chow JM. Rhinologic headaches. Otolaryngol Head Neck Surg 1994;111:211–218.

47. Castellanos J, Axelrod D. Flexible fiberoptic rhinoscopy in the diagnosis of sinusitis. J Allergy Clin Immunol 1989;83:91–94.

48. Cook PR, Nishioka GJ, Davis WE, McKinsey JP. Functional endoscopic sinus surgery in patients with normal computed tomography scans. Otolaryngol Head Neck Surg 1994;110:505–509.

49. Stammberger H, Wolf G. Headaches and sinus disease: the endoscopic approach. Ann Otol Rhinol Laryngol 1988;97(suppl. 134):3–23.

49a. Stammberger H. Functional endoscopic sinus surgery. Philadelphia: BC Decker, 1991; p. 444.

50. Bonaccorsi P. Primary headaches compared with idiopathic rhinogenic headaches: the actual diagnostic misunderstandings. European Rhinologic Society Annual Meeting, 1988.

51. Bonaccorsi P. Surgical therapy (neurovascular decompressive ethmoido-sphenoidectomy) and prophylaxis during developmental age of common, classic, complicated migraine and of cluster headache with rhinogenic pathogenesis. In: The Anatomo-Surgical approach to

Treatment of Migraine. Up-to-Date Meeting on Headache, Florence, Italy. Nov. 23, 1985: pp. 22–44.

52. Hoover S. Nasal pathophysiology of headaches and migraines. Rhinol 1988;26(suppl. 2):111–115.

53. Thomas WC. Obscure sinus infections. Med Times 1960;88:199–206.

54. Sicuteri F, Fusco BM, Marabini S, Campagnolo V, Maggi CA, Geppetti P. Fanciullacci M. Beneficial effect of capsicin application to the nasal mucosa in cluster headache. Clin J Pain 1989;5:49–53.

55. Fusco BM, Geppetti P. Fanciullacci M, Sicuteri F. Local application of capsicin for the treatment of cluster headache and trigeminal neuralgia. Cephalalgia 1991;11 (suppl. 11):234,235.

56. Stone H, Williams B, Carregal EJA. The role of the trigeminal nerve in olfaction. Exp Neurol 1968;21:11–19.

57. Ulrich CE, Haddock MP, Alarie Y. Airborne chemical irritants, role of the trigeminal nerve. Arch Environ Health 1972;24:37–42.

58. Fusco BM, Fiore G, Gallo F, Martelletti P, Giacovazzo M. "Capsaicin-sensitive" sensory neurons in cluster headache: pathophysiological aspects and therapeutic indication. Headache 1994;34:132–137.

59. Lewis JL, Hahn FF, Dahl AR. Transport of inhaled toxicants to the central nervous system: characteristics of a nose-brain barrier. In: Isaacson RL, Jensen KF, eds., The vulnerable brain and environmental risks, Vol 3: Toxins in Air and Water. New York: Plenum, 1994; pp. 77–103.

60. Calderon-Garciduenas L, Osorno-Velazquez A, Bravo-Alvarez H, Delgado-Chavez R, Barrios-Marquez R. Histopathologic changes of the nasal mucosa in southwest metropolitan Mexico City inhabitants. Am J Pathol 1992;140:225–231.

61. Kulle TJ, Cooper GP. Effects of formaldehyde and ozone on the trigeminal nasal sensory system. Arch Environ Health 1975;30:237–243.

62. Blau JN, Solomon F. Smell and other sensory disturbances in migraine. J Neurol 1985;232:275,276.

63. Raffaelli E, Martins O. A role for anticonvulsants in migraine. Funct Neurol 1986;1:495–498.

64. Hirsch AR. Olfaction in migraineurs. Headache 1992; 32:233–236.

65. Bruyn GW. Migraine equivalents. In: Vinken PJ, Bruyn GW, Klawans HL, eds., Handbooks of Clinical Neurology. New York: Elsevier, 1985: pp. 155–171.

66. Adams R, Victor M. Principles of neurology. New York, McGraw-Hill, 1989:183–189.

67. Skillern RH. The accessory sinuses of the nose. Philadelphia, J.B. Lippincott, 1913; p. 57,58.

68. Davidson JP. Indications for and method of operating upon the middle turbinated bone. Atlanta Journal—Record Medicine 1900;2:6–13.

69. Campbell JK, Sakai F. Migraine diagnosis and differential diagnosis. In: Olesen J, Tfelt-Hansen P, Welch KMA, eds., The Headaches. New York: Raven, 1993; p. 281.

22 Smell Disorders

Pathogenesis, Evaluation, and Treatment

Jill Razani, MA, *Terence M. Davidson,* MD, *and Claire Murphy,* PHD

CONTENTS

INTRODUCTION

Although it is estimated that 1–2% of the American population is anosmic (complete smell loss) or severely hyposmic (partial smell loss) and effectively without functional smell, this does not seem to be an issue with which most physicians are familiar or knowledgeable.

Losing one's sense of smell is not as obvious a handicap as losing one's vision or one's hearing. In fact, those who are smell impaired have learned to hide their disability. The fact remains that there are millions of Americans who are smell impaired, and we as physicians who wish to care for these individuals, particularly for their nasal health, have a responsibility to diagnose, treat, and be sensitive to this impairment.

One of the most interesting and informative studies published to date about the sense of smell appeared in *National Geographic (1)*. Those who truly wish to understand olfaction are strongly encouraged to read this article.

Before we begin discussing specific causes or mechanisms for smell loss, we would like to present a case study to give you a flavor for the diversity of the patients typically evaluated at nasal dysfunction clinics.

Case History: J. W.

Mrs. W. presented to the UCSD Nasal Dysfunction Clinic as a 43-yr-old female college counselor

From: *Diseases of the Sinuses* (M. E. Gershwin and G. A. Incaudo, eds.),
©1996 Humana Press Inc., Totowa, NJ.

complaining of nasal airway obstruction, left greater than right, and postnasal drip. History included significant nasal obstruction, rhinorrhea, postnasal discharge, and inhalant allergic symptomatology. The history also suggested a decrease in the sense of smell and parosmias (distorted sense of smell) associated with recurrent sinus infections. There was no history of phantosmia (perception of an odor in the absence of stimuli). The recurrent sinus infections had now occurred monthly over the last 3 yr and, in addition to the smell impairment, gave her a rather sour, unpleasant taste in her mouth.

The past medical history was noncontributory. Physical examination revealed a septum markedly obstructing the airway. Nasal endoscopy confirmed the severely deviated septum as well as identifying very abnormal appearing ethmoid sinuses in both middle meatuses.

Rhinomanometry (airway resistance) before and after Neo-synephrine showed elevated resistance, predominately in the obstructed nasal passage. Her IgE was elevated to twice the normal level. Olfactory threshold and odor identification testing revealed hyposmia.

Surgery was recommended, and the patient agreed. The patient underwent septoplasty and bilateral endoscopic sinus surgery. She made good postoperative recovery and returned to the head and neck surgery clinic several months later for her 3-mo follow-up. It just so happened on this day that the local newspaper had called to ask if we had any recent surgical successes that they could use as a happy Christmas story. Not only had Mrs. W's surgical procedure corrected her airway, decreased her congestion and discharge, and abolished her recurrent sinus infections, but it had also restored her sense of smell. The story in the box below was written by the local newspaper *(The San Diego Union)* and published on December 25, 1993.

"Surgery Lets Her Savor the Wonders of Holiday"

[J. W.] always hoped her Christmas dinners tasted good. This year she will know. An operation on her sinus system has restored her ability to smell and taste—just in time for the most fragrant and tasty time of the year. "I am smelling and tasting things again that I took for granted," she said. "It is so wonderful."

Her problems date to childhood. "I have always been able to taste a little, but not smell very well and I have never been able to correlate the two," she said.

Over time, the problems got worse. When the holidays would roll around, the smell of pine trees, the taste of chocolate—these pleasures, for the most part, escaped her.

She would make batches of hot buttered rum for her friends, who would tell her it was delicious. She would have to take their word for it. Her husband had long told her that an operation might help. Finally, in September, she had one.

Dr. Terence M. Davidson, director of UCSD's Nasal Dysfunction Clinic, performed an endoscopic sinus surgery. He corrected a deviated septum and unblocked her sinuses.

At first there was no change, but about 3 weeks before Christmas she again started smelling and tasting things. Now she is making up for lost time. She and her husband have been visiting fancy restaurants, ordering gourmet foods just to savor the aroma and flavor.

You learn to live with something, and then it changes and you say to yourself, "Why didn't I do this before?"

Today, the college counselor will spend much of her holiday in her kitchen, preparing a feast of turkey, ham, yams, potatoes and Belgian chocolate. "I am looking forward to it for the first time in a long time," she said. She has invited family and friends to celebrate with her. But there also will be the end of a family tradition, she said. Every year she has made Swedish rolls from scratch and every year she has burned them because she could not smell them cooking.

We call Mrs. W. our Happy Christmas patient.

ANATOMY AND PHYSIOLOGY OF OLFACTION

Anatomy

The olfactory epithelium, bulbs, and tract, as well as the olfactory areas in the brain and their communications with other centers constitute the olfactory system. The olfactory receptors are located in the olfactory epithelium, which lines the roof of the nasal cavity and extends to the nasal septum. The epithelium contains ciliated olfactory receptors, microvillar cells, supporting cells, and basal cells *(2)*. The olfactory receptor cells are bipolar neurons extending from the olfactory cleft into the olfactory bulb, and are specialized to detect odorants and transduce olfactory information into electrical impulses *(3)*. These neurons pass through the small openings in the cribriform plate and synapse in the olfactory bulb. The cell bodies of the neurons taper into thin, nonmyelinated axons joining other axons and are then formed into bundles by tubular sheaths of the meninges. These bundles join others to make up the nerve fibers of cranial nerve I (CNI).

Receptors in the olfactory epithelium are not uniform in density, but are interspersed with patches of respiratory epithelium. Receptors have been seen as far from the cleft as the middle turbinate. Volatile chemicals reach the olfactory epithelium by passive diffusion and by active sniffing. Olfactory gland secretions maintain a moist environment, which helps inhaled aromatic molecules to dissolve. Inhalation, exhalation, or retronasal air flow resulting from mouth and pharyngeal movements all enhance nasal air flow and facilitate olfaction *(4)*, presumably by increasing the number of odor molecules in the olfactory cleft. Duration, flow velocity, and volume of a sniff show variability among individuals, but consistency within an individual *(5)*. Altering sniffing strategies does not improve olfactory perception, since a subject's naturally chosen sniff appears to be optimum for him or her *(6)*.

To access the epithelium, an odor molecule must pass through the nasal cavity and diffuse through a mucous layer secreted by both Bowman's glands and by goblet cells in the respiratory mucosa. Thickness and composition of the mucus can influence the diffusion time to the olfactory receptors *(7–11)*. Almost paradoxically, moderately congested, wet, and red epithelium seems to facilitate

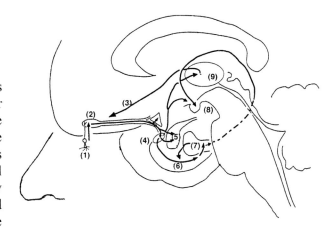

Fig. 1. Numbers in the diagram represent the following brain structures: (1) olfactory receptors; (2) olfactory bulb; (3) orbital frontal cortex; (4) piriform cortex; (5) amygdala; (6) entorhinal cortex; (7) hippocampus; (8) hypothalamus; (9) dorso-medial thalamus.

smell function *(8)*. The olfactory nerve (CNI) projects to the olfactory bulb, which is receptotopically organized. These first-order olfactory nerve fibers synapse with mitral and tufted cells, which are both vertically oriented. Axons from these cells project through the olfactory tracts to the olfactory cortex, which includes the anterior olfactory nucleus, the piriform cortex, the olfactory tubercle, the corticomedial amygdala, and the entorhinal cortex (*see* Fig. 1 for a diagram of these regions). From the olfactory cortex, higher-order fibers project to frontal cortex, thalamus, and limbic system.

In addition to input from the olfactory nerve, free nerve endings of three other cranial nerves (trigeminal, glossopharyngeal, and vagus) provide additional chemoreceptivity in the upper respiratory tract. The burning or irritation from trigeminal stimuli, such as ammonia or hot pepper, interacts with olfactory and gustatory inputs in what has been termed the common chemical sense. Stimulation of these receptors will usually precipitate nasal reflexes, such as sneezing and rhinorrhea, thereby exhaling the noxious stimulus.

Physiology

Transduction of odorant/chemical information into electrical impulses occurs in the receptors on the olfactory cilia. Odor molecules diffuse to the receptor sites in the cell membrane, opening the ionic channels, and electric current flows across the membrane and sets up a receptor potential that spreads from the cilia through the dendrite to the cell body. Depolarization of the cell body triggers action potentials that begin the transmission of electrical information to the olfactory bulb. How the information is coded for thousands of odorants and how that enables the odors to be discriminated are currently a very active area of research. Olfactory cortical areas, the basal forebrain, and the midbrain send efferent projections that modulate the activity in the olfactory bulb.

Within the olfactory cortex, the anterior olfactory nucleus connects the two bulbs together through the anterior commissure; the piriform cortex projects to the mediodorsal thalamus, which then projects to the orbitofrontal cortex. The olfactory tubercle is believed to receive dopaminergic fibers from the midbrain and has been thought to be involved with various functions of the limbic system. The corticomedial areas of the amygdala, believed to mediate emotional and motivational aspects of odor sensations, receive information from the olfactory bulbs. Finally, the entorhinal cortex projects directly into the hippocampus.

EVALUATION

All patients visiting the UCSD Nasal Dysfunction Clinic undergo a complete and thorough evaluation. Our current evaluation form is shown in Table 1. All patients are required to complete a medical history intake, ear, nose, and throat (ENT) examination, and a smell evaluation.

Medical History

Relevant information regarding the patient's medical history is gathered on the form shown on Table 1. The patient's history provides crucial information for making a correct diagnosis. Individuals with sinusitis typically present with the symptoms of nasal obstruction, congestion, postnasal drip, headache, and/or facial pain. Individuals with allergic rhinitis typically know that they have allergies, and may know whether this is seasonal or perennial. Predominant allergic symptoms are nasal congestion, itchy nose, itchy eyes, and sneezing. Sleep abnormalities are a common problem in today's society, and nasal dysfunction certainly contributes to sleep disturbance. In fact, the number of individuals with sleep apnea who are first identified by our nasal dysfunction history is impressive.

During the course of the medical history intake, it is important to consider all psychiatric and stress-related events in the patient's past and current life. Stress plays a major role in the interpretation of one's nasal disability, and although it may not be necessary to perform an extensive psychiatric intake history, it is very useful to consider the patient's stress, and where stress exists to understand how this impacts his or her nasal complaints. The remainder of the history form speaks for itself. History of past and current medications is important information to consider because there are many drugs known to affect the chemical senses, including both smell and taste.

Medical Examination

A general ENT examination is always performed. From a rhinologist's perspective, the middle ear is nothing more than a paranasal sinus adapted for audition. Although our otologic colleagues may not like this perspective, the middle ear is dependent on a healthy nose, and to some degree that which is occurring in the nose is reflected in and is visible at the otoscopic examination. The nasal examination is performed with a light, preferably a coaxial headlight, and with a nasal speculum. Most anatomic obstructions to breathing occur in and around the nasal valve, and these are readily identified at rhinoscopy. Septal deflections are present in virtually everyone, so it is only a question of degree. Where serious anatomic deviations are noted and are obstructive, they can be significant. Tip ptosis, the aging nose, or collapsed nasal valves (from age, surgery, or trauma) should also be noted. The mucosal color reflects nasal health. The normal nasal mucosa is pink. Allergy causes edema and because of increased venous vasculature and engorgement, often takes on a bluish hue. Infected nasal mucosa is typically erythematous with less edema than is seen with allergy. Irritated nasal mucosa is also erythematous and generally not edematous.

Secretions, when present, should be noted. Clear and/or white secretions are found in allergic rhinitis. Mucopurulent secretions are seen when infection is present. The lack of secretion is found in atrophic rhinitis. The oral pharyngeal exam is important, because nasal secretions drain through the nasal pharynx and oral pharynx. Infected secretions leave inflamed mucosa on the lateral pharyngeal walls, and often the only and most readily

Table 1
Sample Evaluation Form

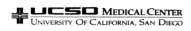 **UCSD** MEDICAL CENTER
UNIVERSITY OF CALIFORNIA, SAN DIEGO

NASAL DYSFUNCTION ASSESSMENT

SEND REPORTS TO
- ❏ HILLCREST (8654)
- ❏ LA JOLLA (0970)
- ❏ MIRA MESA (8217)

Source _____ Date _____

Patient Identification

DATE	REFERRED BY	AGE	SEX	OCCUPATION

COPIES TO	HOME PHONE	BUSINESS PHONE

HISTORY
_____
_____
_____

Scale: 0 = No Disability/Complaint   100 = Maximum Disability/Complaint

_____ Nasal obstruction   _____ Sleep disturbance
_____ Nasal congestion   _____ Stress
_____ Post nasal drip   _____ Itchy eyes
_____ Cough   _____ Hearing loss
_____ Hoarseness   _____ Tinnitus
_____ Itchy nose   _____ Vertigo
_____ Sneezing   _____ # Ear infections

Seasonal allergies: _____ x _____ years
Perennial allergies: _____ x _____ years
Asthma: _____ x _____ years

_____ Nasal Discharge   Color: ❏ clear ❏ white ❏ colored
_____ Irritative Rhinitis
        Sources: ❏ air ❏ home ❏ work ❏ closed building
_____ Stress Induced Rhinitis
_____ Gustatory Rhinitis

Infections: ❏ none   ❏ occasional   ❏ recurrent   ❏ persistent

Head and facial pains: Frequency _____   Intensity _____
    Sites: ❏ forehead ❏ temple ❏ orbital ❏ maxillary
           ❏ other _____

❏ Smell loss   ❏ Parosmia   ❏ Phantosmia   ❏ Dysosmia
❏ Taste loss   ❏ Dysgeusia ❏ Burning mouth

Past Medical History:

Medical Illness _____
_____

Operations _____
_____

Medications _____
_____

Allergies _____
_____

Endoscopy
_____
_____
_____
_____

Examination:

Ears _____
_____

Nose _____
_____

OP _____

Mouth _____
_____

Neck _____
_____

Other _____

Laboratory   RAW SCORES
Olfaction: R; BT _____ + _____ = _____   BT ____ ID ____
            L; BT _____ + _____ = _____   BT ____ ID ____
UPSIT _____   DX _____
Taste: ❏ Normal   ❏ Hypogeusia   ❏ Ageusia

RHINOMANOMETRY		Before	After
	R		
	L		

Cytology   **Rhinologic Diagnosis**
Cells/HPF   ❏ Infection   ❏ Rhino. neuralgia
_____ Goblet   ❏ Allergy   ❏ Smell impairment
_____ Eosinophils   ❏ Irritation   ❏ Inflammatory
_____ Basophils   ❏ Anatomic Obstruction ❏ Trauma
_____ Neutrophils   ❏ Septum   ❏ Post viral
_____ Bacteria   ❏ Valve   ❏ Chemical
                                       ❏ Tip ptosis   ❏ Aging
_____ IgE   ❏ Vasometer (stress)   ❏ Taste impairment
_____ IgA   ❏ Rhinitis medicamentosa ❏ Other
_____ IgG
_____ IgM

Skin Test: ❏ Negative   Positives _____
_____
_____

CT Scan

Scale:	R	L		Stage _____
0 = Normal	___	___	OMC	0 = No disease
1 = Up to ¼ diseased	___	___	Ethmoid	1 = 1 cell
2 = Up to ½ diseased	___	___	Maxillary	2 = > 1 cell on on 1 side
3 = Up to ¾ diseased	___	___	Frontal	3 = Bilateral disease
4 = Opacified	___	___	Sphenoid	4 = Pansinusitis
	___	___	Olfactory Cleft	

available signs of infectious sinusitis are the red streaks coursing down the lateral pharyngeal walls. With allergic rhinitis, the pharyngeal mucosa is often edematous and therefore pale. For those with sleep disorders, the size and position of the uvula and soft palate should be noted. Oral cavity and cervical examination are part of the routine ENT examination, and at least a cursory look and palpation are appropriate.

Nasal endoscopy is crucial to the appropriate evaluation of smell and taste disorders. For those with appropriate skills, the very finest examination is performed with 4- and 2.7-mm rigid, glass rods. The nasal cavity is inspected with these endoscopes. The mucosa is vasoconstricted with a topical decongestant and then anesthetized with a topical, local anesthetic. The entire nasal cavity is examined. This includes the anterior nose, the nasal floor all the way back to and including the posterior choana, and nasal pharynx. The inferior meatus should be examined. Next, the middle meatus is examined and special attention paid to the osteomeatal complex since most sinus disease begins in this area. With careful examination, the hiatus semilunaris containing drainage from the frontal sinus, maxillary sinus, and anterior ethmoid sinuses can be seen. The sphenoid sinus ostium is seen at the back of the nose just medial to the middle turbinate. The superior nasal cavity is then examined, and particular attention is paid to the olfactory cleft. Certainly, large fungating tumors will be diagnosed, as well as polyps and infection. The endoscopist's ability to diagnose olfactory abnormalities is debatable. If the olfactory cleft is obstructed either for anatomic reasons or from tumor, this is readily identified. If inflammation exists, this can often be noted in the olfactory cleft and is certainly consistent with an inflammatory smell impairment. Whether the endoscopist can discern the scarring that may be present with postviral hyposmia or the absence of olfactory epithelium, which occurs in posttraumatic anosmia, is difficult to say. Nonetheless, what one sees must correlate with one's final diagnosis.

Flexible nasal endoscopy is performed by many physicians. However, the clarity of information gathered is not as good as with rigid endoscopes. Nonetheless, it is a far superior examination to a flashlight and nasal speculum. Rigid nasal endoscopy requires training and technical abilities, and those without that training and ability are far less

likely to injure an individual when using the flexible scope.

Anterior rhinomanometry is performed on all patients. Results are reported in units of resistance. Although it is difficult to quantify precisely the relationship of rhinomanometry values to nasal anatomy and function, one develops a certain sense about the individual's nasal air flow. As an example, those who have a marked decrease in resistance after decongestion are certainly suspect for inflammatory illness, most notably, allergic rhinitis or occasionally rhinitis medica mentosa. Those with a marked resistance after decongestion have anatomic obstructions. Another interesting finding is that many times although the air flows fall close to or within normal limits, one will, following decongestion, note an asymmetry from one side to the other. This seems to be a far greater concern to individuals than has been previously discussed or recognized. Individuals expect a certain symmetry in their bodies and will compare one side to another. For example, if the left side is widely patent and the right side is significantly less patent, the individual will feel that either the left or the right side is in one way or another abnormal. One can explain this to the individual. Many will wish the asymmetry to be corrected.

Rhinomanometry is also useful in identifying individuals with atrophic rhinitis or widely patent nasal airways. Individuals require a certain resistance to inspiration, and they like to feel the air sucking into and passing through their nose. If their airways are too widely open or if they have undergone mucosal atrophy from aging or other cause, they no longer perceive the sensory input of inspiration and will often report that they cannot breathe. The fact of the matter is that they breathe too easily. This is extremely important, because if one took the patient's complaint at face value, one might be tempted to open the airway further. This would be a catastrophe. Acoustic rhinomanometry (AR) is another useful analysis of nasal chamber anatomy. We have little experience with AR.

Nasal cytology is performed by taking a small sample of nasal mucus using a rhinoprobe, shown in Fig. 2. The nasal mucus is spread on a glass slide, and prepared with hematoxylin eosin or Giemsa staining. The cytologist then grades the sample for goblet cells, eosinophils, basophils, neutrophils, and bacteria. When more than one or two eosinophils or basophils are seen per high-power field,

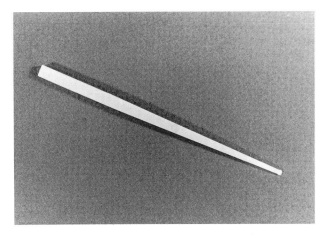

Fig. 2. Rhinoprobe used for nasal cytology examination.

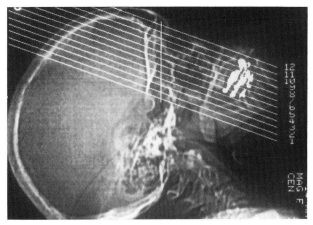

Fig. 3. CT scan of the sinuses.

one must suspect an allergic rhinitis or at least an allergic component to the individual's disease. By the same token, when the eosinophils and basophils are strikingly absent and all that is present are neutrophils and/or bacteria, one must know that there is an infectious process occurring. Fungi are not normally seen in nasal smears. Their presence must point one toward the diagnosis of a fungal rhinitis or sinusitis. Occasionally, malignant cells will be first identified at cytology and then appropriate examination will focus on the malignancy.

Ciliary motility is essential to a healthy nose. Dysmotility certainly impairs respiratory and olfactory function. Can we measure motility changes in inflammatory rhinitis? If so, will this assist in diagnosis and treatment? Some ability to evaluate ciliary function is important. Available options include saccharin motility tests, light microscope inspection, and electron microscopy.

We often measure serum IgE, and our suspicions for IgE-mediated allergy are usually confirmed. Skin testing or radioallergosorbent tests (RAST) looking for IgE-mediated allergy are important. Inhalant allergies are now ubiquitous within our population and so should be closely examined. We typically use a 10-inhalant screening panel. The current data suggest that these will discover 90% of common allergies. More extensive skin testing or RAST panels are only used when indicated for environmental control, specific identification, or when immunotherapy is planned. Other immunoglobulins are not routinely obtained, but there are cases in which they should be considered. A complete blood count (CBC) with differential to look at the percent of eosinophils is an indicator of allergy.

A limited sinus CT scan, when evaluating olfactory dysfunction, is always performed. Contrast media are not required, and with a limited series, both cost and radiation exposure are kept to a minimum. Our typical scan includes 5-mm coronal and 10-mm axials. If the patient cannot extend the head for the coronal scans, 5-mm axials are taken. The scout films are shown in Fig. 3. Although the CT scan is most commonly used to look for sinus disease, we also use it in evaluating smell dysfunction to examine the olfactory cleft. The following case demonstrates this point.

Case Example

Mr. T. is a 33-yr-old man who presented to the UCSD Nasal Dysfunction Clinic with a history that he fell from a height of 14 feet, struck his head, and since that time has had no sense of smell or taste. He will eat the same foods day in and day out because he denies any ability to taste them. He eats less since he has little appetite. He eats to maintain health and to be social. Such foods as ice cream, which he used to enjoy, have no taste, and he eats them with the same indifference that he eats other foods. He can eat the same foods for 5–7 d without any dislike. The patient has on several occasions consumed spoiled milk and either vomited or had diarrhea, mistakes that would not normally be made by individuals with intact smell. He has no other specific nasal symptoms.

On physical examination, his ears, nose, oral pharynx, mouth, and neck are normal. Nasal endoscopy was performed using rigid endoscopes. There was no evidence of inflammatory disease.

The olfactory cleft could be seen anteriorly, and no olfactory epithelium was identified.

Odor threshold and identification testing was performed, and the patient demonstrated bilateral anosmia. He had some trouble identifying ammonia, although he did have trigeminal sensation. A University of Pennsylvania Odor Identification Test (UPSIT) was performed and he scored 5, a score that is on the border between anosmia and malingering. Rhinomanometry was performed before and after Neo-synephrine, and no abnormalities were noted. His cytology as well as his sinus CT scan were normal.

Based on the above information, a diagnosis of posttraumatic anosmia was made, and the patient was counseled about the use of smoke alarms, gas detectors, and spoiled and rotten food precautions.

Smell Evaluation

The following olfactory tests are routinely administered at the UCSD Nasal Dysfunction Clinic. A summary of each of these procedures, as well as procedures used by other clinics, is presented in Table 1. A forced-choice, ascending, olfactory threshold test for the odorant *n*-butyl alcohol is administered to assess smell sensitivity. The patient is presented with a series of odor concentrations in ascending (to avoid adaptation) order. Each bottle containing the odorant is presented with a second bottle containing distilled water (blank). The patient is required to smell the contents of both bottles and decide which of the two contains the stronger odor. The patient's threshold is determined by five successive correct responses (12).

During the smell evaluation, patients are also given odor identification tests. A 10-item forced-choice odor identification test or its analog child version is commonly used for assessing odor identification ability. This odor identification test consists of 10 (the child version consists of 8) common everyday odorants (e.g., chocolate, coffee, baby powder) presented in opaque jars. The patient is required to close his or her eyes and smell the contents of the jar after being familiarized with a cue sheet that contains the names (or pictures for the child version) of the odors presented among a number of distracter odor names (or pictures). This test is designed to produce 90–100% accurate performance in normal subjects.

A second odor identification test is the UPSIT, which is a commercially available examination. The UPSIT consists of a 40-item, microencapsulated (scratch-and-sniff) odor identification test. The patient is asked to scratch the label, sniff, and choose the best answer from a four-alternative list offered for each odor. One advantage of using the UPSIT is the well-developed norms for different age groups. This test may also be sensitive to malingering, since even if a patient cannot identify any of the odors, he or she will score at least 25% correctly owing to chance alone. Thus, a malingering patient may choose to not identify any of the odors correctly, in which case he or she would score lower than the chance level and thus the performance would be suspect. This test may be desirable because of its ease of administration. It is particularly useful for a practicing physician who may want to have a rough idea of olfactory function. In such a case, the UPSIT is a good choice because of its ease of administration and interpretation. However, it should be noted that in some cases, it is important to administer a threshold detection test, since some recent reports suggest that discrepant results can be diagnostic of parosmia and/or phantosmia (13).

Patients with smell dysfunction often complain of taste loss. This is not surprising given the close relationship of the two systems. In fact, a large portion of what we commonly refer to as taste is smell. As explained in the Physiology section, taste and smell are closely related. Odors enhance the flavor of food; thus, patients commonly mistake smell dysfunction for taste problems. In cases where taste abnormalities cannot be ruled out during the medical interview and/or by smell testing, the patient's sense of taste is assessed. Taste testing for all four taste qualities (i.e., sweet, sour, salt, and bitter) is assessed by the method of magnitude estimation (*see* Table 1 for details). The patient's ability to distinguish between (and identify) the different taste qualities, as well as his or her ability to detect differing concentration intensities is assessed by this method. Taste loss and dysgeusia (taste distortions or phantom taste) are assessed by this method.

Evoked response olfactometry is currently being investigated in our clinic. It holds promise for research and possibly for some clinical applications.

DIAGNOSES AND TREATMENT

Based on the above evaluations, we are generally able to make a diagnosis and then recommend an appropriate treatment should such exist. There are times in which we are not certain of the diagnosis, and in these cases, it has become our common practice to prescribe a 7- or 8-d course of systemic prednisone. The usual prescription is 60 mg for 5 d and then a taper of 40, 20, and 10 mg. If there is an element of infection, antibiotics are prescribed concurrently. This will return the sense of smell to those whose smell disorder is potentially reversible, and it identifies those who require treatment for their inflammatory illness. If the patient does not regain smell on prednisone and antibiotics, the only other treatments that have been recommended and have had any success are the administration of some trace metals, such as zinc. It is sometimes reasonable to measure the patient's electrolytes, including trace metals, such as zinc, copper, magnesium, and manganese, and if a deficiency is noted, a prescription for large replacement doses of these minerals is appropriate. The blanket prescription of "buy some vitamins and minerals" does not supply the minerals in sufficient quantities, and since it is such a rare individual who, in fact, responds to this therapy, it is easier and better to measure the serum levels and replace them only in those who are deficient. Those who do not respond and for whom no other obvious correctable lesion is identified can then be so advised and appropriately counseled. Figure 4 is an algorithm we developed at one time to assist the smell disorder evaluator. This is reproduced for the reader's interest.

The majority of patients with smell disorders cannot reasonably expect a return to normal smell function. These patients need to be counseled regarding the fact that their sense of smell will not return to normal. It is important that they recognize their disability. They are unable to smell smoke as an early warning sign of fire. It is therefore important that they have smoke detectors placed in every room in which a fire might develop and in every room in which they sleep. The kitchen and the room with the family fireplace and/or furnace require a smoke detector. The bedroom requires a smoke detector, and if the patient has a favorite chair or couch on which he or she often sits and falls asleep, this room too must have a smoke detector. Patients cannot smell the odorants placed in propane and natural gas. They cannot smell the odor of petroleum and related products. If they have gas appliances, they should be encouraged to switch to electric. If that is not practical, then these rooms should be fitted with gas detectors. The best gas detectors are available at Marine stores. Very acceptable gas detectors are available through recreational vehicle stores, and many gas companies keep information about available gas detectors.

Patients must be counseled about spoiled and rotten food because one's primary forewarning of contaminated food comes from its malodor. The best advice is to befriend a tester. Whether this is a friend or spouse is irrelevant. If all foods are tested by someone with normal olfaction, the smell impaired will save themselves the difficulties of gastrointestinal distress as well as Botulinus poisoning, and so forth. Those who do not have such sniffers available must develop and maintain a spoiled and rotten food patrol. This basically requires throwing out leftovers that are subject to spoilage and being very careful when eating at restaurants.

The greatest pleasure of food is olfactory. Many individuals with smell impairment feel that food has lost its flavor and can never be enjoyed. Although this is to some degree true, there are things one can do to improve this enjoyment. Keep in mind that people who are congenitally anosmic appear to enjoy food every bit as much as those who have a normal sense of smell. These individuals have somehow learned to appreciate the appearance, the texture, the temperature, the consistency, and the contributions of sweet, sour, salt, and bitter. We have found that some of our more positive-thinking patients have learned to enjoy food. They do so by preparing the food carefully and presenting it in an attractive fashion, surrounding the meal with enjoyable input, such as music, candlelight, and pleasant table discussion. We advise people to be careful about the overuse of salt and sugar since these are not healthy. We recommend that individuals can develop and increase enjoyment in trigeminal stimulation by using curry and chili products. Keep in mind that much of the foods eaten in Southeast Asia and India are simply rice with very little added to it. These dishes are made more attractive by adding different curries, and to some degree, the natives enjoy the burn; natives substitute the trigeminal burn for the missing olfactory stimulus. The same can be done for those who have lost their sense of smell,

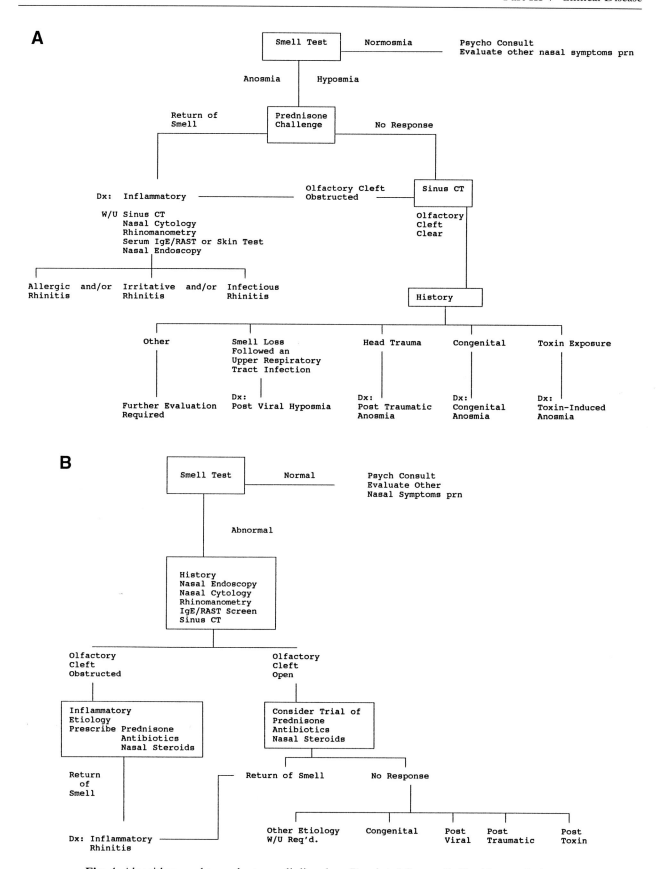

Fig. 4. Algorithm used to evaluate smell disorders. Reprinted from ref. *68* with permission.

and although this is not the solution for all, it has helped a number of patients.

The most exhaustive differential diagnosis known to us for smell disorders was published by Feldman et al. *(14)*. It is included here as Table 2. We have chosen those diagnoses that are either interesting or medically important, and the following pages describe the clinical and psychophysical aspects of these illnesses.

HEAD TRAUMA

The mechanism of posttraumatic olfactory injury can be divided into three general categories: injury to the olfactory nerve fibers, injury to the nose and nasal passages, and injury to olfactory brain centers. The olfactory nerve consists of many fragile fibers that extend from the olfactory epithelium in the nose through the cribriform plate of the ethmoid bone to the cortical cells in the olfactory bulb. It is at the cribriform that the olfactory system is most vulnerable to injury. The amount of force created within the cranium during an injury to the head may cause severing or stretching of the olfactory nerve fibers. When these nerve fibers are damaged, retrograde degeneration of the nerve fibers occurs and causes receptor cell degeneration. It has been hypothesized that, in some cases, the nerve fibers regenerate and reconnect. Although regeneration of severed olfactory fibers has been documented in animals, it has not yet been demonstrated in humans.

Head trauma damaging nasal structures can obstruct the nasal passages, thereby blocking access to the sensory regions of the nose. This can cause olfactory impairment. Provided that more proximal olfactory pathways are not damaged, repair of nasal structures and restoring nasal patency should result in improved olfactory function. Traumatic brain injury, often resulting from closed head injury, can cause contusions, intracranial bleeds, and diffuse axonal injury, all of which can injure olfactory brain centers. Recovery from cortical contusions, brain edema, or intracranial hemorrhage may explain some improvement in olfactory function.

Smell loss owing to head injury was documented as early as the 1800s by Ferrier *(15)* and others. It is currently estimated that approx 1 out of every 400 people in the US suffers from a head injury, and of those, somewhere between 5 and 30% have partial (hyposmia) or complete loss of smell (anosmia) owing to the injury *(16)*. It has been reported that head trauma accounts for approx 14% of all chemosensory disorders in the major chemosensory clinics. However, it should be noted that the proportion of olfactory dysfunction for which head trauma accounts is dependent on the reporting clinic referral base. These data are suggestive, but are no substitute for epidemiological studies and data.

The likelihood of suffering an olfactory loss can be correlated with the severity of the head trauma. Heywood et al. *(17)* used the Glasgow Coma Scale to categorize patients by severity of head trauma. They found that in the mild head-injured group, 40% of the patients suffered some degree of smell loss, whereas in the moderate head-injury group, 78% had smell impairments. They found that the severe injury group had the highest number of smell deficits (92%).

The site of the head injury seems to be an important factor in the development of smell impairment. Sumner *(18)* reported that smell loss resulting from blows to the occipital area resulted in anosmia 21% of the time, but that blows to the frontal or dorsotemporal regions resulted in anosmia only 3.9–10.4% of the time. This study is particularly interesting given that the incidence of frontal region injury was higher (79%), yet the occipital area injury was more likely to result in anosmia.

The different olfactory function tests may aid in diagnosing and locating neural damage. In general, shearing of olfactory nerve fibers results in anosmia, although there is some evidence suggesting that during the recovery and nerve regeneration phase, patients experience only a partial smell loss. Patients with facial trauma often experience partial or unilateral smell loss. Partial smell loss and laterality might also suggest olfactory bulb contusion or damage to higher neural pathways. Furthermore, patients with dysosmia will often show discrepancies between olfactory threshold and odor identification tests. In a recent study, Quionez et al. *(13)* showed that patients suffering from parosmia only and those suffering from both parosmia (distortions in the sense of smell) and phantosmia (smell sensation in the absence of an odor stimuli), but not patients suffering from phantosmia only showed discrepancies between their odor threshold and odor identification results. The data from patients whose olfactory detection threshold falls within the normal range, but are unable to identify

Table 2
List of Possible Differential Diagnoses Known to Cause Smell Impairment[a]

Lesions of the nose/airway
   Structural abnormality
      Deviated septum
      Weakness of alae nasi
Nasal polypi
   Allergic rhinitis
      Seasonal
      Perennial
   Vasomotor rhinitis
   Atrophic rhinitis
   Chronic inflammatory rhinitis
      Syphilis
      Tuberculosis
      Sarcoidosis
      Scleroma
      Leprosy
      Wegener's granulomatosis
      Midline granuloma
   Adenoid hypertrophy
   Sjogrens syndrome
   Hypertrophic rhinitis
   Rhinitis medicamentosa
   Infections and viral
      Influenza or acute viral rhinitis
      Acute viral hepatitis
      Bacterial rhinosinusitus
      Bronchiectasis
      Infected teeth and gums
      Infected tonsils
      Others
         Fungal
         Rickettsial
         Microfilarial
Nutritional/metabolic
   Vitamin deficiency
      Vitamin A
      Vitamin B_6
      Vitamin B_{12}
   Trace metal deficiencies
      Zn
      Cu
   Protein calorie malnutrition
   Total parenteral nutrition (without adequate
      replacement)
   Cystic fibrosis
      Hamartomas
         Scars/previous infarcts
   Myasthenia gravis
   Retinitis pigmentosa
   Vascular insufficiency and anoxia
      Small multiple CVAs
      Transient ischemic attacks
      Subclavian steal syndrome

Others
   Cerebral abscess (esp. frontal or ethmoidal regions)
   Meningitis
   Syphilis
   Syringomyelia
   Paget's disease
   Korsakoff's disease
   Hydrocephalus
   Migraine
Endocrine
   Adrenal cortical insufficiency—Addison's disease
   Congenital adrenal hyperplasia
   Cushing's syndrome
   Hypothyroidism
   Diabetes mellitus
   Primary amenorrheas
      Chromatin negative gonadal dysgenesis—
         Turner's syndrome
      Hypogonadotrophic hypogonadism
      Kallmann's syndrome
   Hypergonadotrophic hypogonadism
   Pseudohypoparathyroidism
   Panhypopituitarism
   Gigantism
   Adiposogenital dystrophy—Froelich's syndrome
Congenital/hereditary etiologies
   Syndrome of hypogeusia and hyposmia
   Triad of:
      Submucous cleft of dorsal hard palate
      Facial hypoplasia
      Stunted growth
   "Red haired disease" with pigmentary abnormality
   Complete and specific anosmias of genetic origin
   Bronchial asthma
Opiates
   Codeine
   Hydromophone HCI
   Morphine
Psychopharmaceuticals (e.g., psilocybin, LSD)
Sympathomimetics
   Amphetamine sulfate
   Phenmetrazine theoclate
   Fenbutrazate HCI
Others
   Antipyrine
   Oral ETOH
   Local vasoconstrictors
   Cimetidine
   L-DOPA
Chemical pollutants (gaseous)
   Sult'uric acid
   Hydrogen selenide
   Phosphorus oxychloride

Table 2 *(continued)*

Pepper and cresol mixture	Other benign or malignant nasal tumors
Benzene	Conductive effect (e.g., adenocarcinoma)
Benzol	Perceptive effect (e.g., schwannoma,
Butyl acetate	neurofibroma)
Carbon disulfide	Nasopharyngeal tumors with extension
Ethyl acetate	Paranasal tumors with extension
Formaldehyde	Leukemic infiltration
Hydrazine	Neoplasms—carcinomas
Oil of peppermint	Lung
Trichloroethylene	Gastrointestinal tract
Hydrogen sulfide	Ovary/breast
Paint solvents	Neurologic
Chlorine	Familial dysautonomia
Benzine	Refsum's syndrome
Nitrous gases	Multiple sclerosis
Industrial dusts (particulate)	Parkinson's disease
Coke/coal	Temporal lobe epilepsy
Grain	Mesial temporal sclerosis
Silicone dioxide	Multiple lentigines syndrome
Spices	Orbital hypertelorism
Flour	Trauma (most common proposed mechanisms:
Cotton	(1) shearing of olfactory nerves; and (2) hemorrhage
Paper	of the basal frontal lobes and bruising of the olfactory
Cement	bulbs and tracts)
Cadmium	Frontal fracture (esp. fronto-ethmoidal fracture)
Ashes	Occipital contrecoup injury
Lead	Nasal fracture
Abetal ipoproteinemia	Drugs
Chronic renal failure	Adrenal steroids (chronic usage)
Cirrhosis of liver	Amino acid excess
Gout	Histidine
Whipple's disease	Cysteine
Neoplasms—intracranial	Anesthetics, local
Osteomas	Procaine HCI
Olfactory groove and cribriform plate	Cocaine HCI
meningiomas	Tetracaine HCI
Frontal lobe tumors (esp. gliomas)	Anticancer agents (e.g., methotrexate)
Paraoptic chiasma tumors	Antihistamines (e.g., chlorpheniramine maleste)
Pituitary tumors (esp. adenomas)	Antimicrobials
Craniopharyngioma	Griseofillvin
Suprasellar meningioma	Lincomycin
Aneurysms	Streptomycin
Suprasellar cholesteatoma	Tetracyclines
Temporal lobe tumors	Intranasal tyrothricin
Midline cranial tumors	Local neomycin
Parasagittal meningiomas	Neoarsphenamine
Tumors of the corpus callosum	Antirheumatics
Neoplasms—intranasal	Mercury or gold salts
Neuro-olfactory	D-Penicillamine
Esthesioneuroepithelioma	Antithyroids
Esthesioneuroblastoma	Methimazole
Esthesioneurocytoma	Propylthiouracil
Esthesioepithelioma	Thiouracil

(continued)

Table 2 *(continued)*

Hyperlipoproteinemia medications	Radiation therapy
Clofibrate	Arteriography
Cholestyramine	Influenza vaccination
Intranasal saline solutions with:	Maintenance hemodialysis
Acetylcholine	Thyridectomy
Acetyl, β-methylcholine	Hypophysectomy
Menthol strychnine	Adrenalectomy
Zinc sulfate	Orchiectomy
Chromium	Oophorectomy
Nickel	Gastrectomy
Chalk	Psychiatric
Potash	Schizophrenic disorders
Iron carboxyl	Olfactory reference syndrome
Medical intervention	Depressive disorders
Laryngectomy	Hysteria
Rhinoplasty	Malingering
Anterior craniotomy	Presbyosmia
Surgical interruption of olfactory tract	Physiological processes
Frontal lobotomy	Circadian variation
Temporal lobotomy	Menses
Paranasal sinus exenteration	Pregnancy
Post anesthesia	Idiopathic

[a]It should be noted that this is an exhaustive list and that most of these diagnoses are quite rare in the general population. Adapted from ref. *14* with permission.

the standard number of odor stimuli, suggest that there are possibly more central types of damage *(19,20)*. In addition, the results from several studies suggest that odor discrimination is associated with the orbital frontal and temporal cortices *(21,22)*.

Parosmia has been reported by a number of patients with head trauma. In some cases, parosmia is a sign of nerve regeneration and the return (at least partially) of the sense of smell *(23)*. In other cases, parosmia can be severe, persistent, and intrusive. As a means of testing whether the parosmia is central or otherwise, the olfactory neuroepithelium can be anesthetized, and if the distorted smell persists, then it is probable that the problem is central *(23)*. Furthermore, patients with temporal lobectomy and temporal lobe epilepsies have displayed impairment in odor recognition *(24,25)*.

The recovery of olfactory function following head injury is thought to depend on the etiology of the olfactory dysfunction. However, in general, it appears that approx one-third of head trauma patients with smell loss recover. Sumner *(18)* reports that 39% of patients that recover do so within the first 10 wk. Data from Sumner *(18)* combined with those of Costanzo and Becker *(26)* suggest that the prognosis for recovery is very poor

for those patients who have not shown signs of improvement in olfactory function within 6–18 mo.

Helping the patient and family members understand the meaning of olfactory losses after head injury, recovery trends, and compensatory strategies is an essential part of the rehabilitative process. Education and reassurance that olfactory impairment is a relatively common sequela of brain injury will help limit patients' frustration and anxiety regarding their olfactory losses.

ALLERGIC RHINITIS

The prevalence of allergic rhinitis is thought to range from 10 to 15% in the general population *(27)* and can be classified in two categories: seasonal and perennial. Persons with symptoms that appear primarily during certain times of the year are considered to have seasonal allergic rhinitis. Ragweed, trees, and grasses are among the most common seasonal allergens. Persons with symptoms that persist for over 2 h/d for more than 9 mo of the year are considered to have perennial allergic rhinitis. Dust mites, indoor molds, and animal danders are among the most prevalent causes of perennial allergic rhinitis.

Pollen's role in initiating allergic rhinitis was discovered as early as the 1800s *(28),* with the role of reaginic antibodies and histamines later discovered. It was found that a histamine-like substance is released from cells in the skin by the interaction of antigen and antibody. In the early 1970s, it was demonstrated that IgE antibodies bind to the surface of basophils and mast cells, which led to the understanding that allergic rhinitis involves the interaction of inhaled pollen antigen with IgE antibodies.

Evaluation

Evaluation of allergic rhinitis, as with all other disorders, should begin with a comprehensive history. The age, gender, and family-related conditions of the patients should be considered carefully, since the incidence with which allergic rhinitis occurs changes with respect to these factors. Once a history has been taken, a complete ENT examination should be performed.

Skin testing and RAST for specific IgE antibodies are the two most widely used methods for confirming the diagnosis of allergic rhinitis. For the skin-testing method, either the surface of the skin is punctured or the antigen extracts are injected intradermally. In a patient experiencing an allergic reaction, histamine is released from the mast cells, causing an inflammatory reaction, classically described as wheal and flare, within minutes.

The RAST is the best known and most widely used in vitro test for measuring IgE levels. Although it has been reported that total IgE levels are elevated in only 40% of patients with allergic rhinitis and that there is considerable overlap between allergic and nonallergic patients in elevation of IgE levels, low levels of IgE can help in excluding allergic disease. The RAST examines specific antibodies that bind to antigen-coated disks, thus making it possible to quantify allergen-specific IgE antibodies.

Smell Disturbances and Treatments

There are few studies on allergic rhinitis and the sense of smell. In an early study, Fein et al. (29) found that anosmia is a problem in many of the more severe cases of nasal allergy (particularly when accompanied by nasal polyps and infection in the sinuses). These authors noted that in order to decrease the incidence of severe anosmia, early therapy for mild allergy should be instituted in order to prevent secondary infection.

The cause of smell loss owing to allergic rhinitis remains unclear. Smell loss may be the result of long-term effects of allergy (not measured by the effects of acute inflammation) or toxicity and/or injury to receptor cells. It is further thought that the anosmia and hyposmia associated with allergic rhinitis may be owing to nasal obstruction, which limits the air flow into the nasal cavity. However, a recent study by Cowart et al. (27) does not substantiate this. Cowart and her colleagues found that even substantial obstruction and low air-flow resistance did not produce clinically significant reductions in the ability to smell.

Some studies have reported that patients with inflammatory related smell disturbances respond to corticosteroid therapy, and others have suggested antimicrobial therapy. In either case, these observations suggest that the inflammatory conditions caused by either infectious or allergic conditions can produce reversible hyposmia.

CHRONIC SINUSITIS AND NASAL POLYPOSIS

It has been estimated that 13% of the population suffer from chronic sinusitis, and approx 9% report having nasal polyps. The major symptoms of chronic sinusitis are nasal obstruction, chronic rhinorrhea, nasal congestion, postnasal drip, headache, and craniofacial pain. These symptoms are often disruptive and, for some incapacitating. In most patients, the condition persists over 3 mo, and 3.5% of the cases require hospitalization.

Chronic Sinusitis

Chronic sinusitis is a result of the interaction between local anatomic factors, host immunocompetence, and sinonasal mucosal reactivity (30). Changes in any or all of these factors may result in the development of chronic inflammatory disease. Maintenance of ventilation in the osteomeatal complex is important for prevention and treatment of chronic sinusitis.

The anterior ethmoid cells are the primary instigators of inflammatory changes in the larger sinuses. In untreated patients, the anterior ethmoid is the area that most often shows chronic mucosal thickening, as shown on computed tomography (CT) scans (30). Inflammation ultimately impairs the mucociliary transport system. The anterior ethmoids are the first to be affected with secondary involvement of the osteomeatal complex and subsequent obstruction and involvement of the maxillary and frontal sinuses. Superior meatal disease involves the postethmoid sinuses and the sphenoid sinus (31,32).

Table 3
Description of the Traditional Olfactory Tests Used for Assessing Smell Loss[a]

Threshold tests
  Staircase procedure
    A threshold measurement that involves testing a series of concentrations of an odorant in a sequence involving
    ascending and descending runs. Typically the patient is asked to choose between two samples, one containing an
    odorant and one a blank. An incorrect response results in increasing the concentration, and a correct response in a
    second presentation, or, after the second presentation, a decrease in concentration.
  Ascending method of limits procedure
    A threshold measurement that is not significantly affected by adaptation, this test involves presentation of a series
    of concentrations of an odorant, in ascending order. Typically, the patient is presented with two samples at a time,
    one containing the odor and one a blank, and forced to choose which contains the odor.
Odor identification testing
  UPSIT
    A 40-item odor test employing microencapsulated (scratch-and-sniff) odors widely used in studies of odor
    identification. The subject scratches the label on each page, sniffs it, reads the four odor names offered, and then
    chooses the correct label from those offered.
  CCCRC odor identification test
    A 10-item odor identification test, designed to produce almost perfect performance in normal adults, this test
    employs natural odors commonly encountered in everyday life. The patient sniffs an odor with the eyes closed and
    then attempts to identify it after familiarizing himself or herself with a cue sheet containing the names of the 10 odor
    items as well as names of items not presented.
  San Diego odor identification test for children
    An eight-item odor test employing natural odors chosen after extensive testing to be well known to most young children
    (e.g., chocolate, peanut butter, Play-Doh, and so forth). These stimuli are presented one by one in opaque jars. The
    children sniff the odors while wearing a "Lone Ranger" mask to prevent visual clues from aiding the identification. They
    then remove the mask and attempt to identify the stimuli. The response mode for this task has also been tailored to the
    young child and has been successfully used with children who have not yet developed reading skills. The children
    are given a cue sheet that contains pictures or line drawings of the items presented in the test as well as pictures of some
    distracter items. The child responds by pointing to the picture of the item that corresponds to the odor smelled.
  Difference threshold
    Determination of the smallest difference between two stimuli that can be discriminated, this measurement typically
    involves a two-alternative, forced-choice presentation of pairs of concentrations of the same odorant with the
    difference between concentrations systematically varied.
  Odor recall task
    To compare recall and recognition memory for odors, odors are presented, either with or without their odor names,
    and the patient is asked to attempt to recall the odors, either with or without a category name as a clue. Odors chosen
    are of the same intensity—common odors whose names are regularly used in everyday life (chocolate, coffee, and
    so on). They are presented to blindfolded subjects at 45-s intervals for inspection, and then again for testing.
  Odor recognition memory test
    Patients are presented with a series of odors. All stimuli are randomly selected and presented for 5 s each, while
    patients are blindfolded. A 45-s interval is maintained between odors to minimize the effects of adaptation. Patients
    do not name the odors and are not informed that they will be tested for memory of these odors. Immediately after
    the familiarity session, patients are presented with another series of odors. Half are randomly selected from the first
    session (old) and half are additional stimuli (new). Patients judge whether stimuli were old or new. The test provides
    information about recognition memory and criterion for reporting detection.

[a]Adapted from ref. 67 with permission.

A thorough and accurate history of the illness, combined with comprehensive nasal endoscopy and CT scans, are key to accurate diagnosis of chronic sinusitis. The impact and manifestations of chronic sinusitis on olfaction have not been thoroughly investigated, although a few studies have shown smell deficits in patients with chronic sinusitis. In a recent study (33), we investigated olfactory threshold sensitivity and odor identification ability of chronic sinusitis patients before and after endoscopic sinus surgery (see Table 3 for description of this procedure). The results indicated a significant impairment in both odor

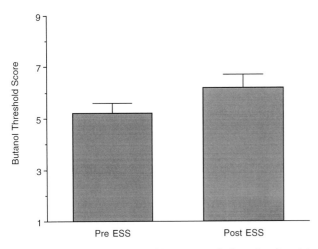

Fig. 5. Olfactory threshold scores of chronic sinusitis patients pre- and postendoscopic sinus surgery.

sensitivity and odor identification ability of the chronic sinusitis patients prior to endoscopic sinus surgery. Furthermore, significant improvement in odor sensitivity and odor identification ability was found after the surgery (*see* Fig. 5). These results also show that endoscopic sinus surgery can be successful in improving olfactory function in patients with chronic sinusitis and may serve as a viable treatment for smell dysfunction in this population.

Parosmia and phantosmia have also been associated with chronic sinusitis. One explanation for these phenomena may be the putrid smelling anaerobic bacteria commonly cultured in patients with chronic sinusitis. Patients often report that the foul-smelling odors seem to originate in their sinuses. Fungal sinusitis and atrophic rhinitis also produce foul-smelling substances.

Polyposis

Nasal polyps usually occur bilaterally, are typically benign in nature, and most commonly arise from ethmoid sinuses. These polyps are fleshy masses with smooth surfaces that extend into the nasal cavity. As of the writing of this chapter, the etiology of nasal polyps is unknown. It is believed that there are a number of etiologies for nasal polyps, although the end product typically appears to be the same. Nasal polyps have traditionally been associated with IgE-mediated atopic rhinosinusitis (affects 5–20% of patients) and with nonallergic sinonasal inflammation *(34)*. It has also been suggested that disorders without a reactive rhinitis or bronchospastic component may be associated with

nasal polyps. Studies of children with cystic fibrosis (CF), a disorder of mucous hyperviscosity, show that they have a 10% frequency of nasal polyposis and this percentage increases to 50 in adulthood *(35)*. It is believed that the sinonasal tract is chronically infected owing to the poor clearing of the nasal mucosal secretions. Microorganisms, such as anaerobes, are commonly cultured from these individuals' sinonasal secretions, and the chronic bacterial infection, as a result of chronic inflammation, may produce polyps.

Regardless of the etiology of the nasal polyps, they all seem to set off a similar chain of events. Mast cells and basophils release inflammatory mediators, which in turn induce ethmoid sinus stromal edema. When the circumference of the mucosa lining the ostia thickens, the ostial diameter becomes smaller and finally obstructed. Obstruction or closure of the ostium interferes with mucociliary transport clearance of secretions containing bacteria and crucial metabolites. It may be that the prolonged contact of vasoactive substances with the mucosa induces more edema and a larger influx of inflammatory cells. When the stimulus persists and causes further triggering of more mediators, the stromal edema appears to become so great that the mucosa prolapses into the nasal cavity.

The presenting symptoms of nasal polyps usually include progressive nasal obstruction, congestion, olfactory dysfunction, rhinorrhea, and on rare occasions, facial discomfort *(36)*. Nasal polyposis can cause significant damage when neglected for prolonged periods. They may cause erosion of the bony facial skeleton, and cause proptosis or widening of the nasal dorsum. Unlike chronic sinusitis, large polyps are easily diagnosed with anterior rhinoscopy. However, when the polyps are large, it is difficult to locate their site of origin, but most frequently they arise from the ethmoid sinuses.

Treatment of nasal polyps is similar to that of chronic sinusitis. Since half of the patients with polyposis respond to medication, the initial treatment should begin with corticosteroids *(37)*. It has been reported that oral corticosteroids are quite effective, in some cases as effective as surgery *(38)*. However, because of the side effects, steroids are usually given intranasally. For those patients who do not respond to medication, surgical removal of the nasal polyps is a good alternative. High-quality nasal endoscopes have markedly improved intraoperative visualization, and thus minimize trauma and operative morbidity. Olfactory dysfunction in this group has not been well characterized. In a recent study, we showed improved olfactory function postendoscopic surgery *(33)*.

CYSTIC FIBROSIS

CF is the most common genetic disorder in the Caucasian population, occurring in approx 1 in 2000 births. CF is an exocrine gland disorder that is inherited as an autosomal recessive trait, and results in viscid mucus and high sodium sweat concentrations. The gene is localized on chromosome 7. CF transmembrane conductance regular (CFTR) is an amino acid protein that functions as a chloride ion-transport channel, the dysfunction of which results in failure to transport chloride ions out of the epithelial lining cells, resulting in a dehydrated and, therefore, viscous mucus. Chronic pulmonary, sinonasal, and pancreatic dysfunctions are the direct result of the viscous mucus.

The life expectancy of patients with CF has increased in the past few decades. In the 1950s, patients with CF were expected to live only a few years. However, subsequent improvements in the antimicrobial therapy and advances in pulmonary medicine have led to improved management of these patients. Survival for CF patients has extended into the second and third decades. Recent advances in lung transplantation and genetically engineered pharmacologic compounds are improving the prospects for long-term survival for these patients.

Patients with CF frequently present with chronic sinusitis. More than 10% of CF patients develop nasal polyposis after the age of three, and in some cases, the polyposis is so extensive as to alter the development of the visceral cranium. These bilateral and multiple polyps usually appear smooth, semitranslucent, and pale yellow.

Since, presumably, the nasal mucus suffers from the same chloride ion-exchange deficiency as the lungs of the CF patient, chronic sinonasal disease is abundant in CF patients. This situation is often exacerbated by such conditions as allergic rhinitis, which occurs with the same frequency in CF patients as it does in the general population (15–30%).

Olfaction has not been well characterized in this population. In a recent study, we examined a number of patients with varying levels of CF disease severity as defined by the Schwachman/Kulczycki

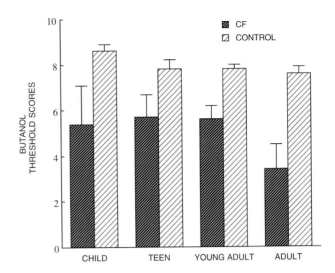

Fig. 6. Olfactory threshold scores of patients with cystic fibrosis and normal age-matched controls. Reprinted from ref. *39* with permission.

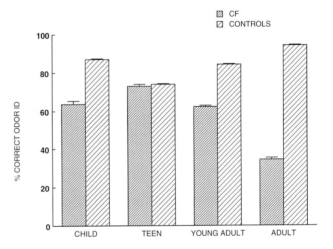

Fig. 7. Odor identification ability of cystic fibrosis patients and normal age-matched controls. Reprinted from ref. *39* with permission.

clinical disease scores. Using the adult or the child odor threshold, sensitivity and odor identification were measured. Figures 6 and 7 show the olfactory impairment of the CF group in comparison to normal age- and gender-matched controls for both smell sensitivity and identification ability *(39)*. Figure 6 also shows that the older adults with CF had poorer odor sensitivity than normal controls, and that adult CF patients showed more impairment on threshold testing than did young adults, teens, or children with CF. This study further found that older adults with more severe clinical disease (i.e., higher Schwachman/Kulczycki scores) showed more severe odor identification impairment, suggesting that olfactory function and disease status of CF patients may be more closely linked than previously thought.

Currently, all CF patients at the UCSD Medical Center awaiting a lung transplant undergo nasal sinus surgery to have polyps removed and to open the sinus ostia. This grants us the unique opportunity to examine smell function in CF patients pre- and postsinus surgery. Preliminary results, with a small number of patients, look promising, with CF patients showing a marked olfactory improvement after surgery. We hope to follow these patients over a number of years in order to characterize their smell disability accurately.

NEURODEGENERATIVE DISORDERS

It has become increasingly apparent that the sense of smell is impaired in a number of patients with neurodegenerative disorders, including Alzheimer's (AD), Parkinson's (PD), and Huntington's disease (HD), and patients with Human Immunodeficiency Virus (HIV)-positive neurocognitive impairment. However, the magnitude of olfactory impairment and the relationship between the degree to which the sense of smell is compromised and progression through the disease process differ for each disorder. Differential diagnosis of dementia can be difficult. For example, definitive diagnosis of AD is only available on autopsy. Thus, the inclusion of smell testing as a diagnostic tool may prove to be helpful.

Alzheimer's Disease

AD is the most frequent neurodegenerative disorder in which the sense of smell has been examined (40). Brains of patients with AD are characterized by cell loss, and increasing neurofibrillary tangles and neuritic plaques. These plaques and tangles are most pronounced in association areas. Anatomical evaluations demonstrate increased plaques and tangles, cell loss and granulovacuolar degeneration in the entorhinal cortex, prepiriform cortex, and the anterior olfactory nucleus (37,38,41), which are all associated regions believed to be involved in olfactory-mediated tasks.

Virtually all studies examining the sense of smell in patients with AD have found deficits (see Doty [42] for a review). Patients with AD have shown deficits in odor identification ability, odor recogni-

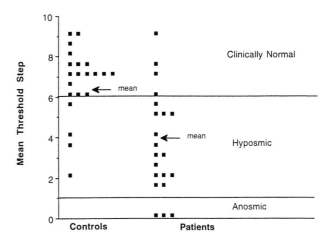

Fig. 8. Individual olfactory thresholds for patients with AD and normal elderly controls. The mean for each group is indicated by an arrow.

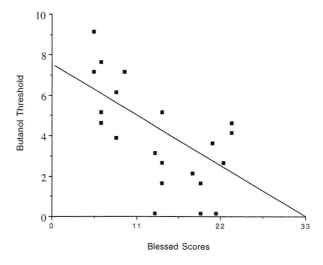

Fig. 9. Scatter diagram illustrating the relationship between olfactory threshold sensitivity and degree of dementia as measured by the number of incorrect responses given on the Blessed Dementia Scale. Reprinted from ref. *43* with permission.

tion ability, and odor detection sensitivity. In a recent study in our laboratory, we found over a 700-fold difference (*see* Fig. 8) between the detection threshold ability of Alzheimer's patients and normal age-matched controls (43). In the same study, it was also found that there is a moderate relationship between the progression of dementia and olfactory loss (*see* Fig. 9). That is, the patients who have progressed farther through the disease show greater smell impairment. A follow-up study with a subset of the same patients revealed that smell impairment in AD patients was not secondary to acute nasal disease, since the patients and age-matched controls had the same degree of rhinologic abnormality *(44)*.

Recently, researchers have been interested in the decline in the sense of smell of patients "at risk" for AD. Schiffman et al. *(45)* compared individuals with a strong family history of AD (with one or more family members affected) with age-, gender-, and race-matched controls, and found that the odor memory of patients of the "at risk" for AD group was impaired. We also found similar results in our laboratory when comparing patients at the very early stages of AD and, thus, classified "at risk" for AD, to normal age- and gender-matched controls *(46)*. Our results revealed that the "at-risk" group showed significant impairment in their smell sensitivity for the odorant butanol. Furthermore, the "at-risk" group was poorer at odor memory than at visual memory tasks when compared to controls. One conclusion that one may draw from these findings is that the regions of the central nervous system (CNS) involved in processing olfactory sensory information are affected early on in the disease process. These data are particularly interesting given that advances for treatment of dementing illnesses are rapidly progressing. As treatment for AD becomes available, procedures for definitive differential diagnosis will need to be well developed so that patients can receive appropriate medical care as early as possible. It appears that olfactory testing may play an important role in the diagnosis of AD.

Other studies have shown impairment in Alzheimer's patients' ability to identify odors. A number of studies using the UPSIT (*see* Table 1 for a description of this test) have revealed decrements in patients' ability to identify the odors *(46a–49)*. The UPSIT is a very useful tool for clinicians because of the ease of administration and interpretation. In addition, it is a self-administered test. Thus, the patient can complete the task alone. However, this test is very cognitively demanding (since the patient's task is to scratch, sniff, read the choice list, recall what each odor choice smells like, and make a decision about the identity of the odor) and should be used with some caution when describing sensory deficits, particularly with demented populations. It may be that patients who cannot name odors or recall what the choices given smell like may, in fact, have normal sensory function, but cognitive difficulties that influence performance on the task. Furthermore, patients with AD show lexical deficits that do not directly involve olfaction, possibly confounding results of odor identification tests that are based on lexical function.

However, results of a recent study from our laboratory suggest that Alzheimer's patients do, in fact, have odor identification deficits *(50)*, even when the odor identification task is not based on lexical function. In this study, patients were presented with common, everyday odors (e.g., chocolate, cinnamon, baby powder) and asked to identify the odors from a list of pictures. We believe this task to be less cognitively demanding than the UPSIT, since tests that are based on lexical function are more difficult for Alzheimer's patients to comprehend and interpret. Results of this study showed that Alzheimer's patients performed more poorly at odor identification than normal elderly age- and gender-matched controls, suggesting that odor identification is impaired in Alzheimer's patients even when the lexical component is eliminated.

Parkinson's Disease

PD is another neurodegenerative disorder for which olfactory deficits have been reported. Patients with PD have documented decreased levels of dopamine (DA) neurotransmitters. However, little information is known about the neuropathology of the olfactory regions of PD patients. We know that in normal persons, there are high levels of DA neurotransmitters in the olfactory tubercle. Therefore, it was thought that the deficit in DA neurotransmitters may be one explanation for the olfactory deficits found in PD. However, olfactory function in these patients does not appear to be a function of antiparkinson medication (L-DOPA, which increases levels of dopamine) *(42)*. Therefore, thus far the etiology for smell deficits in PD patients remains unclear.

PD patients have shown deficits across a number of olfactory tests, including detection threshold, odor discrimination, and odor identification and matching *(51,52)*. However, unlike AD, a relationship between the degree of severity and olfactory impairment has not been demonstrated. In addition, there appears to be no relationship between antiparkinsonian medications and olfactory function *(53)*.

Huntington's Disease

HD is a genetic, autosomal dominant disorder of the brain that is characterized by movement disorders, cognitive impairment, and in some cases, psychiatric problems. The behavioral expression of the disorder typically occurs during late adulthood, as is the case with PD. To date, no detailed neuropathologic studies of the olfactory pathways of patients with HD have been published. Recent data suggest considerable loss of D1, but not D2 receptors, present in the nucleus accumbens and other brain areas of HD patients. However, no abnormalities in the number of DA receptors or the level of DA neurotransmitters in the olfactory tubercle have been reported thus far.

Earlier studies have shown that HD patients have particular difficulties in remembering odor qualities *(53)*. More recent studies have also demonstrated that HD patients have difficulty in odor identification and odor detection *(41)*. In a very recent study, we also found impairments in odor detection thresholds, odor identification abilities, as well as odor memory and odor discrimination *(54)*. Once again, the underlying etiology for the olfactory impairment in HD patients is unclear. However, a recent study by Doty *(41)* suggests that the smell dysfunction occurs close to the time of phenotypic expression of the disorder.

Human Immunodeficiency Virus

It is estimated that 7–28% of patients infected by HIV will develop dementia some time during the course of their illness. Furthermore, an even larger proportion (up to 50%) may develop mild neurocognitive impairment. Autopsies have confirmed direct viral infection of the CNS in a large portion of these patients. In addition, magnetic resonance imaging and CT demonstrate a variety of cortical and subcortical abnormalities in the brains of HIV-positive neurocognitively impaired individuals *(55)*. Yet, it is unclear whether these cognitive deficits are a result of direct HIV infection of the CNS.

One of the first studies examining the effects of HIV on olfaction was conducted by Brody and colleagues *(56)*. These investigators examined odor identification ability of four groups using the UPSIT *(see* Table 1 for description): patients with HIV-associated dementia, asymptomatic HIV-infected patients, patients with clinical evidence for immunosuppression, and HIV-negative con-

trols. They found that the patients with HIV-associated dementia identified significantly fewer odors than the other three groups. Hornung et al. *(57)* in a similar study using the UPSIT found similar results.

A recent study conducted by our laboratory *(58)* found an impairment in odor detection sensitivity for a subset of the HIV-positive population. In this study, we examined HIV-positive patients with neurocognitive impairment, HIV-positive patients with no signs of neurocognitive impairments, and HIV-negative patients. Subjects were given an odor detection threshold test *(see* Table 1 for description) for the odorant butanol. The results indicated that the HIV-positive patients with neurocognitive impairments had lower odor threshold sensitivity than the two control groups. These results may partly be owing to the viral infection in the CNS. However, they may also be partly attributed to nasal disease. High incidence of sinusitis and allergic rhinitis have been reported in patients with HIV. From previous research (parts of which are presented in this chapter), it is clear that nasal disease affects olfaction. Sinusitis appears to occur with a high frequency in patients with HIV-1 infection, with maxillary sinus infection being the most common type *(33,59,60)*. The manifestations of chronic sinusitis and its impact on olfaction have not yet been thoroughly investigated, although smell deficits in patients with chronic sinusitis have been reported *(33)*.

AGING

The perception of food flavor involves a great deal of input from olfaction as well as from taste. The input from olfaction is accomplished by the retronasal stimulation of the olfactory system and thus adds the additional chemosensory stimulation to the flavor of food. It is clear, thus, that the loss of olfactory function can significantly impact the flavor and hedonics of foods. The sense of smell loses considerable functioning over the life-span *(see* refs. *62* and *63* for reviews). Odor threshold sensitivity studies have demonstrated age-related decline in olfactory and trigeminal function *(64–66)*. Figure 10 illustrates the differences in butanol sensitivity for young college students and healthy elderly subjects tested in our laboratory. This figure shows a greater amount of odor variability in odor threshold scores for the eld-

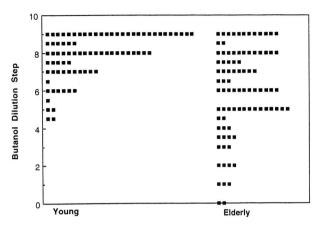

Fig. 10. Individual butanol olfactory threshold scores of young college students and elderly subjects show lower overall sensitivity and higher variability among the elderly. Note that higher butanol threshold steps represent lower concentration of stimuli.

erly population, in addition to overall poorer odor threshold sensitivity.

Weaker perceived intensity and poorer discrimination and odor identification ability have also been demonstrated in the elderly population *(66)*. Therefore, it is not surprising to find that the elderly have more difficulty remembering odors. It is fortunate, however, that most older persons retain a good amount of smell functioning, even though the loss they have experienced may interfere with their enjoyment of foods and nutritional intake. Precipitous, profound smell loss in an elderly patient should not be ascribed to age-related impairment alone, but should be cause for thorough evaluation. As discussed in an earlier section, olfactory dysfunction at the threshold level is especially pronounced in patients with AD, a significant portion of whom reside in nursing homes. Thus, neurodegenerative disease and nasal disease may add to the variability found in smell function of the elderly.

Elderly persons with head injury-related smell loss are usually faced with even greater difficulties, since they have a sensitivity decline characteristic of normal aging in addition to smell loss owing to the head injury *(67)*. It is important for the olfactory examiner to be aware of the poor odor sensitivity and odor identification ability found in the elderly population in order to appropriately assess smell loss resulting from head trauma.

DESCRIPTION OF RESEARCH AND FUTURE DIRECTIONS IN OLFACTION

In addition to the ongoing evaluation and followup of patients with primary complaints of olfactory dysfunction, there are a number of interesting research and clinical practices being conducted by the leading nasal dysfunction clinics in the country. These clinics continue to identify and evaluate the mechanisms underlying human olfactory dysfunction. Some clinics have given specific attention to problems with odorant access to the receptors (odorant conduction problems) and neurologic problems, including both peripheral and central dysfunction. For example, the Syracuse nasal dysfunction clinic is in the process of developing a 3D computer model of the human and rat nose in order to determine regional nasal air flow and the amount of each odorant that is deposited in each position in the nose as a function of odorant mucous solubility, sniff flow rate, and clinically relevant nasal obstructions. Furthermore, the recovery of the olfactory system (physiologically, anatomically, and behaviorally) after olfactory loss is being studied in animals as a model of human olfactory loss seen with head trauma. The olfactory loss seen in certain clinical populations, such as HIV-positive patients and patients with AD, is also being investigated.

One interesting project being conducted at the Rocky Mountain Taste and Smell Center is research designed to investigate whether olfactory biopsy material from probable Alzheimer's patients has consistent pathological changes that may be useful in diagnosis. Special attention is being paid to the possibility of mitochondrial changes associated with AD. In conjunction with this, investigators are involved in an extensive investigation into the qualitative and quantitative changes that may occur in the olfactory epithelium as a result of aging. Researchers intend to test chemosensory function and obtain olfactory epithelium biopsies from 70 control subjects ranging in age from 20 into the 80s and have completed roughly half of the subjects. Data from this project will be used to re-evaluate tissue obtained from a number of pathological cases, including cases of anosmia or hyposmia resulting from head trauma, upper respiratory disease, sinus disease, PD, and many other idiopathic causes. Data that will be obtained from the protocol for the control subjects involve the nature of their biopsy technique. Firm numbers regarding positive biopsies will be used to confirm or deny the technique and possibly allow for statistical inferences regarding negative biopsies.

Researchers are also continuing to study normal and abnormal human olfactory function at the cellular and molecular levels. This is accomplished on human olfactory biopsy material through electrophysiological, biophysical, and molecular biological techniques. In addition to studies of the basic mechanisms of olfactory transduction in normal subjects, studies of the cellular and molecular abnormalities underlying olfactory dysfunction in AD are planned.

Researchers at these centers are also working hard to increase understanding of the relative contributions of olfaction and chemesthesis to the overall perception of volatile chemicals, as well as of the nature and number of chemesthetic qualities. Using the principle that stimulation of the trigeminal nerve can be localized, whereas stimulation of the olfactory nerve cannot, researchers are exploring and defining olfactory detection and nasal chemesthetic lateralization thresholds for a wide range of odorants in both normosmics and anosmics. It is hoped that a clinically relevant test of nasal chemesthetic function and a qualitative measure of the differences among chemesthetic stimuli can be achieved.

The major goal of the Nasal Dysfunction Clinic at the UCSD Medical Center is the evaluation and treatment of olfactory disorders and nasal disease. The clinic maintains a data base with information about patients seen over the past decade that informs our treatment strategies and facilitates chemosensory research. Current research is focused on several questions.

In our research, HIV-positive patients with neurocognitive impairment show olfactory impairment relative to HIV-negative and HIV-positive patients without cognitive problems, and the degree of olfactory impairment is related to neurocognitive impairment. The extent of nasal sinus disease in HIV patients is an area of current exploration that draws on the expertise of all members of our clinical team.

A current assessment of complaints and diagnoses of parosmia and phantosmia among chemo-sensory and nasal/sinus patients is being conducted to determine the prevalence of parosmia and phantosmia among patients whose problems stem from different nasal diseases with a view toward differential diagnosis.

An interest in the different mediators involved in the allergic response drives another research effort on functional assessment of patients following allergic challenge.

A primary interest and another that taps the expertise of the whole team involves the assessment of patients before and after endoscopic sinus surgery. Our current research involves assessment of olfactory function, rhinomanometry, nasal cytology, and patients' reports of symptoms, including nasal obstruction, nasal congestion, and so forth, after endoscopic sinus surgery. In addition, assessment of the health impact of endoscopic sinus surgery, using the Quality of Well-being Scale, is being used to quantify changes in the patient's perceived quality of life following endoscopic sinus surgery.

CONCLUSION

We once wrote a paper titled: "What Happened to Cranial Nerve One," and there are days we again ask ourselves this question. It is amazing how little the medical profession knows about and appreciates the meaning of the sense of smell. It is sometimes incredible how insensitive physicians can be to those who have lost their sense of smell. Comments such as: "So what, lose a little weight" really do little to help these patients. For some people, the sense of smell really is an important sense. People who know their children by their smell, who manage their households by the way it smells, whose talents and enjoyments in life are culinary—for these people their nose is an incredible pleasure, and without it, their life has lost a great deal. These individuals all deserve thorough evaluation and appropriate counseling. For those physicians who choose to perform the evaluation themselves, please be complete and spend the time necessary to make the correct diagnosis and counsel the patient appropriately. For those who feel they do not have the expertise to carry out such a thorough nasal evaluation, referral to one of the clinics listed in Table 4 should be the strategy of choice.

Table 4
List of Smell Dysfunction Centers
in the Country to Which Patients Can Be Referred

Chemosensory Clinical Research Center
Monell Chemical Senses Center
3500 Market Street
Philadelphia, PA 19104-3308

Connecticut Chemosensory Clinical Research Center
University of Connecticut Health Center
Farmington, CT 06032

Clinical Olfactory Research Center
SUNY Health Sciences Center at Syracuse
766 Irving Avenue
Syracuse, NY 13210

MCV Smell and Taste Clinic
Medical College of Virginia
Richmond, VA 23298-0551

Nasal Dysfunction Clinic
University of California, San Diego Medical Center
200 West Arbor Drive
San Diego, CA 92103-8654

National Institute of Dental Research
National Institutes of Health
NIH Building 10, Room 1N-114
Bethesda, MD 20892

Rocky Mountain Taste and Smell Center
University of Colorado Health Science Center
4200 East Ninth Avenue
Denver, CO 80262

University of Cincinnati Taste and Smell Center
University of Cincinnati College of Medicine
231 Bethesda Avenue
Cincinnati, OH 45267-0528

University of Pennsylvania Smell and Taste Center
Hospital of University of Pennsylvania
3400 Spruce Street
Philadelphia, PA 19104-4283

ACKNOWLEDGMENTS

We would like to thank Pam Eller and Beverly J. Cowart, Daniel Kurtz, and April E. Motts for responding to our request for a summary of current research projects at their respective clinics serving patients with nasal dysfunction. This work was supported by NIH Grant No. AG04085 (C. M. and J. R.).

REFERENCES

1. Gibbons B. The intimate sense of smell. National Geographic 1986;170:324–360.
2. Jafek BW. Ultrastructure of human nasal mucosa. Laryngoscope 1983;93:1576–1599.
3. Rowley JC, Moran DT, Jafek BW. Peroxidase backfills suggest the mammalian olfactory epithelium contains a second morphologically distinct class of bipolar sensory neurons: the microvillar cell. Brain Res 1989;502:387–400.
4. Burdach KJ, Doty RL. The effects of mouth movement, swallowing, and spitting on retronasal odor perception. Physiol Behav 1987;41:353–356.
5. Laing DG. Characteristics of human behavior during odor perception. Perception 1982;11:221–230.
6. Laing DG. Natural sniffing gives optimum odor perception for humans. Perception 1983;12:99–117.
7. Getchell TV, Margolis FL, Getchell ML. Perireceptor and receptor events in vertebrate olfaction. Prog Neurobiol 1984;23:317–345.
8. Schneider RA, Wolf S. Relation of olfactory activity to nasal membrane function. J Appl Physiol 1960; 15:914.
9. Youngentob SL, Kurtz DB, Leopold DA, Mozell MM, and Hornung DE. Olfactory sensitivity: is there laterality? Chem Senses 1982;7:11–21.
10. Doty RL, Frye R. Influence of nasal obstruction on smell function. Otolaryngol Clin North Am 1989;22:397–411.
11. Principato JJ, Ozenberger MJ. Cyclical charges in nasal resistance. Arch Otolaryngol 1970;91:71–77.
12. Cain WS, Gent JF, Catalanotto FA, Goodspeed RB. Clinical evaluation of olfaction. Am J Otolaryngol 1993; 4:257–260.
13. Quionez C, Davidson TM, Jaylowayski AA, Nordin S, Murphy C. Dysosmia among patients at the UCSD Nasal Dysfunction Clinic: etiology and effect on olfactory function. Chem Senses (abstract) 1994;19:515.
14. Feldman JL, Wright NH, Leopold DA. The initial evaluation of dysosmia. Am J Otolaryngol 1986;4: 431–444.
15. Ferrier D. The hemispheres considered physiologically. In: The Functions of the Brain. New York: GP Putnam's Sons, 1876; pp. 181–211.
16. Costanzo RM, Zasler ND. Epidemiology and pathophysiology of olfactory and gustatory dysfunction in head trauma. J Head Trauma Rehabil 1992;7:15–24.
17. Heywood PG, Zasler ND, Costanzo RM. Olfactory screening test for assessment of smell loss following traumatic brain injury. Proceedings of the 14th Annual Conference on Rehabilitation of the Brain Injured, Williamsburg, VA, June 7–10, 1990 (abstract).
18. Sumner D. Post-traumatic anosmia. Brain 1964;87: 107–120.
19. Costanzo RM, Heywood PG, Ward JD, Young HF. Neurosurgical applications of clinical olfactory assessment. NY Acad Sci 1987;510:242–244.
20. Cowart BJ, Garrison B, Young IM, Lowry LD. A discrepancy between odor thresholds and identification in dysosmia. Chem Senses (abstract) 1989;14:693.
21. Levin HS, High WM, Eisenberg HM. Impairment of olfactory recognition after closed head injury. Brain 1985;108:579–591.
22. Potter H, Nauta WJH. A note on the problem of olfactory associations of the orbitofrontal cortex in the monkey. J Neurosci 1979;4:361–367.
23. Mott AE. General medical evaluation. J Head Trauma Rehabil 1992;7:25–41.

24. Eskenazi B, Cain WS, Novelly RA, Mattson R. Odor perception in temporal lobe epilepsy patients with and without temporal lobectomy. Neuropsychologia 1986; 24:553–562.

25. Rausch R, Serafetinides EA, Crandall PH. Olfactory memory in patients with anterior temporal lobectomy. Cortex 1977;13:445–452.

26. Costanzo RM, Becker DP. Smell and taste disorders in head injury and neurosurgery patients. In: Meiselman HL, Rivlin RS, eds., Clinical Measurements of Taste and Smell. New York: MacMillan, 1986; pp. 556–578.

27. Cowart BJ, Flnn-Rodden K, McGeady SJ, Lowry LD. Hyposmia in allergic rhinitis. J Allergy Clin Immunol 1993;91:747–751.

28. Blackley C. Experimental Research on the Causes and Nature of Catarrhus Aestivus. Abingdon: Oxford Historical Books, 1898.

29. Fein BT, Kamin PB, Fein NN. The loss of smell in nasal allergy. Ann Allerg 1966;24:278–283.

30. Loury MC, Kennedy DW. Chronic sinusitis and nasal polyposis. In: Getchell TV, Doty RL, Bartoshuk LM, Snow JB, eds., Smell and Taste in Health and Disease. New York: Raven, 1991; pp. 517–528.

31. Stammberger H, Posawetz W. Functional endoscopic sinus surgery: concept, indications and results of the Messerklinger technique. Eur Arch Otorhinolaryngol 1990;247:63–76.

32. Messerklinger W. Endoscopy of the Nose. Baltimore/Munich: Urban & Schwarzenberg, 1978.

33. Maricio M, Davidson TM, Jalowayski AA, Murphy C. Nasal disease and olfaction in chronic sinusitis patients. Chem Senses 1994;19:515.

34. Zeiger RS. Allergic and nonallergic rhinitis: classification and pathogenesis. Part I: allergic rhinitis. Am J Rhinol 1989;3:21–47.

35. Cepero R, Smith RJH, Catlin FI, Bressler KL, Furuta GT, Shandera KC. Cystic fibrosis—an otolaryngological perspective. Otolaryngol Head Neck Surg 1987;97:356–360.

36. Drake-Lee AB, Lowe D, Swanston A, Grace A. Clinical profile and recurrence of nasal polyps. J Laryngol Otol 1984;98:783–793.

37. Lidholdt T, Forgstrup J, Kortholm B, Ulsoe C. Surgical versus medical management of nasal polyps. Acta Otolaryngol (Stockh) 1988;105:140–143.

38. Drake-Lee AB. Medical treatment of nasal polyps. Rhinology 1994;32:1–9.

39. Murphy C, Anderson JA, Markison S. Psychophysical assessment of chemosensory disorders in clinical populations. In: Kurihara K, Suzuki N, Ogawa H, eds. Olfaction and Taste XI. New York: Springer-Verlag, 1994; 609–613.

40. Reyes PF, Golden GT, Fariello RG, Fagel L, Zalewska M. Olfactory pathways in Alzheimer's Disease (AD): neuropathological studies. Soc Neurosci (abstract) 1985; 11:168.

41. Esiri M, Wilcock G. The olfactory bulbs in Alzheimer's disease. J Neurol Neurosurg Psychiatry 1984;47:56–60.

42. Doty RL. Olfactory dysfunction in neurodegenerative disorders. In: Getchell TV, Doty RL, Bartoshuk LM, Snow JB, eds., Smell and Taste in Health and Disease. New York: Raven, 1991; pp. 735–751.

43. Murphy C, Gilmore MM, Seery CS, Salmon DP, Lasker BR. Olfactory thresholds are associated with degree of dementia in alzheimer's disease. Neurobiol Aging 1990; 11:465–469.

44. Feldman JI, Murphy C, Davidson TM, Jalowayski AA, Galindo de Jaime G. The rhinologic evaluation of Alzheimer's disease. Laryngoscope 1991;11:1198–1202.

45. Schiffman SS, Graham BG, Sattely-Miller E, Welch KA. Taste and smell function in persons at risk for Alzheimer's disease. Chem Senses (abstract) 1993; 18:622,623.

46. Nordin S, Murphy C. Olfaction in persons "at risk" for Alzheimer's disease (AD): decline in recognition memory for odors as an early marker for AD. Submitted for publication.

46a. Serby M, Corwin J, Conrad P, Rotrosen J. Olfactory dysfunction in Alzheimer's disease and Parkinson's disease. Am J Psychiat 1985;142:781,782.

47. Knupfer L, Spiegel R. Differences in olfactory test performance between normal aged, Alzheimer's and vascular type dementia individuals. Int J Geriatric Psychiatr 1986;1:3–14.

48. Doty RL, Reyes P, Gregor T. Presence of both odor identification and detection deficits in Alzheimer's disease. Brain Res Bull 1987;18:597–600.

49. Morgan CD, Murphy C, Nordin S. Picture-based odor identification in Alzheimer's patients and normal controls. Chem Senses (abstract) 1994; in press.

50. Ward CD, Hess WA, Calne DB. Olfactory impairment in Parkinson's disease. Neurology 1983;33:943–946.

51. Doty RL, Deems D, Stellar S. Olfactory dysfunction in Parkinson's disease: a general deficit unrelated to neurologic sign, disease stage, or disease duration. Neurology 1988;38:1237–1244.

52. Moberg PJ, Pearlson GD, Speedie LJ, Lipsey JR, Strauss ME, Folstien SE. Olfactory recognition: differential impairments in early and late Huntington's and Alzheimer's diseases. J Clin Exp Neuropsych 1987;9:560–664.

53. Nordin S, Murphy C, Paulsen JS. Sensory- and memory-mediated olfactory dysfunction in Huntington's disease. Submitted.

54. Navia BA, Cho ES, Petito CK, Price RW. The AIDS dementia complex II: neuropathology. Ann Neurol 1986;19:525–535.

55. Brody D, Serby M, Etienne N, Kalkstein DS. Olfactory identification deficits in HIV infection. Am J Psychiatr 1990;148:248–250.

56. Hornung DE, Leopold DC, Clark EC, Youngentob SL. Olfactory deficits in patient's infected with the human immunodeficiency virus. Chem Senses 1991;537.

57. Razani J, Murphy C, Davidson TM, Grant I, McCutchan A. Odor sensitivity is impaired in HIV-positive cognitively impaired patients. Submitted.

58. Zurlo JL, Feuerstein IM. Sinusitis in HIV-1 infection. Am J Med 1992;93:157–162.

59. Meiteles LZ, Lucente FE. Sinus and nasal manifestations of the acquired immunodeficiency syndrome. Ear, Nose Throat J 1990;69:454–458.

60. Small CB, Kaufman A, Armenaka M, Rosenstreich DL. Sinusitis and atopy in Human Immunodeficiency Virus infection. J Infect Dis 1993;167:281–290.

61. Murphy C. Taste and smell in the elderly. In: Meiselman EL, Rivlin RS, eds., Clinical Measurement of Taste and Smell. New York: MacMillan, 1986; pp. 343–347.

62. Schiffman SS. Age related changes in taste and smell and their possible causes. In: Meiselman EL, Rivlin RS, eds., Clinical Measurement of Taste and Smell. New York: MacMillan, 1986; 326–342.

63. Strauss EL. A study on olfactory acuity. Ann Otol Rhinol Laryngol 1970;79:95–104.

64. Schiffman SS, Moss J, Erickson RP. Thresholds of food odors in the elderly. Exp Aging Res 1976;2:389–398.

65. Murphy C. Age-related effects on the threshold, psychophysical function, and pleasantness of menthol. J Gerontol 1983;38:217–222.

66. Murphy C, Davidson TM. Geriatric issues: special considerations. J Head Trauma Rehabil 1992;1:76–82.

67. Davidson TM, Murphy C, Jalowayski AA. Cranial nerve I. Post. Grad. Med., in press.

23 Rhinomanometry

Philip Cole, MD, FRCSC *and Renato Roithmann,* MD

CONTENTS

THEORETICAL CONSIDERATIONS
PRACTICAL CONSIDERATIONS
A RHINOMANOMETRIC SESSION
CONCLUSIONS
REFERENCES

THEORETICAL CONSIDERATIONS

Introduction

Several methods are available for an objective description of how difficult it is to breathe through the nose. In order to simplify comparisons and interpretations of results from different centers, the International Committee on Standardization of Rhinomanometry (1) recommends that this breathing variable be expressed as resistance to respiratory air flow, and determined by the ratio between transnasal pressure and air flow. They advocate that the procedure be termed "rhinomanometry" in place of the more descriptive, but cumbersome term "rhinorheomanometry." The committee recommends further that, if possible, investigators should include in their publications pressure/flow ratios ($\Delta P/\dot{V}$) in Pa/cm³/s in addition to their individual preferences.*

Rhinomanometric measurements, although not directly related to the paranasal sinuses, detect the abnormal nasal air flow, which is a common accompaniment of sinus disease. Details of the ICSR rhinomanometric recommendations are discussed in this chapter together with principles and practice of objective assessment of nasal patency and relevant nasal respiratory physiology.

Characteristics of Nasal Air Flow

(*See also* Chapter 2.) The nasal passages provide complex conduits in parallel for inspiratory and expiratory air flow. During inspiration, convergence of ambient air streams as they enter the nose promotes laminar flow through the narrow nasal valve. Deceleration of the air stream, as it leaves the valve and enters the larger cross-section of the cavum, releases kinetic energy that is dissipated in the generation of inertial disturbances, which disrupt the laminar flow regimen. Mixing and mucosal contact resulting from disturbances induced by the orifice flow enable convective exchanges between air stream and mucosa to cleanse, warm, and moisten inspiratory air during its brief passage through the large cross-section airways leading from the nostrils to the lungs.

In expiration, air-flow disturbances similar to those effected by the nasal valve on inspiration are ensured by expiratory narrowing of the glottis. Resulting orifice flow promotes convective exchanges, and, as a consequence, heat and water

---

*ΔP = pressure differential between points of measurement, e.g., between the nasopharynx and the atmosphere or between the nasopharynx and the inside of a facemask. The use of SI units is recommended by the ICSR. Thus, a pressure of 1.0 cm H_2O = 100 Pa and a resistance of 1.0 cm H_2O/L/s = 0.1 Pa/cm³/s.

From: *Diseases of the Sinuses* (M. E. Gershwin and G. A. Incaudo, eds.), ©1996 Humana Press Inc., Totowa, NJ.

are recovered, mainly in the nasal cavities where temperature and water vapor pressure gradients between expiratory air and mucosa are greater than elsewhere in the airways.

Mathematical Descriptions

(*See also* Chapter 2.) As described, the flow regimens of both inspiratory and expiratory nasal air are nonlaminar, but they do not achieve full turbulence during resting breathing and remain in a transitional phase with varying degrees of flow disturbance. Both laminar and turbulent flow through a regular conduit can be described simply in terms of differential pressure (ΔP) and flow ($\dot{V}$) as $\Delta P = k_1 \dot{V}$ and $\Delta P = k_2 \dot{V}^2$, respectively, where k_1 and k_2 are constants. Neither of these terms alone is adequate for description of nasal respiratory air flow, which, in addition to its varying transitional characteristics, accelerates, decelerates, and reverses through an irregular lumen of constantly changing cross-section and direction.

As fluid begins to move through a regular conduit in response to a pressure gradient, its flow pattern is initially laminar and $\Delta P = k\dot{V}^e$ where exponent e = 1. As flow velocity increases, frictional forces induce disturbances in the air steam and exponent "e" increases also. If velocity and resulting disturbances continue to increase and turbulence is approached, exponent "e" approaches 2. Röhrer's equation $\Delta P = k_1 \dot{V} + k_2 \dot{V}^2$ *(2)* was devised to accommodate differing flow regimens in the respiratory airways, and, despite many critics, it has endured since 1915 and is still widely quoted and employed *(3)*.

Röhrer's critics *(4)* have stated that, in order to describe nasal air flow, an equation requires more than two terms. Röhrer's first term is said to be reduced by a factor of 10 when corrected for a dimensional error. The significance of k_1 and k_2 has been questioned. Gas density and viscosity effects do not fit the equation. Some investigators have applied exponents <2 to flow values and have found an exponent approximating 1.7 to fit nasal respiratory pressure/flow curves. Curve fitting alone has been criticized as insufficient justification. Others have stated that neither Poiseulle's nor Reynold's equation is appropriate for description of nasal respiratory air flow and that it is more adequately described by Bernoulli's equation *(4)*. Principally because these theoretical considerations are incompletely resolved, empirical methods prevail widely,

and use of an empirical standard has been recommended by the ICSR to aid communication between centers.

A distinction between resistance to air flow and resistance to breathing should be recognized. The small nasal airways of a child are more resistive than those of an adult to any designated air flow, and several investigators have reported an inverse ratio between age and nasal air-flow resistance that reaches unity as adult values are attained in the midteens. However, respiratory air flow of a child is less than that of an adult and, as a consequence, differences between child and adult of resistances to breathing are diminished as are the differential transnasal respiratory air-flow pressures.

Transnasal Pressure and Flow Studies

Passive rhinomanometry is a technique in which air is drawn or forced through the nasal passages at a known pressure or flow while breathing is suppressed or diverted. It is widely used in animal experimentation, but is not in general clinical use for human measurements. The method is particularly useful for detecting and recording rapid changes in nasal patency *(5)*, and resistance, as an index of nasal patency, can be calculated from the ratio between a designated pressure and measured flow or vice versa. Active rhinomanometry, in which a subject's nasal breathing provides air flow that is measured concomitantly with transnasal pressure, is in general use worldwide. It is more representative of physiological circumstances than passive rhinomanometry. In some centers, respiratory air flow and/or pressure has been recorded individually against time on a strip chart (Figs. 1 and 2) *(6,7)*. More commonly, nowadays, pressure is plotted against flow in an *x-y* format that produces a sigmoid tracing, but this form of recording lacks the time scale that is a useful feature of strip-chart recording (Fig. 3).

The exponential relationships between transnasal pressure and flow, together with each subject's individual characteristics of breathing (which have complex origins), determine the shape of the sigmoid *x-y* pressure/flow tracing, and its declination varies with nasal patency. A Swedish study of military recruits *(8)* showed that their nasal pressure/flow curves could be arranged in radial order about a common zero and that curves seldom crossed. Each represented an individual subject's nasal respiratory air-flow resistance. Increased

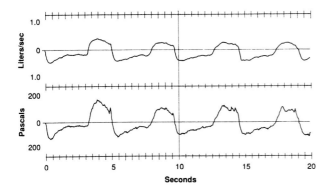

Fig. 1. Strip chart recording of transnasal air flow and pressure during breathing at rest through a healthy nose.

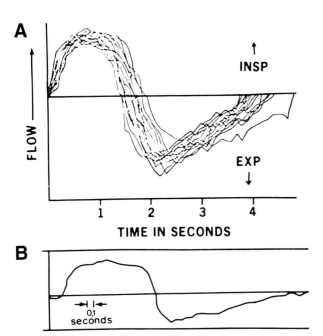

Fig. 2. Nasal air flow during breathing at rest. Note the squarish-wave form of the inspiratory phase in contrast with the gradual slope from peak of the expiratory phase. (A and B reprinted with permission from ref. 6.)

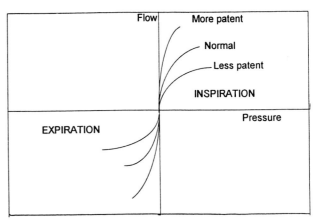

Fig. 3. *x-y* recording of transnasal pressure against flow. Sigmoid curve rotated toward pressure or flow axis by increase or decrease of resistance.

patency rotated curves toward the flow axis and increased resistance toward the pressure axis (Fig. 3).

Although the extremities of an individual subject's pressure/flow tracings are not entirely consistent breath by breath, consistency of the course of the curve over lengthy sequences of breaths is a remarkable characteristic that is exploited in several different forms of resistance calculation. Resistance values can be calculated from the ratio between rectangular coordinates of points on these pressure/flow curves or from polar coordinates *(8)*. Since each curve is sigmoid, calculated resistance values increase as

extremities of the curve are approached from the origin. Common strategies as employed in different centers to obtain useful and reproducible resistance values from the sigmoid pressure/flow curves are as follows:

1. Pressure/flow ratios are calculated at a designated transnasal differential pressure. The ICSR *(1)* suggests 150 Pa (1.50 H₂O), but leaves other options open. A common standard in Japan is 100 Pa. Choices differ widely, at least between 50 and 300 Pa.

   During spontaneous bilateral nasal breathing in adult subjects at rest, a transnasal differential pressure of 150 Pa is seldom achieved; indeed, values <100 Pa are more usual in both Oriental and Caucasian subjects with healthy noses. Artifactual errors associated with voluntary hyperventilation that may be required to elevate transnasal pressure values are discussed later in this chapter (*see* The Patient and Other Centers).

2. The ratios are calculated at a designated transnasal flow of 0.25 L/s, but again choices vary at least between 0.10 and 0.50 L. The close approximation with a straight line of the sigmoid pressure/flow curve in proximity with the origin provides a rationale for designating lesser pressure or flow values since, over this small portion of the curve, the pressure/flow ratio is almost constant for individual tracings over a wide range of nasal patencies. However, during each breath, this portion of the curve is of very brief duration. The longer duration of inspiratory pressure and flow values near the extremity of the curve provides an alternative rationale for designating both greater values and the inspiratory phase (Figs. 1 and 2).

3. As noted above, peak values of pressure or flow at the extremities of the pressure/flow curve are not entirely consistent from breath to breath, but averages obtained from several breaths provide reproducible results. This portion of the curve represents inspiratory pressure/flow values more closely than smaller designated coordinates *(9,10)*. It should be noted also in this regard that respiratory air-flow recordings are not sinusoidal (Figs. 1 and 2). Flow rapidly reaches and maintains a plateau through much of the inspiratory phase (muscular effort), whereas expiratory flow rapidly reaches a peak and then declines (elastic recoil obeys Hook's Law) and may even cease momentarily before the succeeding inspiration.

4. An alternative method that employs multiple pressure/flow points is simplified by digitization of signals with an analog/digital converter and the processing of the digital data by means of a programmed computer. Averaged resistance values representing the whole of one or several curves can be obtained by this form of repeated sampling throughout individual breaths. A 50-Hz sampling rate is adequate for spontaneous breathing, and higher rates do not yield further useful information. The computer-assisted method enables both raw and computed data to be displayed and stored for subsequent processing with the option of hard copy that can be produced as required *(11,12)*. An additional advantage of this method is the ease with which many other concomitant breathing parameters can be computed from the digitized data (Table 1).

It is of interest to note that three commonly employed methods of calculation produce almost identical values at resistances <0.4 Pa/cm^3/s. This range extends well beyond normal adult limits (0.18 ± 0.07 Pa/cm^3/s) *(11)* and calculations of pressure/flow ratios at:

a. 100 Pa;

b. Peak pressure or flow; and

c. Averaged at 50 Hz. All produce similar numerical values *(10)* and detect deviations from normal equally well.

The "normal" adult resistance range cited above was derived intuitively from our own wide practical experience rather than statistics. In an extensive and searching review of rhinomanometry, Pallanch et al. *(13)* have examined the statistical determination and establishment of a normal range of adult resistances.

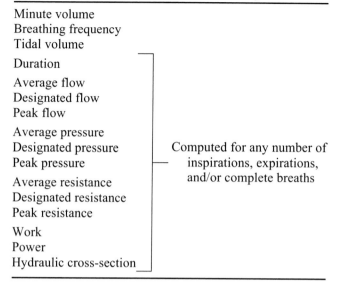

Table 1
Some of the Respiratory Variables
that Can Be Computed Concomitantly
from Digitized Pressure and Flow Signals

Minute volume
Breathing frequency
Tidal volume
Duration
Average flow
Designated flow
Peak flow
Average pressure
Designated pressure   Computed for any number of
Peak pressure   inspirations, expirations,
Average resistance   and/or complete breaths
Designated resistance
Peak resistance
Work
Power
Hydraulic cross-section

In addition to the differing methods that are employed for calculation of nasal resistances, less widely used parameters of nasal patency are derived also from transnasal pressure and flow. Conductance, the reciprocal of resistance, has its advocates. Population studies have shown nasal conductances to attain a more normal distribution than resistances, since the latter are markedly skewed toward higher values *(13)*. Logarithmic and other transforms have been advocated also to provide more normal distribution values that would enable parametric statistical methods to be employed *(13)* in attempts to establish normal limits. Cross-sectional dimensions of the nasal airway have been used by some investigators as measures of nasal patency. They are calculated from pressure and flow by hydraulic engineering formulae, and the derived values are said to vary less than calculated resistances *(11)* (*see also* Acoustic Rhinometry later in this chapter). Power and work of breathing, which have similarities with the computer averaging described above, have been used also. Despite advantages of many alternatives, resistance measurements are most widely used.

Uses of Rhinomanometry

Rhinomanometry has a long and successful history in the study of nasal physiology. Mucovascular volume changes, in the nasal cycle and in response to a variety of local and remote stimuli, have been studied extensively by rhinomanometric assessments of nasal patency *(14)*. Real and simulated structural differences have been investigated *(15,16)*. Rhinomanometric assessments of effects of local and systemic medications and challenges with allergens are currently employed in several centers. Objective documentation of structural and mucosal components of resistance is useful for monitoring nasal therapy *(17)*, and is of medico-legal importance in cases of nasal trauma and of those types of nasal treatment in which risk of patient dissatisfaction is an important factor. In addition, as nasal pathophysiological knowledge and experience increase, rhinomanometry is becoming more firmly established as a useful diagnostic procedure.

Clinical Assessment

Symptoms are the usual cause for patients to seek professional advice and treatment. The sensation of impaired nasal patency is a common symptom, and a careful history and examination by a clinician will provide a diagnosis and indicate appropriate treatment in many cases. In some cases, clinical tests may be undertaken to support a diagnosis.

Recognition of unilateral obstructions by patient and by clinician is fairly well correlated with objective findings, but, as discussed in Chapter 2, a patient's nasal sensation cannot be relied on to provide a dependable estimate of nasal patency. Moreover, subjective estimations by clinicians, even those with experience and skill, may differ. Clinicians' opinions may differ also from objective rhinomanometric assessments; indeed, it has been questioned whether the two techniques assess the same aspects of patency *(18–20)*.

Rhinoscopy has limitations, especially in examination of the leptorrhine nose. Dimensions of the narrow valve are difficult to assess without instrumentation, and instrumentation, e.g., by insertion of a speculum, disturbs tissue relationships in this most critically resistive region of the nose. The major portion of nasal resistance is concentrated in the normally narrowed lumen of the nasal valve (*see also* The Nasal Valve in Chapter 2), and the valve region is the most frequent site of obstruction by mucosal swelling, structural irregularity (e.g., septal deviation), or a combination of these abnormalities. Structural or mucosal displacement of the medial or lateral wall of the valve by as little as 1 mm

is unlikely to be detected by rhinoscopy. Yet, since such small displacements affect resistance or patency exponentially, they can escalate these parameters substantially *(15,16)*, enabling small structural or mucosal variations to be readily detectable by rhinomanometry. Acoustic rhinometric assessments (*see* section on Acoustic Rhinometry later in this chapter), too, can detect these small abnormalities and determine their site without instrumental disturbance of airway dimensions.

The uses of rhinomanometry are extending beyond the research laboratory into the clinical field. In our Toronto ENT Clinics at St. Michael's Hospital, Mount Sinai Hospital, and the Hospital for Sick Children, clinical rhinomanometric assessments have exceeded 2000 annually for several years. In an increasing number of situations, we are finding that, in addition to its proven investigative value, acoustic rhinometry (*see* section on Acoustic Rhinometry later in this chapter) can provide further useful clinical information.

Our patients are accepted on referral by oto-laryngologists, respirologists, allergists, cosmetic surgeons, skull base surgeons, ophthalmologists, dentists and orthodontists, family practitioners, lawyers, and sleep disorder clinicians. Similar rhinomanometric centers are in operation throughout the world and several employ the Toronto system (*see* A Rhinomanometric Session, later in this chapter).

Alternatives to Rhinomanometry

Before discussing technical details of rhino-manometry, objective alternatives to transnasal pressure/flow studies will be considered. Chilled mirrors or other polished surfaces have been used for more than a century to detect asymmetry of nasal expiratory air flow. The subject exhales through the nose against such a surface held close to the nostrils, and dimensions of the two areas of condensation are noted, enabling expiratory air flows through the nostrils to be compared. The technique has been particularly useful in studies of the nasal cycle in humans and in small animals. Refinements of this technique include calibration by concentric markings on the condensing surface and camera recording of thermographic surfaces, but nowadays the method is not widely used in a clinical setting.

Peak flowmeters (Wright type) are modified for nasal use by several investigators in order to obtain a measure of nasal patency. The instruments are inexpensive, easily portable, and simple to use for repeated tests by patients themselves who can be their own control. Peak flows are positively correlated with subjective resistance assessments in individual subjects, but maximized flows are effort dependent and results vary markedly, especially between subjects. The technique has its greatest usefulness in detection of large changes in nasal patency in individual subjects *(21)*. Sniff tests *(22)* promise greater precision.

Oscillometry has been employed in only a few centers. A loudspeaker applied to the nostrils and then to the mouth generates sinusoidal oscillations that are superimposed on normal breathing. The differences between the two impedance measurements provide data for calculation of nasal resistance values *(23)*.

Acoustic rhinometry is a recently developed technique. It is used quite widely in Europe, but, as yet, only infrequently in North America. It provides a promising method for determination of nasal patency that deserves a detailed description in this chapter, since, although it has not yet become well established in the clinician's armamentarium, it has already earned an important place in investigative rhinology.

Acoustic Rhinometry

A technique of acoustic reflection has been exploited by respirologists for several years in the investigation of the large respiratory airways *(24)*. A sound wave generator with a microphonic detector is applied to a respiratory portal (each nasal cavity separately in rhinometry), and reflected sounds are analyzed by a programmed computer and displayed as an area/distance curve representing airway geometry (Figs. 4 and 5) *(25)*. Displayed data can be stored and hard copy obtained as required. The technique enables measurements of the cross-sectional area of the lumen to be made at any point in a nasal cavity, and thus, volume of the lumen between any two points can be computed also. Findings have been validated by means of plastic models and cadavers *(26,27)*. In vivo, human studies in which acoustic cross-sectional areas were compared with cross-sectional areas derived from magnetic resonance imaging have shown close correlation *(28)*.

In our own laboratory, where the techniques described in this chapter were employed, several hundred measurements of nasal patency demonstrated that acoustic reflection compared favorably with rhinomanometry. Results were of at least equal reproducibility and diagnostic sensitivity *(25)*.

Acoustic rhinometric findings in healthy noses confirm air-flow rhinomanometric measurements (Fig. 5) (*see also* Chapter 2) in demonstrating the narrowed and resistive anterior segment of the airway termed the nasal valve and also its dynamic nature. The extended length of the nasal valve lumen is clearly demonstrated in the rhinometer-generated sound path by means of a spring-loaded plastic strip (Breathe Right™) that, by adhesion to the skin overlying the compliant tissues of the anterior nose, dilates the compliant vestibule (Fig. 5) *(25)* (*see also* Chapter 2, The Nasal Valve).

An essential requirement of both rhinometry and rhinomanometry is an adapter that provides a minimally invasive interphase between measuring apparatus and subject. A rhinomanometric technique that avoids invasion at the interphase completely by employment of a head-out body plethysmograph is described later in this chapter, but the technique is, of course, unsuitable for acoustic rhinometric measurements.

The major component of nasal resistance to air flow is situated in the narrowed valve region of the compliant anterior nose (*see also* Chapter 2) where tissue displacements affecting airway lumen bring about exponential changes in air-flow resistance. Thus, small displacements of these yielding tissues, by attempts to create an effective seal between nose and apparatus, risks vestibular tissue malpositioning that can result in substantial measurement errors. The use of nozzles is particularly risky, since an exact fit between nostril and nozzle is unlikely and some tissue displacement is almost inevitable in attaining an airtight seal. The choice of a nozzle of suitable dimensions and its insertion must therefore be undertaken with great care in order to minimize artifactual errors. Indeed, comparisons between different nozzles and connectors have shown substantial measurement differences in both nasal air-flow resistances *(29)* and acoustic cross-sectional areas *(25)*.

Under- or overestimations of valve cross-sectional areas associated with distortion of the nasal vestibule and variability of measurements related to head positioning are minimized by use of a noninvasive nasal adapter and by stabilization of the head with a chin support that also maintains a

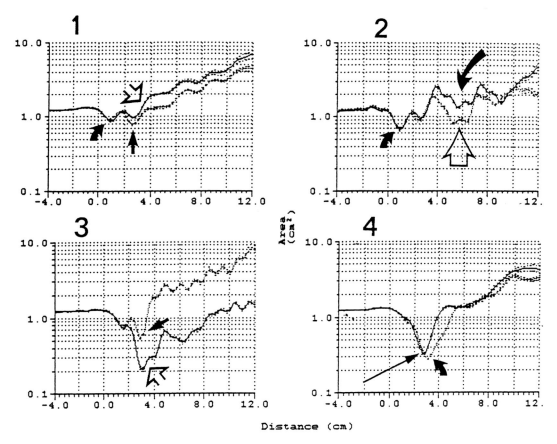

Fig. 4. Acoustic rhinometry printouts. **(A)** Healthy nasal cavity before and after decongestion (open arrow). Entrance to nasal valve area (curved arrow). Piriform aperture and anterior end of inferior turbinate (short straight arrow). **(B)** Nasal polyp and mucosal swelling before (open arrow) and after decongestion (long curved arrow). Entrance to nasal valve area (short curved arrow). **(C)** Mucosal swelling of allergic nose. Open arrow indicates minimal cross-sectional area (MCA) before decongestion. Note increase in MCA after decongestion (solid arrow). From ref. *25*. **(D)** Anterior septal deviation in valve area (curved arrow). Note minimal change with decongestant of MCA after decongestant (long straight arrow).

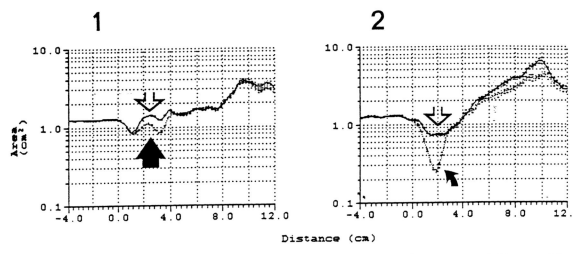

Fig. 5. (A) Acoustic rhinometry printout. Effect of an external dilator (Breathe Right™) on extended lumen of the valve before (solid arrow) and after (open arrow) application. **(B)** Nasal valve collapse (curved arrow). MCA greatly increased (open arrow) by application of external dilator (Breathe Right™). From ref. *25*.

Nasal Adapter

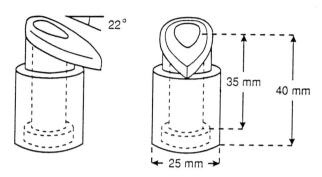

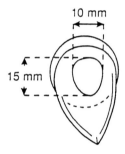

Fig. 6. Plastic connector applied to the rim of the nostril and junction sealed with water soluble jell for minimally invasive conduction of acoustic signals to and from the nasal cavities. (From ref. *25*.)

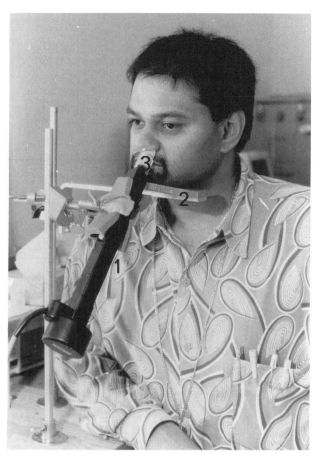

Fig. 7. Subject positioned and stabilized for rhinometric test sound generator wave tube **(A)**, with chin rest **(B)**, and nasal connector **(C)** positioned and stabilized with a clamp. (From ref. *25*.)

constant angle between the wave tube and the subject's head.

In our Toronto laboratories, as an alternative to a nozzle for acoustic rhinometric studies, the end of a plastic tube, molded to form a small oblique disk, (Fig. 6) *(30)*, is positioned to barely touch the margins of the nostril of a subject whose head is stabilized by a chin support. This support also maintains a constant angle between the wave tube and the subject's nasal airway throughout each test. The plastic tube connected to the wave tube of the acoustic rhinometer is fixed in position by a clamp attached to the measuring apparatus (Fig. 7) *(25)*. Water-soluble lubricating gel, expressed from a small syringe with a fine, flexible plastic tube in place of a needle, is used to seal the junction and to complete an acoustic coupling. With practice, a technician is able to accomplish this procedure within a few moments. It causes minimal discomfort for the subject, and integrity of the seal can be checked by a single acoustic test. If the seal is incomplete, addition of gel solves the problem.

Results from single acoustic tests are displayed almost instantaneously. We take averaged values from 10 tests to produce a nasal area-distance graph together with computations of minimal cross-sectional area and nasal volume (Figs. 4 and 5). Four graphs with computations in good agreement complete the series for one side, and the procedure is repeated on the opposite side. In clinical cases, the full procedure is performed again following application of topical decongestant to determine the vascular component of mucosal volume, which enables the clinical investigator to differentiate mucosal from structural components of nasal obstruction (Fig. 4).

For diagnostic purposes, rhinomanometric and acoustic rhinometric findings, in common with results of clinical tests generally, must be considered in association with all clinical findings in order to be correctly interpreted, since different patho-logical conditions can produce similar resistances and similar area/distance curves.

As in many other centers, we have found the acoustic rhinometric technique to be both mini-mally invasive and expeditious. It produces clear and consistent graphical representations and com-puted dimensions of the valve/turbinate complex, mucosal swelling, septal and other structural devia-tions, polyps, and other intrusions on the nasal lumen (Figs. 4 and 5). Mucosal responses to chal-lenge, medication, and vasoactive substances, and results of medical and surgical therapy have been monitored also. Effects of these abnormalities and interventions have been readily and reliably deter-mined in our own and other laboratories by this minimally invasive technique *(31,32)*.

Cross-sectional areas beyond severely narrowed nasal segments are underestimated by acoustic rhinometry *(26)*. The extent of underestimation varies directly with both the degree of narrowing and its length. However, although the precise mag-nitude of posterior obstructions cannot be estimated under these circumstances, their presence can be readily detected (Fig. 4).

Acoustic rhinometry will undoubtedly find an increasingly important niche in rhinology and will add a valuable supplement to existing inves-tigative modalities. We have found it particu-larly useful for precise assessments of nasal valve dimensions, e.g., pre- and postsurgery, and for rapid noninvasive estimations of muco-vascular responses, e.g., in challenge studies. When the method is employed together with rhinomanometry, a comprehensive picture of both respiratory function and geometry of the nasal cavities can be assembled.

PRACTICAL CONSIDERATIONS

Rhinomanometric Methodology

As already described, active rhinomanometry requires concomitant measurements of respiratory air flow, and of differential pressures between the anterior nares and the pharynx during exclusively nasal breathing. There is variety in the details of patient management, instrumentation, signal pro-cessing, data collection, and in presentation of results, but general principles and practices in most rhinomanometric centers are similar. Details are discussed in the following sections.

The Patient

Respiratory air flow through the parallel nasal passages is seldom equal, and inequalities are often severe. They result not only from static structural asymmetries, but also as a consequence of dynamic mucovascular variations on which effects of the spontaneous nasal cycle and of posture are of major importance (*see* Figs. 12 and 13 in Chapter 2). Resistances of the separate nasal cavities vary cyclically over time through a wide range that is dependent on blood content of erectile tissues of the lateral nasal wall and the anterior septum. The magnitude of these cyclical mucovascular changes that determine air-flow resistance reciprocates between sides in such a manner as to maintain a stable resistance of the combined nasal cavities (*see* The Nasal Cycle in Chapter 2). Thus, by contrast with unilateral air-flow resistances, resistances of the combined nasal cavities of healthy individual subjects are relatively stable. When rhinomano-metric measurements were made repeatedly over periods of several months, under comfortable rest-ing conditions, coefficients of variation from the mean of bilateral nasal resistances of healthy indi-vidual subjects were <20% *(33)*.

The resistive cycle is irregular in amplitude and frequency, and, although the latter is measured in hours, change of phase can take place in only a few moments (*see* Fig. 12 in Chapter 2). Furthermore, frequent minor resistive fluctuations of short dura-tion are superimposed on the cycle. Rapid muco-vascular changes are important in rhinological assessments, especially when unilateral rhinoma-nometric measurements are performed as with anterior rhinomanometry (*see* section on Other Centers later in this chapter). Effects of asymmetri-cal pressures on the body cannot be ignored (*see* Chapter 2, Fig. 13), and, as a precaution, patients should be seated symmetrically while assessments are being made.

In addition to spontaneous changes in tone and resulting blood content of the capacitance vessels that reciprocate between sides, mucovascular responses that accompany a wide variety of stimuli affect the nasal airways bilaterally and must be taken into account in rhinological assessments. Among these bilateral responses, consideration should be given to possible effects of nasal and systemic diseases and to medications *(11)*. Several of the latter may be in use for nonnasal conditions

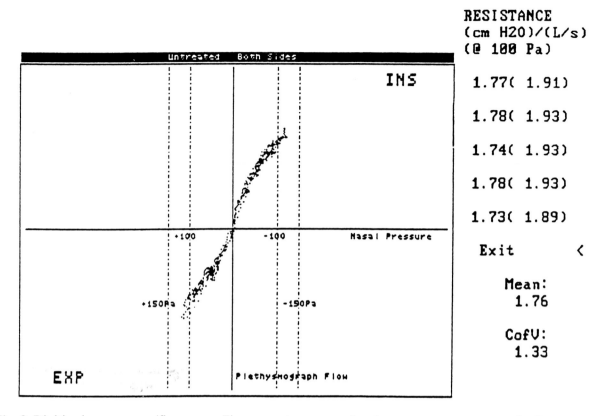

RESISTANCE
(cm H2O)/(L/s)
(@ 100 Pa)

1.77(1.91)

1.78(1.93)

1.74(1.93)

1.78(1.93)

1.73(1.89)

Exit   <

Mean:
1.76

CofV:
1.33

Fig. 8. Digitized *x-y* pressure/flow curve. Five computer-averaged resistance measurements each of two consecutive breaths with a coefficient of variation of 1.33%. Figures in parentheses are resistance values at 1.0 cm H_2O (100 Pa).

(e.g., antihypertensive drugs). It should be noted also that exercise can bring about as substantial a reduction of nasal air-flow resistance as either topical or systemic vasoconstrictors. Effects of exercise on healthy noses are no longer evident following <30 min rest. Allergic noses may show rebound congestion of longer duration, and effects of different therapeutic decongestants vary from <1 h to several hours. By contrast, hyperventilation, vasodilator substances, and irritants (allergens, infection, air pollutants, cold air, and so on) can exert the opposite effect and bring about substantial and, in many cases, prompt congestion *(11)*.

Patterns of breathing are susceptible to psychological disturbances. They are changed markedly by attachment of equipment to the nose or mouth *(34)*, and the altered pattern can affect results of resistance measurement. Minimizing psychological disturbances by reassurance of patients by clinician and auxiliary personnel and a friendly, comfortable environment are of particular importance in rhinomanometric studies. Furthermore, a half-hour of restricted activity should be allowed to

provide the opportunity for patients to achieve a state of respiratory and nasal mucovascular stability in the innocuous environment of the clinic or consulting room before rhinomanometry is performed. Documentation and clinical examination can be undertaken conveniently during this period. Clear explanation of the test to the patient and comfort of the equipment also are of major importance if reliable results are to be obtained.

Equipment Overview

Nasal respiratory air is conducted to and from the nostrils through a flow-measuring device and, concomitantly, transnasal differential pressures are conducted through a small tube from the pharynx to a pressure-measuring device. By means of transducers, whose electrical output is amplified, pressure and flow signals are displayed, most commonly in *x-y* format (as in Figs. 3 and 8 and in Fig. 17 later in this chapter). Calculation of resistance as a pressure/flow ratio is usually automated, and results are displayed.

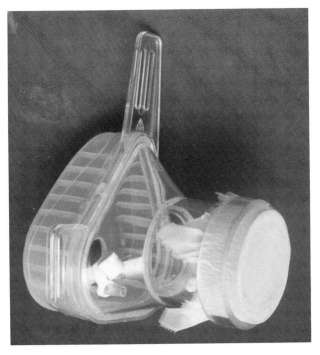

Fig. 9. Modified CPAP mask with 400-mesh dacron resistor as a laminar flow element.

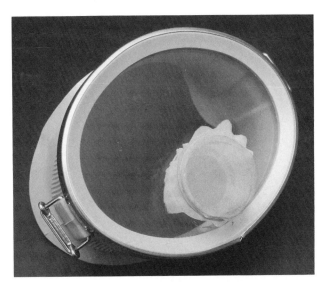

Fig. 10. Modified SCUBA mask. Commonly used, but not recommended by authors.

Airflow

Nasal air flow is customarily measured by means of a pneumotach. This device conducts respiratory air through a laminar flow element of low resistance. Pressure differential across the resistor is directly proportional to flow through it and is detected by a sensitive differential pressure transducer. Responses of the pneumotach, transducer, and associated equipment must be adequate for signals of breathing frequency, and linearity of such a system is not difficult to attain. A lightweight and inexpensive pneumotach resistor can be made from 5-cm diameter, 400-mesh dacron laboratory filter (Fig. 9) and, combined with a Validyne MP45 transducer (Validyne Engineering, Northridge, CA), it provides an electrical signal that bears a linear relationship with air flow well beyond the resting respiratory range. More expensive pneumotachs are readily available commercially.

A nozzle can be used to connect nostril to pneumotach and to conduct respiratory air flow. The risks and precautions attending this type of coupling have been outlined earlier in this chapter (*see* Acoustic Rhinometry), but, despite the limitations of a nozzle, the exercise of exceptional care in choice and insertion has enabled reliable results to be obtained *(35)*. All investigators who use these connecting devices should make doubly sure that precautions to avoid distortion of the vestibular tissues are strictly followed. The coupler recommended above for acoustic rhinometric measurements is unsuitable for air-flow studies and, in many cases, nozzles that are demonstrated in exhibitions of rhinomanometric equipment are unsuitable also. Common faults are external dimensions that distort the vestibule and internal dimensions that impede air flow.

A facemask that includes the nostrils is an alternative to a nozzle. It provides the most widely employed method. There are many types of facemask, and, although the nose may not be affected directly, displacement of mobile facial tissues can displace compliant anterior nasal tissues indirectly and produce misleading artifacts. Displacement of facial tissues as far from the nose as the zygomatic region can affect nasal air-flow resistance substantially.

In addition to discomfort, an ill-fitting mask and pressure of mask against face to achieve a seal risk artifacts. We used modified SCUBA masks (Fig. 10) in our early rhinomanometric work until we recognized them as serious sources of error. Examination of several other types of facemask has demonstrated their potential for error also. The most satisfactory masks we have found are the aviator or fireman type (Fig. 11), which contact the periphery of the face. They usually provide a good seal with-

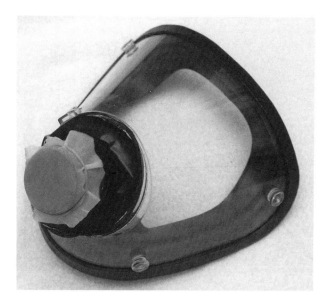

Fig. 11. Fireman- or aviator-type mask satisfactory for adults.

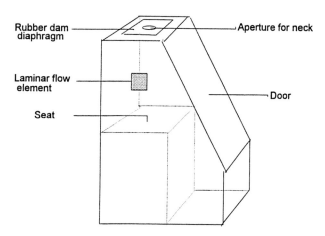

Fig. 12. Diagrammatic representation of the Toronto head-out displacement-type body plethysmograph.

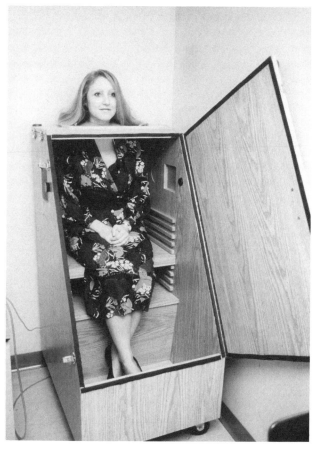

Fig. 13. Subject preparing for rhinomanometric test.

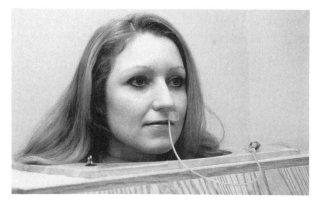

Fig. 14. Pernasal catheter in position.

out the need for firm pressure, but, unfortunately, the range of sizes is limited and is unsuitable for children. We have found that modified CPAP masks (Fig. 9) avoid the major problems noted above. They are light in weight, and provide an effective soft and comfortable seal.

A head-out displacement-type body plethysmogragh (Figs. 12–15), despite its rather formidable bulk, is a stable, reliable, and rugged, yet adequately sensitive, instrument for measuring respiratory air flow *(36)*, and it is simple to calibrate. The crucial advantage of the head-out plethysmograph in rhinomanometry is that disturbing effects of masks and nozzles are avoided by liberating the face entirely from invasive equipment and from the disadvantages discussed earlier. Furthermore, the unencumbered face is available for observation, video studies of nasal, oral, and facial respiratory movements (e.g., oronasal breathing), and for EMG studies. It is available also for assessments of the effects on air-flow resistance of

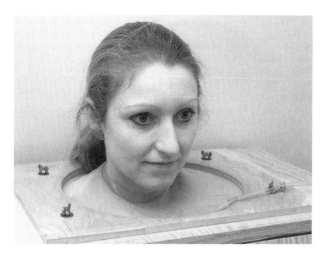

Fig. 15. Rubber dental dam neck seal of plethysmograph.

manipulations of nasal tissues, such as alar retraction, elevation of the nasal tip or effects, of a vestibular dilator (*see* A Rhinomanometric Session, later in this chapter).

Head-out displacement plethysmographs have been used successfully for many years by respirologists for infant studies and by physiologists for small animal studies. Use of the displacement-type plethysmograph, as employed for nasal studies, is far simpler and much less demanding than the more complicated pressure-type that is used in respiratory function laboratories.

The head-out plethysmographs we employ are boxes constructed quite simply from ¾-in laminated particle board (Figs. 12–15). Dimensions are not critical, but volume restriction improves characteristics. A subject sits in the closed box, and the head is passed through a hole in a thin rubber dental dam diaphragm that remains around the neck to form an airtight seal (Fig. 15). When the box is closed and the subject inspires, increase in body volume displaces box air through a laminar flow element in the box wall (400-mesh dacron filter, 12 × 12 cm). In expiration, flow is reversed. Pressure changes in the box that are generated by the subject's respiratory volume change are directly proportional to air flow by displacement through the flow element and are detected by a sensitive differential pressure transducer Validyne MP 101 (Validyne Engineering) between the box and the atmosphere. Thus, respiratory air flow is measured indirectly as box flow by an electrical signal from the transducer. The accuracy, frequency response, and linearity of the system have been determined and found adequate for breathing measurements *(36)*.

Inductive plethysmography provides yet another technique for measurement of respiratory air flow. Although it is probably less precise than the methods described above, the minimally invasive features of this type of equipment are particularly attractive. The technology depends on the property of inductive girdles that enables electronic measurements of volume change of a cylinder to be determined from changes in its circumference. This apparatus is particularly useful in sleep laboratories, where recordings of thoracic and abdominal respiratory volume changes are used to detect and differentiate apneic obstructions in sleeping subjects. It has been used also for nasal air-flow studies *(37)*.

Transnasal Pressure (Fig. 16)

As a subject breathes exclusively through the nose, differential pressures are measured between pharynx and atmosphere by a tube connected to a port of a differential pressure transducer. The other port remains open to the atmosphere when the plethysmograph is used for determination of nasal air flow. When a mask is used, differential pressures are measured between the pharynx and the inside of the mask in place of the atmosphere.

There are three common sites for positioning the open end of the pressure-conducting tubing in a subject's airways. Posterior rhinomanometry is the term applied to the method in which the pressure-conducting tube is passed perorally to the oropharyngeal region. When lips are closed about the tube and the soft palate is relaxed in an intermediate position between tongue and posterior pharyngeal wall, transnasal respiratory pressures can be measured as the subject breathes through the nose.

Despite frequent statements to the contrary, posterior rhinomanometry can be performed successfully in almost all patients. The majority carry out the necessary palato/lingual maneuver with minimal instruction, and, in the remainder, persistence and patience of subject and investigator almost invariably achieve success. We have found failure to be rare in either adults or children in the hands of experienced technicians. Indeed, the posterior method is in general use for children in our laboratories, in preference to other methods, since, in addition to assessment of nasal resistance, it can be employed for measurement of adenoid obstruction of the nasopharyngeal airway *(38)*.

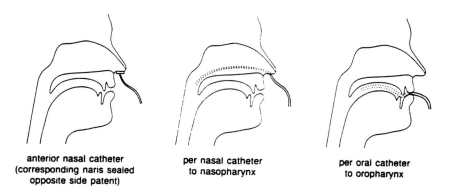

anterior nasal catheter   per nasal catheter   per oral catheter
(corresponding naris sealed   to nasopharynx   to oropharynx
opposite side patent)

Fig. 16. Positioning of pressure-detecting tubing. Anterior, pernasal, and posterior methods.

Anterior rhinomanometry is so called because the pressure-conducting tube is temporarily sealed in the vestibular portion of one side of the nose. As the subject breathes through the unsealed nasal cavity, nasopharyngeal respiratory pressures are conducted through the patent portion of the sealed nasal cavity to the vestibule and the pressure-detecting tube.

Anterior rhinomanometry is probably the most commonly used rhinomanometric method, since, by comparison with posterior rhinomanometry, it requires minimal cooperation from the subject. However, there are disadvantages in that adenoid obstruction cannot be measured by this method, nor can it be used successfully in cases of severe unilateral obstruction or septal perforation.

Unilateral nasal breathing is not natural and unilateral occlusion can reduce contralateral alar dilator muscle tone. Changing the pressure tube and replacing the mask risks redisplacing perinasal facial tissues with resistive consequences, and, furthermore, if the time interval between right and left measurements is protracted, significant spontaneous resistive mucosal changes can occur.

Pernasal rhinomanometry is a method in which a fine, flexible plastic pressure-conducting tube is passed approx 8 cm along the floor of the adult nose to position its open end in the nasopharynx. Infant feeding catheters (8-F [French] gage, 35-cm length) have dimensions and physical characteristics that are entirely suitable. They have lateral openings that avoid dynamic flow artifacts and detect lateral airway pressures, and these openings should be positioned vertically to avoid obstruction by mucosal contact. Validation experiments have shown the catheters to be adequate for conduction of nasopharyngeal pressures and too small to affect nasal

patency significantly when positioned as described. Nasal anesthesia is not necessary if the tube is passed along the nasal floor without hesitation or delay, and any minor patient discomfort ceases as the tube is secured to the upper lip with adhesive tape. A lubricant gel applied to the tube can be used to aid insertion. Patient cooperation is minimized by this method.

An occasional patient has experienced irritation from the tube that has promoted nasal discharge. Usually, in these cases, sniffing and flushing the pressure tube with air from a 50-mL syringe solves the problems, and only rarely must the tube be changed or the procedure abandoned. This problem is so unusual that pernasal measurement is our first choice in all adult patient measurements, and, indeed, these small pernasal catheters are regularly retained *in situ* during lengthy overnight studies of patients in our sleep laboratory without causing problems from nasal irritation.

Signal Processing

Electrical signals resulting from transducer responses to transnasal pressures and flows are amplified for recording purposes. Recordings of concurrent pressure and flow signals against time, separately, on a strip chart (Fig. 1) have been largely displaced by x-y recording of the combined signals with an oscilloscope, which in turn is being displaced by digitized signals and a programmed computer with monitor display (Figs. 8 and 17).

A RHINOMANOMETRIC SESSION

Toronto Clinics (39)

The following description outlines the procedures undertaken in centers where the Toronto sys-

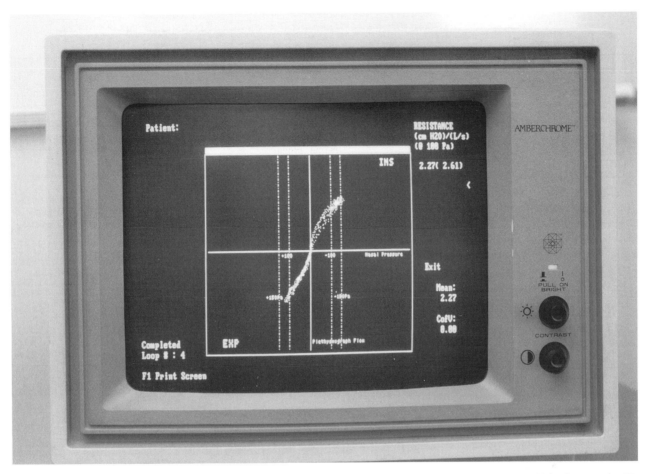

Fig. 17. Computer monitor with *x-y* pressure/flow tracing of four breaths. Normal resistance. (Display not in SI units!) Note accumulation of data points near inspiratory peak and their more even distribution in the expiratory portion of curve.

tem is employed. A head-out body plethysmograph is used together with the posterior rhinomanometric method for children and the pernasal method for adults. Data are acquired as described above by transduction of pressure and flow signals. Analog-to-digital conversion enables processing to be performed by a programmed desk-top IBM or compatible computer.

As an adult patient enters the clinic, documentation is followed by history taking and clinical examination. The rhinomanometric investigation is explained to the patient, who is then seated in the plethysmograph. The neck seal is positioned, and the plethysmograph door is closed (Figs. 13–15).

After assurance that only slight irritation will be experienced, the nasal catheter is inserted 8 cm along the floor of the patient's more patent nasal cavity without hesitation or delay, and fixed in position by adhesive tape. It remains in this posi-

tion, detecting postnasal pressures, until all testing is concluded.

Transducer connections are completed, a computer program is activated, and the patient is instructed to breathe normally and exclusively through the nose. When a typical regularly repeating sigmoid tracing on the computer monitor screen indicates that subject and system are performing in a satisfactory manner, the data-acquisition portion of the computer program is activated. Resistances are computed at a 50-Hz sampling rate and averaged over several breaths (two regular consecutive breaths are accepted as adequate for clinical purposes), and the result is displayed on the monitor screen. Measurements are repeated until five results with a computed coefficient of variation from the mean of <8% are obtained. Research may require greater precision and, in order to attain a better average, a larger number of consecutive breaths

Table 2
Typical Nasal Airflow Resistances of Normal and Abnormal Noses Obtained
by Clinical Testing as Described in the Text

| Nasal cavities, comment | Sides | Resistance, $Pa/cm^3/s$ | | | |
		Unremarkable findings	Mucovascular swelling	Right anterior structural obstruction	Approximate normal range
Untreated	Both	0.21	0.37	0.25	0.18 ± 0.07
Untreated	Left	0.40	1.69	0.44	Varies with cycle
Untreated	Right	0.51	0.50	1.01	Varies with cycle
Decongested	Both	0.13	0.11	0.24	Untreated halved
Decongested	Left	0.26	0.31	0.35	0.30 ± 0.10
Decongested	Right	0.35	0.22	0.96	Untreated halved
Retracted	Left	0.12	0.14	0.15	Decongested halved
Retracted	Right	0.18	0.17	0.17	Decongested halved

can be measured and a <5% coefficient of variation is not difficult to attain.

The next step is to measure resistance of each nasal cavity separately while the opposite side is occluded, and the routine that has just been described for the combined nasal cavities is repeated for left and right sides.

When this has been accomplished, each nasal cavity is sprayed 3× with 0.1% xylometazoline hydrochloride, and the plethysmograph door is opened for the patient's comfort during the 10 min allowed for nasal mucosal decongestion. The routine is then repeated with the combined nasal cavities and with each side separately. Finally, resistances of each of the decongested nasal cavities are measured separately during alar retraction. A printout of results with clinical comment can be ready for reporting to the referring practitioner by phone, fax, or mail in <30 min from commencement of the measurements. There are many days in which our rhinomanometric clinic assessments exceed 10 patients.

Typical results are shown in Table 2, and a few explanatory comments are presented here in order to clarify details of the procedure. Initial measurement of the combined and untreated nasal cavities indicates the nasal resistance the patient is experiencing at the time of examination. Resistances of the separate and untreated nasal cavities almost invariably differ, not only from structural or mucosal abnormalities, but also from continual mucosal changes of the nasal cycle, and although the measurements are therefore of limited diagnos-

tic value, they may confirm or deny the symptom or rhinoscopic finding of unilateral obstruction.

Decongested resistance values of the combined nasal cavities indicate the contribution of mucovascular swelling to air-flow resistance, and measurements from separate sides can demonstrate residual structural components of resistance. Finally, since alar retraction relieves obstruction in the compliant anterior nose, it enables resistance measurements to determine the anterior or posterior site of an obstruction. Rhinoscopy is repeated while the mucosa is decongested. Thus, the structural and mucosal components of nasal obstruction and their side, site, and severity can be determined.

It should be noted also that relief of nasal obstruction by means of a decongestant does not exclude the possibility of a structural abnormality. It may be obstructive only when the mucosa is not decongested.

The procedure with children differs only in the employment of posterior rhinometric pressure measurement by means of a mouth tube (in place of a pernasal tube in adults) to detect and determine the extent of adenoid obstruction in addition to nasal cavity resistance. It is usual for children to perform the necessary palato-lingual maneuver spontaneously or to learn it more readily than some adults. Feedback from the tracing on the monitor screen, encouragement from a friendly and experienced technician, and a nonthreatening atmosphere almost invariably produce success. It should be noted also that children prefer the plethysmograph by far to the discomfort of a facemask and, rather than being intimidated by the plethysmograph, they find it fun *(38)*.

Calibration of the complete system is checked weekly by means of an electrically driven piston pump and resistor that simulate nasal breathing. The system is stable, but occasionally the check may indicate that a calibration adjustment is necessary, which is easily performed. It requires only a few moments with a flowmeter and a manometer to recalibrate the complete system.

Field trials, involving nasal air-flow resistance measurements, require portable equipment, and we use a facemask in place of the more cumbersome plethysmograph, together with a customized and compact computerized system *(39)*. We have attempted breathing studies of sleeping subjects in a coffin-shaped head-out body plethysmograph that we used for posture studies (The Nasal Cycle in Chapter 2), but have found the portable equipment and modified CPAP mask/pneumotachs to be more convenient (Fig. 9).

Other Centers

In most other centers, nasal air flow is measured with a facemask or, more rarely, a nozzle in place of a plethysmograph. Transnasal pressures are measured by either anterior or, less commonly, posterior rhinomanometric methods. Methods of data acquisition and processing vary, but digitization of signals and programmed computer processing are increasingly popular.

The most common rhinomanometric procedure in other centers is anterior rhinomanometry. Prior to application of a facemask that incorporates a pneumotach for measurement of nasal air flow, a fine plastic tube is inserted for pressure measurement in a nasal vestibule and sealed in position with adhesive tape, which occludes the intubated nostril. The mask is then adjusted and secured in a position that ensures an airtight seal, and measurements of pressure and flow are obtained as the subject breathes exclusively through the unoccluded nasal cavity. When representative results have been acquired, the mask is removed, the pressure tubing is replaced in the opposite side, the mask is replaced, and the procedure is repeated. In many centers, the above left and right routine is repeated following decongestion of the nasal mucosa and, in at least one center, alar retraction is accomplished by insertion of small nasal vestibular dilators to determine the anterior or posterior site of obstruction *(40)*.

Some investigators apply Ohm's Law for resistors in parallel in order to calculate resistance of the combined nasal cavities. Ohm's Law is applicable to laminar flow conditions, and although differences in results between anterior and posterior rhinomanometry might be a consequence of nonlaminar flow (and other factors also [11]), they are accepted by many investigators as adequate for clinical work.

A designated transnasal pressure of 150 Pa, as used in several centers, is not achieved by all subjects during spontaneous unobstructed unilateral breathing at rest and by few subjects during bilateral breathing. In these cases, hyperventilation may be necessary to achieve 150 Pa. Calculation of resistances at a transnasal pressure of 150 Pa produces greater values than calculation at lesser pressures and, furthermore, marked hyperventilation promptly elevates nasal resistance by reflex increase in mucovascular volume. Results obtained at 150 Pa usually exceed those obtained at 100 Pa, at peak and by computer averaging by 25–30%.

CONCLUSIONS

Rhinomanometry provides an important objective gage of nasal patency. It is useful in many rhinological situations, including investigation of nasal mucosal responses, medicolegal documentation, monitoring of therapy, as a diagnostic procedure to support clinical findings, and to help avoid inappropriate therapeutic measures. An agreed format for presentation of results, as recommended by the International Committee on Standardization of Rhinomanometry, can aid comparison and interpretation of reports from different centers.

The dynamic air-flow findings of rhinomanometry, supplemented by the dimensional findings of acoustic rhinometry, provide an objective and comprehensive assessment of function and form of the nasal cavities, and add invaluable support to clinical diagnosis and appraisal of the extent of nasal dysfunction.

Sinus diseases are commonly associated with nasal abnormalities (e.g., mucosal swelling) that are reflected in rhinometric and rhinomanometric findings, but, since the existence of paranasal sinuses is incompletely explained, there are no objective tests of their function. Assessments of maxillary ostial patency are performed following antral puncture by injection of air or saline or by manometry and in many centers by endoscopy.

REFERENCES

(Several references in this list have been chosen for their own extensive reference lists and included for the convenience of readers who wish to refer to original work on which this chapter is based.)

1. Clement PAR. Committee report on standardization of rhinomanometry. Rhinology 1984;22:151–155.
2. Röhrer F. Der Stromungwiderstand in den menschlichen Atemwegen und der Einfluss der unregelmassigen Verzweigung des bronchial Systems auf den Atmungsverlauf in verschiedenen Lungenbezirken. Arch Ges Physiol 1915;162:225–299.
3. Schumacher M. Rhinomanometry. J Allerg Clin Immunol 1989;83(4):711–718.
4. Cole P. The Respiratory Role of the Upper Airways. St. Louis: Mosby-Year Book 1993; pp. 91–123.
5. Syabbalo NC, Bundgaard A, Entholm P, et al. Measurement and regulation of nasal airflow resistance in man. Rhinology 1986;24:87–101.
6. Proctor DF, Hardy JB. Studies of respiratory airflow. Bull Johns Hopkins Hosp 1949;85:253.
7. Cottle MH. Rhino-sphygmo-manometry: an aid in physical diagnosis. Int Rhinol 1968;6:7–26.
8. Broms P. Rhinomanometry. Thesis, University of Lund, Sweden, 1980.
9. McCaffrey TV, Kern EB. Clinical evaluation nasal obstruction: a study of 1000 patients. Arch Otolaryngol 1979;105:542–545.
10. Naito K, Iwata S, Ohoka E, Kondo Y, Takeuchi M. A comparison of current expressions of nasal patency. Eur Arch Otorhinolaryngol 1993;250:249–252.
11. Cole P. The Respiratory Role of the Upper Airways. St. Louis: Mosby-Year Book, 1993; pp. 125–158.
12. Naito K, Cole P, Chaban R, Humphrey D. Computer averaged nasal resistance. Rhinology 1989;27:45–52.
13. Pallanch JF, McCaffrey TV, Kern EB. Evaluation of nasal breathing function. In: Cummings CW, Fredrickson JM, Harher LA, Krause CJ, Shuller DE, eds., Otolaryngology—Head and Neck Surgery, 2nd ed., vol. 1. St. Louis: Mosby-Year Book, 1993; pp. 665–686.
14. Cole P. The Respiratory Role of the Upper Airways. St Louis: Mosby-Year Book, 1993; pp. 1–59.
15. Chaban R, Cole P, Naito K. Simulated septal deviations (2). Arch Otolaryngol Head Neck Surg 1988;114:413–415.
16. Cole P, Chaban R, Naito K, Oprysk D. The obstructive nasal septum: effect of simulated deviations on nasal airflow resistance. Arch Otolaryngol—Head Neck Surg 1988;114:410–412.
17. Gordon ASD, McCaffrey TV, Kern EB, Pallanch JF. Rhinomanometry for preoperative and postoperative assessment of nasal obstruction. Otolaryngol Head Neck Surg 1989;101:20–26.
18. Hardcastle PF, Haake von N, Murray JAM. Observer variation in clinical examination of the nasal airway. Clin Otolaryngol 1985;10:3–7.
19. Keay D, Smith I, White A, Hardcastle PF. The nasal cycle and clinical examination of the nose. Clin Otolaryngol 1987;12:345–348.
20. Hardcastle PF, et al. Clinical or rhinometric assessment of the nasal airway—which is better? Clin Otolaryngol 1988;13:381–385.
21. Holmstrom M, Scadding GK, Lund VJ, Darby YC. Assessment of nasal obstruction. A comparison between rhinomanometry and nasal inspiratory peak flow. Rhinology 1990;28:191–196.
22. Pertuze J, Watson A, Pride NB. Maximum airflow through the nose in humans. J Appl Physiol 1991;70(3):1369–1376.
23. Shelton DM, Pertuze J, Gleeson MJ, Thomson J, Denman WT, Goff J, Eiser NM, Pride NB. Comparison of oscillation with three other methods for measuring nasal airways resistance. Resp Med 1990;84:101–106.
24. Hoffstein V, Fredberg JJ. The acoustic reflection technique for non-invasive assessment of upper airway area. Eur Respir J 1991;4:601–611.
25. Roithmann R, Cole P, Chapnik J, et al. Acoustic rhinometry in the evaluation of nasal obstruction. Laryngoscope 1995;105:275–281.
26. Hilberg AC, Swift DL, Pedersen OF. Acoustic rhinometry: Evaluation of nasal cavity geometry by acoustic reflection. J Appl Physiol 1989;66(1):295–303.
27. Mayhew TM, O'Flynn P. Validation of acoustic rhinometry by using the Cavalieri principle to estimate nasal cavity volume in cadavers. Clin Otolaryngol 1993;18:220–225.
28. Hilberg O, Jensen FT, Pedersen OF. Nasal airway geometry: comparison between acoustic reflections and magnetic resonance scanning. J Appl Physiol 1993;75:2811–2819.
29. Cole P, Havas T. Nasal resistance to respiratory air flow: a plethysmographic alternative to the face mask. Rhinology 1987;25:159–166.
30. Hansen BJ, et al. Morphometrical evaluation of nosecasts to acoustic rhinometry and the noseadapter in acoustic rhinometry. J Jap Rhinol Soc 1991;30:124,125.
31. Lenders H, Persig W. Diagnostic value of acoustic rhinometry: patients with allergic and vasomotor rhinitis compared with normal controls. Rhinology 1990;28:5–16.
32. Grymer LF, Hilberg O, Pedersen OF, Rasmussen TR. Acoustic rhinometry: values from adults with subjective normal nasal patency. Rhinology 1991;29:35–47.
33. Cole P. Stability of nasal airflow resistance. Clin Otolaryngol Allied Sci 1989;14:177–182.
34. Askanazi J, Silverberg PA, Foster RJ, Hyman AI, Milic-Emili J, Kinney JM. Effects of respiratory apparatus on breathing pattern. J Appl Physiol 1980;48(4):577–580.
35. Naito K, Iwata S, Kato R. The influence of face masks and a nasal nozzle on nasal airflow. J Otolaryngol Jpn 1990;93(3):393–397.
36. Niinimaa V, Cole P, Mintz S, Shephard RJ. A head-out exercise body plethysmograph. J Appl Physiol 1979;47:1336–1339.
37. Warren DW, Hinton VA, Hairfield WM. Measurement of nasal and oral respiration using inductive plethysmography. Am J Orthod 1986;89(6):480–484.
38. Parker LP, Crysdale WS, Cole P, Woodside DW. Rhinomanometry in children. Int J Paed Otorhinolaryngol 1989;17:127–137.
39. Cole P. Toronto rhinomanometry: laboratory, field and clinical studies. J Otolaryngol 1988;17:331–335.
40. Guillette B, Perry CJ. Use of nasal valve stent with anterior rhinomanometry to quantitate nasal valve obstruction. Ann Otol Rhinol Laryngol 1990;99:175–178.

24 Upper Airway Endoscopy

William K. Dolen, MD and John C. Selner, MD

Contents

INTRODUCTION

The interpretation of upper airway symptoms is usually based on a partial evaluation of these structures. Routine examination of the nasal passage is generally performed by inspection of the anterior nasal passage with an otoscope, or at best, with a nasal speculum. Physical examination of the paranasal sinuses consists of percussion and transillumination. These traditional methods limit the extent to which physicians can evaluate symptoms in the nose and paranasal sinuses, resulting in therapeutic decisions often made on the basis of presenting symptoms and signs *(1)*. A more complete examination is possible with an otolaryngologist's mirrors, but most physicians have not developed this skill *(2)*, and most who have are rewarded with only a fleeting glance at these complex structures *(3)*. The intricate bony structure of the skull can make interpretation of plane X-rays difficult, and even computed tomography offers only a static glimpse of the dynamic function of these areas. The medical and industrial development of instruments specifically designed for upper airway endoscopy has made a safe, convenient, and affordable alternative to previous practice available to any physician interested in comprehensive evaluation of the upper airway. This places him or her at the same advantage as his or her pulmonary and gastroenterology colleagues who routinely perform endoscopic examinations, assuming a willingness to master the technique *(4)*.

As with any diagnostic skill, appropriate use of upper airway endoscopy requires discipline and commitment to the understanding of the basic anatomy and physiology of the upper airway. Although many medical school curricula do not emphasize these areas, the upper airway has immediate relevance to both the understanding of potential mechanisms operating in host defense and the homeostatic functions of respiration. Humidification, heat regulation, air filtration, and flow dynamics involved in the presentation of air for pulmonary gas exchange are fundamental considerations in the disciplines of otolaryngology, allergy, pulmonary medicine, environmental illness, neurotoxicology, and sleep physiology.

From: *Diseases of the Sinuses* (M. E. Gershwin and G. A. Incaudo, eds.), ©1996 Humana Press Inc., Totowa, NJ.

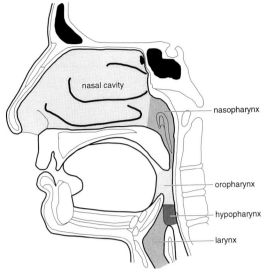

Fig. 1. The upper airway. The five major divisions are indicated. Adapted from ref. *(4)*.

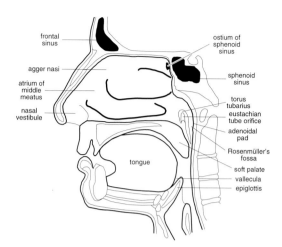

Fig. 2. Sagittal section of the upper airway, demonstrating the lateral structures of the nasal cavity and pharynx. Adapted from ref. *(4)*.

ENDOSCOPIC UPPER AIRWAY ANATOMY

For convenience in the study of anatomy and pathology, the upper airway *(4,5)* may be divided into sections (Fig. 1). In adults, each nasal cavity is a channel approx 9 or 10 cm in length from the nostril to the choana. The choana (posterior naris) separates the nasal cavity from the nasopharynx. The oropharynx, in which the palatine tonsils are located, extends from the inferior margin of the soft palate to the valleculae at the base of the tongue. The hypopharynx is located below the oropharynx at the level of the larynx. The triangular inlet of the larynx (aditus laryngis) is formed by the superior margin of the epiglottis, the aryepiglottic folds, and the arytenoid cartilages. The larynx is continuous with the trachea below the cricoid.

Anterior Nasal Structures

The nasal septum divides the nasal cavity into right and left chambers. The nasal vestibule is the most anterior and inferior portion of the nasal cavity (Fig. 2). It is bounded medially and laterally by the lower lateral cartilages and extends to the inferior border of the upper lateral nasal cartilage. The vestibule is lined by skin, rather than by mucosa, which gives rise to the vibrissae—coarse nasal hairs that serve as a protective mechanism. Above the vestibule and in front of the middle meatus is the nasal atrium, and above this is the agger nasi, an area that generally contains anterior ethmoid air

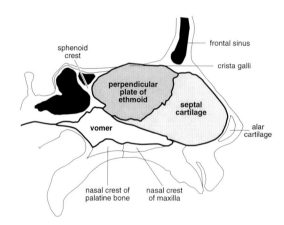

Fig. 3. Cartilaginous and bony structures of the nasal septum. Adapted from ref. *(4)*.

cells. The nasal valve is located at the junction of the vestibule and the nasal cavity. This structure, whose cross-sectional area is regulated by the dilator naris muscle, provides limiting resistance to air flow. The nasal floor is formed anteriorly by the maxillary bone and posteriorly by the palatine bone. It is slightly concave and passes horizontally from the vestibule to the choana. The nasal cavity narrows superiorly to form the roof of the nose. The middle portion of the nasal roof is approximately parallel to the nasal floor, but the anterior and posterior parts slope inferiorly.

Nasal Septum

The septum consists of both cartilaginous and bony components (Fig. 3), with mucous membrane

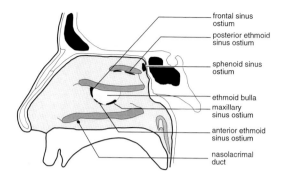

Fig. 4. Sagittal section of the upper airway with the turbinates removed, demonstrating the paranasal sinus ostia and the nasolacrimal duct. Adapted from ref. *(4)*.

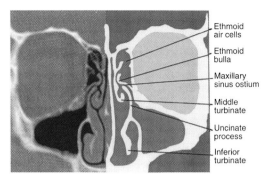

Fig. 5. Composite frontal section of the skull demonstrating the ethmoid and maxillary sinuses. A CT image is on the left; a drawing of the structures seen in the CT image is on the right. Adapted from ref. *(4)*.

overlying perichondrium or periosteum of the underlying cartilage or bone. The mobile, anterior portion of the septum is composed of a quadrangular septal cartilage resting on a ridge on the maxillary bone and articulating posteriorly with the thin, delicate bone of the perpendicular plate of the ethmoid and inferiorly with the thicker, more rigid bone of the vomer. The vomer forms the medial border of the choanae, and rests on the crest of the maxillary bone anteriorly and the crest of the palatine bone posteriorly. The perpendicular plate of the ethmoid extends superiorly, attaching to the cribriform plate (lamina cribosa). A superior projection of the hard palate, the maxillary ridge (crista nasalis maxillae; nasal crest of maxilla) often forms a "T" anteriorly at the base of the septum. The lateral wings of the "T" may project into the nasal cavity and be mistaken for a septal deviation.

Turbinates

Three or four turbinates on each lateral side provide filtration, heating and cooling, and humidification of inspired air, and offer resistance to air flow. The turbinates are comprised of a scroll-shaped egg-shell-thin bony supporting structure (the concha) and overlying mucosa. Clefting of the turbinates may occur both horizontally and sagittally; clefting of a middle turbinate may be difficult to distinguish from a nasal polyp on anterior examination. The space created by a turbinate and the lateral wall of the nose is called a meatus.

INFERIOR TURBINATE AND INFERIOR MEATUS

The inferior concha is a separate bone sitting in an opening in the maxilla and resting in the lateral wall of the nasal passage. The turbinate follows the lower lateral wall of the nose in a course parallel to

that of the nasal floor. In patients with deviation of the septum, the inferior turbinates are not the same size. The only normal opening in the inferior meatus is that of the nasolacrimal duct, which drains tears through a large opening in the anterior roof of the meatus (Fig. 4), located about 1 cm from the anterior margin of the turbinate. Compromise of the nasolacrimal duct can lead to tearing and acute or chronic dacryocystitis. The orifice is almost never seen by fiberoptic rhinoscopy, but can be viewed with a rigid endoscope. An opening found in the lateral wall at this location is most likely a classic antral window surgically placed in the inferior meatus to provide drainage for the maxillary sinus (Fig. 5).

MIDDLE TURBINATE AND MIDDLE MEATUS

The middle turbinate, like the superior turbinate, is part of the ethmoid bone and is suspended from the roof of the nose rather than from the lateral wall. The anterior edge is superior and posterior to that of the inferior turbinate. A crescent-shaped cleft, the semilunar hiatus (hiatus semilunaris), is located in the middle meatus (Fig. 4). The ostium of the nasofrontal duct and the anterior ethmoid ostia typically are located in the anterior and mid portions of the hiatus. Frequently, the nasofrontal duct will have a separate opening anterior to the semilunar hiatus. The maxillary sinuses open into the postero-inferior portion of the hiatus. In normals, the ostium of the maxillary sinus varies in size from pinpoint to several millimeters in diameter. Large accessory ostia may be present; it is often possible to advance the endoscope into the maxillary sinus itself in a patient with a large ostium or a large accessory ostium. The ethmoid bulla (bulla ethmoidalis), which contains anterior and middle ethmoid air cells, is posterior and superior to the semilunar hiatus.

SUPERIOR AND SUPREME TURBINATES

The superior turbinate is a short structure obliquely located superior and posterior to the middle turbinate. The posterior ethmoid sinuses drain into the superior meatus (Fig. 4). A supreme turbinate medial to the superior turbinate is occasionally noted.

SPHENOETHMOIDAL RECESS

The sphenoethmoidal recess is a relatively inaccessible region located superior, posterior, and medial to the superior turbinate. It contains the ostia of the sphenoid and posterior ethmoid sinuses (Fig. 4).

Paranasal Sinuses

Thin bony partitions separate the sinus cavities from other structures of the head. The frontal, ethmoid, and maxillary sinuses comprise three walls of the orbit, and the sphenoid sinus is posterior to the orbit. The sella turcica is superior to the sphenoid sinus; other adjacent structures include the internal carotid artery, the optic nerve, and the brain. The frontal sinus is also juxtaposed to the brain; infection could extend posteriorly into the dura and brain, inferiorly into the orbit, or anteriorly into bone and periostium, resulting in a subperiosteal abscess (Pott's Puffy Tumor) *(6)*.

The maxillary sinuses (antra of Highmore) are the largest of the paranasal sinuses (Fig. 5). The roots of the maxillary molar teeth often extend into the floor of the maxillary sinus. The floor of the sinus may extend down into the alveolar process. The ostium draining the sinus is located superiorly on the posterior medial wall of the sinus; accessory sinus ostia are commonly found. Ciliary action sweeps secretions and bacteria against the force of gravity up to the small ostium and out into the middle meatus.

Three to twelve ethmoid air cells comprise each side of the delicate ethmoid labyrinth, located along the medial wall of each orbit (Fig. 5). Those with ostia emptying into the middle meatus are defined as anterior ethmoid cells, and those that have ostia that empty into the superior or supreme meatus are defined as posterior. A few air cells that might drain in or superior to the ethmoid bulla would be designated by some anatomists as middle ethmoid air cells. Posterior ethmoid sinuses may also drain into the sphenoid sinus. The fovea ethmoidalis, the roof of the ethmoid sinuses, extends above the level of

the cribriform plate by about 1 cm. The ethmoid labyrinth is separated from the orbit by the lamina papyracea (lamina orbitalis ossis ethmoidalis). The middle ethmoid air cells medially form the ethmoid bulla (bulla ethmoidalis ossis ethmoidalis). On occasion, a misplaced posterior ethmoid cell will locate in the middle turbinate, forming a concha bullosa. Anterior ethmoid cells may be found in the agger nasi and uncinate process. Ethmoid cells that have migrated into the superior roof of the maxillary sinuses are called Haller cells.

The sphenoid sinus is a posterior extension of the ethmoid labyrinth (Figs. 4 and 5). It is centrally placed in the skull, and pain originating from the sinus may be referred behind the eyes, to the temples, or to the occiput. An irregularly shaped bony septum forms two or more often asymmetrical structures. Each portion of the sphenoid sinus empties into the sphenoethmoidal recess through an ostium in its superior anterior wall.

If the ethmoid labyrinth is followed anteriorly and superiorly, it is evident that the frontal sinus (Fig. 4), like the sphenoid sinus, is actually an enlarged, septated ethmoid air cell. The extent of the frontal sinus is variable. Some individuals have only a rudimentary frontal sinus; in others, the sinus may be so large that it extends out over the orbit or almost back to the temporal bone. A large frontal sinus causes the frontal bossing characteristic of some adults. The frontal sinus drains to the middle meatus through the nasofrontal duct.

Nasopharynx

The torus tubarius is located on the lateral wall of the nasopharynx, defining and protecting the orifice of the Eustachian tube or tympanopharyngeal duct (Fig. 2). Rosenmüller's fossa is a vertical cleft, a potential space, between the posterior lip of the torus tubarius and the adenoidal pad. It is of considerable importance because many of the insidious malignancies of the pharynx have their origin in this space. The adenoid, or pharyngeal tonsil, is the first collection of lymphoid tissue downstream from the nasal passages and sinuses.

Oropharynx and Hypopharynx

The lingual tonsils are located on either side of the dorsum of the base of the tongue anterior to the epiglottis (Fig. 6). The median glossoepiglottic fold and the two lateral glossoepiglottic folds extend from the epiglottis to the base of the tongue. The val-

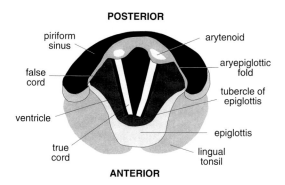

POSTERIOR

piriform sinus

arytenoid

false cord

aryepiglottic fold

tubercle of epiglottis

ventricle

true cord

epiglottis

lingual tonsil

ANTERIOR

Fig. 6. Structures of the larynx, oriented as they would be seen through a flexible fiberoptic endoscope. Adapted from ref. *(4)*.

leculae are cup-shaped spaces, separated by the median glossoepiglottic fold, posterior to the base of the tongue and anterior to the epiglottis. To the right and to the left of the larynx are the piriform sinuses, gutter-like structures that direct food to the esophagus.

Larynx

The framework of the larynx is formed by the thyroid, cricoid, and epiglottic cartilages and by pairs of arytenoid, corniculate, and cuneiform cartilages. The aryepiglottic folds and the arytenoids are located immediately behind the epiglottis (Fig. 6). The nodular swellings located medially in the aryepiglottic folds are the corniculate cartilages, which sit on top of the arytenoid cartilages. Lateral to the corniculate cartilages are the cuneiform cartilages. The aperture of the glottis (rima glottidis) is formed by the true vocal cords (vocal folds; plicae vocales) and the posterior commissure between the arytenoids. The anterior ligament of the true vocal cords is located at the anterior angle of the vocal cords. Between the true vocal cords and the false vocal cords (vestibular folds; plicae ventriculares) are the laryngeal ventricles.

The true vocal cords are anteriorly attached to the thyroid cartilage. The posterior attachment is to the vocal processes of the arytenoid cartilages. The true cords are relatively less vascular and are therefore whiter appearing than the surrounding mucosa. The strong vocal ligaments are covered by connective tissue and a thin layer of epithelium. Reinke's space is the potential space between the vocal ligaments and the subepithelial connective tissue layer. The mobile arytenoid cartilages move in and out with respiration and phonation.

UPPER AIRWAY PATHOLOGY

Too often, a patient complaining of nasal congestion or other upper airway symptoms will be placed on decongestant therapy, antibiotics, or allergen immunotherapy when symptoms are largely owing to anatomic obstruction of the nasal passage or other conditions primarily managed by surgery. By routine examination, it is difficult to diagnose posterior deviation of the nasal septum, or to detect nasopharyngeal obstruction by a choanal polyp or hypertrophied adenoidal tissue. Endoscopy is a convenient tool for direct inspection of nearly all portions of the upper airway. This section will summarize pathology of the upper airway as it might be encountered using flexible fiberoptic endoscopy in an outpatient allergy-immunology practice.

Mucosa

In health, the upper airway mucosa are moist and pink; the nasal mucosa shrink easily when topical decongestants are applied. Dryness of the mucosa may accompany various systemic diseases (such as "sicca syndrome"), may result from living in a low-humidity environment, or may be a feature of atrophic rhinitis or rhinitis sicca. Allergic rhinitis classically produces a pale bluish discoloration of the nasal mucosa associated with clear rhinorrhea. Mucosal "cobblestoning" is a sign of chronic inflammation. When an exudate is present, its consistency and clarity may be evaluated by rhinoscopy. Although presence of a purulent exudate draining from a paranasal sinus orifice is evidence of sinusitis *(7)*, this observation does not permit differentiation of bacterial, viral, or inflammatory etiologies.

Nasal Cavity

SEPTUM

The septum is rarely straight in normal adults and may deviate considerably from the midline even in asymptomatic individuals. In normals, one side of the nasal cavity may be larger than the other, but differences are not perceived, except in patients with chronic rhinitis or an exaggerated nasal cycle. More prominent septal deviations result in obstructive symptoms, and complex deviations may produce bilateral obstruction. A blow to the tip of the nose will cause telescoping, dislocation, or other types of distortion of these delicate bones and cartilages without external signs of a fractured nose. Trauma may produce a septal hematoma with separation of mucoperichondrium from the septal cartilage, resulting in a septal abscess and subsequent perforation. Other injuries may result in chronic nasal obstruction, abnormal nasal function, and change in voice quality. Severe septal deviations can present an insurmountable obstacle to the rigid endoscope and, on occasion, preclude fiberoptic endoscopy as well. Septal deviation may compress the nasal turbinates and cause facial pain in the trigeminal (V) nerve distribution. A variety of conditions, such as infection of a posttraumatic septal hematoma and abuse of cocaine or the topical nasal decongestants, can result in septal perforation. Patients with septal perforation may complain of nasal crusting, intermittent bleeding, and a whistling sound with nasal breathing. A septal spur is a displacement of the perpendicular plate of the ethmoid bone and the quadrangular septal cartilage into the nasal cavity. If this spur impinges on adjacent mucosal tissues, facial pain will result. Occasionally, the lateral process of the maxillary ridge will form a shelf on which the cartilaginous portion of the septum rests. This maxillary ridge is a common finding, but may be sufficiently large to cause symptomatic obstruction.

TURBINATES

Hypertrophy of the nasal turbinates may occur secondary to chronic inflammation of the nasal mucosa, especially that of the paranasal sinuses, or in cases of septal deviation as a compensatory mechanism in the nasal passage opposite to the obstructed side. Primary turbinate hypertrophy may also occur without obvious underlying cause. Complete or partial turbinectomy may have been performed in an attempt to relieve obstructive symptoms or as an adjunct in more complicated nasal surgery. Horizontal or sagittal clefting of a turbinate is a normal anatomic variant, which may be confused with polypoidal degeneration. It may also be difficult to distinguish polypoidal degeneration of a turbinate from polyps that are emanating from the anterior group of ethmoid air cells and entering the nose through the middle meatus. In either case, manipulation of the suspected polyps under direct visualization may be useful. A concha bullosa may produce significant obstruction of the nasal airway and is associated with obstruction of other sinus ostia.

NASAL POLYPS

Typically, polyps are hyperplastic mucosa originating in the ethmoid sinuses and prolapsing into the nasal cavity. Polypoid degeneration of the mucosa of the turbinates is less common, but can result in formation of polyps on the turbinates themselves. Polyps characteristically are slightly yellow or translucent, smooth, gelatinous appearing, avascular structures. They can often be moved with a cotton-tipped applicator so that their origin may more clearly be defined. Squamous metaplasia results as a consequence of dry air inducing keratinization of the mucosa covering the polyp, producing an opaque pink appearance. Polyps from the anterior and middle ethmoid air cells enter the nasal cavity from the middle meatus. They are usually easy to visualize on routine anterior examination of the nose, may extend anteriorly, and can produce total nasal obstruction. It is not possible to detect posterior ethmoid polyps on routine speculum examination unless they have become large. Polyps located in the middle meatus have their origin from anterior ethmoid or maxillary sinuses. Polyps extending from the sphenoethmoidal recess originate from the sphenoid or posterior ethmoid sinuses.

NEOPLASMS

Malignancy in the nose is an uncommon finding, but initially can produce complaints, such as pain, burning, or rhinorrhea, typically masquerading as chronic sinusitis. Any lesion suspicious for malignancy should be evaluated by an otolaryngologist.

Nasopharynx, Superior Oropharynx

CHOANA

Although complete bilateral choanal atresia almost always presents at birth, unilateral atresia or choanal stenosis might not be diagnosed until adulthood. Stenosis may be membranous or bony.

TORUS TUBARIUS

The torus is a partial ring of tissue surrounding the Eustachian tube ostium. A variety of conditions involving the torus could produce symptoms and signs of Eustachian tube dysfunction. A cyst of the torus blocking the Eustachian tube orifice would be evident on fiberoptic endoscopy, as would lymphoid infiltration or edema from chronic inflammation. Since adenoidectomy is often done by blind curettage, damage to the Eustachian tube and torus with resulting formation of scar tissue and adhesions could lead to Eustachian tube dysfunction. Additionally, the torus contains lymphatic tissue, the "tubal tonsils," which forms part of Waldeyer's ring; hyperplasia of the tubal tonsils might play a role in the etiology of chronic otitis media *(8)*.

ROSENMÜLLER'S FOSSA

This vertical cleft, a potential space between the posterior lip of the torus tubarius and the adenoidal pad, is of considerable importance because many of the insidious malignancies of the pharynx have their origin here. It is impossible to visualize this area on routine speculum examination.

ADENOID

Although it lacks the afferent lymphatic vessels that would permit its classification as a lymph node, the adenoid is the first major collection of lymphoid tissue in the upper airway. It varies in size in response to regional inflammation and is near the torus tubarius and Eustachian tube orifice. Hyperplasia of the adenoid is a common cause of nasal obstruction and rhinorrhea in children; in extreme cases, anterior herniation of adenoidal tissue through the choanae may result in total upper airway obstruction. In addition to producing discomfort, obstruction may result in hyponasal speech, other variations in voice quality, orthodontic difficulties owing to abnormal development of facial bones (adenoidal facies), and sleep disturbances including obstructive sleep apnea *(8)*. Whether adenoidal hyperplasia plays a direct role in the pathogenesis of Eustachian tube dysfunction is less clear *(9)*. A nasopharyngeal angiofibroma may mimic the obstruction of adenoidal hypertrophy and may be associated with recurrent epistaxis; these typically present in adolescence.

Anterior rhinorrhea may result from severe adenoidal hypertrophy or other obstructing lesions of the nasopharynx. Chronic adenoiditis may cause posterior rhinorrhea and halitosis; adenoidal tissue may block the orifice of the Eustachian tube producing otitis media with effusion, acute purulent otitis media, otalgia, and variation in hearing. Adenoidal tissue is frequently removed in patients with chronic rhinosinusitis. Since obstruction may recur within a few months of adenoidectomy, re-examination is indicated if symptoms return.

PHARYNGEAL WALL

Direct observation of the pharyngeal walls can reveal a variety of abnormalities. One of the most striking is spasm of the pharyngeal constrictor muscles associated with anxiety or chemical irritation of the upper airway. The patient complaining of a tight throat may indeed have a tight throat; this might be difficult to appreciate on direct pharyngeal examination, and the symptoms and signs might otherwise be confused with those of asthma. Anterior bony protrusions (osteophytes) from the vertebral bodies behind the posterior pharyngeal wall can also cause obstruction; mucus collecting on these projections can lead to chronic pharyngeal symptoms. The pulsations of a carotid aneurysm might be noted on examination of the oropharynx. Cobblestoning of the mucosa results from hypertrophy of lymphoid tissue and is a sign of upstream inflammatory reaction. An infected Tornwaldt's cyst can produce postnasal drip, occipital headache, halitosis, otalgia or hearing loss, and posterior cervical lympadenopathy *(10)*. Other causes of pharyngeal wall masses include retention cysts, persistence of Rathke's pouch, branchial cleft cysts, and neoplasms *(11)*.

MALIGNANCIES

Since most of the pathology originating in the nasopharynx is painless, insidious development of malignancies is possible. The first sign of pathology may be metastasis to the regional lymph nodes. Trigeminal neuralgia may result from malignancy involving the trigeminal nerve (V). Palsy of cranial nerves III, IV, and VI is also an ominous sign of nasopharyngeal malignancy.

Oropharynx, Hypopharynx, Larynx

Perhaps the most common sign of hypopharyngeal and laryngeal pathology is hoarseness or other changes in voice quality. These are often the result of vocal cord polyps, nodules, contact ulcerations, and granulomas. Other symptoms include odynophagia, dysphagia, hoarseness, a weak cough, and aspiration. A sensation of tightness in the throat or dysphagia may be the direct result of hypertrophy of lymphatic tissue, edema, or muscle spasm. Gastroesophageal reflux can result in chronic inflammation of the airway, chronic cough, and dysphagia. Patients presenting with a history of severe asthma with an atypical clinical course may have dysfunction of the vocal cords. Examination of the upper airway during an acute episode will be diagnostic.

POSTERIOR TONGUE, LINGUAL TONSILS

The circumvallate papillae form prominent pink nodules on the posterior tongue. The filiform papillae may appear white, a normal variant owing to mucosal keratinization, or black as the result of drinking coffee, smoking tobacco, or other exposures. White discoloration of the filiform papillae can be confused with *Candida* infection. Hypertrophy of the lingual tonsils may cause dysphagia, a globus sensation, or a feeling that something is stuck in the throat.

EPIGLOTTIS

A variety of circumstances can lead to irritation, with hypervascularity and edema, of the epiglottis. Gastroesophageal reflux, chronic sinusitis, and irritants, such as chemicals and tobacco smoke, may produce irritation of the epiglottis. Edema of the glottic structures may be present in patients with acute urticaria and angioedema of the buccal mucosa, tongue, and pharynx. When facilities for intubation or tracheotomy are available, the fiberoptic endoscope may be used to diagnose acute epiglottitis *(12)*.

GLOTTIS

Any change in voice quality, including hoarseness, is an indication for examination of the hypopharynx and larynx. In dysphonia plicae ventriculares, abnormal voice quality results from use of the false vocal cords for speech. Laryngoceles may produce a muffled voice; infection of laryngoceles may produce acute airway obstruction *(13)*.

TRUE VOCAL CORDS

Vocal cord nodules and polyps are characteristically found at the junction of the anterior and middle third of the membranous vocal cord. A nodule is a small sessile callus, which may be hemorrhagic or pale gray in color. It is an accumulation of fibrous tissue in the submucosa. The surface mucosa covering the nodule is usually intact and indistinguishable from surrounding mucosa. Often the mucosa over the nodule may appear hypertrophied. When a nodule is present, a vocal polyp may be located on the opposite cord at the position of contact with the nodule when the cords are adducted. The most common cause of nodules is voice abuse, common in teachers, singers, and screamers. Reinke's edema, or diffuse polyposis of the vocal cords, results from filling of Reinke's space with fluid, usually as the result of voice abuse or smoking. It is characterized by harsh, low-pitched dysphonia, often in a middle-aged individual. Contact ulcers and granulomas are the result of trauma to the areas involved. Persons screaming at sporting events may damage the vocal processes of the arytenoids; this can also occur as a complication of intubation. The mucosa overlying the cartilaginous structures are denuded. Usually, contact ulcers are on the inner surface of the vocal process of the arytenoids. Ulcers are most often seen as the result of loud talking, oversinging, or shouting for prolonged periods, and result from the vocal process being forcefully pushed together. Drug abuse, such as the smoking of crack cocaine, can result in unrestrained voice use and cough, producing contact ulceration. Mucosal integrity is compromised, and infection of the underlying tissue may follow. Granulomas may form in association with the ulcers. Paralysis of one or both vocal cords should prompt further investigation. Paralysis of the left cord may be associated with dysfunction of the left recurrent laryngeal nerve and mediastinal malignancy.

Christopher et al. reported a peculiar vocal cord dysfunction syndrome in patients diagnosed as having asthma *(14)*. Each patient had a history of paroxysmal wheezing and dyspnea despite bronchodilator therapy, but on auscultation had laryngeal stridor transmitted to the chest. Each patient had a negative methacholine or histamine challenge test, but evidence of variable extrathoracic obstruction on flow-volume loop during episodes. Endoscopy was normal during asymptomatic periods, but during an episode of wheezing, revealed nearly total adduction of the vocal cords during inspiration and expiration, producing a "small posterior diamond-shaped chink." The arytenoids remained in a normal lateral position, and "the false vocal cords tended to bunch together to a variable degree, obscuring the laryngeal ventricles." When the patients and normal subjects were asked to reproduce the sound voluntarily, they were not able to produce the small posterior chink, bunching of the false cords, or maintain the arytenoids in abduction. Similar reports in the literature suggest that vocal cord dysfunction may not be a rare condition and that in some cases vocal cord dysfunction can coexist with asthma *(15–18)*.

Many patients with well-characterized asthma note tightness in the throat as well as in the chest during episodes. Collett and associates have described expiratory constriction of the glottis during histamine or nebulized water bronchial challenge in 10 of 12 asymptomatic asthmatic patients *(19)*. Administration of continuous positive airway pressure relieved this expiratory glottic constriction. This apparently normal phenomenon, perhaps the vocal cord equivalent of pursed lip breathing, is distinct from the vocal cord dysfunction syndrome.

INSTRUMENTATION

Routine examination of the upper airway usually consists of inspection of the anterior nares with a nasal speculum and examination of the pharynx with a tongue depressor. Many physicians use an otoscope as a light source; this instrument has a focal length of approx 2.5 cm with a depth of focus of only 1 cm, permitting examination of only the proximal portion of the nasal cavity. The standard otolaryngologist's head mirror, with a focal length of 10–12 in, allows the examiner to focus a pinpoint beam of light on the structures to be examined. With adequate vasoconstriction and by skillful manipulation of the patient's head, it is possible to examine large portions of the nasal cavity as well as part of the nasopharynx. Use of a tongue depressor permits evaluation of parts of the posterior pharyngeal wall, but an indirect mirror examination allows a more complete inspection of the nasopharynx, hypopharynx, and the glottic structures. An experienced examiner can evaluate many children and most adults without use of topical anesthesia or sedation. In practice, however, this method has remained unsatisfactory for many situations. Even under optimum conditions, these conventional methods do not permit examination of the recessed structures of the upper airway, such as the sinus ostia, sphenoethmoidal recess, and Eustachian tube ostium.

The field of endoscopy dates from 1868, when Kussmaul examined the esophagus and stomach of sword swallowers with a rigid metal tube. By the turn of the century, endoscopes illuminated by incandescent lights were in occasional clinical use. Maltz described use of an endoscope specifically designed for sinuscopy in 1925 *(20)*. These primitive instruments were uncomfortable for patients, difficult to use, and provided only limited views of recessed structures. By 1956, the medical and industrial development of fiberoptic technology

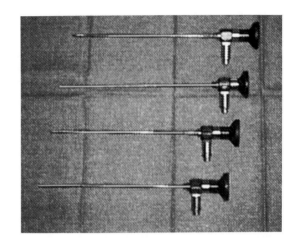

Fig. 7. Rigid endoscopes.

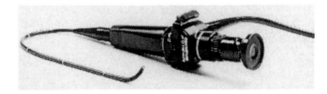

Fig. 8. A flexible fiberoptic endoscope. (Photograph courtesy of Olympus Corporation, Melville, NY.)

had produced a flexible gastroscope; miniaturized instruments designed for nasal endoscopy came into wide use in the late 1970s.

Rigid nasal endoscopes, such as the Hopkins telescope (Fig. 7), are optically excellent instruments that permit exhaustive inspection of the nasal cavity and are used for functional endoscopic sinus surgery. Because the tip of these instruments is not flexible, a set of at least three or four separate instruments with different viewing angles is required for a complete examination. Because it can be used in patients of all ages *(21)*, is simpler, and is less expensive, the flexible fiberoptic endoscope (Fig. 8) is used by most allergists *(22–24)* and primary care physicians *(25)* (as well as by many otolaryngologists *[26]*) for office examinations. Although office endoscopy suites can be quite elaborate, a minimal and satisfactory setup consists only of a portable light source and the endoscope itself. These can be taken from room to room and used for hospital consultations.

Photodocumentation

With either type of instrument, findings can be photographed or videotaped. Although not essential for office endoscopy, photodocumentation is very useful for academic purposes, for communicating results to other physicians, for patient education, and for comparison evaluation of therapeutic interventions. Still photography generally requires a relatively expensive high-intensity xenon light source; a conventional light source usually suffices for video recording. The choice of 35mm camera or video camera is limited to those that are compatible with the mounting system of the camera adapters available from the endoscope manufacturer. Some expensive still photography systems feature automatic exposure control; less complex setups work well, but require considerable photographic expertise. Home and commercial quality video cameras work well for video documentation, as do the more expensive miniaturized instruments. Home video monitors and videocassette recorders are sufficient for routine office use. A video printer interfaced to the videocassette recorder can provide reasonably good quality color prints of examination findings.

EXAMINATION TECHNIQUE

Preparation for Examination

Other than explanation of the procedure to the patient, the only special preparation usually required is decongestion and topical anesthesia, which are generally needed for adequate examination of recessed structures. Fasting is not necessary.

The patient is seated in an examining chair, preferably one with an adjustable headrest. A small child may sit in a parent's lap. Before administration of decongestant and topical anesthetic, the examiner should perform a preliminary speculum inspection of the anterior nasal cavity to determine patency of the nose and to identify pathology that might be eliminated by vasoconstrictor. The patient is then asked to clear nasal secretions by gentle blowing of the nose; on occasion, saline irrigation may be necessary to clear the nasal passage of mucus and debris.

Different topical decongestants may be used to shrink the nasal mucosa. Oxymetazoline is usually satisfactory. Many clinicians use 0.5% cocaine in a 1.0% ephedrine solution or 4% cocaine solution, which produces both decongestion and anesthesia, and should not produce psychotropic effects. Use of cocaine, however, requires disciplined record keeping; the physician may be asked to produce

usage records. Conceivably, traces of cocaine could be detected in a urine drug screen performed after the examination. Other topical decongestants include 3% ephedrine, phenylephrine, and xylometazoline. The selected decongestant is delivered by a standard nasal atomizer. Anesthesia of the pharynx and larynx is not necessary. Nasal mucosal anesthesia is readily achieved with 4% xylocaine solution, also delivered by a nasal atomizer. The anesthetic has an unpleasant taste, takes a few moments to take effect, and may produce an uncomfortable, but transient globus sensation if swallowed. If desired, the rhinoscope may be lubricated with 2% viscous xylocaine or a water-based lubricant.

In administering decongestant and topical anesthetic, it is important to recall that the nasal cavity is relatively small anteriorly and posteriorly with its largest dimension at the midpoint. In general, one or two sprays of each drug should be directed straight back, and the same amount superiorly and posteriorly at about a 45° angle.

Examination Sequence

Examination should proceed in a consistent, logical sequence, varied when needed for individual patients. It is usually convenient to examine structures of the anterior nasal cavity first, followed by examination of the pharynx and larynx. The sphenoethmoidal recess and middle meatus are more difficult to examine and may be less well anesthetized than other structures. Thus, they are generally examined last.

The patient is reminded that he or she may talk to the examiner during the examination. With proper decongestion and topical anesthesia, the procedure should not be at all painful; the patient should be asked to communicate any discomfort (other than pressure) to the examiner so that the endoscope may be withdrawn from that area. The scope may be defogged by placing it into the patient's mouth for a moment. After lubrication, the endoscope is placed into the nasal vestibule. The examiner's left hand is placed against the patient's forehead approximately at the base of the nose, and the thumb and index finger are used to hold the endoscope at the patient's nostril. Because the examining chair has a headrest, the examiner can control the patient's head and can also monitor variations in the patient's head position. Since many patients will tense the frontalis muscle when more sensitive areas of the airway are examined, one can often perceive patient discomfort before anything is said. Changes in skin temperature may be an early sign of a vasovagal reaction.

The right hand is used to manipulate the endoscope, and the left hand is used to support the endoscope and the patient's head. The fingers of the right hand should grasp and support the endoscope, leaving the thumb free to manipulate the tip of the endoscope. The endoscope is maintained in a straight anterior-posterior position, allowing it to adjust to the contours of the nasal passage as it is advanced, perhaps with slight manipulation of the endoscope tip. The endoscope tip may be flexed with the lever controlled by the thumb of the right hand or moved by altering the position of the endoscope in the nasal passage using the index finger and thumb of the left hand. It is important to remember that, in general, the endoscope will travel toward whatever structure is in the center of the eyepiece or video screen as it is advanced, and that slight flexing or moving the endoscope tip can result in a marked change in the direction of travel. All movements should be performed gently, and the endoscope should not be advanced when distant structures are not visible. A white flashback indicates contact of the endoscope with the nasal mucosa. Rather than advancing blindly, the examiner should withdraw the endoscope slightly, until anatomic landmarks can be seen and recognized.

With the endoscope at the nostril, the nasal vestibule with its vibrissae will be encountered and often a medial protrusion on the floor of the nose (the feet of the medial crura of the lower lateral cartilages) will be noted. After one has advanced about 1 cm, the inferior turbinate, floor of the nose, and septum will be in view (Fig. 9). If the endoscope tip is flexed slightly upward, the middle turbinate will be seen in the distance; with upward flexion to 60–90°, the superior portion of the anterior nose (agger nasi) can be evaluated. If the inferior turbinate is large or swollen, it may be necessary to advance the tip of the endoscope over the anterior margin of the inferior turbinate to view the middle turbinate. A large maxillary ridge or displaced septal cartilage may similarly impede advancement of the endoscope. With the endoscope placed in the middle portion of the nasal cavity, the roof of the nose may be viewed by directing the endoscope upwards; this is the region of the cribriform plate. It is not usually possible to advance the endoscope toward the superior turbinate from this position.

To view the anterior portion of the middle turbinate, the tip of the endoscope is directed over the inferior turbinate (Fig. 10). The endoscope is usually advanced to the choana along the floor of the nose, but the middle meatus approach may be alternatively used if the lower route is obstructed. The structures of the middle meatus may be inspected at this point.

Having been returned to the floor of the nose, the endoscope is directed posteriorly along the nasal floor until it is approx 4–5 cm into the nasal passage. At this point, the choana of the nose (posterior naris) is usually in view, although depending on the size and status of the inferior turbinate, this may not be well visualized. Deviation of the septum may also interfere with observation of the posterior recesses of the nasal passage. At this point, the tip of the endoscope is directed upward (Fig. 11), and the inferior margin of the middle turbinate comes into view. It is usually possible to direct the endoscope superiorly and laterally into the middle meatus either at this point in the examination, or later after examination of the larynx and sphenoethmoidal recess. At this point, identification of the uncinate process and ethmoid bulla, which define the semilunar hiatus, is often possible. The ostium, or accessory ostia, of the maxillary sinus may be identified. The ostia of the nasofrontal duct and the anterior and middle ethmoid air cells are more difficult to locate, and ordinarily will not be seen on routine fiberoptic examination of the nose.

Again, the endoscope tip is returned to the floor of the nose and advanced to the posterior margin of the inferior turbinate with the choana clearly in view. It is advanced slightly so that structures of the nasopharynx may be viewed through the choana (Fig. 12). The adenoidal pad appears on the posterior wall of the nasopharynx, and the torus tubarius, which surrounds the orifice of the Eustachian tube, is well visualized. The endoscope is advanced into the nasopharynx. Once the posterior margin of the septum (vomer) is lost from view, the tip of the endoscope may be flexed slightly and rotated 90° toward the ipsilateral torus to examine the Eustachian tube orifice. The patient may be asked to sing "eeee" or say "k-k-k-k" to make the orifice more visible. If the endoscope is advanced slightly into the nasopharynx, rotated, and the tip is flexed 180° behind the septum, the contralateral Eustachian tube orifice may be examined. Between the posterior margin of the torus and the adenoidal pad is a vertical cleft known as Rosenmüller's fossa. This space begins at the top of the nasopharynx coincident with the adenoidal tissue and proceeds caudad between the torus and the adenoidal pad into the inferior portion of the nasopharynx. After these structures have been examined, the endoscope is rotated back to the midline, and the tip is flexed inferiorly. The patient is asked to breathe through the nose to keep the soft palate from obstructing the view. The lateral and posterior walls of the pharynx, the soft palate, and uvula are inspected for mucosal irregularities, pulsations, and protrusions into the pharynx.

The endoscope is advanced into the oropharynx (Fig. 13). Structures of the posterior tongue, the palatine tonsils, the epiglottis, the valleculae, and glosso-epiglottic and lateral epiglottic folds are examined.

The endoscope is kept close to the posterior wall of the pharynx as it is directed into the hypopharynx and oropharynx (Fig. 13). The patient is encouraged to breathe quietly and asked not to swallow, but reassured that swallowing will merely result in the sensation of attempting to swallow the endoscope, not in discomfort. In the process of swallowing, the epiglottis can strike the endoscope; should this happen, the endoscope may be withdrawn slightly until the sensation of swallowing the endoscope has been lost. At this point, the examination may continue.

The endoscope is directed along the posterior pharyngeal wall in the midline, over the epiglottis (Fig. 14). In this position, the arytenoids, the superior projections of the corniculate and cuneiform cartilages, the aryepiglottic folds, the true and false vocal cords, and the ventricles are well visualized. Slight rotations of the endoscope in this position will reveal the piriform sinuses. From this position, the examiner often will see well into the trachea.

The vocal cords should be examined during quiet and deep breathing, and in phonation. To examine the cords in adduction, the patient is asked to sing "eeee." Often polypoidal changes and edematous distortion of the vocal cords can be identified with this maneuver. Displacement of the bony structures of the glottis, asymmetrical functioning (including paralysis) of the cords, and pathology, such as nodules, polypoidal changes, granulomas, and contact ulcerations, will be apparent at this stage of the examination. Sometimes the endoscope must be withdrawn to just above the epiglottis before the patient is asked to phonate.

The endoscope is withdrawn under direct visualization to a position just anterior to the choana. As the endoscope is directed superiorly, the anterior margin of the sphenoid bone comes into view. As the endoscope is advanced superiorly and anteriorly by flexing the tip 90–120°, the posterior and then the anterior margins of the superior turbinate may be examined (Fig. 15). Medial to the superior turbinate, the ostium of the sphenoid sinus will often be visualized. The ostia of the posterior ethmoid air cells are less likely to be seen. Since this area may not be well anesthetized in some patients, this portion of the examination should be done after examination of the laryngeal structures.

If structures of the middle meatus were not previously examined, they are studied at this time. It is usually easier to examine the middle meatus from posterior to anterior.

Following withdrawal of the endoscope under direct visualization, examination of the other side of the nose is carried out. When possible, a video-tape of the examination may be replayed and explained to the patient. Afterward, the equipment is cleaned and disinfected in preparation for the next examination. It is our practice to clean the flexible fiberoptic endoscope with soap and water, rinse it with water, and wipe it with a pad soaked in isopropyl alcohol. Next, it is disinfected by soaking for 20–60 min in full-strength Cidex. After it is rinsed with water, the endoscope is allowed to air-dry. In cleaning and disinfecting the endoscope, care should be taken not to bend it at the point at which the flexible insertion tube attaches to the rigid control section; doing so will break the fiberoptic bundles.

INDICATIONS FOR EXAMINATION

Nearly any symptom referable to the upper airway is a relative indication for upper airway endoscopy, particularly when routine clinical evaluation does not yield a satisfactory diagnosis or when response to management is suboptimal. The information obtained will almost always directly influence interpretation of patient complaints, establishment of a diagnosis, and selection of treatment strategies.

Routine use of endoscopy in physical examination has been advocated by some (2) and discouraged by others (27), primarily because of concerns that routine endoscopy would not be cost effective.

Table 1
Selected Indications for Upper Airway Endoscopy *(4)*

General
   Any symptom or complaint referable to the upper airway
Nose, nasopharynx
   Nasal obstruction, particularly if unilateral
   Snoring, mouth breathing
   Anosmia
   Headaches, facial pain
   Epistaxis
   Rhinorrhea
   Acute or chronic sinusitis
   Earache; recurrent or chronic otitis media
   Regional lymphadenopathy
   Assessment of results of surgical intervention
Hypopharynx, larynx
   Dysphagia, globus
   Hoarseness, other changes in voice quality
   Chronic cough
   Atypical asthma, laryngeal dysfunction

The diagnostic yield of unselective use of endoscopy in primary care, otolaryngology, or allergy-immunology practices has not been adequately studied. Selected examples of direct indications for endoscopy are listed in Table 1. Although the utility of nasal endoscopy in the evaluation of patients with acute sinusitis is not well defined, the combination of endoscopy and computed tomography (CT) is essential in the evaluation of patients with chronic sinusitis.

Nose

Complaints that might prompt fiberoptic examination of the nose include nasal obstruction (particularly if unilateral), anosmia, headaches, facial pain, epistaxis, rhinorrhea, sinusitis, earache, recurrent or chronic otitis media, and regional adenopathy. One may also assess the result of surgical intervention.

Nasopharynx

Many common complaints originate in the nasopharynx. These can result in posterior nasal obstruction, anterior facial pain, headaches, epistaxis, rhinorrhea, ear pain, recurrent sinusitis, recurrent otitis media, and regional adenopathy, particularly of the posterior cervical lymph nodes. Examination of the nasopharynx is essential in evaluating these complaints, particularly in patients with nasal obstruction and Eustachian tube dysfunction.

Hypopharynx and Larynx

Patients with dysphagia, odynophagia, and globus may have distinct pathology of the hypopharynx or larynx. Disorders of these areas may cause referred ear pain. Hoarseness or changes in voice quality may signal pathology in these areas. Gastroesophageal reflux may produce chronic inflammation of the airway, resulting in chronic cough and painful swallowing. Patients with upper airway obstruction may present with a history of atypical asthma refractory to usual treatment *(14)*.

Endoscopy in Sinusitis

In evaluating patients with unrelenting symptoms of sinusitis, but normal X-rays or CT, other conditions warrant consideration. Other causes of nasal congestion with facial pain include severe mucosal congestion, nasal polyposis, simple and complex septal deviation, septal spurs (Fig. 16), turbinate hypertrophy, and tumors. In all of these, nasal endoscopy will rapidly resolve the differential diagnosis.

Several approaches to the diagnosis of acute sinusitis (e.g., history and physical examination alone, culture of pus aspirated from a sinus, plain X-rays, computed tomography, ultrasound) are available, and each has its advocates. Although some clinicians intuitively consider the finding of purulent drainage from a sinus orifice (Fig. 17) as diagnostic of infectious sinusitis, this assumption has not been verified. Fiberoptic nasal endoscopy and plain sinus X-rays were performed in a study of 246 patients referred to an internal medicine clinic for evaluation of headache, after electroencephalogram and cranial CT had been normal *(7)*. The endoscopic finding of purulent material "emanating from the sinus drainage regions," and the radiologic finding of "clouding, fluid levels, and mucosal thickening" were considered evidence of infectious sinusitis. Of these, 98 (40%) had endoscopic evidence of sinusitis with normal X-rays, 84 (34%) had both endoscopic and radiologic evidence of sinusitis, and 64 (26%) had no evidence of sinusitis by endoscopy or X-rays. No patients had radiologic evidence of sinusitis alone. Nearly all patients diagnosed with sinusitis returned reporting relief of headache after a 2-wk course of amoxicillin-clavulinate or trimethoprim-sulfamethoxazole and had normal endoscopic examination at a return visit. Only four of the patients with

Fig. 9.

Fig. 13.

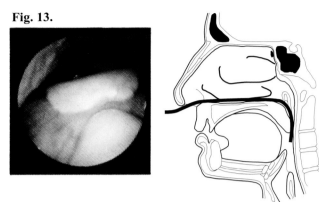

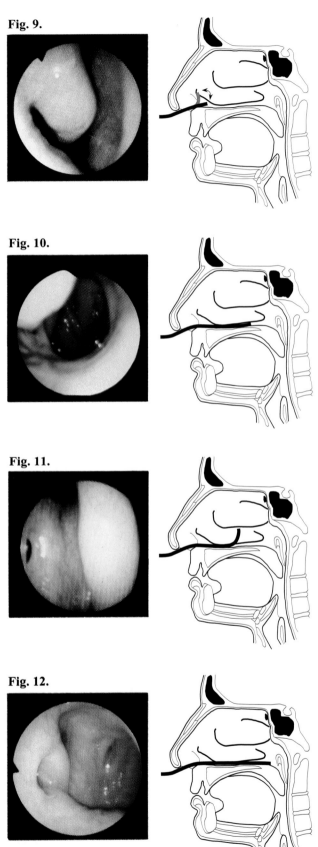

Fig. 10.

Fig. 11.

Fig. 12.

normal endoscopy and X-rays reported relief from headache. Even though this single study has generated considerable enthusiasm for endoscopic diagnosis of infectious sinusitis, one must remember that the patient population studied consisted of individuals presenting with chronic headaches. The sensitivity and specificity of endoscopy in the diagnosis of acute or chronic sinusitis in more usual clinical circumstances awaits definition, as does correlation with other diagnostic methods, especially CT and antral puncture.

In the evaluation of sinus disease, one rarely has the opportunity to examine the sinuses themselves by endoscopy. Occasionally, an accessory ostium of the maxillary sinus or a sphenoid sinus ostium will permit inspection of the sinus mucosa. Surgically created antral windows are routinely large enough to allow direct examination of the maxillary sinuses. Nonetheless, endoscopy is extremely

---

Fig. 9. The anterior structures of the right nasal passage viewed with a flexible fiberoptic endoscope. The septum is on the right, and the inferior turbinate is on the left. Adapted from ref. *(4)*.

Fig. 10. The floor of the right nasal passage viewed with a flexible fiberoptic endoscope. The structure at 10 o'clock is the right inferior turbinate. Adapted from ref. *(4)*.

Fig. 11. The right middle meatus viewed from below with a flexible fiberoptic endoscope. The middle turbinate is on the right and an accessory ostium of the right maxillary sinus is at 9 o'clock. Although endoscopy does not usually permit a direct view of the paranasal sinuses, it is possible to assess general condition of the nasal mucosa and to evaluate for gross structural abnormalities. Adapted from ref. *(4)*.

Fig. 12. Nasopharyngeal structures. The Eustachian tube orifice surrounded by the torus tubarius is seen at 9 o'clock. Adapted from ref. *(4)*.

Fig. 13. Oropharyngeal structures. The uvula is seen at 5 o'clock, resting on the lingual tonsil. The epiglottis is posterior to the lingual tonsil. Adapted from ref. *(4)*.

Fig. 14.

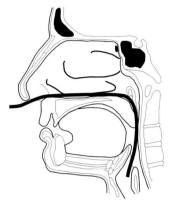
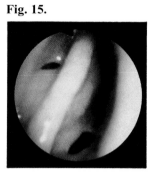

Fig. 15.

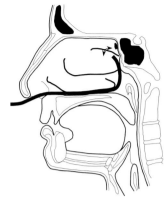

useful in the evaluation of patients with chronic sinusitis, because these structures drain into the nasal passage itself and disease of the nasal passage can underlie or complicate sinusitis.

Endoscopic examination of the recessed areas of the nasal passage has reshaped concepts of the pathogenesis and surgical treatment of chronic sinusitis, with particular emphasis on surgery of the ostiomeatal complex to promote adequate mucociliary clearance *(28)*. Complete preoperative coronal CT combined with nasal endoscopy is essential for defining anatomy and planning surgery in this narrow area, as well as for ruling out gross pathology in the nasal cavity. At the time of surgery, endoscopic visualization will have both reduced surgical complications and permitted accurate and precise dissection of involved structures.

Fig. 16.

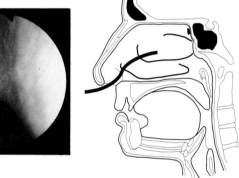

Fig. 17.

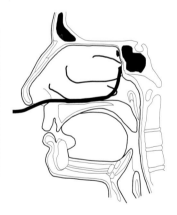

Fig. 18.

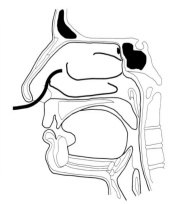

Fig. 14. The larynx *(see* Fig. 6). The true and false vocal cords are shown anteriorly. Adapted from ref. *(4)*.

Fig. 15. The right superior meatus and sphenoethmoidal recess viewed from below with a flexible fiberoptic endoscope. The septum is on the right. A posterior ethmoid sinus ostium is located at 10 o'clock, and the right sphenoid sinus ostium is located at 6 o'clock. Adapted from ref. *(4)*.

Fig. 16. A septal spur in the right nasal cavity. This structure, the result of an old injury, forms a sharp edge impacting on the middle turbinate and causes facial pain mimicking sinusitis. Adapted from ref. *(4)*.

Fig. 17. A view of the right sphenoethmoidal recess using a flexible fiberoptic endoscope. The nasal septum is located on the right portion of the picture. On the left, at 10 o'clock, a stream of creamy appearing mucopurulent pus is seen, with presumptive origin in the posterior ethmoid or sphenoid sinuses. Adapted from ref. *(4)*.

Fig. 18. A widely patent antral window in the right middle meatus. The septum is on the right at 3 o'clock, and the middle turbinate is at 12 o'clock. The mucosa of the right maxillary sinus appear in the distance at 9 o'clock. Adapted from ref. *(4)*.

In addition to evaluating the need for surgery, endoscopy can assess results of medical and surgical interventions. The reduction of mucosal congestion, produced either by oral decongestants or topical corticosteroids, is obvious. Likewise, one may easily assess the anatomic outcome of sinus surgery by follow-up nasal endoscopy (Fig. 18).

Research Applications

The rhinoscope permits direct visualization of the nasal mucosa. When examinations are videotaped or photographed, results of therapeutic intervention may be compared before and after therapy. A quantitative modification of the basic rhinoscopic technique permits measurement of cross-sectional nasal airway in the anterior nose, resulting in the ability to estimate nasal patency *(29)*.

SUMMARY

The thought of developing competence in upper airway examination may be intimidating. One need only recall first awkward attempts to drive a car, a medical student's anxiety in examining the tympanic membrane of a struggling 12-mo-old, or the difficulty in distinguishing a split S1 from an S4 gallop in order to realize that skill in endoscopy requires not only a basic understanding of related anatomy, physiology, and pathology, but also relatively frequent use of the endoscope, ideally in collaboration with professional colleagues also experienced in the examination of the upper airway.

Although rigid endoscopy requires considerable manual dexterity, nearly any motivated physician can learn to use flexible fiberoptic endoscopy in an office practice. These examinations contribute significantly to the interpretation of patient complaints and influence therapeutic decision making. Upper airway endoscopy should be taught early in the course of training in allergy or otolaryngology, where the procedure can be used as a means of teaching upper airway anatomy and pathology as well as a way to facilitate collaboration, rather than competition, with other specialists. Intelligent use of upper airway endoscopy will result in early and appropriate requests for consultation.

In known or suspected paranasal sinus disease, diagnostic nasal endoscopy is useful in addressing differential diagnosis, evaluating for factors underlying or predisposing to chronic sinusitis, and in planning and evaluating results of surgery. A role for endoscopy in diagnosis of sinusitis has been proposed, but not convincingly validated in comparison studies with other methods. Endoscopy is a simple office procedure suitable for use by any physician interested in disorders of the upper airways.

REFERENCES

1. Williams JW, Simel DL. Does this patient have sinusitis? Diagnosing sinusitis by history and physical examination. JAMA 1993;270:1242–1246.
2. Klein HC. Why can't physicians examine the larynx? JAMA 1982;247:2111.
3. Selkin SG. Flexible fiberoptics and pediatric otolaryngology. A simple technique for examination and photodocumentation. Pediatr Otorhinolaryngol 1983;5: 325–333.
4. Selner JC, Dolen WK, Spofford B, Koepke JW. Rhinolaryngoscopy, 2nd ed. Denver: Allergy Respiratory Institute, 1989.
5. Messerklinger W. Endoscopy of the nose. Baltimore: Urban & Schwarzenberg, 1978.
6. Feder HM, Cates KL, Cementina AM. Pott puffy tumor: a serious occult infection. Pediatrics 1987;79:625–629.
7. Castellanos J, Axelrod D. Flexible fiberoptic rhinoscopy in the diagnosis of sinusitis. J Allergy Clin Immunol 1989;83:91–94.
8. Dolen WK, Spofford B, Selner JC. The hidden tonsils of Waldeyer's ring. Ann Allergy 1990;65:244–248.
9. Holliday MJ. Ear disease in patients with inflammation of Waldeyer's ring. Otolaryngol Clin North Am 1987;20: 287–294.
10. Miller RH, Sneed WF. Tornwaldt's bursa. Clin Otolaryngol 1985;10:21–25.
11. Guggenheim P. Cysts of the nasopharynx. Laryngoscope 1967;77:2147–2168.
12. Cox GJ, Bates GJ, Drake-Lee AB, Watson DJ. The use of flexible nasopharyngoscopy in adults with acute epiglottitis. Ann R Coll Surg Engl 1988;70:361,362.
13. Melnick HB, Sumerson J. Laryngocele: an uncommon entity. Trans Pa Acad Ophthalmol Otolaryngol 1987; 39:610–613.
14. Christopher KL, Wood RP, Eckert C, et al. Vocal cord dysfunction presenting as asthma. N Engl J Med 1983; 308:1566–1570.
15. Rogers JH, Stell PM. Paradoxical movement of the vocal cords as a cause of stridor. J Laryngol Otol 1978;92:157,158.
16. Appleblatt NH, Baker SR. Functional upper airway obstruction: a new syndrome. Arch Otolaryngol 1981; 107:305,306.
17. Rodenstein DO, Francis C, Stanescu DC. Emotional laryngeal wheezing: a new syndrome. Am Rev Respir Dis 1983;127:354–356.
18. Kattan M, Ben-Zvi Z. Stridor caused by vocal cord malfunction associated with emotional factors. Clin Pediatr 1985;24:158–160.
19. Collett PW, Brancatisano T, Engel LA. Changes in the glottic aperture during bronchial asthma. Am Rev Respir Dis 1983;128:719–723.
20. Maltz M. New instrument: the sinuscope. Laryngoscope 1925;35:805–811.

21. Silberman HD. The use of the flexible fiberoptic naso-pharyngoscope in the pediatric upper airway. Otolaryngol Clin N Am 1978;11:365–370.

22. Rohr A, Hassner A, Saxon A. Rhinopharyngoscopy for the evaluation of allergic-immunologic disorders. Ann Allergy 1983;50:380–384.

23. Selner JC, Koepke JW. Rhinolaryngoscopy in the allergy office. Ann Allergy 1985;1985:479–482.

24. Ransom JH, Kavel KK. Diagnostic fiberoptic rhino-laryngoscopy. Kans Med 1989;90:105–115.

25. Dewitt DE. Fiberoptic rhinolaryngoscopy in primary care. Postgrad Med 1988;84:125,126.

26. Lancer JM, Jones AS. Flexible fiberoptic rhinolaryn-goscopy: results of 338 consecutive examinations. J Laryngol Otol 1985;99:771–773.

27. Schumacher MJ. Fiberoptic nasopharyngoscopy: a proce-dure for allergists? J Allergy Clin Immunol 1988;81: 960–962.

28. Stammberger H. Endoscopic endonasal surgery—con-cepts in treatment of recurring sinusitis. Otolaryngol Head Neck Surg 1986;94:143–147.

29. Zedalis D, Dolen WK, Selner JC, Weber RW. Evaluation of nasal patency by fiberoptic rhinoscopy. J Allergy Clin Immunol 1989;83:973–978.

PART IV SURGICAL MANAGEMENT

25 Sinusitis in Children

Principles of Surgical Management

Mark A. Richardson, MD

CONTENTS

We are very reluctant to perform sinus surgery in children; children under 10 years of age account for less than 2% of our surgical cases. In contrast to adults, many other than just ethmoidal causes usually can be identified and treated in children's sinusitis (adenoids, allergies). Functional endoscopic surgery in children requires expert knowledge and experience and we strongly recommend that novices not start with pediatric cases.—Heinz Stammberger (1).

INTRODUCTION

Sinusitis as an acute process in children must be a frequent occurrence given the number of upper respiratory illnesses they are subject to in their early

From: *Diseases of the Sinuses* (M. E. Gershwin and G. A. Incaudo, eds.), ©1996 Humana Press Inc., Totowa, NJ.

childhood, as well as the relative lack of immunity present. In most cases, these episodes of inflammation within the nose and paranasal sinuses probably resolve without any treatment or respond quickly and appropriately to antibiotic management. In rare cases, additional antibiotics may need to be administered for an infection that does not respond appropriately to initial management, and it is an exceptional event if chronic sinusitis develops, which is unresponsive to multiple-drug therapy. Those patients who do not respond to long-term courses of antibiotics and who persist in showing signs of inflammation or infection symptomatically and objectively present on a computer tomographic (CT) scan would seem to be candidates for surgical treatment. The place for functional endoscopic sinus surgery in children who have recurrent infections that clear in response to therapy is not clear.

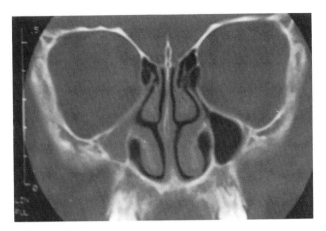

Fig. 1. Absent uncinate and hypoplastic sinus.

In addition, the effect of adenoidectomy or limited drainage of the sinuses in not well documented. Despite these unknowns, selection of the appropriate patient who would benefit from endoscopic sinus surgery and adjunctive procedures, such as adenoidectomy, septoplasty, and turbinoplasty, is critical to a successful result.

ANATOMY

Neonates and infants are born with small, poorly developed ethmoid and maxillary sinuses, which gradually enlarge and extend to the frontal and sphenoid areas. The uncinate process begins as a hypoplastic ridge that gradually extends itself superiorly as the child grows gradually increasing the depth of the infundibular area (2). This development of the uncinate process may act as a protective device in older children and adults to shield the maxillary sinus from inflammation and secretions within the nose. In the process, once inflammation does occur, the infundibulum could act as a site of obstruction of adequate clearance of secretions from the maxillary sinus ostea and anterior ethmoid area. The vertical range and degree of complexity of the ethmoid sinuses also increases with advancing age (3). There are developmental anomalies of the sinuses that can lead to hypoplastic development, poor drainage, and abnormal function. These abnormalities should be searched for in any child who has persistent opacification or other abnormalities on routine radiographic evaluations (4). (See Fig. 1.)

Clearance of secretions naturally produced by glandular epithelium within the paranasal sinuses takes place via the action of ciliated epithelia. All secretions are directed through this mucociliary action to the natural ostea of the paranasal sinuses. Any factor that thickens secretions or impairs ciliary motility can alter effective transport, as can swelling or edema at the osteal site. Diminished partial pressure of oxygen within the sinus cavities can affect the qualities of glandular secretions, causing thicker and more viscid mucus to be formed (5).

A variety of factors can increase ciliary beat frequency. Theophylline, caffeine, Neo-Synephrine, and other drugs, as well as exercise, raise the frequency of ciliary activity, which, in combination with agents that thin mucus or may diminish edema at the ostea site, would facilitate clearance of secretions (6,7). Surgical treatment is also directed toward facilitating secretion, clearance, and ventilation of the paranasal sinuses through elimination of gross anatomic obstacles. (Diagnosis and treatment have been covered in other portions of the text and will not be mentioned here.)

It is important to note for appropriate surgical planning any underlying conditions, such as cystic fibrosis (CF), ciliary dyskinesia, immunologic deficiency, and so on. A CT scan is mandatory prior to the consideration of endoscopic sinus surgery for the treatment of sinusitis. Once a CT scan has been obtained, an assessment of the level of involvement of the sinuses can be made that would generally be relegated to one of four categories:

1. Normal;
2. Disease limited to the maxillary sinuses;
3. Ethmoid and varying degrees of maxillary involvement; and
4. Pan-sinusitis.

Assessment of disease extent is necessary for the surgical decision-making process as well as the prognosis postoperatively. Staging systems have been proposed by a variety of authors, which may be used prognostically to estimate long-term success rate. One such system uses four stages as follows (8):

Stage 1: Anatomic abnormalities, unilateral sinus disease, and bilateral ethmoid disease;
Stage 2: Bilateral ethmoid disease with one dependent sinus involved;
Stage 3: Bilateral ethmoid disease with two dependent sinuses involved; and
Stage 4: Diffuse sinus polyposis.

These categories obviously progress from best to worst and are not applied strictly to pediatrics, but are primarily estimates that relate to adult disease. It is helpful to set reasonable expectations for parents and patients as to the results of the surgery based on objective findings on the CT scan.

TIMING OF OBJECTIVE EVALUATION

Some controversy exists over the timing of radiographic evaluation of sinusitis. Generally in my practice, when patients are referred, they have been evaluated in some fashion, either through a Water's view or CT scan, prior to their actual appointment. This allows some reference point so that if further radiographic procedures are performed, improvement or nonresponse can be documented. I feel that it is most important to obtain the CT scan at the completion of a maximal trial of medical therapy, so that I can make sure that everything has been done to normalize the radiographic appearances of the sinuses. This would include at least two trials of prolonged antibiotic coverage of 21 d to 1 mo. The incidence of abnormalities on CT, both anatomic and inflammation related to upper respiratory illness, are high enough so that taken as independent factors, they alone cannot be used as indicators for surgery. In a study by Gwaltney et al. (9), identifying the effect of upper respiratory illnesses on the appearance of sinuses on CT, approx 70% of patients with an upper respiratory illness demonstrated changes on CT indicating sinusitis. These changes were not permanent and, in fact, disappeared with the passage of time and treatment of the underlying upper respiratory infection if necessary. A clinical history of more than 3 mo duration of sinusitis is a minimum criteria for referral for the majority of my patients. At the time of their examination and evaluation, additional treatment with third-generation cephalosporins or generic may be performed if their use has not already preceded my evaluation. In patients under the age of 2 yr, it would be extremely unusual to proceed with endoscopic sinus surgery without having first performed an adenoidectomy in conjunction with drainage and/or culturing of the sinuses to see if its effect would be beneficial enough to reduce the frequency of sinusitis.

INSTRUMENTATION

Endoscopic sinus surgery in the pediatric population does require special instrumentation. Instruments that are commonly used in adults may be found excessively large and difficult to manipulate in the child's nose. Accordingly, attempts at endoscopic sinus surgery should only be undertaken when appropriate tools are available, which usually means a separate set of instruments and telescopes. The author's own preference is for a 25° angle scope permitting both straight-ahead and angled visualization with a suction irrigating device in order to keep the lens clear. A separate suction device is used on the field in addition to the suction irrigating sheath in case there is significant enough bleeding to obstruct the field of view. Since endotracheal tubes are commonly used without cuffs in pediatrics, it is important to make sure that the tube has a small leak rather than a large one. Otherwise, there will be a continuous reflux of air and secretions into the nose and nasopharynx, which will prevent good visualization. Packing placed inside the oral cavity can sometimes minimize excessive air leak, or an oral airway can at least divert the stream of air and secretions away from the nasal cavity, if visualization is impaired.

Additional devices that can be used in the sinus would include the laser, which would generally be of the KTP type (10). This delivers a small amount of power, but is generally adequate to make incisions within the nasal cavity that remain relatively bloodless. The arthroscopic shaver, using an oscillating head of the smallest diameter, which is usually used for temporomandibular joint surgery, can be used to remove mucosa without stripping or exposing bone in a limited and relatively bloodless fashion. This "hummer" is particularly useful for the removal of polyps within the nasal cavity and is extremely beneficial when used to treat patients with CF. When performing endoscopic surgery, the objective should be a clean surgical field with minimal bleeding, preservation of all normal mucosa, and removal of all bits and irregular portions of bone created by the surgical process.

MAXILLARY ANTROSTOMY: INFERIOR MEATAL ANTROSTOMY

Placement of an inferior antrostomy has been a procedure performed historically for a variety of reasons. In the past, it has been used in association with Caldwell-Luc procedures to provide immediate and gravitational drainage of the blood that may accumulate in the sinus after removal of diseased

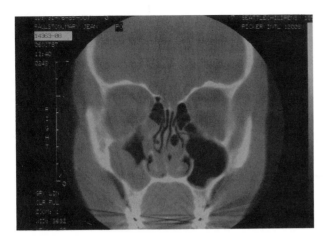

Fig. 2. Patient inferior antrostomy with persistent chronic sinusitis.

mucosa. It has also been used intermittently for the treatment of chronic sinusitis in order to provide ventilation and drainage. The use of inferiorly placed antrostomies, however, is nonphysiologic, based on a variety of authors' experiences looking at mucociliary clearance mechanisms from within the sinus *(11)*. Other authors have indicated the low rate of successful amelioration of sinusitis via inferior antrostomy and the high rate of spontaneous closure at 6 and 12 mo follow-up *(12)*. Additionally, many have speculated that placement of an inferior antrostomy may, in fact, lead to the development of sinusitis in certain individuals through certain patterns of mucosal clearance that might lead to bacteria actually contaminating the maxillary sinus. (*See* Fig. 2.)

The overall response rate for chronic sinusitis to the inferiorly placed antrostomy ranges from 20 to 50% in different series *(11,12)*. This low rate of response, I think, indicates the overall failure of inferiorly placed antrostomies to remain patent, and also to provide anything beyond ventilation and gravitational elimination of thick secretions that may be present in the maxillary sinus. The use of inferiorly placed antrostomies should probably be limited to patients with ciliary dyskinesia or other abnormalities of mucociliary clearance, such as CF, or where access to the maxillary sinus through an inferiorly placed antrostomy would seem to be reasonable, such as those immunocompromised patients with fungal disease.

Historical perspectives on the use of antrostomies are revealing. It is certainly a time-honored procedure that has been used in a variety of clinical situations. A detailed review by Lund *(13)* has revealed that the rate of spontaneous closure of the inferior antrostomy in children is probably related to continued bony growth and the limitation of oversizing the inferior antrostomy in younger patients. She did show that inferior antrostomy did result in symptomatic improvement in most individuals, and in specifically looking at goblet cell hypoplasia, there was a reduction in the number of goblet cells in those patients with moderate disease processes. Interestingly, however, patients with severe goblet cell hypoplasia did not seem to respond to inferior antrostomy.

Regarding inferior meatal antrostomy, at least in the pediatric population, it can be concluded that there is a high rate of spontaneous closure, there may be symptomatic benefit in a limited number of patients, but overall it should be reserved for short-term aeration and access to the maxillary sinus rather than a permanent resolution to chronic sinus disease.

MAXILLARY ANTROSTOMY: MIDDLE MEATAL OSTIAPLASTY

Those patients who have isolated maxillary sinus disease owing to congenital abnormalities of the infundibulum or uncinate process could obviously have their problems resolved through relatively simple enlargement of the natural ostea within the middle meatus. In those patients who have abnormalities of the uncinate process identified on CT scan, the orbit may be in a slightly lower position, and it can be inadvertently traumatized during surgery. Other patients with isolated maxillary sinusitis could also benefit from simple middle meatal ostiaplasty.

PROCEDURE: MIDDLE MEATAL MAXILLARY SINUS OSTIAPLASTY

The CT scan obtained preoperatively should be in view and should be referred to during the course of the surgery to act as a road map. Extensive removal of the lateral aspect of the nasal wall has, in unpublished reports, resulted in abnormal nasomaxillary growth in snouted animals. For this reason, when approaching the maxillary sinus ostea, it is best to be as conservative as possible in terms of removal of excess tissue when performing a simple maxillary antrostomy (Fig. 3). In general, after the nose has been topically vasoconstricted,

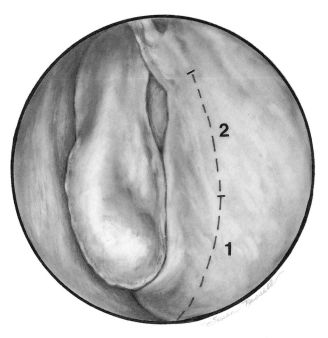

Fig. 3. Site of incision for limited or complete uncinectomy.

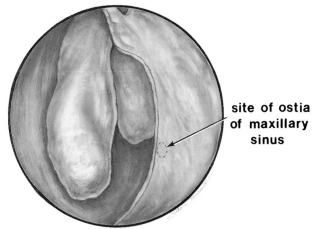

Fig. 4. Uncinate removed with ethmoid Bullae visualized.

the middle turbinate is medialized in order to expose the middle meatus and the area of the maxillary sinus ostea. The uncinate can be injected with a solution of 1% xylocaine with 1–100,000 epinephrine, and only its most inferior aspect removed in order to visualize the maxillary sinus ostea. In some cases, it is possible to cannulate the ostea gently with a blunt right-angle probe without removal of the uncinate and also to visualize it well enough with an angled telescope to enlarge the ostea without any uncinectomy being performed. It is important to make sure that the natural ostea is included in the opening, since all mucociliary clearance is directed to only one area. In special circumstances where access to cystic lesions in the maxillary sinus cannot otherwise be reached through the middle meatus, an inferior antrostomy is performed. It is placed midway posteriorly underneath the inferior turbinate in order to avoid damage to any dental roots or the nasolacrimal opening present in the anterior inferior portion of the meatus. Since the inferior meatal opening has a high rate of spontaneous closure, it should be made relatively large if any hope of a permanent opening remaining functional is expected. In general, subsequent to both middle meatal maxillary antrostomies and inferior antrostomies with appropriate avoidance of mucosal injury, the operator will avoid the necessity for any type of secondary procedure or significant concern regarding scar formation. Stenting with absorbable material is generally not necessary, and on postoperative evaluations, the patient's antrostomies can be cannulated with a small 2.2-mm flexible endoscope in order to visualize the maxillary sinus and check the patency of the ostea.

ETHMOIDECTOMY

Ethmoid disease present on the CT scan would indicate the potential need for anterior ethmoidectomy alone or in combination with posterior exenteration. Again, using the CT scan as an atlas for dissection, the nose, after being topically vasoconstricted with oxymetazoline nasal spray, is then examined and the attachment of the middle turbinate to the lateral nasal wall is injected with xylocaine with 1:100,000 adrenaline. The turbinate itself and the uncinate process are also injected with the same solution. When performing an ethmoidectomy, the uncinate process is removed in order to visualize the ethmoid bulla and the maxillary sinus ostea. (*See* Fig. 4.) Once the maxillary sinus ostea has been enlarged (if necessary), the anterior ethmoid air cells can be approached, extending the maxillary antrostomy superiorly, visualizing the bone surrounding the orbit directly, or by opening the ethmoid bulla and removing the anterior ethmoid air cells step by step until the nasofrontal area is visualized and all polypoid disease has been removed. In the course of the dissection, fracture of the lamina papyracea can easily occur with the extrusion of orbital fat into the operative field. This in and of itself, as long as it is recognized immediately, does not constitute a significant problem, although it should be avoided with careful technique. If, however, the fatty contents of the periorbita are grasped, significant injury may take place. During the course of the surgery, the patient's eyes are always left uncovered so that intraoperative complications related to the periorbita can be monitored continuously. Normal mucosa should be left alone, and only diseased or polypoid tissue should be removed. Once the anterior ethmoidal dissection has been completed, a rolled stent of Gelfilm™ is placed within the ethmoid cavity in order to prevent synechiae. In some cases, coating the Gelfilm with a steroid solution, such as Kenalog®, may diminish inflammation present at the operative site. If the posterior ethmoid area is involved with the inflammatory process, the basal lamella of the middle turbinate is perforated carefully, and the posterior ethmoid cells removed stepwise until the anterior wall of the sphenoid sinus and its ostea are identified. The Gelfilm stent can also be extended into the posterior ethmoid cavity in order to prevent synechiae in that area. Normal mucosa should be preserved when possible to promulgate rapid healing.

ADENOIDS

The efficacy of adenoidectomy for treatment of both recurrent and chronic paranasal sinusitis in children is unknown, although a variety of investigative attempts are under way to try to identify linkage between adenoid pathology and the development of inflammation in the nose and paranasal sinuses. Differentiating chronic adenoid infection from paranasal sinusitis is sometimes difficult and is a diagnosis that is often made by exclusion.

The function of the lymphoid tissue present in the oral and nasopharynx is thought to be related to the development of an immune response locally to exogenous microorganisms or other inhaled or ingested antigenetic substances (14). In a normal individual, a balance must be maintained between the processing of antigenetic material and the clearance of such material. Alterations in the balance between normal colonization with nonpathogens and pathogens lead to pathologic states that have been targeted in the development of adenoid hyperplasia and adenoid infection. Recently, such alterations have been implicated in the development and persistence of middle ear effusions, and

removal of the adenoid tissue has been found in specific age groups to allow for resolution of middle ear fluid (15). Culture analysis of altered flora of adenoid tissue identified isolates of pathogens (*Haemophilus influenzae, Streptococcus, pneumoniae, Staphylococcus aureus, Moraxella*) that are the most common organisms found in acute and chronic sinusitis. It would seem that a link then might exist between adenoids and the development of paranasal sinusitis, but the exact nature of this connection is unknown.

Obstruction of mucociliary clearance through simple adenoid hyperplasia is one means by which mucous flow could be altered, thereby increasing the risk of inflammation in the nose, which could alter or affect mucociliary clearance of the sinuses. Additionally, the altered immunologic status state of the adenoids and the existence of pathogenic bacteria could allow for spread of an infection to the paranasal sinus areas in the absence of antibiotic coverage. The decision to perform an adenoidectomy as an adjunctive procedure for the treatment of chronic sinusitis in children, then, would seem to be reasonable if:

1. Adenoid hyperplasia is producing symptoms that in and of themselves would potentially indicate the need for adenoidectomy;
2. Symptoms of purulent nasal discharge, nasal congestion, and obstruction are present unaccompanied by pathologic changes in the sinuses; or
3. Deep nasopharyngeal culture analysis reveals pathogenic bacteria unresponsive to antibiotic treatment.

Unfortunately, this does not cover all patients in whom an adenoidectomy may be of benefit, and certainly in patients who have not undergone adenoidectomy as prior treatment, adenoidectomy may be a potential factor that may positively influence the chronic nature of their sinusitis. In cases where minimal or limited maxillary disease is present, an initial stage of surgical management would include adenoidectomy and maxillary antrostomy as a therapeutic alternative.

POSTOPERATIVE MANAGEMENT

Once the surgery has been completed and the Gelfilm roll placed in the appropriate location in order to prevent synechiae, the most difficult portion of the performance of endoscopic sinus surgery begins, namely, the assurance that healing takes place in an appropriate fashion without excessive scarring causing a redevelopment of infection. Cultures are taken at the time of surgery in order to ensure appropriate antibiotic management postoperatively. This is generally continued for 2–3 wk and longer if healing is inadequate at that point in time. The patients are seen back at approx 10 d postoperatively having been maintained on antibiotics, saline rinses to the nose, and, in some cases, topical antibiotics to the nares to help reduce any crusting that may be occurring within the nasal cavity. At the initial postoperative visit in those patients who will permit it, the crusts are cleaned, and the nose is carefully inspected for any significant granulation tissue or problems with healing. In those patients in whom examination or inspection of the nasal cavity is impossible, it is sometimes necessary to use a brief anesthetic in order to examine the ethmoid cavity and ascertain that healing is taking place in an adequate fashion. There may be no significant difference in overall success rates through routine examination of postoperative patients under anesthesia vs those patients who are merely observed and treated carefully in an outpatient setting. Overall, recurrence rates range from 10–15% using both methods of postoperative management (16–19).

The small 2.2-mm flexible endoscope can be used in order to visualize the ethmoid cavity and maxillary sinus ostea with a minimum of discomfort for even the youngest of patients. Subsequent to the initial visit, the patients may be continued on their antibiotics and begun on beclomethasone aqueous spray in order to reduce the amount of inflammation and granulation tissue present. The patients are seen again in another 10 d, and, at this point, the decision of whether or not to remain on antibiotics can be made depending on the status of the surgical site. In general, it may take 6–8 wk or longer for complete resolution of the inflammatory process surrounding both the chronic sinusitis and surgery to resolve completely. This also should be carefully explained to the parents preoperatively in order to avoid any excessive expectations they may have regarding the results.

SPECIAL CIRCUMSTANCES

Cystic Fibrosis

CF is a genetic disease with autosomal recessive inheritance that affects exocrine gland function.

Any child presenting with chronic sinusitis and the development of nasal polyposis should be evaluated for the possibility of carrying this genetic disorder. The pathophysiology has been identified as abnormal ion transport in epithelial cells lining the exocrine glands of the respiratory tract. Reduced chloride permeability across the apical membrane of these cells leads to a net flow of sodium chloride into the epithelial cells with passive water absorption (20). Resulting secretions within the sinuses become progressively thickened and less able to be transported in a normal fashion. Pan-opacification of the paranasal sinuses is present on X-ray films in 90–100% in patients over 8 mo of age. The frontal sinuses rarely develop in these patients, probably because of chronic inflammation, which inhibits normal pneumatization. The incidence of nasal polyposis ranges from 10–32% in varying series. The most common age for presentation of symptoms is between 5 and 14 yr. The CF polyps are distinct in that there is a delicate relatively normal basement membrane, few eosinophils, and the mucous glands contain acid mucins rather than neutral mucins. The most common pathogens retrieved from cultures of the sinuses include *Pseudomonas aeruginosa, H. influenzae, S. pneumoniae,* and *S. aureus (21).*

If after intense medical treatment including long-term antibiotics, nasal steroids, and other means has been unsuccessful in eliminating:

1. Chronic nasal obstruction with mouth breathing;
2. Chronic purulent drainage; or
3. Persistent pain or tenderness then operative treatment should be considered (22).

A CT scan is obtained and after the appropriate preparation for surgery with the CF specialist who is managing that particular individual, surgery may be planned. (*See* Fig. 5.) Endoscopic surgery with complete removal of all polyps and their origin from the ethmoid or maxillary sinuses generally provides a longer interval between surgical procedures, which may be needed on a repetitive basis. A complete ethmoidectomy is performed with a sphenoidotomy if indicated, and a large middle meatal antral window is created at the site of the natural ostea. In addition, because of the lack of normal physiologic clearance of secretions (*see* Fig. 6), a large inferior meatal window is made to permit gravitational drainage of some secretions and adequate moisturization through irrigation of

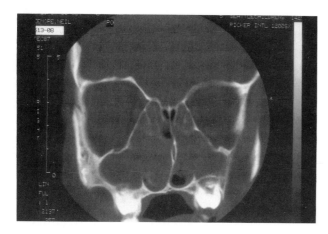

Fig. 5. Characteristic changes of cystic fibrosis.

the nasal cavity. Also, irrigation of the maxillary sinus with flexible catheters or curved probes can be more easily accomplished if wide drainage has been established. Topical antibiotic irrigation may also be useful in reducing infection.

Fungal Sinusitis

The incidence of mycotic infections of the nose and paranasal sinuses or at least their recognition seems to be on the increase. Those factors that predispose to fungal infections (diabetes, immune incompetence, radiation treatment for malignancy, long-term antibiotic and steroid therapy) all may predispose patients to develop paranasal sinus mycosis. *Aspergillus* is by far the most common fungal organism identified and probably occurs as a secondary disease process superimposed on a chronic sinusitis *(6)*. The underlying inflammatory process creates an ideal environment for fungal growth with stasis of secretions, diminished oxygen content, and abundant nutrients present. The diagnosis can usually be made after radiographic evaluations reveal granular opaque areas on CT scan. On magnetic resonance (MR) scanning, the mycotic growth on T2-weighted images will not be visualized, but on T1-weighted images will easily be seen. Occasionally, inspection of the nose will reveal thick viscid brownish secretions exuding from the middle meatus. In cases of fungal sinusitis, surgical management should include removal of all fungal debris with establishment of appropriate drainage in order to allow residual mucosa to return to its normal state. In immunocompromised patients, it may be necessary to biopsy mucosa in order to ascertain whether or not the fungus is inva-

sive. If there is tissue invasion, treatment with systemic medication, such as Amphotericin, may be necessary in combination with more aggressive surgical debridement *(22)*.

Acute Sinusitis with Complications

Abscess formation in the orbital space secondary to complications of ethmoid sinusitis has only recently been treated through endoscopic management. However, if the surgeon is experienced and has the confidence necessary to attempt endoscopic drainage of an abscess, there is certainly no technical reason why it cannot be performed. In general, the only limiting factor is the amount of edema and inflammation present in the nose owing to the presence of the acute sinusitis and if there is excessive bleeding, which would prevent adequate visualization of the space to be drained.

The same would be true for air–fluid levels in the frontal and sphenoid sinuses, which are producing pain or other evidence of toxicity, which are not responding appropriately to antibiotic management.

Anatomic Abnormalities— Maxillary Sinus Hypoplasia

In a review of 136 pediatric patients operated on for chronic sinusitis, 20 patients were found to have hypoplasia of the maxillary sinus for an approximate incidence of 17.5% in our population. This is a higher prevalence rate than is found in other series, which have a range of 6.3–10.4%. In association with maxillary sinus hypoplasia, there was deviation or absence of the uncinate process, which would lead to the conclusion that perhaps the hypoplastic sinus is more prone to infection. Among the 20 children with hypoplasia, the sinus mucosal disease was limited to or most severe in that abnormal sinus. Eleven of the 20 patients had lateral deviation of the uncinate process. At surgery, the uncinate process was frequently indistinguishable from the lateral nasal wall, and invariably a thick viscid mucus was removed from the affected sinus. In some cases, the surgeon may find only a membranous covering over the area of the maxillary sinus ostea. Orbital volume is increased on the side of the hypoplastic sinus, and the orbital floor actually is lower on this side and more prone to injury during osteoplasty *(4)*. (*See* Fig. 7.)

When no distinct uncinate process or maxillary sinus ostea can be identified (*see* Fig. 8), direct puncture into the maxillary sinus is necessary to

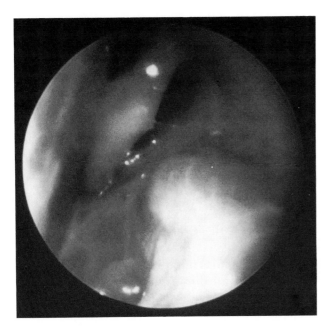

Fig. 6. Cystic fibrosis patient with expansion of medial maxillary wall.

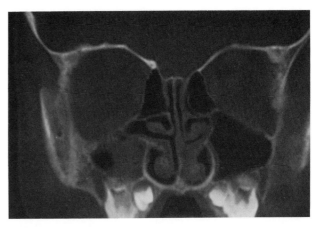

Fig. 7. Lateral deviation of uncinate with maxillary sinus disease.

achieve an opening. In some cases, it is necessary to make an inferior antrostomy, pass a right-angle probe through the inferior antrostomy, and use that probe to identify where the middle antrostomy should be placed. With appropriate care, injury to the lamina papyracea is unusual. After creation of a large antrostomy, results have been excellent in patients who have no other underlying or concomitant disease process, such as allergy or nasal polyposis.

Many other abnormalities were identified in patients with chronic sinusitis with a slight propensity of involvement toward the site of disease. Despite this, the relatively common finding of anatomic abnormalities that are not associated with chronic sinusitis should not lead to surgery in nonsymptomatic individuals.

Revision Surgery

Since the widespread application of endoscopic sinus surgery to chronic sinusitis both in the pediatric and the adult population, there is now a category of patients who continue to have problems postoperatively and require revision surgery. Revision surgery is the most difficult type of endoscopic procedure to be performed, because typically anatomic relationships have been altered, and scarring and fibrosis at the previous surgical site impair visualization and the normal "feel" that takes place at the initial operation. In some cases,

it may be necessary to use external approaches to the ethmoid sinuses in order to clear out residual disease adequately with the most safety for the patient. Maintenance of appropriate anatomic landmarks during the initial surgery obviously permits the accomplishment of revision surgery with the least amount of difficulty.

Allergy with Nasal Polyposis

Significant allergy with the resultant development of sinusitis and nasal polyposis is an unfavorable prognostic indicator for the eventual outcome for endoscopic surgery. In all cases of children who have nasal polyps and in whom a sweat chloride examination for CF has been negative, an evaluation of the immunologic status of the patient, especially regarding allergy, should be performed. If there is any indication that the polyps are related to aspirin sensitivity, it should be discontinued. There is no confirming evidence that treatment of the underlying inhalant allergy will actually eliminate or prohibit the development of nasal polyposis, although a search for antigenic stimuli should be undertaken at least in order to enable the patient or his or her parents to begin treatment.

This patient population may specifically benefit from the use of intranasal inhaled steroids, such as beclomethasone, and in some cases when acute infection accompanies nasal polyposis, brief courses of oral steroids in conjunction with antibiotics may provide significant benefit for clearance of the infection and reduction in the overall extent of nasal polyposis. Should surgery become necessary because of chronic infection, nasal obstruction, or

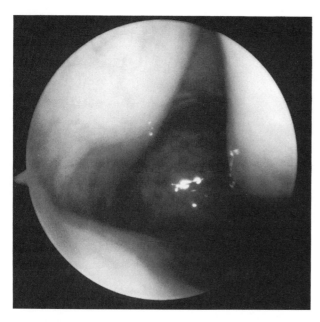

Fig. 8. Absent uncinate processes Bulla Ethmoidalis in background.

facial pain, newer strategies for the removal of the polyps, including lasers or the "hummer," an oscillating shaver more commonly used for arthroscopic surgery may be used to remove the polyps with minimum bleeding and discomfort for the patient, allowing further endoscopic surgery to take place in a field uncompromised by significant bleeding.

Immune Deficiency

Elsewhere in this text, the medical work-up for patients with chronic sinus disease has been mentioned. The potential for immune deficiency certainly exists to a significant degree in any chronic sinus population, and the evidence of significance of any immune deficiency should be searched for and treated if possible. The results of endoscopic sinus surgery for those patients who are truly immune deficient are not as successful in stages 1 to 3, but certainly approach the success rate achieved by those patients at stage 4 levels *(23)*.

COMPLICATIONS

A thorough comprehension of anatomy, distances, and complete review of the preoperative CT scan will prevent significant complications in most cases. Adequate visualization with appropriate instrumentation for pediatric patients is essential as well in the prevention of significant

complications. Minor complications, such as scarring in the ethmoid cavity, dehiscence of the lamina papyracea, bleeding, or contraction of the maxillary sinus osteoplasty, take place with a frequency of 8–20% *(24,25)*. Major complications, such as intraorbital hematoma, cerebral spinal fluid leaks, blindness, and anosmia, are uncommon, but should always be mentioned in the preoperative counseling with the patient's parents.

SUMMARY

Endoscopic sinus surgery for pediatric patients is an option for those patients who have sinus disease objectively confirmed by CT scan that has been resistant to prolonged medical treatment. Complications are diminished through experience, a knowledge of anatomy, and appropriate instrumentation, which permits excellent visualization of the anatomic spaces involved. Use of endoscopic sinus surgery for recurrent sinusitis is unclear, and certainly in the absence of demonstrated anatomic abnormalities, which would increase the possibility of sinusitis, adenoidectomy alone or in combination with maxillary osteoplasty may be a more preferable and conservative option. Any disease factors that underlie or contribute to the development of sinusitis should be searched for, since they can affect surgical planning. The prognosis for any individual patient can be estimated based on the extent of sinus disease on CT scan and then any underlying factors that may be present. Endoscopic sinus surgery is a safe and effective means of dealing with chronic sinusitis in the pediatric population.

REFERENCES

1. Stammberger H. Functional Endoscopic Sinus Surgery. Philadelphia: BC Decker, 1991.
2. Myerson MC. The natural orifice of the maxillary sinus. I. Anatomic studies. Arch Otolaryngol. 1932;15:80.
3. Rice OH, Schaefer SD. Endoscopic Paranasal Sinus Surgery. New York: Raven, 1988.
4. Milczuk H, Dalley R, Nessbacher FW, Richardson MA. Nasal and paranasal sinus anomalies in children with chronic sinusitis. Laryngoscope 1993;103(3):46,47.
5. Carenfelt C, Wodberg C. Purulent and non-purulent maxillary sinus secretions with respect to PO$_2$, PO$_2$, and pH. ACTA Otolaryngol (Stock H) 1977;84:138–144.
6. Ingels KJ, Kortman MJ. Factors influencing ciliary beat measurements. Rhinology 1991;29:17–26.
7. Phillips PP, McCaffrey TV. The effect of phenylephrine on nasal mucociliary transport. Otolaryngol Head and Neck Surgery 1990;103:558–565.

8. Kennedy DW. Prognostic factors, outcomes and staging in ethmoid sinus surgery. Laryngoscope 1992; 102:1–18.

9. Gwaltney JM, Phillips CD, Miller RD, Riker DK. Computer tomographic Study of the common cold. NEJM 1994;330(1):25–30.

10. Weisberger EC. Lasers in Head and Neck Surgery. Tokyo: Igaku-Shoin, 1991.

11. Muntz HR, Lusk RP. Nasal antral windows in children: a retrospective study. Laryngoscope 1990;100: 643–646.

12. Lusk R. Pediatric Sinusitis. New York: Raven, 1992.

13. Lund VJ. Inferior meatal antrostomy. J Laryngol Otol 1988;15:1–18.

14. Brodsky L, Koch J. Bacteriology and immunology of normal and diseased adenoids in children. Arch Otolaryngol Head Neck Surg 1993;119:821–829.

15. Gates GA, Avery CA, Cooper JC, Prihoag TJ. Effectiveness of adenoidectomy and tympanostomy tubes in the treatment of chronic otitis media with effusion. WEJM 1987;317:1444–1451.

16. Levine HL. Functional endoscopic sinus surgery: evaluation, surgery and followup of 250 patients. Laryngoscope 1990;100:79–83.

17. Lusk RP, Muntz HR. Endoscopic sinus surgery in children with cardiac sinusitis: a pilot study. Laryngoscope 1990;100:654–658.

18. Maniglia A, Chandler I, Goodwin W, Flynn J. Rare complications following ethmoidectomies. A report of eleven cases. Laryngoscope 1981;91:1239–1244.

19. Serdahl C, Berris C, Chole R. Nasolacrimal duct obstruction after endoscopic sinus surgery. Arch Ophthalmol 1990;108:391,392.

20. Quinton M. Chloride in permeability in cystic fibrosis. Nature 1983;301:421,422.

21. Shapiro ED, Milmoe GJ, Wald ER, Rodnan JB, Bowen AD. Bacteriology of the maxillary sinuses in patients with cystic fibrosis. J Infect Dis 1982;146:589–593.

22. Ramsey B, Richardson MA. Impact of sinusitis in cystic fibrosis. J Allergy Clin Immunol 1992;90(no. 3):547–552.

23. Wiatrak BJ, Willging P, Myer CM, Cohon RT. Functional endoscopic sinus surgery in the immunocompromised child. Otolaryngol Head Neck Surg 1991;105:818–825.

24. Stankiewicz JA. Blindness and intranasal endoscopic ethmoidectomy. Otolaryngol Head Neck Surg 1989; 101:320–329.

25. Weymuller EA. Complications of endoscopic sinus surgery. Operative Techniques Oto/HNS. 1990; 149–152.

26 Sinusitis in Children

An Overview of Nonendoscopic and Endoscopic Techniques

Rodney P. Lusk, MD

INTRODUCTION

The literature regarding the surgical management of chronic sinusitis is confusing at best. Ancillary surgical procedures, such as tonsillectomy, adenoidectomy, and antral lavage, are discussed extensively in the older literature, but opinion as to the efficacy varies widely, and recent literature focuses primarily on endoscopic sinus surgery. This chapter will examine the efficacy of nonendoscopic and endoscopic procedures used to manage chronic sinusitis.

This chapter does not focus on the diagnosis of chronic sinusitis, but a few comments on that subject are appropriate before surgical treatment is discussed. Infections of the sinuses are thought to originate in the nose *(1–4)*. Most episodes of acute sinusitis resolve spontaneously or with antibiotics, but a small percentage proceed to chronic infection. It is generally believed that sinusitis should be documented with coronal CT scans, after a prolonged course of medical management, before the diagnosis can be confirmed. If there is evidence of failure to control or treat the infection, then it is appropriate to consider surgical intervention. The following surgical procedures have been proposed as effective in the management of chronic sinusitis.

REMOVAL OF FOREIGN BODY

In the pediatric population, it is not rare that foreign bodies are placed into the nasal passage. This is usually associated with a foul-smelling unilateral purulent nasal drainage; other symptoms include nasal airway obstruction and occasional

From: *Diseases of the Sinuses* (M. E. Gershwin and G. A. Incaudo, eds.),
©1996 Humana Press Inc., Totowa, NJ.

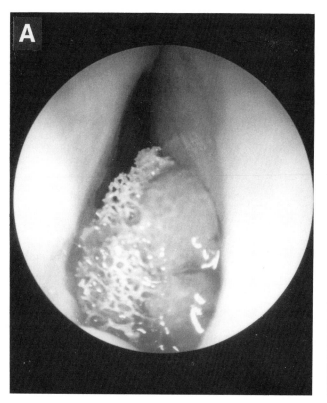 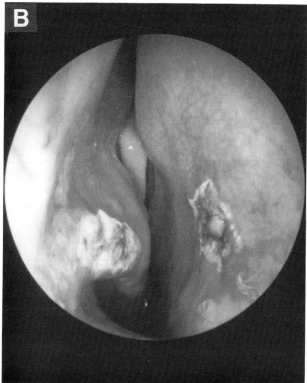

Fig. 1. (A) Foreign body in the nose. **(B)** Nose after foreign body removal.

headaches. It is rare that chronic sinusitis is unilateral, so if the symptoms are unilateral, a foreign body should be considered in the differential diagnosis. On occasion, lesions caused by a foreign body can be confused with a tumor because of the exuberant granulation tissue that forms (Fig. 1 A,B).

TONSILLOADENOIDECTOMY

Obstruction of the nose and nasopharynx caused by tonsil and adenoid hypertrophy has been shown to be associated with many of the symptoms of chronic sinusitis. Most of these studies used symptoms only or symptoms and plain sinus films to make the diagnosis of chronic sinusitis. In most cases, there was no effort to use aggressive medical management, and diagnoses were retrospective. For these reasons, the studies must be interpreted with caution. Preston (5) found that purulent rhinorrhea was associated with hypertrophied tonsils in 65% of the patients. He thought rhinorrhea was indicative of chronic sinusitis, but it is not necessarily appropriate to base the diagnosis on this one symptom. (Wilson [6], for example, identified purulent rhinorrhea in 27% of newborns,

and it is difficult to know if this symptom is secondary to sinusitis [7–9]). There is some indication of a higher incidence of sinusitis in patients with enlarged tonsils. Merck (10) evaluated the size of the adenoid pad with lateral sinus films and assessed the incidence of maxillary sinusitis on plain sinus films. McAlister et al. (11) have shown that plain films are not as accurate as CT scans in assessing the status of the sinuses, but concluded that the correlation was greatest in the maxillary sinus. This means that Merck's data should be interpreted with caution, but his findings are of interest, because, the incidence of sinusitis increased as the size of the adenoid pad increased: Abnormal maxillary sinuses were noted in 13% of children with small adenoid pads, 24% with medium-sized adenoid pads, and 34% with large pads.

Other investigators have noted an association between maxillary sinusitis and adenoid or tonsil disease. Most of the evidence was acquired through antral puncture of the maxillary sinus. The indications for tonsilloadenoidectomy (T&A) appear to be a combination of tonsil and adenoid hypertrophy and recurrent infections. We now know that the indications for T&A in the past were too liberal.

Realizing that there was a lack of well-defined criteria for T&A, Mollison and Kendall *(12)* noted maxillary sinusitis in 22%, Crooks and Signy *(13)* in 24%, and Gerrie *(14)* in 9% of their patients undergoing tonsillectomy. Carmack *(15)* attempted to rule out allergy and sinusitis in patients that he performed T&As on and still found 14.2% of his patients had diseased maxillary sinuses. There are no good studies assessing the incidence of sinusitis in normal children as documented by maxillary antrostomy.

It follows that if the tonsils and adenoids are associated with disease, removing them may be associated with a lower incidence of sinusitis. Most investigators *(9,15–19)*, however, have found that T&A has not consistently corrected symptoms of chronic sinusitis. Paul *(9)* noted that disease cleared with almost equal frequency when treated with medical management and with T&A. His medical management and the duration of follow-up are not well defined, but this was one of the first studies to call into question the efficacy of T&A in treating chronic sinusitis. Fujita et al. *(20)* noted, in a study on Eustachian tube function, that following T&A, sinusitis "improved" in 56% of patients with sinusitis, but in only 24% of nonadenoidectomy patients. This represents a significant improvement, but is certainly far from complete resolution.

The causal relationship between the tonsils and adenoids and chronic sinusitis remains unclear. It would seem that if the adenoids were large enough to cause stasis of secretions, then the symptoms of sinusitis could be mimicked. It is also conceivable that this stasis can cause inflammation of the sinus ostia, which can then result in sinusitis. As Birrell *(21)* stated over 40 yr ago, "No sinus can remain free from secretion when the nasal cavity, with which it communicates, contains a plentiful supply of secretion."

Our current state of knowledge does not allow us to predict which patients will symptomatically improve with an adenoidectomy. If there is significant stasis of secretions secondary to adenoid hypertrophy, it would appear that adenoidectomy would be the first logical step. Studies have not been performed that assess the effect of adenoidectomy on CT-diagnosed chronic sinusitis which has failed aggressive medical management by current standards. Some evidence, however, suggests that adenoidectomy does not have an effect by our current standards of treatment. Parsons and Phillips

(22) evaluated 14 patients who had medically resistant sinusitis diagnosed with CT scan, and adenoidectomy failed to control their symptoms in all cases. This is consistent with our experience as well.

ANTRAL LAVAGE

The maxillary sinus has been most frequently studied because of its accessibility. The ostium, however, is hidden by the uncinate process, so one cannot look directly into the maxillary sinus. The physical manifestation of sinusitis is purulence from the middle meatus (Fig. 2A). If the middle meatus is clear (Fig. 2B), it is suggestive, but not assured, that there is no infection of the maxillary sinus. In patients with evidence of chronic maxillary sinusitis, antral lavage is performed to irrigate or suction the debris from the sinus.

The sinus can be entered in one of three ways (Fig. 3). The oldest technique is to enter through the natural ostium. In adults, this can be performed under local anesthesia, but children require a general anesthetic. A curved cannula is inserted into the middle meatus along the posterior half of the middle turbinate. It is then rotated laterally and pulled forward in an attempt to cannulate the ostium. In the pediatric age group, the ostium is small and difficult to palpate or cannulate. It cannot be visualized without an uncinectomy. The ostium is not parallel to the medial wall of the middle turbinate and cannot be cannulated in all patients *(23,24)*. If the cannula is forced into the lateral wall of the nose, it will most likely push through the lamina papyracea and into the orbit at the inferior medial wall. Once the irrigation has started, if the secretions are clear, there is always the question about the placement of the cannula: Is it in a normal sinus, or in the nose and not irrigating the sinus?

Lund *(25)* credits Gooch with the first description of an intranasal inferior meatal puncture, but Myerson *(24)* indicates the procedure was popularized by Lichtwitz (1886), Krause (1887) *(26)*, and Mikulicz (1887) *(27)*. This procedure was developed because of concern about trauma to the ostium of the maxillary sinus, and because cannulation of the natural ostium was not always possible *(27,28)*, trauma to the sphenopalatine artery could result in significant bleeding *(27)*, and the close proximity of the ostium to the orbit could result in orbital complications *(27)*. This method of evaluation may not be successful in the younger patient because the

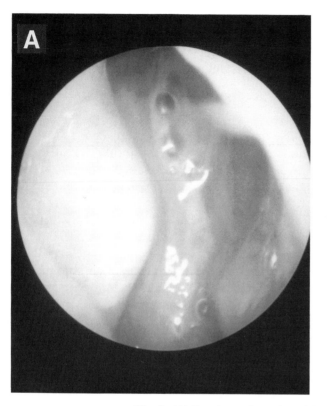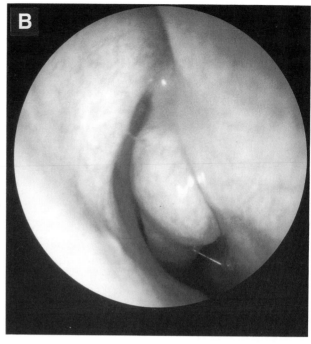

Fig. 2. (A) Purulence from the middle meatus. **(B)** Clear middle meatus.

sinus may not be developed below the inferior turbinate. Cannulation of the inferior meatal puncture and repeated postoperative irrigations have also been suggested *(15,18,29,30)*. Huggill and Ballantyne *(31)* irrigated the sinus with antibiotics several times a day through a polyethylene cannula. Over time, these methods of treatment have proven to be unsuccessful and are now infrequently used.

Penetrating the anterior wall of the maxillary sinus (the canine fossa puncture) is likely the most direct route into the sinus. It was first introduced in 1743 and was repopularized in the early 1970s *(32)*. In the child, this approach is likely the safest *(33)*, but is compromised by the high floor of the maxillary sinus, the possibility of trauma to the tooth roots, and the thick anterior maxillary sinus wall. Stammberger *(34)* does not recommend this approach in children <9 yr old because of the risk of traumatizing the tooth roots. It does have the fullest arch for visualization of the sinus with a telescope.

Cannulation of the sinus by any of these methods may be associated with significant risk of complication. The trocar can penetrate the orbit, the posterior wall of the maxillary sinus, or the lateral wall of the nose, each of which can be associated with

significant morbidity. Lavage via the inferior meatal and canine fossa route can be combined with sinoscopy to document the sinus contents. Kim et al. *(35)* reported that the first effort to perform sinoscopy was in 1903 by Hirschmann through the canine fossa approach. Kim et al. *(35)* also found that sinoscopy was more accurate in assessing the sinus contents than plain sinus films.

The efficacy of antral lavage has had mixed reviews in the literature. Carmack *(15)* recommended early intervention and suggested it should be used as a primary mode of therapy. Rarely will one lavage be successful, and many surgeons recommend multiple lavages *(13,18,36,37)* before proceeding to a Caldwell-Luc procedure. Crooks and Signy *(13)* recommended as many as 10 lavages before abandoning it, and Dean *(29)* was quoted by Alden as recommending lavage 6–20 times in children. This frequency of surgical intervention would not be tolerated in our current medical system. Medical decongestion of the nose and ostium has been felt by Stammberger to be equally successful *(34)*.

Antral lavage continues to be practiced today, but is used selectively in patients who are usually having other procedures, such as a tonsillectomy

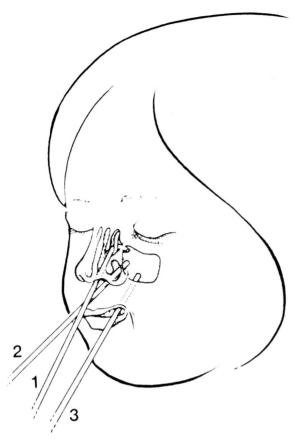

Fig. 3. Three methods of entering the maxillary sinus: (1) natural ostia, (2) inferior meatus, and (3) canine fossa.

and/or adenoidectomy. Good prospective studies are not available to guide us about which patients are best treated in this manner. In most pediatric patients, a general anesthetic will be required. In adult patients, the canine fossa is associated with considerable pain, and there is little doubt that the same will be true in children. The inferior meatal puncture or antrostomy is traumatic, and the maxillary sinus may be too small to be entered. The most significant factor contributing to the interior antrostomy's efficacy in resolving chronic sinusitis is likely the persistence of untreated ethmoid disease. The ethmoid sinuses are known to be involved with almost equal frequency *(11)*.

INFERIOR MEATAL ANTROSTOMY

Inferior meatal antrostomies reflect a natural progression in the effort to aerate and drain the maxillary sinus. This procedure became a popular surgical technique in the management of maxillary sinus disease and therefore in the management of chronic sinusitis *(25)*. It gained wide acceptance

until the Caldwell-Luc procedure was introduced. In the inferior meatal antrostomy, the maxillary sinus was opened through the anterior wall, and usually the mucosa was stripped from the sinus cavity.

Fortunately, this procedure was never widely used in the pediatric population. Lund *(25)* reports a steady decline in the incidence of inferior meatal antrostomy and Caldwell-Luc procedures at the Royal National Throat, Nose, and Ear Hospital from 1950 to 1985. There is little scientific evidence that the inferior meatal antrostomy is efficacious, particularly in the pediatric age group. In the older literature *(27)*, this procedure was thought to be safer than the middle meatal antrostomy, but with today's instrumentation, this idea no longer holds. The procedure is based on assumptions that a patent hole in the inferior portion of the maxillary sinus will aerate the sinus and that gravity will allow the purulence and secretions to drain into the nose. Neither of these assumptions is valid.

Maintaining patency of the inferior antrostomy in the pediatric age group is particularly problematic. Lund *(25)* did both retrospective and prospective evaluations of window patency in adults and children. In a retrospective study of 216 patients, she found the antrostomy closed in 45% and patent in 50%, with 5% that could not be assessed. Of the 15 patients who were younger than 16 yr, only two had patent antrostomies, and these were in 14- and 15-yr-old patients. Surgical technique was thought to be a factor in maintaining patency, so a prospective study was performed to assess how large the opening had to be to remain patent. Lund found that the antrostomy had to be >1 cm in length and .5 cm in height to remain patent. In the pediatric age group, the medial wall of the maxillary sinus is frequently not large enough to allow a window of this size. In the prospective study, six antrostomies were performed in four children, and all failed.

The other fallacious assumption was that gravity would allow the secretions to egress through a patent antrostomy *(38)*. We now know that the ciliary blanket lining the sinuses is a very powerful organ *(4,39,40)*. The presence of a patent antrostomy does not alter the ciliary flow, and if the natural ostium is occluded, secretions will continue to accumulate. Gravity does not appear to have any appreciable effect on the clearance of secretions. Indeed, secretions can circulate from the nose through the inferior meatal antrostomy, into the maxillary sinus, and out through the natural ostium.

Since it is difficult to maintain patency of the inferior meatal antrostomy in children, one would expect a correspondingly low success rate in clearing maxillary sinus disease. Muntz and Lusk *(41)* performed a retrospective evaluation of 39 children (mean age 6.3 yr) who had documented chronic sinusitis and had undergone bilateral inferior maxillary antrostomy. Finding a failure rate of 60% at 1 mo and 73% at 6 mo, they concluded that the inferior meatal antrostomy was not a viable option for treating chronic maxillary sinusitis in the pediatric age group.

MIDDLE MEATAL ANTROSTOMY

Obstruction of the osteomeatal complex has become a central theme in our current thinking about the cause of chronic sinusitis. The obstruction can occur at the sinus ostium or in a more common drainage pathway known as the osteomeatal complex. Relieving these sites of obstruction improves sinus clearing and physiology. Another mechanism of draining the maxillary sinus is to enlarge the obstructed maxillary ostium and allow the cilia to clear the sinuses normally.

Around the turn of the century, Freer *(42)*, Sluder *(43)*, and Canfield *(44)* recommended removing most of the medial wall of the maxillary sinus through the middle and inferior meatal antrostomy. Wilkerson *(45)* cites Ostrum as the first to recommend a limited middle meatal antrostomy to treat maxillary sinus disease. The procedure was controversial because it was thought the primary nerves and vascular supply to the maxillary sinus coursed through the natural ostium *(46)*. Trauma to these structures would then result in irreparable damage to the sinus and risk protracted pain and paresthesia. Hilding *(47)* performed antrostomies in various sites in rabbits. Using three rabbits in each of three groups (total of nine rabbits), he found that all three animals in which the natural ostium was widened became infected, and two of the three animals became infected if an inferior antrostomy was performed, but none of the animals became infected if the antrostomy were performed as far away from the ostium as possible. He cautioned about transferring this practice to humans, but based on this study, the middle meatal antrostomy was abandoned as a surgical procedure. Wilkerson *(45)* reported that in spite of good results with the middle meatal antrostomy, he abandoned the procedure because

of the widespread sentiment against it. He later returned to the approach, and through his work, interest was rekindled in middle meatal surgery.

With current instrumentation, middle meatal antrostomy is more precisely performed and has significantly less morbidity associated with it. Kennedy et al. *(2)* retrospectively evaluated 117 antrostomies in 75 adult patients. Three of the ostia could not be identified, and in 20 cases, there were problems in seeing the ostia. Four months after surgery, 98% of the ostia was patent. Lavelle and Harrison *(49)* reported a patency rate of 94% in 150 patients over a 20-yr period. Davis found patency between 87 and 94% *(50,51)*. It appears that the major complication aside from failure to clear the infection is epiphora, secondary to lacrimal duct trauma. The risk is not high, however; our group have yet to see this complication in approx 1000 separate procedures (500 patients) performed.

Middle meatal antrostomy carries a high patency rate and appears to be the most efficacious way of treating maxillary sinus disease to date. The approach allows removal of the osteomeatal disease or anatomical abnormalities that predispose the sinus to disease. The remaining factor to be investigated is how large the created ostium should be. This is particularly important in the pediatric age group since minimal surgery is likely the most prudent course to follow.

SUMMARY

This discussion has addressed primarily the maxillary sinus—the largest of the sinuses and the easiest to treat. We know, however, that the ethmoid sinus is involved with equal frequency, and the failure to treat it in chronic infections is a frequent cause of failure to resolve the disease.

ENDOSCOPIC MANAGEMENT OF PEDIATRIC CHRONIC SINUSITIS: INTRODUCTION

Endoscopic sinus surgery is possible because of the Hopkin's rod lens telescope, which was originally designed as a diagnostic instrument. Endoscopic sinus surgery was initially performed in adults *(1–4,52–54)*, then as smaller instruments and telescopes became available, the same techniques were used in children.

The goal of endoscopic sinus surgery is to create a wider opening in the middle meatus. Limited endoscopic ethmoidectomy and maxillary antrostomy in children has theoretical advantages because it can be much less traumatic to developing tissues. The principles to be followed in adult endoscopic sinus surgery were described by Messerklinger *(55)*, and the procedure was popularized by Kennedy *(2,52,54,56)* and Stammberger *(1,3,4, 34,57)*. These same principles were applied in pediatric endoscopic surgery by Lusk and Muntz *(58–60)*, Parsons *(22)*, Gross *(61,62)*, and others *(63,64)*. The most important principle, particularly in the pediatric population, is preservation of normal structures and mucosa. Chronic sinusitis is located primarily in the anterior ethmoid and maxillary sinuses, therefore it seems best to remove the anterior disease directly through the middle meatus, in the method popularized by Kennedy and Stammberger. Frequently the ethmoid dissection is extended into the posterior ethmoid cells, but every attempt is made to preserve normal mucosa. Newer instruments, like mechanical debriders and through-cutting forceps, allow for greater preservation of the mucosa.

INDICATIONS

Candidates for endoscopic sinus surgery should have been symptomatic for at least several months; therefore, surgical intervention is not recommended for children with symptoms for only a few months. Prior to any consideration of surgery, an appropriate work-up should be performed for systemic disease, allergies, and local anatomical problems, and thorough trial of medical management should be instituted. As indicated early in this chapter, the optimum antibiotic dosage and duration of therapy need further study. At this time it appears that several courses of long-term (4–6 wk) broad-spectrum antibiotics and probably topical nasal steroid spray are appropriate. A CT scan should be performed at the end of a prolonged course of antibiotics.

The allergy evaluation is essential. It is our impression that highly allergic patients are less likely to be cured with surgery alone. This is important information to have when counseling parents about realistic expectations. If the symptoms are mild and the amount of disease documented on CT scan is mild to moderate, then it may be prudent to first treat the allergies.

Systemic disease should be considered in patients with sinusitis, otitis media, and pneumo-

nia or bronchiectasis. Cystic fibrosis, immune deficiency, and ciliary dyskinesia should be ruled out. A chest X-ray should be performed to rule out situs inversus and Kartagener's syndrome. A cilia biopsy is best performed in the trachea instead of the nose because chronic infection of the nose may cause abnormal cilia. Screening immunoglobulins (IgG, IgM, IgA, and possibly IgE) should be obtained in patients being considered for surgery, but the need for IgG subclasses is debatable because 10% of the population has abnormal results on these tests *(65,66)* but are asymptomatic. If an underlying immune deficiency is identified, it should be treated. Endoscopic sinus surgery should be considered in such cases because many of the symptoms will be improved *(60)*. For the patients with pansinusitis, it is particularly important to obtain a sweat test to rule out cystic fibrosis. The indications for endoscopic sinus surgery will continue to undergo refinement.

TECHNIQUE

The technique of pediatric endoscopic sinus surgery is described in detail in other texts *(67)* and is beyond the scope of this chapter. A few comments, however, are appropriate.

A general anesthetic is used in pediatric patients; 0.05% oxymetazoline has been found to be a better vasoconstrictor than cocaine or phenylephrine *(68)*. Transoral sphenopalatine blocks with 0.5 cc of 1% lidocaine with 1/100,000 epinephrine are now routinely used for better vasoconstriction.

Examination of the pediatric nasal cavity is best performed with a 2.7-mm 0° telescope. The 0° telescope can be more accurately manipulated minimizing trauma to the mucosa. It is very difficult to roll the telescope into the middle meatus of a child in the manner described by Kennedy *(54)*. The middle meatus of children is best examined through displacement of the middle turbinate with a Freer elevator. Examination of the sphenoid recess in children is also difficult to perform. Some surgeons recommend that the 4.0-mm telescope be used in almost all children *(61,63)*, but the 2.7-mm telescope should be used more frequently to decrease trauma to the tissues. With practice, the view is not restrictive, and the illumination is adequate.

The uncinate process is initially removed with a sickle knife or back-biting forceps. Either technique is satisfactory, but the back-biter has been

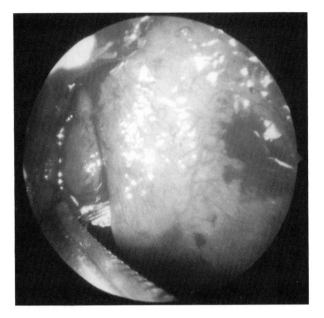

Fig. 4. Back-biting forceps used to remove the uncinate process.

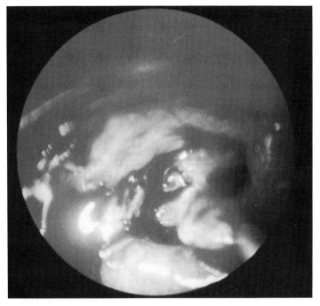

Fig. 5. Ostium of the maxillary sinus visualized through a 30° telescope.

found to be less traumatic. The back-biter is a necessity in the case of hypoplastic maxillary sinuses (Fig. 4). It is crucial to remove all of the uncinate process to expose the natural ostium of the maxillary sinus. When the entire uncinate process is removed, the middle meatus is maximally opened, and the chance of traumatizing the lateral surface of the middle turbinate is minimized.

The ostium of the maxillary sinus is easiest to identify with a seeker and a 30° telescope immediately after the uncinate process has been removed (Fig. 5). The ostium is best opened into the posterior fontanel. Attempt to keep the mucosa intact superiorly and anteriorly. It is appropriate to culture fluid in the maxillary sinus at this time. If the mucosal flap can be created, the ostium will remain patent and heal quickly (Fig. 6). If infraorbital cells are present, the decision to open them will have to be made at the time of antrostomy since they are a frequent cause of failure to keep the ostium patent (Fig. 7).

Once the maxillary antrostomy has been performed, the ethmoid bulla is entered. It is safest to enter at the anterior inferior medial border. Anaerobic, aerobic, and fungal mucosal cultures are taken at this time. As the medial wall of the ethmoid bulla is removed, care is taken not to traumatize the mucosa on the lateral border of the middle turbinate. The lateral border of the middle turbinate is

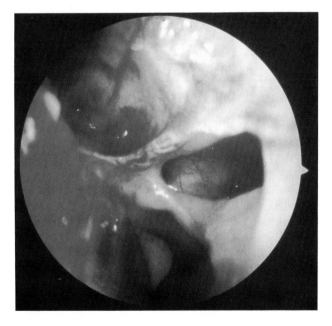

Fig. 6. Maxillary ostium well healed 2 wk postoperatively.

followed posteriorly to the basal lamina. The mucosa over the basal lamina can be kept intact if an anterior ethmoidectomy is all that is necessary. A 30° telescope is used to identify the lamina papyracea (Fig. 8). As a general rule, dissection into the frontal recess is not performed unless disease is extensive. The appropriate management of the developing frontal recess is not clear. Scarring

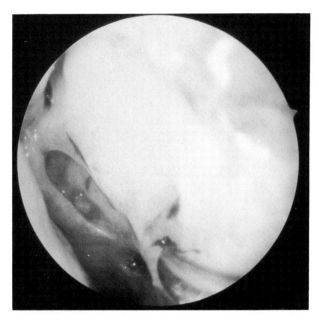

Fig. 7. Obstructed postoperative maxillary antrostomy.

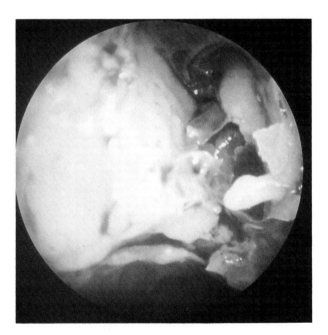

Fig. 8. View of the lamina papyracea through a 30° telescope.

in this area can cause life-long morbidity. It would seem prudent to be very conservative in the frontal recess until more is known about its development.

If there is disease in the posterior ethmoid cells, the basal lamina is penetrated. The posterior cells are large, and the roof of the ethmoid is easiest to identify posteriorly. The cells are best entered inferiorly, and the forceps are directed along the lateral

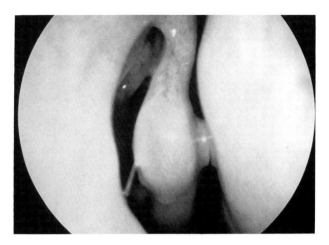

Fig. 9. Postoperative patent middle meatus.

roof toward the thicker frontal bone. The mucosa from the posterior cells should be removed carefully in an attempt to leave as much mucosa as possible. Care is taken during the posterior dissection not to injure the optic nerve. The sphenoid sinus is not as frequently diseased in children as in adults and therefore is not frequently opened. In children, the sphenoid must be entered through the ethmoid cells because there is not enough room to enlarge the sphenoid ostium through the sphenoid recess.

POSTOPERATIVE CARE

The usual postoperative care for sinus endoscopy must be modified for the pediatric age group. It is recommended to stent the ethmoid cavity with rolled Gelfilm (Upjohn, Kalamazoo, MI), which is removed 2 wk later under a second general anesthetic. Granulation tissue in the frontal recess and the ostium of the maxillary sinus is carefully removed. Another half roll of Gelfilm is placed back into the middle meatus and is allowed to absorb over the next 2–3 wk. During the postoperative phase, the patient remains on full-dose antibiotics. Using this technique, scarring has been very limited (Fig. 9).

RESULTS

Several groups have reported that endoscopic ethmoidectomy can be performed safely in children (22,59,61,63,69). Gross et al. (61) reported follow-up data on 57 children ranging in age from 3–13 mo for an overall success rate of 92%, with 64% of patients improved and 28% resolved (or cured).

Lusk and Muntz *(59)* reported on 31 patients in a pilot study. These patients had a minimum of 1-yr follow-up. All the patients in this study had failed prolonged medical management, and 48% of the children had undergone multiple surgical procedures for their sinusitis. The mean presurgical duration of symptoms in these children was 26 mo. At 1 yr postoperatively, the parents were asked to assess the efficacy of the surgical procedure in their children by rating the outcome on a scale of 1–10, with 10 being normal and 1 the worst ever. Seventy-one percent of all the parents gave their child a rating of 8–10 1 yr postoperatively. If children with systemic disease, such as immunodeficiency disease and cystic fibrosis, were excluded, 81% of the parents rated the children between 8 and 10. Twenty-three percent of the parents gave a rating between 5 and 7 (improved but not normal), and 6% were rated at 4 or less. None of the children, according to the parents, were worse following the surgical procedure.

Lazar et al. *(63)* retrospectively evaluated 210 pediatric patients with 420 endoscopic sinus surgery procedures, which were not further characterized. Many of these children had failed tonsillectomy and adenoidectomy (54%) and nasal antral windows (29%). Follow-up through questionnaires was reported for 49% of the patients' parents. Eighty-eight percent of those responding thought their children were significantly better with respect to their headaches, nasal discharge, nasal obstruction, and cough, and would recommend the surgery to others. The authors, however, stated that these responses probably reflect a significant bias.

Duplechain et al. *(69)* found that there was a significant reduction in missed school days in 88% of the children who had undergone endoscopic sinus surgery. They found endoscopic surgery to be safe and effective in the pediatric population. In a retrospective study of 52 patients followed for an average of 21.8 mo, Parsons *(22)* found significant improvement in all symptoms after endoscopic sinus surgery.

The most frequent procedure performed by this author's group was bilateral anterior ethmoidectomy and maxillary antrostomy with the next most frequent procedure being total ethmoidectomy and maxillary antrostomy. In the experience of a number of surgeons, the overall degree of improvement is in the 80% range and is remarkably consistent *(22,59,61,63,69)*.

There is little information about the incidence and effectiveness of revision surgery in children. Lazar *(70)* reported an overall success rate of 78%, but only a small percentage of their revision surgery patients were children. The overall revision rate of this author's group is currently 11%. Data were prospectively collected on symptoms in 22 of 45 patients and demonstrated significant reduction ($p < .002$) in rhinorrhea, nasal obstruction, irritability, day cough, and night cough. There was a trend toward resolution of headaches ($p = 0.27$) but it was not significant. When the parents were asked to subjectively rate their child's symptoms on a 1 (worst ever) to 10 (normal) scale, 14 were improved, 2 unchanged, and 7 worse according to their last visit. Overall this represents a significant improvement ($p = 0.02$).

CONCLUSION

The pathophysiology of pediatric chronic sinusitis is not yet well understood. Contributing factors likely include a developing immune system and small ostia to the sinuses. Prospective assessment of the medical and surgical management of sinusitis is necessary. As more is understood about the pathophysiology of sinusitis, better medical and surgical intervention will be adopted.

REFERENCES

1. Stammberger H. Endoscopic endonasal surgery—concepts in treatment of recurring rhinosinusitis. Part II. Surgical technique. Otolaryngol Head Neck Surg 1986; 94:147–156.
2. Kennedy DW, Zinreich SJ, Rosenbaum AE, Johns ME. Functional endoscopic sinus surgery. Theory and diagnostic evaluation. Arch Otolaryngol 1985;111:576–582.
3. Stammberger H. Nasal and paranasal sinus endoscopy. A diagnostic and surgical approach to recurrent sinusitis. Endoscopy 1986;18:213–218.
4. Stammberger H. Endoscopic endonasal surgery—concepts in treatment of recurring rhinosinusitis. Part I. Anatomic and pathophysiologic considerations. Otolaryngol Head Neck Surg 1986;94:143–147.
5. Preston HG. Maxillary sinusitis in children, its relation to coryza, tonsillectomy and adenoidectomy. Va Med Mon 1955;82:229–232.
6. Wilson TG. Surgical anatomy of ENT in the newborn. J Laryngol Otol 1955;69:229.
7. Shone GR. Maxillary sinus aspiration in children. What are the indications. J Laryngol Otol 1987;101:461–464.
8. Clark WD, Bailey BJ. Sinusitis in children. Tex Med 1983;79:44–47.
9. Paul D. Sinus infection and adenotonsillitis in pediatric patients. Laryngoscope 1981;91:997–1000.

10. Merck W. Relationship between adenoidal enlargement and maxillary sinusitis. HNO 1974;6:198,199.
11. McAlister WH, Lusk RP, Muntz HR. Comparison of plain radiographs and coronal CT scans in infants and children with recurrent sinusitis. Am J Roentgenol 1989;153:1259–1264.
12. Mollison WM, Kendall NE. Frequency of antral infection in children. Guy's Hosp Rep 1922;72:225–228.
13. Crooks J, Signy AG. Accessory nasal sinusitis in childhood. Arch Dis Child 1936;11:281–306.
14. Gerrie J. Sinusitis in children. Br Med J 1939;2:363,364.
15. Carmack JW. Sinusitis in children. Ann Otol Rhinol Laryngol 1931;40:515–521.
16. Hoshaw TC, Nickman NJ. Sinusitis and otitis in children. Arch Otolaryngol 1974;100:194,195.
17. Walker FM. Tonsillectomy and adenoidectomy: unsatisfactory results due to chronic maxillary sinusitis. Br Med J 1947;908–910.
18. Stevenson RS. The treatment of subacute maxillary sinusitis especially in children. Proc R Soc Med 1947;40:854–858.
19. Cleminson FJ. Nasal sinusitis in children. J Laryngol Otol 1921;36:505–513.
20. Fujita A, Takahashi H, Honjo I. Etiological role of adenoids upon otitis media with effusion. Acta Otolaryngol Suppl (Stockh) 1988;454:210–213.
21. Birrell JF. Chronic maxillary sinusitis in children. Arch Dis Child 1952;27:1–9.
22. Parsons DS, Phillips SE. Functional endoscopic surgery in children: a retrospective analysis of results. Laryngoscope 1993;103:899–903.
23. Van Alyea OE. Nasal Sinus and Anatomical and Clinical Considerations. Baltimore, MD: Williams and Wilkins, 1942.
24. Myerson MC. The natural orifice of the maxillary sinus. Arch Otolaryngol 1932;80–91.
25. Lund VJ. Inferior meatal antrostomy. Fundamental considerations of design and function. J Laryngol Otol Suppl 1988;15:1–18.
26. Krause H. Instrumente rach Dr. Krause. Monztschrift fur Ohrenheilkunde 1887;21:70.
27. Mikulicz J. Zur operativen Behandlung das Kempyens der Highmorshohle. Lagenbeck's Archiv fur Klinische Chirurgie 1887;34:626–634.
28. Proetz AW. Essays on the Applied Physiology of the Nose. St. Louis: Annals Publishing, 1941.
29. Alden AM. A new procedure in the treatment of chronic maxillary sinus suppuration in children. Arch Otolaryngol 1926;4:521–525.
30. Asherson N. Intubation of the maxillary antrum for acute empyema. Lancet 1937;1399,1400.
31. Huggill PH, Ballantyne JC. An investigation into the relationship between adenoids and sinusitis in children. J Otolaryngol 1952;66:84–91.
32. Peterson RJ. Canine fossa puncture. Laryngoscope 1973;83:369–371.
33. Ritter FN. A clinical and anatomical study of the various techniques of irrigation of the maxillary sinus. Laryngoscope 1977;87:215–223.
34. Stammberger H. Functional Endoscopic Sinus Surgery. Philadelphia: B. C. Decker, 1991.
35. Kim HN, Kim YM, Choi HS. Diagnostic and therapeutic significance of sinoscopy in maxillary sinusitis. Yonsei Med J 1985;26:59–67.
36. Maes JJ, Clement PA. The usefulness of irrigation of the maxillary sinus in children with maxillary sinusitis on the basis of the Water's X-ray. Rhinology 1987;25:259–264.
37. StClair T, Negus VE. Diseases of the Nose and Throat. London: 1937.
38. Hajek M. Pathology and Treatment of the Inflammatory Diseases of the Nasal Accessory Sinuses. St. Louis: Mosby, 1926.
39. Pedersen M, Mygind N. Rhinitis, sinusitis and otitis media in Kartagener's syndrome (primary ciliary dyskinesia). Clin Otolaryngol 1982;7:373–380.
40. Yarnal JR, Golish JA, Ahmad M, Tomashefski JF. The immotile cilia syndrome: explanation for many a clinical mystery. Postgrad Med 1982;71:195–197, 200–202.
41. Muntz HR, Lusk RP. Nasal antral windows in children: a retrospective study. Laryngoscope 1990;100:643–646.
42. Freer OT. The antrum of highmore: the removal of the greater part of its inner wall through the nostril for empyema. Laryngoscope 1905;15:343–349.
43. Sluder G. A modified mikulicz operation whereby the entire lower turbinate is sawed in intranasal operations on the antrum of highmore, with presentation of a patient. Laryngoscope 1909;19:904–910.
44. Canfield RB. The submucous resection of the lateral nasal wall in chronic empyema of the antrum, ethmoid and sphenoid. JAMA 1908;51:1136–1141.
45. Wilkerson WW. Antral window in the middle meatus. Arch Ophthalmol 1949;49:463–489.
46. Proetz AW. The Displacement Method of Sinus Diagnosis and Treatment. St. Louis: Annals Publishing, 1931.
47. Hilding AC. Experimental sinus surgery: effects of operative windows on normal sinuses. Ann Otol Rhinol Laryngol 1941;50:379–392.
48. Schroeckenstein DC, Busse WW. Viral "bronchitis" in childhood: relationship to asthma and obstructive lung disease. Semin Respir Infect 1988;3:40–48.
49. Lavelle RJ, Harrison MS. Infection of the maxillary sinus: the case for the middle meatal antrostomy. Laryngoscope 1971;81:90–106.
50. Davis WE, Templer JW, LaMear WR. Patency rate of endoscopic middle meatus antrostomy. Laryngoscope 1991;101:416–420.
51. Davis WE, Templer JW, LaMear WR, Davis WE Jr, Craig SB. Middle meatus anstrostomy: patency rates and risk factors. Otolaryngol Head Neck Surg 1991;104:467–472.
52. Kennedy DW. Serious misconceptions regarding functional endoscopic sinus surgery [letter]. Laryngoscope 1986;96:1170,1171.
53. Kennedy DW, Kennedy EM. Endoscopic sinus surgery. AORN J 1985;42:932,934.
54. Kennedy DW, Zinreich SJ, Shaalan H, Kuhn F, Naclerio R, Loch E. Endoscopic middle meatal antrostomy: theory, technique, and patency. Laryngoscope 1987;97:1–9.
55. Messerklinger W. Endoscopy of the Nose. Baltimore-Munich: Urban & Schwarzenberg, 1978.
56. Friedman M, Josephson JS, Kennedy DW, Kelly DR, Rice DH, Sisson GA. Difficult decisions in endoscopic sinus surgery. Otolaryngologic Clin North Am 1989;22:777–799.

57. Stammberger H, Posawetz W. Functional endoscopic sinus surgery. Concept, indications and results of the Messerklinger technique. Eur Arch Oto-rhino-laryngology 1990;247:63–76.

58. Lusk RP, Lazar RH, Muntz HR. The diagnosis and treatment of recurrent and chronic sinusitis in children. Pediatric Clin North Am 1989;36:1411–1421.

59. Lusk RP, Muntz HR. Endoscopic sinus surgery in children with chronic sinusitis—a pilot study. Laryngoscope 1990;100:654–658.

60. Lusk RP, Polmar SH, Muntz HR. Endoscopic ethmoidectomy and maxillary antrostomy in immunodeficient patients. Arch Otolaryngol Head Neck Surg 1991;117:60–63.

61. Gross CW, Gurucharri MJ, Lazar RH, Long TE. Functional endonasal sinus surgery (FESS) in the pediatric age group. Laryngoscope 1989;99:272–275.

62. Gross CW, Lazar RH, Gurucharri MJ. Pediatric functional endonasal sinus surgery. Otolaryngologic Clin North Am 1989;22:733–738.

63. Lazar RH, Younis RT, Gross CW. Pediatric functional endonasal sinus surgery: review of 210 cases. Head Neck 1992;14:92–98.

64. Younis RT, Lazar RH. The approach to acute and chronic sinusitis in children. Ear Nose Throat J 1991;70:35–39.

65. Diaz JD, Nelson RP, Lockey RF. IgG subclass deficiency and recurrent infections [clinical conference]. Ann Allergy 1988;61:333,375–378.

66. Morell A, Skvaril F, Hitzig WH. IgG subclasses: development of the serum concentrations in "normal" infants and children. J Pediatr 1972;80:960–964.

67. Lusk RP. Surgical Management of Chronic Sinusitis. In: Lusk RP, ed., Pediatric Sinusitis. New York: Raven, 1992; pp. 77–126.

68. Riegle EV, Gunter JB, Lusk RP, Muntz HR, Weiss KL. Comparison of vasoconstrictors for functional endoscopic sinus surgery in children. Laryngoscope 1992; 102:820–823.

69. Duplechain JK, White JA, Miller RH. Pediatric sinusitis. The role of endoscopic sinus surgery in cystic fibrosis and other forms of sinonasal disease. Arch Otolaryngol Head Neck Surg 1991;117:422–426.

70. Lazar RH, Younis RT, Long TE, Gross CW. Revision functional endonasal sinus surgery. Ear Nose Throat J 1992;71:131–133.

27 Sinusitis in Adults
Principles of Surgical Management and Overview of Techniques

Renato Roithmann, MD, Ian Witterick, MD, FRCSC,
Philip Cole, MD, FRCSC, and Michael Hawke, MD, FRCSC

Contents

INTRODUCTION

Half a century ago when it was customary for the operating aural surgeon to use a head mirror or headlight, mallet, and gouge, technology made a major contribution to this field of surgery by introducing the operating microscope and microinstrumentation. Within a very few years, their use became universal in the otological centers of developed countries, and the quality and possibilities of aural surgery were greatly enhanced.

More recently and within a similarly short period, technological advances of endoscopes and instrumentation have enable comparable strides to be made in many surgical fields, not the least of which is surgery of the paranasal sinuses and, concomitantly, advances in diagnostic imaging have added powerful weapons to the armamentarium of the sinus surgeon.

As the basic studies of Messerklinger, Wigand, Stammberger, and others have emphasized,

health of the paranasal sinuses is dependent on unobstructed mucociliary transport via the ostiomeatal complex (OMC), and this essential principle is now widely recognized. Close examination of the constricted ostiomeatal region can be accomplished much more readily by tomography and nasal endoscopy, and the presence and extent of obstruction can be more accurately determined than by older methods. Although skilled otolaryngology—head and neck surgeons achieved successful results with sinus surgery before the advent of computed tomography (CT) and endoscopic techniques, the advantages offered by these recent advances have led to their wide acceptance and employment for treatment of types of sinus disease that are becoming increasingly more clearly defined.

Anatomic development of the paranasal sinuses is inconsistent. Moreover, their anatomy can be altered by disease and by previous surgery. Current techniques help minimize surgical risks to the orbital contents, optic nerve, intracranial contents, and carotid artery, which are separated from sinus cavities by thin, and sometimes eroded, sinus walls.

From: *Diseases of the Sinuses* (M. E. Gershwin and G. A. Incaudo, eds.),
©1996 Humana Press Inc., Totowa, NJ.

The head mirror, nasal speculum, and plain sinus X-ray examinations have been superseded by endoscopes, video displays, and CT. Coakley curets, Kerrison rongeurs, and large bone and tissue biting forceps are increasingly displaced by microequivalents.

In many cases of sinus disease, re-establishment of adequate drainage in the ostiomeatal region by endoscopic surgery enables more widely extended sinus disease to resolve and can thus avoid the need for the more radical sinus procedures, such as the Caldwell-Luc, transantral and external ethmoidectomy, and osteoplastic frontal flaps. However, the need for more radical measures remains for some patients who suffer from sinus disease.

A further important advantage of current technology is the facility for video display and taping of endoscopic examination and surgery. In addition to furnishing a permanent record of the procedure, video and surgical commentary by the operating surgeon can provide an excellent teaching medium.

The following sections of this chapter outline the principles of management, and provide an overview of the techniques of diagnosis and treatment of sinusitis in adult patients.

PRINCIPLES OF SURGICAL MANAGEMENT

Mucociliary Clearance (Messerklinger's Concepts)

In the past, it was believed that chronic sinusitis was an infectious process arising primarily from abnormalities within the affected sinus itself. Conventional sinus operations for chronic infection are directed at removing diseased mucosa in the sinus. Based on studies of mucociliary clearance, Messerklinger demonstrated that the etiology of most cases of chronic recurring sinusitis in the maxillary and frontal sinuses is related to anatomical variations or mucosal pathology obstructing the natural drainage pathways of these sinuses (1).

Drainage openings surgically created in a sinus at locations distant from the natural ostia are bypassed by the mucous blanket produced in the sinus as it is preferentially transported by the cilia of the respiratory epithelia to the natural ostium. The mucus produced in the anterior ethmoid, frontal, and maxillary sinuses drains into an anatomically complex region of the lateral nasal wall under the middle meatus called the OMC (Fig. 1A,B).

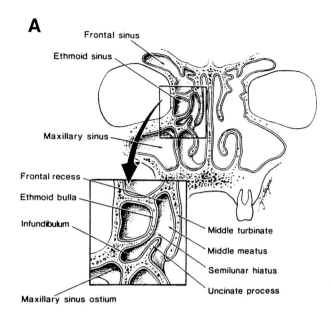

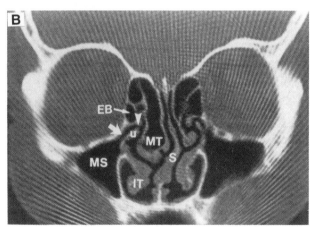

Fig. 1. (A) Anatomy of the OMC. Reprinted from ref. *49* with permission. **(B)** OMC—CT appearance (coronal view): EB = ethmoid bulla; u = uncinate process; MT = middle turbinate; IT = inferior turbinate; ethmoid infundibulum (arrow); hiatus semilunaris (arrowhead); MS = maxillary sinus. The nasal septum (S) is deviated to the left side. The vertical plate and the free margin of the right middle turbinate are pneumatized. Reprinted from ref. *30* with permission.

The OMC is bounded by the middle turbinate medially, the root of the ethmoid sinus superiorly, and the medial wall of the orbit (lamina papyracea) laterally, and it opens into the middle meatus inferiorly.

Mucus from the anterior ethmoid, frontal, and maxillary sinuses drains into the ethmoidal infundibulum and then into the middle meatus through the hiatus semilunaris. The hiatus semilunaris is located between the posterior edge of the sickle-shaped uncinate process anteriorly and the bulla ethmoidalis (largest air cell of the anterior ethmoid sinus) posteriorly.

The OMC is an anatomically narrow region. Small variations in the size or shape of the structures or minor mucosal edema can cause opposing mucosal layers to come into contact with each other. This mucosal contact impairs the mucociliary clearance and ventilation of the sinuses draining into the OMC.

Messerklinger pioneered the concept that re-establishment of ventilation and drainage via the physiologic routes can bring about resolution of even extensive pathological changes in the dependent sinuses (maxillary and frontal) without touching the mucosa in the sinus itself (2,3). Surgery to achieve this goal has been termed "functional endoscopic sinus surgery" (FESS) by Kennedy (3).

There are several other acronyms for this type of surgery, including endoscopic sinus surgery (ESS), conservative endoscopic sinus surgery (CESS), and minimal endoscopic sinus surgery (MESS). FESS will be used for the purposes of this chapter. Restoration of mucociliary clearance and ventilation through the OMC is now considered essential in managing most patients with chronic recurring sinusitis.

Precise Knowledge at Nasal/Sinus Anatomy and Diagnosis

Recognition of anatomical landmarks that provide surgical guidance are essential for safe sinus surgery. The surgeon must be aware of the high intrasubject and intersubject variability in anatomy and the critical relationships with adjacent vital structures, such as the orbit and anterior cranial fossa. The anatomy of each individual patient should be clearly established by careful nasal endoscopy and radiologic imaging prior to any proposed surgical procedure on the sinuses.

Nasal endoscopy is performed in the outpatient setting with fiberoptic telescopes (rigid or flexible) and topical nasal decongestant, often in combination with a topical anesthetic agent. Rigid telescopes are available in a variety of diameters (e.g., 4 mm and 2.7 mm) and angles of view (e.g., 0, 30, 70, and 120°). The 0 and 30° 4-mm rigid telescopes provide an excellent field of view in most instances, but may be too wide to access the narrow nasal cavities found in some patients. In these cases, a 2.7-mm rigid telescope or a flexible telescope may be useful. The goal of nasal endoscopy is to visualize and document the anatomy (normal and abnormal) and pathologic processes of the nasal cavity. Particular attention is paid to the lateral wall of the nose in the region of the middle turbinate and middle meatus where the anterior ethmoid, frontal, and maxillary sinuses drain. In addition, CT scans of the sinuses are indispensable to evaluate further the extent of disease and clarify anatomical relationships (see preoperative considerations).

Management of Systemic Disease

The pathogenesis and natural course of chronic hypertrophic inflammatory sinusitis are incompletely understood, and many patients (e.g., those with diffuse nasal polyposis, aspirin sensitivity, and asthma) require continued medical therapy (e.g., topical nasal steroids, immunotherapy) following OMC surgery in order to maintain control of their symptoms and to decrease the risks of recurrence of disease (4–6).

Surgery alone will not solve the problem of recurring and chronic sinusitis in all circumstances, and it must be recognized that systemic host factors contribute to nasal mucosal edema and obstruction of the OMC. These factors include allergies as well as immunological, environmental (e.g., pollution, smoking), and genetic influences (4,7,8).

Surgical Planning

Current concepts of sinus surgery direct the surgeon to tailor the operation to the disease with maximal preservation of healthy tissue and to re-establish the sinus drainage system via their respective natural ostia (9,10). The critical role of the anterior ethmoid cells and the OMC in the pathogenesis of maxillary and frontal sinusitis must be kept in mind in surgical treatment planning. It is essential to consider the type and extension of the disease, the training background of the surgeon, and the general condition of the patient. Patient symptoms together with endoscopic and imaging findings must all be taken into account in precise surgical planning.

There are wide regional variations in the indications for surgery and the type of surgical procedure performed for chronic sinusitis. Over the last decade, there has been increasing interest and movement toward the adoption of "minimal access surgery." In otolaryngology—head and neck surgery, the interest in FESS has grown exponentially since its introduction to North America in 1985 *(3,6,9–17)*. This is not to say that patients with chronic or recurrent sinusitis cannot be managed with equally good results by "traditional" or conventional sinus operations *(5,18)*.

Factors considered in the choice of procedure include the type and extent of disease, and the patient's physical condition and ability to withstand anesthesia. In addition, the expectations and wishes of the patient must be considered. In reality, for many patients with chronic sinusitis, the choice between a traditional or endoscopic technique may largely depend on the training, experience, and skill of the surgeon.

Clear advantages of FESS include minimal trauma to normal nondiseased tissue and the ability to remove often subtle pathology. Endoscopic techniques are well suited to opening the natural ostia of the maxillary and frontal sinuses. In addition, illumination and visualization with an endoscope are superior to a head light and nasal speculum, and endoscopes with deflected angles of view allow the evaluation and removal of disease from recesses that could not be seen by previously used methods. Both conventional and newer endoscopic techniques are discussed below.

CONVENTIONAL TECHNIQUES

The foundations of conventional sinus surgery were developed toward the end of the 19th century. Operations were developed to open into the sinuses (trephination) and curet diseased mucosa out of every sinus either intranasally or via an external incision. The priorities of conventional sinus surgery include complete removal of all diseased tissue and opening of the natural drainage pathways. If opening of the natural pathways is not feasible, wide communication into the nose at another site is created to permit gravitational drainage, or the sinus is obliterated to prevent ingrowth of mucosa and possible recurrence of disease. Cosmetic factors with external procedures are also of concern, particularly to the patient.

Conventional Maxillary Sinus Operations

Antral irrigation or lavage is a procedure intended to clear infected purulent material from the maxillary sinus. Sinuses with thickened membranes only are not appropriate for irrigation. Antral lavage may help some patients with acute maxillary sinusitis that is not responding to medical management and is useful for obtaining culture material. In our experience, antral lavage is rarely helpful in managing patients with chronic sinusitis. The procedure is typically carried out in the physician's office with local anesthesia. A trocar is placed into the sinus either through the canine fossa or under the inferior turbinate. Sterile saline or some other solution is gently irrigated into the nose.

Intranasal antrostomy involves creating a large window into the maxillary sinus under the inferior turbinate. The window needs to be large to preclude subsequent closure during the healing phases. This procedure usually provides ventilation of the sinus, but may not provide adequate drainage as the cilia continue to transport mucus to the natural ostia bypassing the antrostomy.

Prior to the development of FESS, the Caldwell-Luc was the standard procedure for patients with recurrent or chronic maxillary sinusitis. Even with endoscopic techniques, it is still useful for removing fungal disease, massive polyposis, and some mucoceles or cysts from the sinus. It can be performed under local or general anesthesia. An incision is made in the upper gingivobuccal sulcus over the canine fossa and an opening created in the anterior wall of the sinus large enough to inspect the entire sinus and remove diseased tissue. A nasoantral window is made under the inferior turbinate or the natural ostium is enlarged.

Conventional Frontal Sinus Operations

Trephination of the frontal sinus is performed for acute frontal sinusitis unresponsive to medical management. An incision is made in the superior and medial aspect of orbit immediately below the brow. The sinus is entered through the inferior edge of supraorbital rim, the purulent material is evacuated and a drain is placed. Postoperatively, the sinus may be irrigated daily through the drain until the return is clear.

There are several external operations available for patients with chronic frontal sinusitis, including mucosal-preserving and mucosal-eliminating procedures. Both types of mucosal-preserving techniques begin with an external ethmoidectomy. The Lynch procedure removes a large part of the medial floor of the frontal sinus, and the Boyden procedure extends this to enlarging the nasofrontal duct and attempts to reconstruct it with a mucosal flap, usually pedicled from the septum. The disadvantages of these procedures are the required external incision, and the potential for the orbital soft tissues to collapse medially and obstruct the nasofrontal duct once the stent is removed.

There are three basic types of mucosal-eliminating procedures that remove variable portions of the frontal bone and all of the sinus mucosa. In the Reidel operation, the anterior wall and floor of the frontal sinus are removed, and the sinus obliterated by redraping the forehead skin over the posterior table, leaving a major cosmetic deformity. The Killian procedure is similar, but spares the supraorbital rim and approx 1 cm of the adjacent inferior frontal bone so the postoperative appearance is more acceptable. These two procedures are rarely performed, but may be indicated for severe frontal sinusitis with osteomyelitis of the anterior table.

The third option is the osteoplastic flap, which is the external mucosal-eliminating procedure of choice in most circumstances. This is particularly suited for symptomatic mucoceles placed laterally in the frontal sinus away from endoscopic access or in cases of stenosis of the frontal recess and/or ostia. The osteoplastic flap procedure involves creating an anterior frontal bone flap through a bicoronal or brow incision. The bicoronal incision is preferable because it can usually be concealed by hair (but this may recede later in life, exposing the incision), whereas the brow incision leaves a noticeable scar and usually some postoperative numbness of the forehead. A posteroanterior (PA) plain sinus X-ray is used as a template intraoperatively to define the frontal bone flap, which is fractured inferiorly attached by periosteum. The mucosa of the entire sinus is removed, and several options exist for managing the frontal ostium/recess and the sinus cavity. Traditionally, the frontonasal ducts were plugged, for example with fascia, and the sinus "obliterated" with fat obtained from another site (e.g., abdomen, thigh, submental region). The fat is nonvascularized and may reabsorb over time. Another technique enlarges the frontal ostium/recess with a drill and stents the area for a variable period postoperatively. If one frontal recess is patent and functional, another option is to remove the intersinus septum so that mucus from both frontal sinuses can drain through the functional side.

Conventional Ethmoid Sinus Operations

The ethmoid sinus may be approached through the nose, through the maxillary sinus, or by external incisions. A frequent indication for intranasal ethmoidectomy has been recurrent obstructive nasal polyposis in which a patent nasal airway could not be maintained by office polypectomy. The transantral approach to the ethmoid sinus gives good visualization of the floor of the orbit, which the surgeon can follow medially and superiorly as it becomes the lamina papyracea. If the goal of surgery is to open only the ethmoid sinuses, then this approach would seem to offer little over intranasal ethmoidectomy owing to the requirements for a sublabial incision and Caldwell-Luc-type approach. The transantral approach may be preferable when portions of the orbital floor are also removed for thyroid orbitopathy. External ethmoidectomy can be used for treatment of extensive polypoid sinus and nasal disease, chronic ethmoiditis, and as an approach to neoplasms and cerebrospinal fluid leaks of the frontoethmoid region. The advantage of external ethmoidectomy is excellent visualization, but at the price of an external incision and the removal of the lamina papyracea, which may be important as a barrier to protect the eye from future sinus inflammation.

Intranasal ethmoidectomy in the presence of extensive nasal polyposis can be a difficult and dangerous procedure because of the problems visualizing the anatomy with a headlight and mirror, the bleeding associated with removal of the polyps, and the distortion of landmarks from the polyps themselves or from previous polypectomies. Following removal of any nasal polyps, the anterior half of the middle turbinate is usually resected to gain access to the ethmoid sinuses, which are then removed. The associated bleeding can be profuse at times such that intermittent packing is required for control.

External ethmoidectomy is usually performed through a gently curved vertical incision placed midway between the inner canthus and the dorsum of the nose. Elevation of the periosteum off of the lamina papyracea identifies the frontoethmoid suture line, which serves as a landmark for the level of the cribriform plate and the uppermost extent of the posterior ethmoidal cells. The anterior and sometimes the posterior ethmoid arteries are ligated or cauterized as they exit through the frontoethmoid suture line. The close proximity of the optic nerve to the posterior ethmoid artery must always be kept in mind. The lamina papyracea is removed and the ethmoidal cells exenterated.

Conventional Sphenoid Sinus Operations

The sphenoid sinus can be reached by transeptal, transnasal, and transethmoid (intranasal, transantral, or external) approaches. The preferred procedure depends on the preference and experience of the surgeon and the coexistence of ethmoid disease. If ethmoid disease is absent, a direct route (transeptal or transnasal) is preferable, but if there is co-existent ethmoid disease that needs to be dealt with as well, then one of the other approaches may be selected.

FUNCTIONAL ENDOSCOPIC SINUS SURGERY

There are two important variations in endoscopic surgical techniques. Sphenoethmoidectomy under endoscopic control is similar to traditional intranasal ethmoidectomy with planned radical removal of tissue to open all of the sinuses. On the other hand, the guiding concept of FESS, and the subject of the rest of this section, is to remove tissue obstructing the OMC and facilitate drainage while conserving normal nonobstructing anatomy and mucous membrane (*see* section on Mucociliary Clearance [Messerklinger's Concepts]) *(3,16)*. The rigid fiberoptic nasal telescope provides superb intraoperative visualization of the OMC, allowing the surgery to be focused and precise. Bleeding is minimized by vasoconstricting the mucosa and atraumatic technique. The 0° (forward-viewing) 4-mm telescope is the endoscope of first choice, and the 30 and 70° telescopes have special uses, such as examining the frontal recess or maxillary sinus through the natural ostium. The image may be projected to a television monitor through a small camera attached to the eyepiece of the endoscope. The surgeon has the choice of performing the operation while looking through the endoscope, from the monitor, or a combination of both.

Proper equipment and training are required to identify the important anatomical landmarks and perform the directed surgical techniques.

Indications

Surgery is indicated and planned in accordance with patient history, endoscopic examination, and

CT. The main established indications for FESS include:

1. Continued chronic and/or recurrent sinusitis despite appropriate medical treatment or previous surgical treatment;
2. Recurrent sinusitis secondary to nasal polyposis; and
3. Correction of anatomic variations predisposing to chronic and/or recurrent sinusitis.

The ideal candidate for FESS is the patient who remains symptomatic despite appropriate medical treatment and whose OMC shows persistent inflammation and/or anatomic obstruction on nasal diagnostic endoscopy, associated or not with pathological CT findings *(19,20)*. The significance of CT-scan abnormalities must be evaluated in conjunction with the patient's symptoms and endoscopic findings, since approx 30% of patients without sinus symptoms or signs have been found to exhibit sinus "abnormalities" on CT scanning performed for reasons other than suspected sinus disease *(21,22)*.

The vast majority of patients with acute sinusitis are managed medically, with surgery being reserved for those who fail to respond or who are threatened by complications (e.g., orbital, intracranial). Cotton pledgets soaked with vasoconstrictor can be placed endoscopically in the middle meatus for 20–30 min to reduce edema around the ostia and promote drainage of purulent secretions. This form of therapy, repeated two to three times each day together with systemic antibiotic, may avert an impending complication and bring about resolution of even severe cases of acute sinusitis. Experienced surgeons have reported using endoscopic measures to drain periorbital abscesses caused by acute ethmoiditis *(9,23)* and in the management of empyema of the frontal or maxillary sinus *(9)*.

Fungal sinusitis, mucoceles, and nasal polyps have also been successfully managed through FESS *(9)*. Extended applications of the endoscopic technique include the management of cerebrospinal fluid leak, nasal meningoceles and some benign neoplasms, orbital decompression for thyroid orbitopathy, choanal atresia, lacrimal obstruction, optic nerve decompression, and pituitary tumor surgery *(24–27)*.

Contraindications

According to Stammberger and Hawke *(9),* the Messerklinger technique is inappropriate for the surgical approach to extensive, invasive disease involving the paranasal sinuses or skull base. Examples include osteomyelitis, malignant neoplasms, and benign fibrosseous lesions. In addition, ESS is contraindicated in patients with an incipient central nervous system complication related to acute sinusitis. Endoscopic techniques may be unsatisfactory for accessing laterally positioned disease in the frontal or maxillary sinuses, or opening post-inflammatory stenoses of the ostium of the frontal sinus (9,10).

Preoperative Considerations

Radiological assessment before any surgical procedure is contemplated is essential for surgical planning, and careful nasal endoscopy enables the otolaryngologist to delineate mucosal surfaces and identify middle meatal soft tissue abnormalities that are not diagnosed from imaging studies (28). Plain sinus radiographs are of little value in assessment of the OMC, because they do not show this critical region in enough detail to differentiate subtle anatomical and mucosal changes (29). CT scans clearly demonstrate and differentiate soft tissues, bone, and air (29,30), and are the imaging modality of choice for clinical evaluation and planning of FESS. Ideally, the CT examination should be performed when the patient is least symptomatic and after antibiotics have been administered to control acute exacerbations. The coronal plane without contrast is selected because the images are displayed in the anatomic plane encountered during endoscopic surgery, and this view affords optimal demonstration of the anterior ethmoid and ostiomeatal structures (Fig. 1B). The CT scans are scrutinized for anatomical variations, relationship of the OMC to the skull base and lamina papyracea, evidence of inflammation, mucoperiosteal thickening, and the patency of the ostia and ethmoidal prechambers. In previously operated patients or those where posterior ethmoid or sphenoid sinus surgery is contemplated, biplanar (coronal + axial) CT scanning is helpful in order to determine relationships of important surrounding structures, including the optic nerve and internal carotid artery.

Informed consent is obtained after detailed discussion with the patient of the disease process, alternative management strategies, and the proposed surgery, including the type of anesthesia (local or general), the risks of surgery (see complications), realistic expectations, and the importance of post-

operative follow-up. Patients are instructed to avoid aspirin and other nonsteroidal anti-inflammatory drugs for at least 1 wk before the procedure. Some patients with diffuse mucosal edema and nasal polyposis benefit from a short (7–14 d) course of systemic corticosteroids preoperatively to reduce tissue edema and bleeding at the time of surgery. The CT scans are displayed in the operating room during FESS, so the surgeon can easily review them during surgery.

Surgical Techniques

It is critical for all surgeons to see what they are doing, and although the rigid nasal telescope gives an excellent view of intranasal structures, even small quantities of blood can obscure landmarks, making the procedure more difficult and sometimes dangerous. It is therefore essential to minimize trauma to nondiseased tissue and maintain excellent hemostasis. Various techniques to control bleeding include topical mucosal vasoconstriction, infiltration of vasoconstricting drugs locally or via a greater palatine canal block, and hypotensive anesthesia.

Patients undergoing surgery under local anesthesia tend to bleed less than those undergoing the same procedure under general anesthesia. In most adults, local anesthesia with iv sedation provides excellent hemostasis (31) and appropriate visibility. Other advantages of local anesthesia include less risk of cardiorespiratory complications than with general anesthesia, and intraoperative pain can provide an important early warning to the surgeon of impending injury to the roof of the ethmoidal sinus, orbit, or optic nerve. If an orbital complication develops (e.g., orbital hematoma), it may be recognized earlier and appropriate treatment and follow-up initiated (10). Local anesthesia is generally associated with a shorter and easier post-operative recovery than general anesthesia. The anesthesiologist plays an important role in sedating and monitoring the patient during local anesthesia. The advantages of general anesthesia include immobilization of the patient and easier instrumentation because of the reduction of intraoperative pain and anxiety.

The medications used for topical anesthesia and vasoconstriction differ between centers. A single agent, such as topical cocaine (e.g., 4–10%), or a combination of agents (e.g., 1:1000 epinephrine combined with 2% tetracaine or 0.1% xylometazoline) may be used for these purposes. Although dosages based on patient weight must be adhered to, cocaine has been associated with cardiac arrhythmias using submaximal dosages, particularly when used in combination with epinephrine and some inhalational anesthetic agents (e.g., halothane). Cottonoids with the topical agents are placed in the OMC region for 5–10 min followed by infiltration of the lateral nasal wall (uncinate process) with an anesthetic/vasoconstricting agent (e.g., 1 or 2% xylocaine with 1:100,000 or 1:200,000 epinephrine) (9,32). The mucosa of the middle turbinate is injected when partial or total turbinectomy is contemplated. Inadvertent damage to the mucous membrane of the anterior nose from the tip of the needle must be avoided, and the number of injected sites should be minimized to limit oozing from puncture sites. If the patient reports pain during the course of the surgical procedure, topical anesthetic is reapplied. Injection of the sphenopalatine nerve either by the intranasal or transpalatal route when total sphenoethmoidectomy is planned complements the local anesthesia protocol (4).

Functional ESS is generally tailored to the clinical and radiologic findings. Although it is possible to perform total sphenoethmoidectomy by the Messerklinger technique, such radical procedures are avoided as a routine by most surgeons. According to Stammberger and Hawke (9), "Under no circumstances should extensive bony surfaces be denuded of their mucosal covering, because this will increase the chance of postoperative osteitis."

In order to minimize the risk of disorientation, experienced endoscopic surgeons recommend using the 0° (straightforward viewing) telescope as much as possible (4,9,33). The 30 or 70° nasal endoscopes are more safely used after the important topographic landmarks have been identified and usually are required only in special situations (e.g., for viewing the frontal recess or the cavity of the maxillary sinus).

Although the most common endoscopic technique utilizes anterior-to-posterior dissection (Messerklinger approach), a posterior-to-anterior dissection is preferred by some surgeons (see Posterior-to-Anterior Dissection [Wigand Approach]) (17).

Anterior-to-Posterior Dissection

The first step consists of opening the ethmoidal infundibulum by resecting the uncinate process

in its entirety. If a sickle knife is used for this purpose, it is important to keep the blade parallel with the lateral nasal wall to avoid injuring the lamina papyracea and orbital contents. Commonly, superior and inferior remnants of the uncinate process obscure access to the frontal recess, and the maxillary sinus ostium and should be removed.

The ethmoidal bulla and anterior ethmoid air cells are removed until the basal lamella is identified. The basal lamella is the lateral attachment of the middle turbinate and is also referred to as the "ground" and "grand" lamella. If the ethmoidal bulla and adjacent cells are completely removed, the operative field will be bordered medially by the middle turbinate, laterally by the lamina papyracea, superiorly by the roof of the ethmoid sinus, and posteriorly by the vertical portion of the basal lamella of the middle turbinate. The posterior ethmoidal sinus is then approached, if diseased, through the basal lamella as far medially and inferiorly as possible. Removing the entire basal lamella should be avoided to prevent destabilizing the middle turbinate. The optic nerve may lie in intimate contact with posterior ethmoid air cells (cells of Onodi) laterally. A further important point to note is the angle of the endoscope, which must change, usually from a 45 to a 30° angle to the hard palate, as the surgeon proceeds more deeply into the ethmoidal labyrinth (Fig. 2A,B). This maneuver allows the endoscopist to follow a path along the base of the skull. In the minority of cases in which it is necessary to open the sphenoid sinus (9), entry should be as far medially and inferiorly as possible to decrease the risk of injury to the optic nerve and internal carotid artery. Careful review of coronal and axial CT scans is essential before the sphenoid is approached surgically in order to determine the anatomic relationships of these important structures (Fig. 3A,B).

The surgical steps that follow include inspection of the frontal recess and the maxillary sinus ostium. The frontal recess should be cleared of disease, but in most cases, the sinus does not need to be entered nor is the ostium of the frontal sinus routinely enlarged. The entrance to the frontal sinus is manipulated as little as possible with the Messerklinger technique, and although there are specific techniques described for safe dissection of the frontal recess (34,35), this is a technically challenging area to manage by endoscopic means. The frontal recess is anterior to the anterior ethmoidal

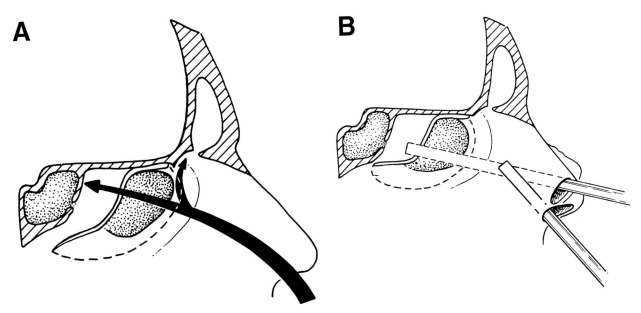

Fig. 2. (A) Schematic drawing of the endoscopic procedure. The path of the instruments is shown as a gray arrow assuming that an advance to the sphenoid sinus is necessary or that the frontal recess needs to be entered for some manipulation anterior to the bulla and in an anterosuperior direction. Reprinted from ref. *9* with permission. **(B)** Schematic drawing illustrating the change in angulation of the endoscope required as it advances into the ethmoidal sinus. Initially, the endoscope is introduced at an angle of about 45° to the hard palate. This angle decreases as the instrument is advanced posteriorly. Depending on the anatomic conditions, the final angle of the endoscope at the anterior wall of the sphenoid sinus is in the range of 15–25° to the hard palate. Reprinted from ref. *9* with permission.

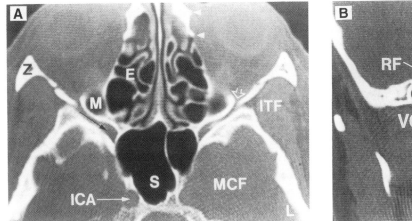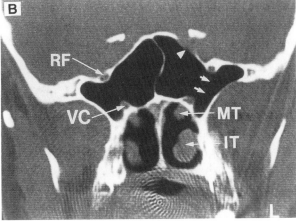

Fig. 3. (A) Normal axial CT scan demonstrating the anterior and posterior lacrimal crests (arrowheads), the ethmoid labyrinth (E), the superior recess of the maxillary sinus (M), the zygoma (Z), the pterygopalatine fossa (black arrow), the inferior orbital foramen (open arrow), the infratemporal fossa (ITF), the middle cranial fossa (MCF), the sphenoid sinus (S), and the internal carotid artery (ICA). Reprinted from ref. *50* with permission. **(B)** Coronal CT scan of the sphenoid sinus. The lateral recesses of the sphenoid sinus (arrows) and dehiscence of the roof of the sphenoid close to the optic nerve on the left side (arrowhead) can be seen, as well as the foramen rotundum (RF), pterygoid (vidian) canal (VC), and the posterior ends of the inferior turbinate (IT) and of the middle turbinate (MT). Reprinted from ref. *50* with permission.

artery, and many surgeons use this artery as a land-mark for the posterior-to-anterior approach. One must be extremely careful, particularly medially, because the skull base is very thin and easily perfo-rated at this point. The supraorbital ethmoid air cell that lies lateral to the frontal recess should be iden-

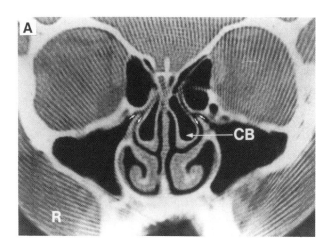 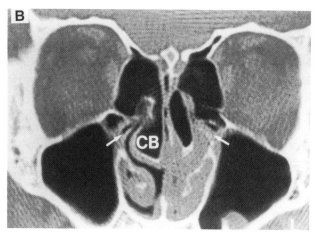

Fig. 4. (A) This coronal CT scan demonstrates bilateral large concha bullosa (CB) with attendant narrowing of the ostiomeatal complexes and turbinate sinuses (small arrows). Reprinted from ref. *50* with permission. **(B)** Coronal CT scan showing bilateral concha bullosa. The large air cell in the left middle turbinate (CB) has produced apposition of the middle and the inferior turbinates. The large ethmoid bulla together with the concha bullosa has occluded the left middle meatus; the ethmoid infundibulum is shown by the white arrows. Reprinted from ref. *50* with permission.

tified. It may be necessary to remove a superior remnant of the uncinate process to localize the frontal recess. If it is obscured by an enlarged agger nasi cell, we use Kuhn curets (45 and 90°) and angled Blakesley-Weil forceps to explore this intricate region. Severe and long-standing sinus disease may cause frontal recess contraction and bony obstruction, which can make endoscopic enlargement difficult or impossible *(9)*, and is often better managed through traditional external frontal sinus procedures. If the frontal recess cannot be identified accurately from the nose, a burr-hole (trephination) in the anterior frontal sinus can be placed to visualize the progress of the endoscopic procedure from above *(9)*.

The ostium of the maxillary sinus is typically lateral to an inferior remnant of the uncinate process. Palpation with a bent spoon or curved suction along the bony insertion of the inferior turbinate will help to locate the ostium. If the natural ostium is stenosed, enlargement is performed posteriorly and inferiorly. The extent to which the surgeon enlarges the ostium depends on the severity of the condition, but extension too far anteriorly risks damage to the nasolacrimal duct and should be avoided. Although its benefit has not been conclusively established, surgically connecting accessory ostia with the natural ostium is routinely performed in an attempt to prevent the circular transportation of secretions shown by Messerklinger's studies *(1)*. Under the guidance of 30 or 70° scopes, the interior

of the maxillary sinus is inspected through the natural ostium, but it is not a routine to interfere surgically with mucosal disease.

Middle turbinate surgery is usually not necessary, although some surgeons perform this as a routine part of endoscopic surgery. Total turbinectomy should be avoided if possible, because the middle turbinate has an important role in nasal physiology, and furthermore, it is an essential anatomical landmark *(36)*. Removal of the lateral half of a concha bullosa that contributes to ethmoidal disease or is itself diseased (Fig. 4A,B) is, in many cases, the first surgical step of the endoscopic procedure. Severe polyposis of the middle turbinate constricting the middle meatus or cases where the middle turbinate prevents surgical access are additional indications for turbinectomy.

Turbinate surgery increases the risk of adhesions between the middle turbinate and lateral nasal wall from denuded mucosal surfaces and weakening of the support of the turbinate. A Merocel sponge moistened with beclomethasone inserted into the middle meatus for 24–48 h has been used to prevent adhesions *(9)*, but it is our current practice to place silastic sheeting in the middle meatus and leave it in position for at least a week with promising results.

Following endoscopic surgery under local anesthesia, we do not pack the middle meatus as a routine. In some cases, a strip of gauze soaked in vasoconstrictor is left *in situ* for 2–4 h and removed before the patient is discharged. An overnight gauze pack impregnated with bismuth-iodoform-paraf-fin paste (BIPP) is a useful hemostatic measure when bleeding is severe during surgery or if at the end of the procedure there is a persistent bleeding. In these cases, the patient's discharge from the hospital is delayed.

Some surgeons successfully employ a "two-handed" video-endoscopic technique (20). The principles of surgery are the same as in the procedure described above, but a well-trained assistant guides the endoscope, leaving the operating surgeon's hands free to manipulate the suction canula while holding surgical instruments. Both surgeon and assistant monitor the procedure by video.

Posterior-to-Anterior Dissection (Wigand Technique) (17)

The first step is to identify the sphenoid sinus by partial resection of the posterior end of the middle turbinate. The sphenoid ostium is then located, and the anterior wall of the sphenoid is penetrated followed by dissection of the posterior ethmoid. The skull base is identified posteriorly, and dissection is completed from posterior to anterior. The procedure offers some advantages in the endoscopic management of extensive sinus disease and is usually performed under general anesthesia.

Microscopic Endonasal Surgery

Some sinus surgeons use a microscopic endonasal technique to perform functional sinus surgery and report finding it advantageous, especially when there is diffuse disease involving all paranasal sinuses (37). A three-dimensional binocular view with various magnifications, the use of a self-retaining speculum, bimanual surgery, and convenient control of bleeding during the procedure are advantages stressed by surgeons using this technique (37,38). One disadvantage is the need for general anesthesia because of the pain caused by the constant pressure exerted by the self-retaining nasal speculum. The indications for microscopic endonasal surgery are similar to those for FESS, and some surgeons combine the two techniques, which they regard as especially useful in the evaluation of the maxillary sinus ostium, frontal recess, and their respective sinuses.

Postoperative Care

The patient should be informed that nasal obstruction secondary to reactive swelling of the nasal mucosa is to be expected during the first few postoperative days and to use acetaminophen for pain relief if necessary. Patients are instructed not to blow their nose during the first 48 h after surgery because of the risk of surgical emphysema of the facial tissues, the orbit, and the cranial cavity (especially if the lamina papyracea or bone of the skull base was breached during the procedure). A systemic antibiotic (e.g., penicillin or cephalosporin) is commonly prescribed for at least 1 wk postoperatively. The thick crusts that form in the ethmoid cavity can be removed with greater ease if softened by saline spray and mineral oil, and it is our usual practice to have patients sniff a homemade solution consisting of 1 tsp each of sugar, salt, and sodium bicarbonate dissolved in 240 mL of warm water. Between the first and fourth postoperative days, judicious removal of secretions, clots, and crusts from the nasal cavity and middle meatus is undertaken, and, in some cases, it may be possible to remove secretions from maxillary and frontal sinuses by means of a curved aspirator (e.g., Eustachian tube catheter).

The healing phase, although not entirely predictable, requires at least 2–3 wk, and careful nasal endoscopy to clean the ethmoid cavity and to identify residual (e.g., remaining polyps, bone fragments) or developing problems (e.g., synechia, ostial stenosis) is essential on a regular basis during the months following surgery. Topical nasal corticosteroids or short courses of systemic corticosteroids help to prevent or delay the recurrence of diffuse polypoid rhinosinusitis. Imaging is not a routine in the first months postoperatively, unless there are complications requiring it.

Success depends not only on the procedural expertise and competence of the endoscopic surgeon, but also on meticulous postoperative endoscopic follow-up and, in many cases, medical therapy. Long-term medical therapy owing to mucosal hyperreactivity is essential in many patients (e.g., cystic fibrosis, ASA triad: asthma-polyposis and aspirin-sensitivity).

Complications

The complications of ESS are similar to those associated with traditional techniques. Stankiewicz (39) has shown that as the endoscopic surgeon's experience increases, the complication rate decreases. Endoscopic surgical treatment should be restricted to patients with limited disease until

Table 1
Complications of ESS

Minor	Major
Synechia	Intracranial injury and/or bleeding
Ostial stenosis	Cerebrospinal fluid leak
Minor hemorrhage	Persistent diplopia
Periorbital ecchymosis	Blindness
Orbital emphysema	Carotid artery injury
Transient diplopia	Orbital hematoma
Tooth numbness and pain	Severe hemorrhage
Nasolacrimal duct injury	Meningitis and brain abscess
Disturbance of olfaction	

experience enables the operating surgeon to become fully confident with the instrumentation and technique before extending this type of surgery to more complicated cases (e.g., disease involving the posterior ethmoid or sphenoid sinuses).

Nevertheless, complications occur even in competent hands, and surgeons must be prepared to recognize and to manage such problems at an early stage, especially those involving the orbit and the brain *(40,41)*. Major and minor complications are summarized in Table 1.

Early identification of the lamina papyracea during ESS is very important for orientation and to minimize the risk of orbital injury. Dehiscence of the lamina papyracea and/or the presence of orbital fat can be assessed by direct external pressure on the orbit while the surgeon looks through the endoscope to note bulging of orbital fat into the ethmoid cavity *(41)*. The surgeon must not manipulate herniated orbital fat, since such a maneuver risks an orbital hematoma. Usually any complications that follow exposure of periorbita or orbital fat are minor and consist of ecchymosis or emphysema of the eyelids. However, any visual complaint should be carefully evaluated. Damage to the anterior or posterior ethmoid arteries can result in intraorbital or retrobulbar hematomas, and immediate measures to reduce intraorbital pressure (e.g., mannitol, lateral canthotomy, and opening of the orbital septum in the area of the lower eyelid) and an ophthalmology consultation are mandatory, since irreversible blindness can occur if the complication does not receive urgent attention. Injury to the medial rectus muscle through an unrecognized perforation of the lamina papyracea can result in diplopia, and if this does not resolve spontaneously, it is usually amenable to surgical correction.

Injury to the optic nerve, which is particularly vulnerable in the region lateral to the posterior ethmoid and sphenoid sinuses, can result in permanent visual impairment.

Cerebrospinal fluid fistula is the most frequent intracranial complication. A common point of injury is the roof of the ethmoid sinus near the anterior ethmoid artery. The surgeon must avoid invasion of the region superiorly and medially in the roof of the ethmoid and anteriorly in the area of the anterior ethmoid artery *(42)*. The bone of the skull base is very thin at these points, and the dura is adherent to the cribriform plate and fovea ethmoidalis *(43)*. If an intraoperative fistula occurs and is identified, it should be repaired immediately. When a fistula is noted postoperatively, conservative treatment may be successful. Surgical repair is indicated in persistent cases, either by intranasal endoscopy and/or microscopy (leak visible), or through an external or intracranial approach (leak not visible) *(42)*.

Mucosal bleeding during surgery is usually controlled by topical application of a vasoconstrictor on a cottonoid. Arterial bleeding (e.g., from the posterior septal artery) may require unipolar or bipolar coagulation for control. Use of suction might help the surgeon to continue, but as a general principle, it is better to pack the nose and abandon the surgery in order to avoid complications if the operative field cannot be clearly visualized. The bone covering the cavernous portion of the internal carotid artery may be thin or absent in the sphenoid sinus, and the surgeon must be extremely careful while dissecting in the lateral recess of the sphenoid sinus to avoid damage to either the carotid artery or the optic nerve.

Synechia between the lateral wall and the middle turbinate can develop postoperatively. The best prophylaxis against their development is minimally traumatic surgery and prevention of damage to the mucosa of the middle turbinate as much as possible. We routinely place a piece of silastic in the middle meatus at the end of the endoscopic procedure when it is very narrow or the middle turbinate is unstable. The silastic is removed after 1–2 wk following surgery, and it seems to decrease scarring and the development of synechia. According to Lanza and Kennedy *(44)*, frontal recess stenosis occurs in approx 12% of all patients who undergo surgery in this region and can be a difficult postoperative complication to correct.

Nasolacrimal duct damage can result from excessive anterior enlargement of the maxillary sinus ostium with back-biting forceps *(45)*. The lacrimal sac is vulnerable during the initial lateral nasal wall incision with the sickle knife, and bone removal should not be extended anteriorly into the thick cortical bone surrounding the nasolacrimal duct. The ensuing epiphora may resolve spontaneously, but some cases require dacryocystorhinostomy.

Results

It is our own and others' experience that the best results with the Messerklinger technique are achieved in patients with limited disease in the OMC *(4,9)*. Patients with diffuse nasal polyposis or hyperplastic sinusitis, allergic rhinitis, reactive airway disease (e.g., asthma), ASA triad (aspirin, asthma, nasal polyps), immune disorders, cystic fibrosis, and previous endonasal sinus surgery respond less well. They do not experience the same rate of symptom improvement as the group described above *(9,15)* and require continued medical therapy.

It is difficult and probably inappropriate to compare results published from different centers because no uniform rhinosinusitis staging system and reporting criteria of success and failure exist *(4)*. The situation is further complicated, since subjective symptomatology correlates weakly with objective information (nasal endoscopy and/or CT) *(21,22,46)*. Should a patient who is asymptomatic postoperatively be considered successfully treated when nasal endoscopy shows clearly residual or recurrent disease in the OMC? Should a symptomatic patient with normal findings on nasal endoscopy and CT be considered a failure? These questions are as yet not fully answered.

Lund and Mackay have reported a simple staging system based on subjective (visual analogue scale) and objective findings (CT and endoscopy) *(13)*. Kennedy *(4)* has proposed a staging system based on the extent of disease (CT and endoscopic surgical findings). Schaitkin et al. *(15)* use patients' subjective reports of symptom improvement as the basis for deciding whether the operation was successful. In the absence of a standardized staging system or outcome measure for rhinosinusitis, the success rate is reported as >80% in adult patients. FESS has substantially improved patient symptoms and their health status *(47,48)*.

SUMMARY

FESS and its indications, limitations, complications, and success are becoming increasingly well established in the otolaryngologist's clinical practice. Concurrent developments in imaging techniques have contributed substantially to accurate diagnosis and follow-up, and to surgical precision and safety. Patients remain who suffer from extensive sinus disease for whom FESS is unsuitable. These patients may benefit from traditional sinus surgery. Training of the otolaryngologist—head and neck surgeon should include acquisition of skills in both the newer endoscopic procedures and the traditional sinus procedures that have been tested by time.

REFERENCES

1. Messerklinger W. Endoscopy of the Nose. Baltimore: Urban & Schwarzenberg, 1978.
2. Stammberger H. Endoscopic endonasal surgery—concepts in treatment of recurring rhinosinusitis. Part I. Anatomic and pathophysiologic considerations. Otolaryngol Head Neck Surg 1986;94:134–136.
3. Kennedy DW, Zinreich SJ, Rosenbaum A, Johns ME. Functional endoscopic sinus surgery: theory and diagnosis. Arch Otolaryngol 1985;111:576–582.
4. Kennedy DW. Prognostic factors, outcomes and staging in ethmoid sinus surgery. Laryngoscope 1992; 102:1–18.
5. Lawson W. The intranasal ethmoidectomy: an experience with 1,077 procedures. Laryngoscope 1991;101: 367–371.
6. Stammberger H, Posawetz W. Functional endoscopic sinus surgery: concepts, indications and results of the Messerklinger technique. Eur Arch Otorhinolaryngol 1990;247:6376.
7. Lund VJ. Surgery of the ethmoids—past, present and future: a review. J Royal Soc Med 1990;83:451–455.
8. Huerter J. Functional endoscopic sinus surgery and allergy. Otolaryngol Clin North Am 1992;25: 231–237.
9. Stammberger H, Hawke M. Essentials of functional endoscopic sinus surgery. St. Louis, MO: Mosby-Year Book, 1993.
10. Lanza DC, Kennedy DW. Current concepts in the surgical management of chronic and recurrent acute sinusitis. J Allergy Clin Immunol 1992;90:505–511.
11. Schaefer SD, Manning S, Close LG. Endoscopic paranasal sinus surgery: indications and considerations. Laryngoscope 1989;99:1–5.
12. Vleming M, Middelweerd RJ, de Vries N. Complications of endoscopic sinus surgery. Arch Otolaryngol Head Neck Surg 1992;118:617–623.
13. Lund V, Mackay IS. Staging in rhinosinus. Rhinology 1993;31:183,184.
14. Rice DH. Endoscopic sinus surgery. Otolaryngol Clin North Am 1993;26:613–618.

15. Schaitkin B, May M, Shapiro A, Fucci M, Mester SJ. Endoscopic sinus surgery: 4-year follow-up on the first 100 patients. Laryngoscope 1993;103:1117–1120.

16. Stammberger H. Endoscopic endonasal surgery: concepts in treatment of recurring rhinosinusitis. Part II—Surgical technique. Otolaryngol Head Neck Surg 1986;94: 147–156.

17. Wigand ME. Endoscopic Surgery of the Paranasal Sinuses and Anterior Base Skull Bone. New York: G. Thieme, 1990.

18. Friedman WH, Katsantonis GP. Intranasal and transantral ethmoidectomy: a 20-year experience. Laryngoscope 1990;100:343–348.

19. Kennedy DW. First-line management of sinusitis: a national problem? Otolaryngol Head Neck Surg 1990; 103:847–888.

20. Levine H, May M. Endoscopic sinus surgery. New York: Thieme Medical, 1993.

21. Havas TE, Motbey JA, Gullane PJ. Prevalence of incidental abnormalities on computed tomography scans of the paranasal sinuses. Arch Otolaryngol 1988;114: 856–859.

22. Bolger WE, Butzin CA, Parsons DS. Paranasal sinus bony anatomic variations and mucosal abnormalities: CT analysis for endoscopic sinus surgery. Laryngoscope 1991;101:56–64.

23. Elverland HH, Melheim I, Anke IM. Acute orbit from ethmoiditis drained by endoscopic sinus surgery. Acta Otolaryngol (Stockh) 1992;492:147–151.

24. Metson R. Endoscopic surgery for lacrimal obstruction. Otolaryngol Head Neck Surg 1991;104:473–479.

25. Kennedy DW, Goodstein ML, Miller NR, Zinreich SJ. Endoscopic transnasal orbital decompression. Arch Otolaryngol Head Neck Surg 1990;116:275–282.

26. Jankowski R, Auque J, Simon C, Marchal JC, Hepner H, Wayoff M. Endoscopic pituitary tumor surgery. Laryngoscope 1992;102:198–202.

27. Mattox DE, Kennedy DW. Endoscopic management of cerebrospinal fluid leaks and cephaloceles. Laryngoscope 1990;100:857–859.

28. Vining EM, Yanagisawa K, Yanagisawa E. The importance of preoperative nasal endoscopy in patients with sinonasal disease. Laryngoscope 1993;103:512–519.

29. Zinreich SJ. Imaging of chronic sinusitis in adults: X-ray, computed tomography, and magnetic resonance imaging. J Allergy Clin Immunol 1992;90:445–451.

30. Roithmann R, Shankar L, Hawke M, Kassel E, Noyek A. CT imaging in the diagnosis and treatment of sinus disease: a partnership between the radiologist and the otolaryngologist. J Otolaryngol 1993;22:253–260.

31. Gittelman PD, Jacobs JB, Skorina J. Comparison of functional endoscopic sinus surgery under local and general anesthesia. Ann Otol Rhinol Laryngol 1993; 102:289–293.

32. Riegle EV, Gunter JB, Lusk RP, Muntz HR, Weiss KL. Comparison of vasoconstrictors for functional endoscopic sinus surgery in children. Laryngoscope 1992; 102:712–716.

33. Sillers MJ, Kuhn FA, Owen RG. Surgery of the nose and paranasal sinuses. Cur Opinion Otolaryngol Head Neck Surg 1994;2:42–47.

34. Loury MC. Frontal recess dissection: endoscopic frontal recess and frontal sinus ostium dissection. Laryngoscope 1993;103:455–458.

35. Metson R. Endoscopic treatment of frontal sinusitis. Laryngoscope 1992;102:712–716.

36. Lamear WR, Davis WE, Templer JW, McKinsey JP, Del Porto H. Partial endoscopic middle turbinectomy augmenting functional endoscopic sinus surgery. Otolaryngol Head Neck Surg 1992;107:382–389.

37. Amedee RG, Mann WJ, Gilsbach JM. Microscopic endonasal surgery of the paranasal sinuses and the parasellar region. Arch Otolaryngol Head Neck Surg 1989;115:1103–1106.

38. Draf W, Weber R. Endonasal micro-endoscopic pansinus operation in chronic sinusitis I. Indications and operation technique. Am J Otolaryngol 1993;14:394–398.

39. Stankiewicz JA. Complications in endoscopic intranasal ethmoidectomy: an update. Laryngoscope 1989;99: 686–690.

40. Maniglia AJ. Fatal and other major complications of endoscopic sinus surgery. Laryngoscope 1991;101: 349–354.

41. Stankiewicz JA. Blindness and intranasal endoscopic ethmoidectomy: prevention and management. Otolaryngol Head Neck Surg 1989;101:320–329.

42. Stankiewicz JA. Cerebrospinal fluid fistula and endoscopic sinus surgery. Laryngoscope 1991;101:250–256.

43. Kainz J, Stammberger H. The roof of the anterior ethmoid: a place of least resistance in the skull base. Am J Rhinol 1990;4:7–12.

44. Lanza DC, Kennedy DW. Endoscopic sinus surgery. In: Bailey BJ, ed., Head and Neck Surgery—Otolaryngology, Philadelphia: J. B. Lippincott, 1993; pp. 389–401.

45. Serdahl CL, Berris CE, Chole RA. Nasolacrimal duct obstruction after endoscopic sinus surgery. Arch Ophtalmol 1990;108:391,392.

46. Lund VJ, Holmstrom M, Scadding GK. Functional endoscopic sinus surgery in the management of chronic rhinosinusitis. An objective assessment. J Laryngol Otol 1991;105:832–835.

47. Hoffman SR, Mahoney MC, Chmiel JF, Stinziano GD, Hoffman KN. Symptom relief after endoscopic sinus surgery: an outcome based study. ENT J 1993;72: 413–420.

48. Piccirillo JF, Edwards D, Haiduk A, Thawley SE. Psychometric and clinimetric validity of the 31-item rhinosinusitis outcome measure (RSOM). Abstract book of the 40th Annual Scientific Meeting of the American Rhinologic Society, 1994; p. 16.

49. Facer GW, Kern E. Sinusitis: current concepts and management. In: Bailey BJ, ed., Head and Neck Surgery-Otolaryngology, Philadelphia: J. B. Lippincott, 1993.

50. Shankar L, Evans K, Hawke M, Stammberger H. An atlas of imaging of the paranasal sinuses. London: Martin Dunitz, 1994.

28 Soft Tissue Masses of the Paranasal Sinuses

Principles of Surgical Management and Overview of Techniques

Peter Clement, MD, PHD
and Andrzej Roman Halama, MD, PHD

CONTENTS

Since the introduction of endoscopes and the easy access to high-resolution imaging techniques, the management of most of the soft tissue masses has shown a dramatic change. The combination of modern rigid wide-angle endoscopes with a diameter of <4 mm assisted by very powerful light fountains (up to 450 W) not only offers a perfect visualization of the deepest endonasal structures, which can never be seen accurately by the naked eye, but also allows permanent recording of the endoscopic findings on tape or film for educational or medicolegal purposes. Those parts of the nasal cavity and paranasal sinuses that are not directly accessible to endoscopes can still be visualized in detail by the latest generation of high-resolution CT or MRI scanners.

Before any decision is made for an imaging technique procedure in a patient with nasal complaints, a thorough endoscopy of the nasal cavity is mandatory. In most of the cases, this endoscopy will already differentiate between inflammatory disease or a tumor-like process. Inflammatory disease is responsible for the greatest part of all soft tissue masses found in the paranasal sinuses. If such inflammatory disease is suspected, a CT scan is the imaging technique of choice, because it allows a good visualization of the soft tissues as well as of the fine bony structures. The work of Messerklinger *(1)* initiated a revival of all kinds of anatomical variations of the lateral nasal wall, already described by Zuckerkandel at the turn of the century, and their importance to the drainage of the ostiomeatal unit *(2)*. These anomalies are responsible for most cases of chronic and recurrent rhinosinusitis. MRI does not have any major role in the diagnosis of soft tissue masses induced by inflammatory disease, because it does not show at all the fine bony structures that can be visualized so well by high-resolution CT scanning (Fig. 1). Only in cases of fungal disease (*Aspergillus* infection) does MRI allow immediate diagnosis because of the typical high-density signal and in cases of recent mucoceles because of the typical low-density signal, on the T_1-weighted images. If, on the other hand, the history and endoscopy are suggestive of a soft tissue tumor, CT as well as MRI with and without contrast are necessary to evaluate the extent of the process. Soft tissue tumors are no indication for endoscopic paranasal sinus surgery, except in not very extensive cases of inverted papilloma. Most of the soft tissue tumors still need the more classical surgical approaches, where initially the total removal of the tumor is the major goal.

From: *Diseases of the Sinuses* (M. E. Gershwin and G. A. Incaudo, eds.), ©1996 Humana Press Inc., Totowa, NJ.

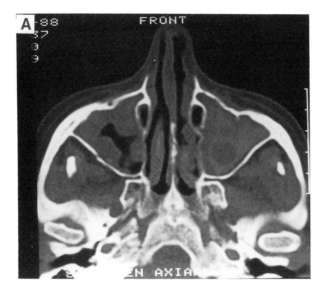

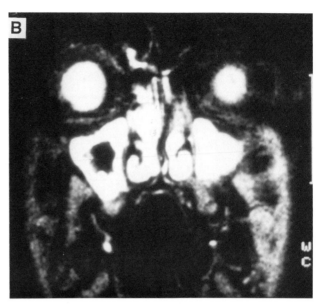

Fig. 1. (A) Axial CT scan of a patient with chronic pan-sinusitis. The CT scans show clearly the fine bony structures, and the presence of a big polyp in the right maxillary surrounded by pus, and a swollen mucosa of the left maxillary sinus with persistent lumen. **(B)** T_2-weighted coronal MRI image of the same patient. The soft tissue mass (swollen mucosa) is clearly demonstrated, but the bony structures are not visible.

SOFT TISSUE MASSES AND ENDOSCOPIC SURGICAL TECHNIQUES

Indications

Soft tissue masses that can be treated via endoscopic techniques are mostly of inflammatory origin. When a sinus is completely opaque, CT scan does not always allow differentiation between real soft tissue mass (edema, polyps, or cysts) and fluid stasis (mucus, pus) owing to a blocked ostium. This differentiation can be made only during surgery or endoscopic examination of the involved sinus.

Acute infections of the sinuses are not very often seen by the otolaryngologist because of the frequent and widespread use of broad-spectrum antibiotics by general physicians in the treatment of common infections of the upper respiratory tract. In our country, patients are referred to the ear, nose, and throat (ENT) specialist only when complications of acute sinusitis occur (orbital phlegmon, intracranial abscesses, or osteomyelitis).

Inflammatory mucosal changes are mostly induced by chronic or recurrent infections of the sinuses. Most of the infections are of bacterial origin, perhaps initiated by viral infection, but a considerable percentage (up to 10%) *(3,4)* is also caused by fungal infection (90% by *Aspergillus*

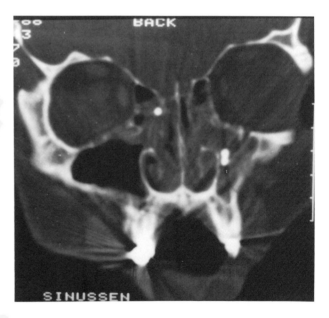

Fig. 2. Coronal scan of a bilateral *Aspergillus* pan-sinusitis with the concrements typical for this type of infection.

fumigatus) (5). These noninvasive mycotic infections (Fig. 2) of the sinuses can be effectively treated by endoscopic techniques. This high percentage of fungus disease seen in recent years may be the result of better diagnosis procedures or the increased use of broad-spectrum antibiotics and/or corticosteroids in the treatment of chronic rhino-

Table 1
CT-Scan Findings
of the Paranasal Sinuses in a Population
of Patients with Chronic Nasal Complaints

Without signs of paranasal sinus inflammation, n = 149 (42%)	
With anatomical anomalies	67%
Without anatomical anomalies	33%
Without signs of paranasal sinus inflammation, n = 201 (58%)	
Maxillary sinus disease	73%
Anterior ethmoid disease	35%
Posterior ethmoid disease	19%
Frontal sinus disease	13%
Sphenoid disease	13%

Table 2
Percentage of Patients with CT-Scan Signs
of Anatomical Abnormalities in a Population
of 350 Adult Patients with Chronic Nasal Complaints

Signs of soft tissue disease	No, 42% (n = 149)	Yes, 58% (n = 201)
Septal deviation	45%	75%
Concha bullosa	44%	33%
"Haller" cell	10%	1%
Processus uncinatus bullosa	2%	1%

sinusitis. Because of the frequent use of such antibiotics, it often becomes very difficult to find pathogenic microorganisms in chronic rhinosinusitis with important inflammatory changes of the mucosa. The key to the treatment of these chronic rhinosinusitis cases, however, is not the use of antibiotic therapy, but the restoration of the drainage and ventilation of the paranasal sinuses, especially in the region of the ostiomeatal complex. Therefore, correction of the anatomical variations of the nasal lateral wall and septum is most important, since it restores an adequate drainage and ventilation of the paranasal sinuses. Posterior septal deviations interfere with sinus drainage and can be corrected using modern septoplastic techniques restoring a normal sinus and nasal ventilation. Anomalies of the nasal lateral wall, such as overdeveloped lacrimal or agger nasi cells, anomalies of the uncinate process, ethmoid bulla, or turbinates, can be corrected endoscopically. Only when these anomalies are associated with important chronic soft tissue reaction interfering with sinus drainage, not responding to medical treatment, is surgery indicated.

In a CT scan study of 350 adults with chronic nasal complaints, the authors (6) showed that 58% of these patients had soft tissue disease (Table 1). In these 350 patients, the authors compared the percentage of occurrence of anatomical variations on one hand to the number of patients showing mucosal disease on the other hand. In the group with mucosal disease only, the percentage of occurrence of septal deviations was definitely higher (75 vs 45%). The other anomalies were found to be evenly distributed in the groups of patients with and without sinus disease (Table 2). Looking at the maxillary sinus, only 23% of the patients showed minimal edema of the mucosa, 12% showed 50% of the maxillary sinus to be opaque, 4% showed 75% of the maxillary sinus to be opaque, and 3% showed a complete shadow of the sinus. A clear-cut solitary polyp of the maxillary sinus was found in 22%, and multiple polyps only in 3% (6).

In 196 children (3–14 yr) with chronic nasal complaints (6), 64% had CT scan signs of mucosal sinus disease. The total number with chronic nasal complaints was higher in the younger children (3–8 yr), with a marked drop at the age of 7–8 yr. In younger children, the disease was more severe, with a higher degree of opacity and more frequent bilateralism. It seems, therefore, that the natural history of chronic rhinosinusitis in children shows a tendency to resolve spontaneously in at least 50% of the cases after the age of 7–8 yr. Therefore, the authors are very reluctant to operate on young children, because they believe that chronic rhinosinusitis in children is an expression of a temporary immune immaturity that does not need surgery, unless sinus complications develop or the quality of life is at risk. According to Lusk and Muntz (7), 80% of the children in their study benefited from surgery. However, because the average age of their operated children was 6.6 yr, their percentage of 80% successful procedures needs to be evaluated taking into consideration the natural history of the disease.

Chronic rhinosinusitis can also be caused by such diseases as the immotile cilia syndrome, Kartagener's syndrome (bronchiectasis, chronic sinusitis, and situs inversus), and congenital or acquired immune deficiency (8,9). In these cases, endoscopic sinus surgery can reopen the access to the different sinuses, so that the postoperative ven-

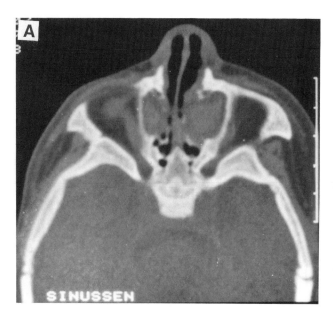

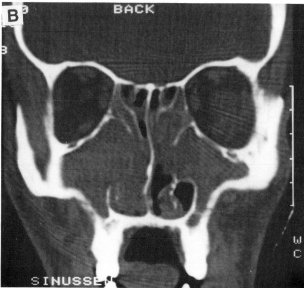

Fig. 3. (A) Axial CT scan of a 3-mo-old child with cystic fibrosis. The sphenoidal sinuses are clear, as well as the ethmoids (not seen on the scan), but the lateral nasal wall is displaced medially blocking completely the nasal cavity. **(B)** Coronal CT scan of a 13-yr-old child with cystic fibrosis and massive polyposis.

tilation and cleaning becomes possible, but it will not, of course, improve the drainage, since this is the result of the impaired mucociliary function or the suppressed immune system.

A special entity of chronic rhinosinusitis is described as polyposis nasi. In these cases, the major part of the paranasal sinus is opaque, and endoscopy of the nose reveals massive polyposis protruding from the middle meatus, sometimes leading to complete nasal obstruction. According to the literature, 14% *(10)* of the patients with nasal polyposis have aspirin intolerance. On the other hand, 36–60% of the patients *(5–10)* suffering from aspirin intolerance will develop nasal polyposis and 39% have the triad of aspirin intolerance, asthma, and nasal polyposis (Samter's syndrome). According to Settipane *(10)*, 65% of the patients with nasal polyposis show positive allergy skin tests.

In a group of 57 atopic children (positive history, allergy skin test, and radio allergosorbent test (RAST) for at least one major allergy), 56% showed soft tissue inflammation on the CT scans *(6)*. Of these 57 children, 63% showed mild involvement of the maxillary sinus mucosa and 37% severe soft tissue disease (more than 50% of the lumen of the maxillary sinus was opaque).

In 25 adult patients with massive nasal polyposis *(11)* and after oral prednisolone treatment (60 mg for 4 d followed by gradual reduction of the dose by

5 mg/d), 72% showed subjective improvement owing to the involution of their polyposis, and in 52%, there was a dramatic improvement as evidenced on the CT scans. Especially good results were seen in the ASA-intolerant patients, and not as good results in the allergic group. There existed, however, a strong tendency toward recurrence within 5 mo. Therefore, the authors treat all their cases of massive nasal polyposis with prednisolone preoperatively, because this will bring about in at least 50% of the cases a dramatic involution of the polyposis, which will facilitate the surgery considerably.

All children under the age of 5 yr with real nasal polyps proved to have cystic fibrosis *(12)*. In 84 patients (age 3 mo to 34 yr) with cystic fibrosis, 12% of the children had nasal obstruction because of mucopyosinusitis with medial displacement of the lateral nasal wall (Fig. 3). In 45%, the nasal obstruction was the result of nasal polyposis. In 28 of the latter patients, CT scans were performed and showed in all cases massive involvement of the anterior and middle ethmoid, maxillary, and frontal sinus (if present). In 42%, the posterior ethmoid and sphenoid were free of disease *(13)*. In 18 children with cystic fibrosis and total nasal obstruction, the authors performed 29 endoscopic total sphenoethmoidectomies, with an average follow-up of 4 yr. In all these children, the quality of life

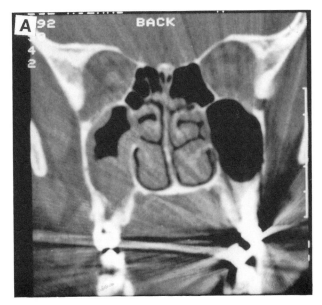
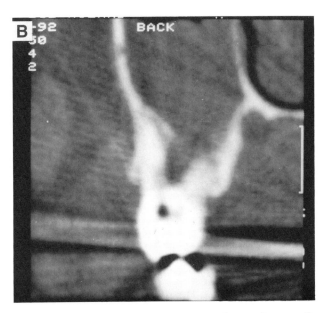

Fig. 4. (A) Coronal CT scan of a patient with a left-sided pan-sinusitis after antibiotic treatment. Note the persistent soft tissue mass on the floor of the maxillary sinus, whereas the ethmoid and infundibulum region are clear. This is typical for a dentogenous maxillary sinusitis. **(B)** Close-up view of the left molar showing a bony dehiscence over the palatal root.

improved dramatically after surgery. In 44%, however, recurrences occurred, making revision surgery necessary. On average, 1.6 surgical procedures/child were necessary, going from 1 to 3 (only 1 child) revision surgeries. All the cases with multiple massive recurrences were children operated on for the first time below the age of 6 yr.

In some cases of Wegener's granulomatosis and after failure of medical treatment, endoscopic sinus surgery can drain the obstructed sinuses *(14)*, but persistent scaring and crusting can be expected, requiring meticulous postoperative care. According to Maran and Lund *(5)*, nasal sarcoidosis is not a good indication for endoscopic surgery, since it may exacerbate the condition.

Chronic maxillary sinusitis can be caused by dental disease (apical abscess, periapical infection, infected dentiginous cyst, dental filling). In these cases, most of the tissue inflammation is at the level of the floor of the maxillary sinus, decreasing toward the ostium (Fig. 4), with no or minimal involvement of the ethmoid region, in contrast to maxillary disease caused by ostium problems, where the majority of the soft tissue inflammation is around the ostiomeatal complex.

A very good indication for endonasal endoscopic sinus surgery is mucoceles, since this technique dramatically reduces operative morbidity *(15)* by offering a minimally invasive approach and allowing accurate follow-up under direct endoscopic vision. Only those mucoceles that cannot be approached satisfactorily require an external approach.

Benign (especially osteoma) and malign tumors can also lead to ostial obstruction and consequent chronic rhinosinusitis. If the osteoma can be exposed adequately, it can be removed endoscopically. If not, or in cases of malignant tumors, more classical approaches are needed for adequate exposure and complete removal of the tumor.

Finally, inverted papilloma can be treated quite well endoscopically when the location of the tumor allows easy access and complete removal (involvement on the frontal sinus by the tumor is certainly a contraindication to endoscopic removal). Furthermore, all signs of malignancy must be absent, and the patient must be compliant to a good follow-up *(16)*. Under these conditions, the morbidity of lateral rhinotomy and/or maxillectomy can be avoided, considerably increasing patient comfort and aesthetic aspect.

Techniques

Based on a better understanding of the pathophysiology of chronic rhinosinusitis, the importance of the ostiomeatal complex *(2)* as the key area in the pathogenesis of this disease has been stressed during the last decade by many authors. This area

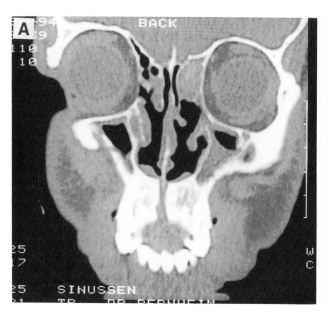 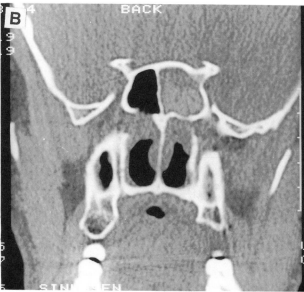

Fig. 5. (A) Coronal CT scan of a typical post-Caldwell-Luc condition. Isolated soft tissue mass in the right frontal recess and blocked infundibulum on the same side, resulting in chronic maxillary sinusitis with fluid level. **(B)** Coronal CT scan of the same patient showing an isolated soft tissue mass in the right sphenoid. During surgery, both soft tissue masses proved to be the result of fungal infection.

contains the most narrow clefts of the paranasal sinus system, and contact between opposite mucosa layers (1–4) in this isthmus area leads to disruption of the mucociliary clearance, causing retention of secretions creating increased potential for infection (17,18). Wigand (18) showed that restoration of ventilation and drainage after removal of cysts and polyps initiates the recovery of diseased mucosa. The concept was introduced to preserve as much mucosa as possible, because most of the mucosal disease seemed to be reversible after adequate drainage and ventilation. This newer insight contradicts the older concept of the Caldwell-Luc operation, which stressed the importance of total exenteration of the mucosa. This new concept drastically changed the surgery for chronic and recurrent sinusitis in such a way that indications for the more classical techniques, such as the Caldwell-Luc approach, external ethmoidectomy, collapsing procedures (removal of the anterior table bone or "Ridel" technique), and osteoplastic flap approach, with or without obliteration of the frontal sinus, have become extremely rare. The current state of the art is the "endoscopic technique." The success of the technique is owing not only to equally satisfactory results or even superior percentage of better results, but also to marked better postoperative comfort for the patient (18).

In a group of patients in whom the classical Caldwell-Luc procedure failed to relieve initial symptoms, it was shown (19) that in all cases there existed residual disease in the anterior ethmoidal area, demonstrating again the importance of this region in the pathophysiology of the disease (Fig. 5). Some authors (20,21) perform most of their endonasal surgery with the microscope, but the inability to "see around corners" (22) in this way will always force the surgeons to use an endoscope at a certain stage of the surgery if they need lateral or retrograde vision (23).

From the foregoing, it is clear that, in the majority of the cases of endoscopic surgery, one has to focus on the ostiomeatal complex of the middle meatus to restore drainage and ventilation of the maxillary sinus, frontal sinus, and anterior and middle ethmoid. If the pathology of the soft tissue extends into the posterior ethmoid, the superior turbinate will be displaced medially, closing the sphenoethmoidal recess and impeding the ventilation and drainage of not only the posterior ethmoid, but also the sphenoidal sinus. In these cases, the basal lamella of the middle turbinate needs to be perforated and removed so that these last two sinuses can be widely exposed as well. Endoscopic surgical techniques can thus range from limited surgery, such as sinoscopy, inferior and middle meatal antrostomy, and turbinoplasty, to more

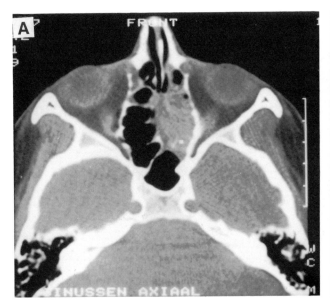 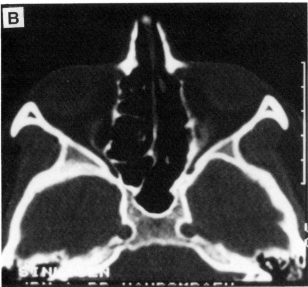

Fig. 6. (A) Preoperative axial CT scan of a right isolated posterior ethmoiditis. **(B)** Postoperative scan of the same patient (partial ethmoidectomy or in this case posterior ethmoidectomy).

extended surgery, such as anterior or partial ethmoidectomy, total ethmoidectomy, and total spheno-ethmoidectomy (Fig. 6) *(4,18,23–25)*.

All these procedures can be performed under local anesthesia. The authors, however, prefer for the more extensive surgery in adults, and for all pediatric cases, general anesthesia with hypotension (systolic blood pressure around 90 mmHg). When using general anesthesia and hypotension, one needs only to decongest the mucosa of the nasal cavity, whereas infiltration with a combination of local anesthetic and a vasoconstrictor is unnecessary. Even in the most extensive cases of massive polyposis, blood loss will seldom exceed 400 mL. When minor procedures without general anesthesia are performed, decongestion and surface anesthesia of the nasal mucosa with or without infiltration can be used.

MINOR PROCEDURES

Sinoscopy. Although antral lavage was a very popular procedure in the routine ENT practice, it has now become quite exceptional, since with the better understanding of the pathophysiology of chronic rhinosinusitis, it is obvious that, in the majority of cases, the pathological changes of the soft tissue in the maxillary sinus are secondary to ostiomeatal pathology.

Fifteen years ago, with the introduction of rigid endoscopes, the repetitive antral puncture and

lavage were replaced by an inspection of the maxillary sinus through a 4-mm trocar and placement of a permanent drainage tube allowing daily lavage, avoiding the repetitive punctures that were unpleasant for the patient. CT-scan studies showed, however, that the recurrence rate of chronic maxillary sinusitis was quite high if there persisted residual disease in the anterior ethmoid. Therefore, indication for sinoscopy followed by antral lavage has become rather exceptional. In children with chronic rhinosinusitis, the authors *(26)* were not able to demonstrate better cure rates after 3 wk on standard X-ray examination in a group of children with irrigation of the maxillary sinus via a drainage tube compared to a control group without drainage. Sinoscopy is mainly indicated for diagnostic purposes, and combined with lavage, it is also indicated in acute conditions where drainage of the sinus gives immediate relief of the discomfort and pain. In children with purulent ethmoiditis complicated by an orbital extension of the infection (beginning orbital phlegmon), concomitant presence of a complete shadow of the maxillary sinus and absence of response to iv broad-spectrum antibiotic treatment within 2 d, antral lavage can be a good indication (Fig. 7). In these cases, the authors observed during nasal endoscopy before the sinoscopy with drainage of the maxillary sinus a bulging of the fontanel region, indicating pus under pressure. After drainage and daily lavage via

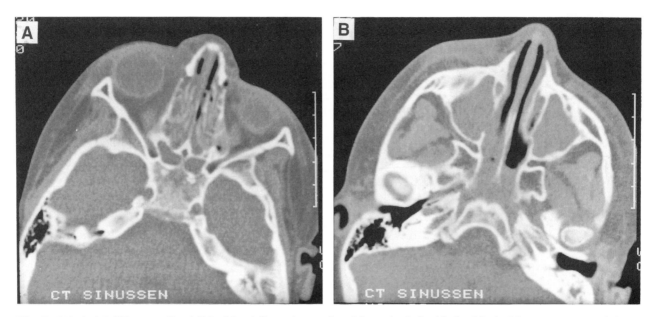

Fig. 7. (A) Axial CT scan of a child with a bilateral pan-sinusitis and a left-sided orbital phlegmon. **(B)** Axial CT scan of the same patient. Note the bilateral maxillary sinusitis with a bulging of the posterior fontanel region indicating pus under pressure in this sinus.

a plastic tube in the inferior meatus, the symptoms resolved within 24 h. However, if CT-scan signs of subperiostal abscess formation are observed, then more extensive surgery is required, such as endoscopic removal of the lamina papyracea and incision of the periorbita, or a lateral rhinotomy in both cases with drainage of the abscess. In all these cases, the sinoscopy and drainage is performed via the inferior meatus. Sometimes this route or a fossa canina approach can be indicated for biopsies of suspected lesions, removal of foreign bodies, and marsupialization of cysts.

Inferior Meatal Antrostomy. This procedure was routinely performed in the Caldwell-Luc approach and was once quite popular in the treatment of chronic rhinosinusitis in children. Critical evaluation of the results, however, showed that in spite of a wide antral window in the inferior meatus, mucociliary clearance was still directed toward the natural ostium in the middle meatus *(4).* In view of the tendency for spontaneous closure of the inferior meatal window, some authors even developed a permanent silastic prosthesis that at times itself started to act as a foreign body after some time, resulting in an increased morbidity and poor outcome *(27),* and according to Muntz and Lusk *(28),* showed a 76% failure rate after 6 mo of follow-up. A patent inferior meatal window will only prevent

the development of pus under pressure and will allow easy access to the maxillary antrum for examination or cleansing. Sometimes it can be indicated when there exists a compartmentalization of the maxillary sinus after Caldwell-Luc procedures, where an inferior meatal antrostomy is the only way for adequate drainage of an isolated inferior compartment.

Middle Meatal Antrostomy. This antral window is located in a more physiological location than the inferior meatal window, if one considers the natural pathway of maxillary sinus mucociliary clearance. To prevent stenosis, it is wise to make a wide middle meatal window, extending the opening inferiorly by removing the horizontal part of the uncinate process and posteriorly by removing a part of the perpendicular plate of the palatal bone. This procedure is performed in an isolated way for any pathology confined to the maxillary sinus without any ethmoid involvement, such as a foreign body, isolated cysts of mucoceles, chronic or recurrent infection, or *Aspergillus* infection accompanied or not by ostial stenosis. This middle meatal antrostomy is performed routinely in all cases of ethmoidectomy or sphenoethmoidectomy. A middle meatal window affords good conditions of inspection of the state of the maxillary sinus mucosa during the followup and allows wide access for removal of possible postoperative recurrence.

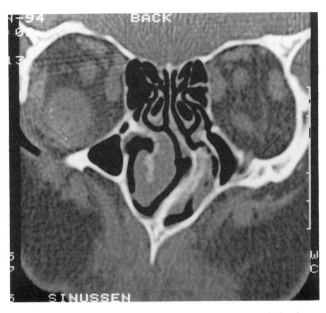

Fig. 8. Coronal CT scan showing a huge septal deviation to the right side and a concha media bullosa on both sides without any sign of mucosal inflammation. Note the compensatory oversized left inferior turbinate. This CT scan is of considerable help in the surgical planning. This patient needs a septoplasty, trimming of the left inferior turbinate (mainly soft tissue swelling) with lateralization of the same turbinate. A submucous partial resection of the bony structure of this turbinate is not necessary.

Turbinoplasty. Depending on the endoscopic and CT findings, the inferior turbinate can be reshaped by performing a submucosal bony resection, if there exists a bulla or an oversized bony part of the turbinate. It needs to be luxated laterally if the inferior turbinate extends too much medially because of compensation for septal concavity or needs to be luxated medially if there exists a lateralization of the turbinate blocking the inferior meatal window as frequently observed after Caldwell-Luc procedures. Finally, any hyperplastic tissue of the turbinate can be removed endoscopically (partial resection or trimming of the turbinate), and cauterization, submucous diathermy, cryosurgery, or laser vaporization of hypercongestive tissue is also performed more accurately under direct vision (Fig. 8). Total turbinectomy should be avoided under any circumstances because of the irreversible disastrous consequences involved (no compensation possible, atrophy with crust formation, granulation tissue leading to epistaxis, headache, fetor, and sensation of nasal obstruction).

The most common pathology of the middle turbinate is a concha bullosa impeding the drainage and ventilation of the middle meatus. Endoscopic removal of the most lateral part of the bulla will restore the normal physiology of the middle meatus and preserve the lateral part of the olfactory mucosa. This procedure is very often carried out in combination with more extensive ethmoidectomies. In cases of polypous degeneration of the mucosa or hyperplasia, the middle turbinate can be trimmed. In extensive cases complete removal can be considered, but one must realize that this turbinate is a very important landmark, and a complete removal will increase the risks of serious complications in revision surgery (16).

Isolated removal of the superior turbinate is rarely necessary, but in extensive disease, this turbinate is very often displaced medially, showing an extreme hyperplasia or polypous degeneration of the mucosa. On the other hand, it is a very important landmark in order to find the ostium of the sphenoidal sinus. This ostium is always located medially of this turbinate in the sphenoethmoidal recess. After identification of this turbinate and total removal, the sphenoidal ostium can be identified easily. Entering the sphenoidal sinus via the natural ostium is the only way that one can be 100% sure to be in the sphenoidal sinus, and it is also the safest way.

MAJOR PROCEDURES

Anterior Ethmoidectomy, Posterior Ethmoidectomy, Total Ethmoidectomy, and Total Sphenoethmoidectomy. The Messerklinger (*see* ref. *4*) and Wigand *(18)* approaches for total sphenoethmoidectomy are the two best-known techniques. With the Messerklinger technique, anterior ethmoidectomy is first performed starting with the removal of the vertical part of the uncinate process, opening the infundibulum ethmoidalis, and cleaning the frontal recess superiorly, followed by the removal of the bulla ethmoidalis. The skull base or the roof of the ethmoid (fovea) is identified in its anterior part, which is the most difficult and dangerous location for the identification of this structure. If maxillary disease is also present, which is mostly the case, then the natural ostium of this sinus is enlarged anteriorly. If posterior disease is present as well, then the basal lamella of the middle turbinate is perforated, and the posterior ethmoid entered and cleared of disease. This operation can also be extended to the sphenoidal sinus that is entered via the posterior ethmoid. Since in the beginning Wigand mostly operated massive polyposis, a total sphenoethmoidectomy was developed by him. After removal of the inferior border and the tail of the middle turbinate, the posterior ethmoid is entered as well as the sphenoidal sinus. Once the sphenoidal sinus is opened, it is easy to identify the roof of the posterior ethmoid as well. According to the authors, the identification of the skull base in the posterior part of the ethmoid or the sphenoid is safer because the roof of the ethmoid and the nasal cavity are more in one plane. Furthermore, at this posterior level, the depth of the fossa olfactoria is smaller than in the anterior ethmoid (3.18 vs 4.79 mm) and there are fewer dehiscences (58.9 vs 92.8%) *(29)*. Then the lamina papyracea is identified and the posterior and anterior ethmoid completely cleaned. Finally, the agger nasi is opened, the frontal recess freed from disease, and the middle meatus fenestrated toward the maxillary sinus.

Many variations on these two techniques exist, so that one of the authors (Clement) has developed his own technique. The concept of his technique consists of using easily recognizable landmarks throughout the whole surgery. It consists of the following steps:

- Step 1: Identify the inferior and middle turbinate (in massive polyposis, one has to remove the polyps first to be able to identify these structures). It is striking to see that even in extreme cases of polyposis, the middle turbinate is mostly intact and does not show major polypoid degeneration, so that it can be identified easily if one proceeds carefully with the polypectomy.
- Step 2: Medialize the middle turbinate and identify the uncinate process and the bulla ethmoidalis. Because of the edema of these two structures completely closing the hiatus semi-lunaris inferior, the ostium of the maxillary sinus very often cannot be identified.
- Step 3: Incise with a Freer elevator, laterally of the vertical part of the uncinate process, and extend this incision inferiorly of the uncinate process through the anterior and posterior fontanel (Fig. 9A). If the disease is confined to the frontal sinus and frontal recess only, the incision does not need to be extended horizontally. Since the Freer is curved, it is impossible in this way to damage the nasolacrimal duct.

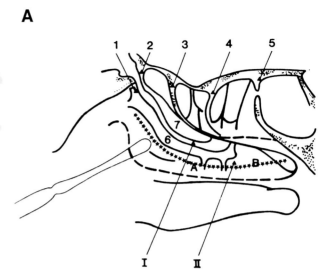

A

Fig. 9. (A) Incision laterally and inferiorly to the uncinate process (stars) starting high up the infundibulum ethmoidalis and extending through the fontanel region until the posterior wall of the maxillary sinus is reached. Dotted line: contour of the middle turbinate. I: ostium of the maxillary sinus in the hiatus semilunaris inferior. II: most frequent location of an accessory ostium: A-region of the anterior fontanelm B-region of the posterior fontanel, 1. basal lamella of uncinate process, 2. basal lamella of bulla ethmoidalis, 3. basal lamella of middle turbinate, 4. basal lamella of superior turbinate, 5. anterior wall of sphenoidal sinus, 6. uncinate process, and 7. bulla ethmoidalis.

Furthermore, this instrument is quite sturdy, so it allows easy luxation of the whole uncinate process medially.
- Step 4: At this point, the uncinate process can be removed by opening the infundibulum ethmoidale superiorly and giving a wide access to the maxillary sinus posteriorly. The perpendicular plate of the palatine bone can be removed with Blakesley-Weil forceps extending the fenestration of the maxillary sinus posteriorly, while with the back-biting Ostrum forceps, the antral window is widened in an anterior-superior direction.
- Step 5: Next, the maxillary sinus is cleared of disease with a curved Blakesley Weil (45 or 90°), and the roof of this sinus is identified as well as its posterior wall. These two landmarks are very important. The roof of the maxillary sinus will considerably facilitate the identification of the lamina papyracea later on. The posterior wall of the maxillary sinus gives the level, in a frontal plane, of the anterior wall of the sphenoidal sinus and the most posterior cell of the posterior eth-

moid (if this cell is not protruding above the sphenoidal sinus).

- Step 6: After removal of the vertical part of the uncinate process, the frontal recess can be inspected and cleaned. The drainage of the frontal sinus is mostly impeded by a medialization of the upper part of the uncinate process or by an extension of the lacrimal cell into this frontal recess. This lacrimal cell can be called an "agger nasi" cell when it extends laterally and anteriorly of the medial turbinate, a "nasal" cell when it extends laterally and toward the nasal bones, or a "frontal" cell when it goes into the frontal sinus. Especially when this cell is extending toward the frontal sinus, it can mislead the surgeon into thinking that the frontal sinus is already opened, although in fact one has a huge recessus terminalis. In any case, when the cleaning of this region becomes problematic, the author prefers to proceed to step 7 first. Once the roof of the anterior ethmoid and the relief of the anterior ethmoidal artery have been identified, one can return to this step to clean the frontal recess completely, exposing widely the ostium of the frontal sinus. If there exists any problem in this region, it is safer to work from posterior to anterior, starting from a well-identified skull base.

- Step 7: Open and completely remove the bulla ethmoidalis. Once the bulla is opened, it is not so difficult to find the lamina papyracea laterally, especially because the floor of the orbit has already been identified during step 5. After removal of the medial part of the bulla and identification of the lamina papyracea, one can try to look for the roof of the anterior ethmoid. In extensive disease, however, again it can still be difficult and hazardous to find the skull base in this quite anterior region because of the variability of the depth of the fossa olfactoria *(29)*. If in doubt, it is better to proceed to step 8 before going toward the skull base.

- Step 8: After identification of the basal lamella of the middle turbinate, this structure is perforated in its medial inferior part, opening the posterior ethmoid. Then the posterior ethmoid is cleaned of polyps, and, even in cases of extensive disease, the skull base can be identified more safely in this region for the previously mentioned reasons (Fig. 9B). In exceptional cases where it is still difficult to find the skull base or when one knows from the CT scan that the optic nerve is bulging

B

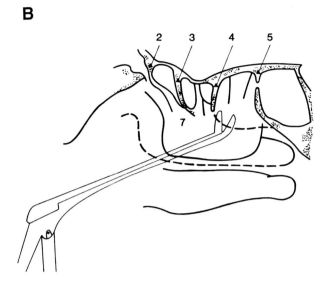

Fig. 9. (B) After removal of the major part of the uncinate process and bulla ethmoidalis, and after perforation of the basal lamella of the middle turbinate the skull base is identified in the posterior ethmoid region.

into the posterior ethmoidal cell ("Onodi" cell), one can go for the next most important landmark, which is the superior turbinate.

- Step 9: At this stage of the operation, lateralization of the middle turbinate becomes necessary in order to identify the superior turbinate and to open the sphenoethmoidal recess. Contrary to the middle turbinate, the superior turbinate very often shows polypous degeneration. This turbinate is mostly pushed medially toward the septum by the polyposis in the posterior ethmoid, closing any access to the sphenoethmoidal recess. After removal of this turbinate, which can be done safely in this region, one gets a good view into the sphenoidal recess. At this time of the operation, one has to palpate with a straight suction canula (Frazier No. 8 or No. 10) the anterior wall of the sphenoidal sinus, medially to the attachment of the superior turbinate. One will always find the ostium of the sphenoidal sinus medially to the attachment of this superior turbinate. The ostium can be high up (89.5%) or low (10.5%) into the sphenoethmoidal recess *(29)*.

- Step 10: Once the ostium of the sphenoidal sinus has been identified, it will be widened in an inferior lateral direction with a 90° angled bone-biting Hajek forceps (Fig. 9C). The only safe way to open the sphenoidal sinus is via its natural ostium. The author thinks that entering the sphenoidal

C

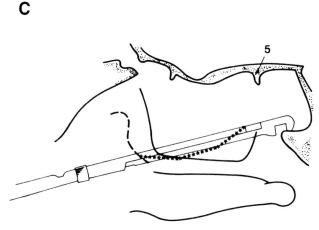

5

Fig. 9. (C) Following the skull base, the ethmoid and the frontal recess are completely cleared of bony structures, leaving a wide-open frontal ostium. Finally, the anterior wall of the sphenoid sinus is removed, starting from the ostium downward, and the inferior border and tail of the middle turbinate are removed as well (stars).

sinus via the posterior ethmoid is less safe, and sometimes a posterior ethmoidal cell, extending above the sphenoidal sinus, can mislead the surgeon, assuming that he or she has already entered the sphenoidal sinus. When extensive disease exists, it is not always very clear on a CT scan how far the most posterior ethmoidal cell reaches. Once the sphenoidal sinus is widely opened, the posterior ethmoidal cells and especially the lateral wall of these cells as well as the skull base can also be identified in a safer way. Once the skull base is completely freed in its anterior and posterior part and after identification of the anterior ethmoidal artery (not always possible [29]), the ostium of the frontal sinus can be exposed.

- Step 11: In most cases, the author prefers at this stage of the operation to remove the inferior border and the tail of the middle turbinate. He prefers to remove the structure only at the end of the operation because it is an important landmark during the surgery.

Depending on the extent of the soft tissue disease, endoscopic ethmoidectomy can be limited to anterior ethmoidectomy (steps 1–3 and/or 4), total ethmoidectomy (steps 1–7), or total sphenoethmoidectomy (steps 1–11). Using this safe technique, proceeding from one landmark to another, the author did not have any major complication (i.e., blind eye, diplopia, CSF leak, or an internal carotid lesion) on a

total of more than 800 ethmoidectomies (90% of these operations consisted of total sphenoethmoidectomy; 25% were revision cases, mostly post-Caldwell-Luc). According to the author, the most difficult postoperative challenge is to keep a good long-term drainage and ventilation of all the sinuses and especially of the frontal sinus. The frontal recess is the most narrow passage in the postoperative cavity, and because of the tendency of scar tissue and synechiae formation in this region, it needs a good postoperative follow-up.

In conclusion, one can state that endoscopic paranasal sinus surgery is the technique of choice in nearly all cases of chronic or recurrent sinusitis. It has replaced in less than a decade the more classical techniques because it respects more the normal physiology of the sinuses. In experienced hands, it has proven to give better and longer-lasting good results with less morbidity to the patient. The complication rate is certainly not higher than with the conventional techniques.

SOFT TISSUE MASSES AND EXTERNAL SURGICAL APPROACHES

A discussion of soft tissue tumor epidemiology, pathology, and staging was already presented in Chapter 13. In the following section, external approaches and procedures commonly used in surgical treatment of paranasal soft tissue masses will be reviewed. For technical details, the reader is referred to a surgical atlas.

Essentially all soft tissue tumors except lymphoma—non-Hodgkin type—and multiple myloma (plasmocytoma) are eligible for surgical resection. The choice of extranasal surgical approach and procedures for removal of sinonasal tumors is determined by localization and extent of the lesion. This information can be obtained from clinical evaluation, i.e., physical examination, imaging techniques, and biopsy. In order to avoid surgical artifacts, the imaging should preferably be completed before the biopsy. As a rule, the biopsy should be obtained through the intranasal route. With the recent advances in nasal endoscopy, the Caldwell-Luc procedure intended primarily for tissue diagnosis and tumor staging should be avoided. Breaking through the anterior bony wall in a patient with a malignant tumor will inevitably cause the spread of the tumor cells in the cheek.

The lateral rhinotomy and midfacial degloving are the basic approaches to expose surgically tumors of the nasal cavity and paranasal sinuses.

Lateral Rhinotomy

Lateral rhinotomy is merely a skin incision along the side of the nose, historically ascribed to Moure, but actually first used by Gensoul in 1827 *(30)*. The incision begins midway between the medial canthus and the bridge of the nose; it continues downward on the lateral edge of the nose and curves medially below the lower ala to the midline at the columella. A common extension of the basic lateral rhinotomy incision is the Weber-Ferguson incision. This incision through the external surface of the lower eyelid just below the lashes and through the upper lip in the midline opens the surgical field laterally with an infraorbital extension and prevents retraction of the lower eyelid. Recently, however, Stell suggested that the so-called Weber-Ferguson incision would be more accurately termed the Blondin-Gensoul incision *(30)*.

A temporal extension over the zygoma to the pretragal area was described by Barbosa (cited in ref. *31*). A lateral rhinotomy incision extending superiorly up to the eyebrow can be used to improve access to the frontoethmoid region. This is helpful in exposing lesions involving the cribriform plate, the frontal sinus, and anterior cranial fossa. In 1979, de Fries et al. *(32)* developed a transfacial approach in which two large midfacial flaps, one containing the entire external nose, were raised, exposing the maxillae, both medial orbital walls, and the nasal and paranasal cavities. Through this panoramic approach, large lesions of the nasal cavity that involve the ethmoid and maxillary sinuses as well as the anterior skull base can be easily exposed. The complication rate of lateral rhinotomy and its modifications are approx 10–15%, including epiphora, ectropion, nasal collapse, synechiae, and unacceptable scars.

Midfacial Degloving Approach

The midfacial degloving approach to the nose and paranasal sinuses first described by Portmann and Retrouvey in 1927 has been increasingly utilized during the past decade as an alternative approach to lateral rhinotomy because of the cosmetic advantage *(33)*. This approach is accomplished through a lateral gingivo-buccal incision performed from the midline to the maxillary tuber-

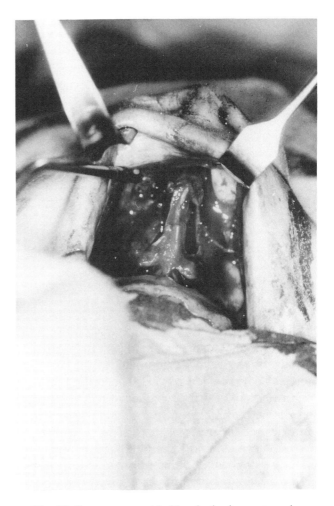

Fig. 10. Exposure provided by degloving approach.

osity combined with nasal intercartilaginous and transfixion incisions. The entire midface can be retracted upward exposing both nasal cavities and maxillary sinuses (Fig. 10). Although these exposures superiorly may be slightly limited, this approach has been used successfully in the management of benign sinonasal tumors, including inverted papillomas, low-grade malignancies of the ethmoid, and high-grade malignancies limited anteriorly and inferiorly to the maxillary sinus. With this approach, access to the lateral maxilla is also somewhat restricted compared to that of extended lateral rhinotomy. Nevertheless, Maniglia *(34)* has used this approach routinely for total maxillectomy. Price et al. proposed the use of the midfacial degloving approach to the central skull base for craniofacial resections *(33)*. Complications of the midfacial degloving are hypoesthesia, moderate vestibular stenosis, and epiphora (5–15%).

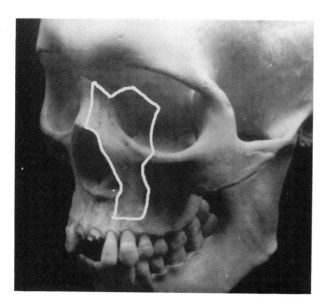

Fig. 11. The bone cuts for medial maxillectomy.

In the surgical management of benign maxillary neoplasms, the Lefort I approach to the maxilla should also be considered *(35)*. The Lefort I down-fracture technique offers excellent direct visualization of the maxillary antrum bilaterally and the entire lesion. There is no loss of bone with fast return to normal maxillomandibular function.

During the past decades, surgical treatment of malignant sinusal tumors has evolved toward an aggressive, *en bloc* removal of all involved bone and soft tissue with free margins. The following surgical procedures are commonly used for treatment of paranasal tumors.

MEDIAL MAXILLECTOMY

This procedure was originally described by Sessions and Larson in 1977 and subsequently modified by Sessions and Humphreys in 1983 *(36)*.

Medial maxillectomy is indicated for low-grade malignant and benign lesions involving the ethmoid, in addition to the lateral nasal wall and maxillary sinus. Tumor extension to the lateral maxilla, orbit, or anterior cranial fossa requires more extensive surgical procedure. The better exposure provided by lateral rhinotomy incision of the anterior superior nasal cavity, frontal, and ethmoid sinuses, as well as the medial orbit offers an oncologic advantage over the degloving approach for the removal of neoplasms. In medial maxillectomy, block resection contains the entire lateral nasal wall with the inferior middle turbinates, the ethmoid labyrinth, and the lamina papyracea (Fig. 11). This

procedure is especially suitable for management of inverted papilloma. The unique biology of these tumors is characterized by bone destruction, tendency to recur, and a 6–30% incidence of malignancy. Since inverting papillomas tend to spread by metaplasia of the adjacent mucosa, excision of a wide tissue margin is indicated. It has been proven that the technique of lateral rhinotomy with block resection of the lateral nasal wall, combined with removal of all mucosa of the ipsilateral maxillary antrum, ethmoid, and sphenoid sinuses should remain as a standard of care, particularly in advanced-stage inverting papilloma of the sino-nasal tract *(37)*. With this approach, the recurrence rate of these tumors is 8 vs 70% after endonasal removal *(38)*. In general, after lateral rhinotomy with medial maxillectomy, there is a 9% recurrence for benign tumors and 15% for malignant neoplasms, the latter only in the patients with non-melanoma malignant neoplasms not receiving postoperative radiotherapy *(39)*.

The most frequent complications after this procedure are cavity crusting, epicanthal scarring, and epiphora.

TOTAL MAXILLECTOMY

Total maxillectomy was first performed by Gensoul in 1827 and simultaneously by Lizars in Edinburgh *(30)*. Total maxillectomy is the standard operation for advanced malignant tumors of the maxillary sinus and ethmoids. A close relationship between ethmoids and antrum often results in early invasion of the ethmoid labyrinth. Therefore, many antral lesions are in fact antroethmoid. Superior extension of the lesion in the ethmoid roof or posterior involvement of the orbital apex is beyond the limits of this procedure. Involvement of the facial soft tissue, orbit, or alveolar bridge will require modification of the total maxillectomy accordingly.

During the last decade, there has been discussion regarding the strict application of total maxillectomy. The amount of tissue to be removed depends on the site and extension of the tumor, which can be precisely preoperatively assessed by imaging. A recent study by Lund et al. *(40)* found that CT alone offered a 78% accuracy in depicting tumor extent compared with operative and histological findings. The addition of MRI increased the accuracy to 94%, and adding MRI with gadolinium to 98%. Therefore, in certain centers, a clear shift

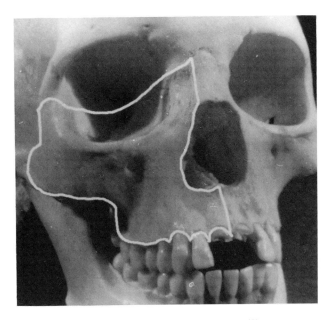

Fig. 12. Limits of resection for total maxillectomy.

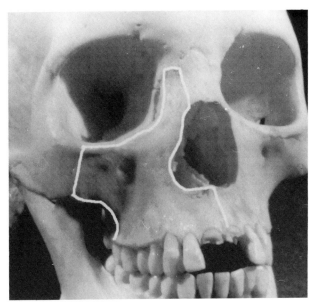

Fig. 13. The bone cuts for partial maxillectomy.

can be observed toward performing individually tailored subtotal maxillectomies combined with radiotherapy instead of standard total maxillectomy. The rationale of this policy is only to resect the diseased segment and its surrounding tissue, rather than a large block of tissue, which includes a not-diseased tissue. Also, some controversy exists on strict indications for orbital exenteration in combination with total maxillectomy. However, in view of recent reports, indications for orbital exenteration are: bone erosion, invasion of the periorbita, posterior ethmoids, or orbital apex (41). However, bone erosion does not constitute an absolute indication for orbital exenteration (37).

The approach for total maxillectomy depends on whether exenteration is planned. Midfacial degloving approach or Weber-Ferguson lateral rhinotomy incision may be used, respectively of tumor extension. In total maxillectomy with orbital exenteration, the block resection specimen includes the orbital contents, the floor and the medial wall of the orbit, the malar bone and a portion of the zygomatic arc, the antrum, ethmoid labyrinth, anterior wall of the sphenoid sinus, the pterygoid plates, and the hard palate. If the ethmoid or nasal cavity is involved with the tumor, the nasal septum is included in the specimen (Fig. 12). Reconstruction of the orbital wall (contour) may be accomplished with the use of a pericranial or temporalis muscle flap, or a split-thickness graft. However, an orbital

prosthesis is the only cosmetic rehabilitation available to the patient with orbital exenteration. If the orbita is preserved, reconstruction of the resected orbital floor may be achieved with fascia, dermis, split-thickness skin graft, Marlex mesh, and tantalum mesh. Anniko et al. (42) have recently reported a technique to restore the maxilla contour using one to three microvascular flaps, including bone transplants from the fibula. This improves the results cosmetically, and, after 1–1.5 yr, reconstruction of the bite function becomes feasible using dental implant with titanium. No surgical attempt should be made to reconstruct the palatal defect after maxillectomy. A preoperatively prepared palatal prosthesis is the best choice for the patient.

Malignant tumors involving only the floor of the maxillary sinus or the hard palate may be managed by partial maxillectomy. This procedure differs from total maxillectomy on the preservation of the orbital floor (Fig. 13). The midfacial degloving approach is very suitable for this procedure. The resected area includes the lower two-thirds of the maxilla with the hard palate. The lower turbinate is included into the specimen, whereas the superior and middle turbinates are excised separately. Postoperative complications following total maxillectomy include infection, skin graft failure, flap contraction or necrosis, and lower eyelid edema. When the eye is preserved, ocular ptosis enophtalmus and epiphora may occur.

CRANIOFACIAL RESECTION

Craniofacial surgery for *en block* resection of advanced frontoethmoidal-orbital cancer was first reported in 1954 by Smith et al. *(43)*. The subsequent work of Malecki in 1959 added improvements to the technique of combined resection of frontal sinus tumors *(44)*. However, it was only in 1963 that the work of Ketcham et al. *(45)* stimulated, especially in the USA, the interest in performing craniofacial resections for advanced paranasal and orbital cancers. Since then, many modifications of the surgical technique as well as improvements in the morbidity and mortality from this operation have been reported. Nevertheless, as Shah et al. *(46)* stated, "no clear consensus exists currently in the literature with regard to the applicability of various techniques in any given circumstance." The indications for anterior cranial facial resection are benign and malignant tumors originating in the superior nasal cavity, paranasal sinus, and orbita extending beyond the limits of resection possible by partial or total maxillectomies. The extent of craniofacial resection is usually individually tailored according to the tumor extent, but involvement of the nasopharynx, superior or posterior sphenoid, clivus, foramen lacerum, or significant intracranial or intracerebral extension is unlikely to result in cure, although a palliative effect may be obtained *(47)*. Strict contraindications for anterior craniofacial resection are: involvement of the cavernous sinus, intracranial carotid artery, optic chiasm, or temporal lobe *(46)*. For *en block* resection of ethmoid tumors eroding the roof of the sinus with no transdural extension, a single otolaryngologic approach through frontal window craniotomy for exposure of the central floor of the anterior fossa may be used (Fig. 14). For more extensive tumors, a combined team approach of an otolaryngologist—head and neck surgeon and neurosurgeon is necessary. A bifrontal craniotomy with bone flap is usually performed. This approach ensures wide exposure of the intracranial tumor extension and effective control of intracranial CSF leaks or hemorrhage. Usually for the facial resection of the tumor through extended lateral rhinotomy or the transfacial approach, a medial maxillectomy or a total maxillectomy is performed with or without orbital exenteration.

After craniofacial resection, the *en bloc* bone specimen should contain the ipsilateral ethmoid labyrinth, superior and lateral walls of the sphe-

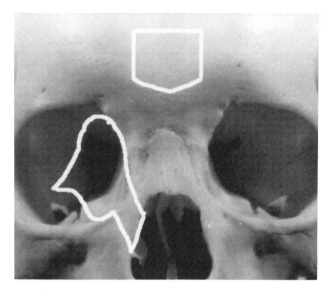

Fig. 14. Craniofacial resection for ethmoidal tumors. Exposure of the floor of the anterior cranial fossa through a "window" craniotomy.

noid, anterior cranial fossa, and cribriform plate. It can be extended to include the orbital roof, the opposite ethmoid, or the frontal sinus and maxilla. After resection, the reconstruction of the anterior skull base and dura should be kept as simple as possible *(47)*. All exposed soft tissue is grafted with split-thickness skin graft. When the patient had preoperative radiotherapy, sometimes a pedical galea pericranial flap is used. The split-thickness skin graft is also used to line the nasal cavity and maxilla defect. It offers good wound healing and facilitates early fitting of a dental prosthesis.

The expected sequelae of craniofacial resection are facial and forehead anesthesia and permanent anosmia. The complication rate of this procedure varies between 10 and 15%. The most common complications of craniofacial resections are infection and CSF leakage. Ophthalmological complications occur in patients with and without orbital exenteration (mononuclear blindness, diplopia, paralytic ptosis). Cerebral complications include headache, acute brain syndrome, hemiplegia, and transient confusion. In our last 10 craniofacial resections, only 1 patient developed infection and CSF leak requiring removal of the bone flap. In contrast, Cheesman et al. *(48)* reported no complications in a series of 60 patients with craniofacial resections.

Long-term survival rates of craniofacial resections seem to be encouraging. In 1973, Ketcham et al. *(49)* reported a 5-yr survival in 49% of the patients, and Schramm *(47)* in 1991 reported a 75% 4-year survival and an 8% recurrence rate. In 1988, Lund and Harrison *(50)* reported 5-yr survival in 45%. Recently, Shah et al. *(46)* in 1992 presented a series of 71 patients who underwent craniofacial resection with a 5-yr overall survival of 56%. The long-term survival varies considerably among the various pathological diagnoses *(51)*. The best local control was achieved with well-differentiated tumors, including well-differentiated squamous cell carcinoma, adenocarcinoma, and chondrosarcoma. Poor local control was achieved in differentiated carcinoma and melanoma. Patient's survival after craniofacial resection is related to the extent of the disease. Patients with either dural or brain invasion have a significantly decreased survival rate in comparison to no dural invasion. Orbital invasion has a less significant effect on long term survival than those with dural invasion. Those patients requiring orbital exenteration experienced a 40% survival rate, whereas those requiring dural resection showed a 22% survival rate *(51)*. It appears that the majority of patients who require dural resections develop local recurrences or spinal cord metastasis. This was presumably from direct siding of the tumor to the CSF.

Nevertheless, in view of the series of various authors, it appears that craniofacial resection is not only a palliative, but also a curative procedure in a selected group of patients with malignant paranasal soft tissue masses.

The treatment of paranasal sinus malignant tumors is challenging owing to its rarity and the difficulty of diagnosing in the early stage, before it involves contiguous structures and important organs, such as the eye and brain. It is known that 9–12% of the patients with sinonasal tumors are asymptomatic *(37)*. Moreover, in spite of recent advances in diagnostic techniques and availability of health care, the average delay between the onset of symptoms and final diagnosis of sinusal tumors remains approx 1 yr. Therefore, at the time of diagnosis, nearly every second patient with sinonasal cancer has involvement of the orbit and 10–20% have extension to the pterygo-palatina fossa *(37)*. Approximately 10% of the patients with ethmoid and maxillary cancer have cervical metastases on the initial presentation *(52)*. This situation must not lead to the treatment policy of despair; however, if the tumor is not removed, it will grow further, causing much more deformity and pain than any surgery.

Nearly 80% of sinus malignancies rise in the antrum, 20% in the ethmoid sinus, and <1% in the frontal and the sphenoid sinuses *(53)*. Squamous cell carcinoma is the most common malignancy of the maxillary sinus, but adenocarcinoma predominates in ethmoid sinus cancers. Knegt et al. *(54)* noted that 20 of 32 ethmoid sinus lesions were adenocarcinoma, and a squamous cell carcinoma was present in only 9 patients. Other series have shown a predominance of squamous cell carcinoma in the ethmoid sinus *(53)*.

Although there is no standard method of treatment of sinusal cancers, the best patient survival would appear to be from a combination of surgery and radiotherapy. Surgical procedures can be radical, i.e., total maxillectomy with orbital exenteration and anterior craniofacial resection, or less radical, in which preservation of the orbita or other structures is attempted. Whether the radiotherapy should be delivered preoperatively or postoperatively remains controversial. Preoperative radiotherapy is preferred when the globe is a low-to-moderate risk for invasion. Following Sisson et al. *(55)*, the use of preoperative radiation therapy for antral and ethmoid sinus cancers increases the globe salvage rate. However, preoperative radiation therapy is associated with delayed wound healing and increased duration of hospital stay. Postoperative radiation therapy has the theoretical advantage of localization of high-risk resection margins and less impact on wound healing.

Evaluation of various treatment results is difficult because of the relative rarity of paranasal malignant tumors, lack of uniform staging system, use of different treatment modalities, and evaluation criteria. Lee and Ogura *(56)* reported that of 96 patients with maxillary sinus carcinomas, 54 (77%) had squamous cell carcinoma. After preoperative radiation (mostly 5000–7000 cGy) and surgery, 5 yr of absolutely no evidence of disease, survival rates were 60, 45, 28, and 38% in patients with T_1, T_2, T_3, and T_4 tumors, respectively. Radiation therapy alone (mostly 6000–7400 cGy) failed to produce a single survival among 23 patients (2 with T_2, 6 with T_3, and 15 with T4 tumors). In one of the recent series of Anniko et al. *(42)*, 77 patients with paranasal carcinoma (clinically considered to have their primary location in the maxillary sinus) were treated by primary surgery and postoperative radiotherapy. Five-year survival rates of patients with T_3 and T_4 carcinomas were 42 and 40%, respectively, and the 10-yr survival rates were 40 and 14%, respectively.

In view of existing studies on the combined treatment of maxillary carcinoma, it is reasonable to expect a 5-yr survival rate of about 60–70% for T_1 and T_2 lesions, and 30–40% for T_3 and T_4 lesions after resection and postoperative radiation. Poor prognostic factors in patients with maxillary sinus carcinoma includes positive neck lymph nodes, erosion of the pterygoid plates, pterygo palatina fossa invasion, and orbital invasion. None of the patients with lymph node metastases to the neck at the time of initial diagnosis could be cured in the series of Hordijk and Brons (52). For advanced unresectable disease, average 5-yr survival rates of 10–15% are achieved with high-dose irradiation alone.

The use of anterior craniofacial resection has improved the prognosis of ethmoid tumors. Craniofacial resection with subsequent radiotherapy is a treatment of choice for advanced tumors. The average 5-yr survival rate for ethmoid malignancies seems to be 50–60% (37). Some of the best results have been achieved in patients with advanced sinus cancers with a combination of chemotherapy, surgery, and aggressive radiation therapy. Preoperative radiotherapy, surgical tumor debulking, and postoperative radiotherapy and topical 5-fluorouracil were used in 32 patients with ethmoid sinus cancer (54). In 20 of these patients with adenocarcinoma, the actual 5-yr survival was 100%. The remaining 12 patients had squamous cell carcinoma and/or undifferentiated carcinoma, and the actual 2-yr and 5-yr survival rates were 75 and 43%, respectively. This report awaits further confirmation. Primary malignancy of the sphenoid and frontal sinuses is extremely rare; therefore, except for the case reports, no reliable information exists. From a literature review of 42 cases of malignant neoplasms of the sphenoid sinus, it seems that a debulking with radiation therapy may be used in these cases (57). The overall survival rate in these patients varied from 5–25% (37).

Fortunately, malignant soft tissue masses are quite uncommon in children, the most frequent being undifferentiated carcinoma and rhabdomyosarcoma. The diagnostic and surgical approaches are similar to those in adults. Disturbances of facial growth have not been seen with lateral rhinotomy or degloving surgery either in infants or in young children. However, during the last 20 yr, the role of aggressive *en bloc* surgery in children has been reduced with the advent of chemotherapy and modern radiation therapy.

REFERENCES

1. Messerklinger W. In: Endoscopy of the Nose. Urband and Schwarzenberg Baltimore-Munich, 1987; pp. 1–179.
2. Flottes L, Clerc P, Riur R, Devilla F. La Physiologie des sinus. Librairie Arnette, Paris 1960—quoted by Nauman HH, Naumann WH. 10 Kurze Pathophysiologie der Nase und ihrer Nebenhöhlen. Hals-Nasen-Ohren Heilkunde in Praxis und Klinik. Band 1 Obere und untere Luftwege I Berendes J, Link R, Zöllner F, eds., Stuttgart: Georg Thieme Verlag, 1977; pp. 10.1–10.55.
3. Zinreich SJ, Kennedy DW, Malat J, Curtin HD, Epstein JI, Huff LC, Kumar AJ, Johns ME, Rosenbaum AE. Fungal sinusitis: diagnosis with CT and MR imaging. Radiology 1988;169:439–444.
4. Stammberger H. Functional Endoscopic Sinus Surgery. Philadelphia: B. C. Decker, 1991; pp. 1–529.
5. Maran AGD, Lund VJ. Infections and nonneoplastic disease. In: Clinical Rhinology, Stuttgart: Georg Thieme Verlag—New York: Thieme Medical Publishers 1990; pp. 59–108.
6. Clement P, Van der Veken P, Iwens P, Buisseret Th. X-ray, CT-scan, MR-imaging. In: Mygind N, Naclerio RM, eds., Allergic and Non-Allergic Rhinitis, Copenhagen: Munksgaard, 1993; pp. 58–65.
7. Lusk RP, Muntz HR. A pilot study. Laryngoscope 1990;100:654–658.
8. Marshall KG, Attia EL. Nasal polyps. In: Disorders of the Nose and Paranasal Sinuses. Diagnosis and Management, Littleton, MA: PSG Publishing, 1987; pp. 217–233.
9. Manning SC, Wasserman RL, Leach J, Truelson J. Chronic sinusitis as a manifestation of primary immunodeficiency in adults. Am J Rhinol 1994;8,1:29–34.
10. Settipane GA. Nasal polyps. In: Settipane GA, ed., Rhinitis, 2nd ed., Providence, RI: Oceanside Publications, 1991; pp. 173–195.
11. Van Camp C, Clement PAR. Results of oral steroid treatment in nasal polyposis. Rhinology 1994;32:5–9.
12. Schramm VL. Inflammatory and neoplastic masses of the nose and paranasal sinus in children. Laryngoscope 1979;89, 12:1887–1897.
13. Brihaye P, Clement PAR, Dab I, Desprechin B. Pathological changes of the lateral nasal wall in patients with cystic fibrosis (mucoviscidosis). Int J Pediatr Otorhinolaryngol 1994;28:141–147.
14. Park AH, Stankiewicz JA. Wegener's granulomatosis: the role of endoscopic sinus surgery. Am J Rhinology 1993;7, 6:261–265.
15. Kennedy DW, Josephson JS, Zinreich J, Mattox DE, Goldsmith MM. Endoscopic sinus surgery for mucoceles: a variable alternative. Laryngoscope 1989;99:885–895.
16. Vleming M. Papiloma inversum. In: Endoscopische neusbijholte chirurgie. Thesis Drukkerij Elinkwijk bv Utrecht 1991; 7–2: pp. 102–108.
17. Kennedy DW, Zinreich SJ, Rosenbaum AE, Johns ME. Functional Endoscopic Sinus Surgery. Theory and diagnostic evaluation. Arch Otolaryngol 1985;111:576–582.
18. Wigand ME. Transnasale, endoscopische Chirurgie der Nasennebenhöhlen bei chronischer Sinusitis. I. Ein biomechanisches Konzept der Schleimhautchirurgie. H.N.O.

1981;29:215–221. II. Die endonasale Kieferhöhlen—Operation. H.N.O. 1981;29:263–269. III. Die endonasale Siebbeinausräumung H.N.O. 1981;29:287–293.

19. Stammberger H, Zinreich SJ, Kopp W, Kennedy DW, Johns ME, Rosenbaum AE. Zur operativen Behandlung der chronisch rezidivierenden sinusitis—Caldwell-Luc versus funktionelle endoskopische Technik. H.N.O. 1987;35:93–105.

20. Heerman J. Endonasale mirkrochirurgische Siebbeinausräuming bei Blutdrucksenkung am halbsitzende Patienten. H.N.O. 1982;30:180–185.

21. Draf W. Die chirurgische Behandlung entzundlicher Erkrankungen der Nasennebenhöhlen. Arch Otorhinolaryngol 1982;235:133–305.

22. King HC, Mabry RL. Surgical management of sinusitis. In: A Practical Guide to the Management of Nasal and Sinus Disorders, New York: Thieme Medical Publishers, 1993; pp. 133–160.

23. Terrier G. Surgery. In: Rhinosinusal Endoscopy. Diagnostic and Surgery. Milan, Italy: Morell Arti Grafiche S.r.l. Osnago (Co). 1991; pp. 141–248.

24. Mehta D. In: Atlas of Endoscopic Sinonasal Surgery. Philadelphia: Lea and Febiger, 1993; pp. 1–118.

25. Rice DH, Schaefer SD. Endoscopic Paranasal Sinus Surgery. New York: Raven, 1988; pp. 1–29.

26. Maes JJ, Clement PAR. The usefulness of irrigation of the maxillary sinus in children with maxillary sinusitis on the basis of Water's X-Ray. Rhinology 1987;25:259–264.

27. Parsons DS, Philips SE. Functional endoscopic surgery in children: a retrospective analysis of results. Laryngoscope 1990;100:643–646.

28. Muntz HR, Lusk RP. Nasal antral windows in children: a retrospective study. Laryngoscope 1990;100: 643–646.

29. Lang J. In: Klinische Anatomie der Nase, Nasenhöhle und Nebenhöhlen. Grundlagen für Diagnostiek und Operation. Aktuelle Oto-Rhino-Laryngologie Band 11. Stuttgart: Georg Thieme Verlag, 1988; pp. 1–133.

30. Stell PM. History of surgery of the upper jaw. In: Harrison D, Lund VJ, eds., Tumours of the Upper Jaw. New York: Churchill-Livingstone, 1993; pp. 1–15.

31. Mertz JS, Pearson BW, Kern EB. Lateral rhinotomy. Indications technique and review of 226 patients. Arch Otolaryngol 1983;230–235.

32. de Fries H, Deeb ZE, Hudkins CP. A transfacial approach to the nasal-paranasal cavities and anterior skull base. Arch Otolaryngol Head Neck Surg 1988;144:766–769.

33. Price JX, Hollidar H, Johns ME, Kennedy DW, Richtsmeier WJ, Mattor DE. The versatile midface degloving approach. Laryngoscope 1988;98:291–295.

34. Maniglia JA. Indications and techniques of midfacial degloving. Arch Otolaryngol Head Neck Surg 1986;112:750–752.

35. Armstrong JE, Bhardwaj AK, Lefort I. Down fracture of the maxilla application to benign antral neoplasm. Otolaryngol 1988;17,6:288–292.

36. Sessions RB, Humphreys DM. Technical modifications of the medial maxillectomy. Arch Otolaryngol 1983;109: 575–577.

37. Myers EN, Carrau RL. Neoplasms of the nose and paranasal sinuses. In: Bailey BJ, ed., Head and Neck Surgery—Otolaryngology, Philadelphia: J. B. Lippincott, 1993; pp. 1091–1109.

38. Myers EN, Petruzelli GJ. Endoscopic sinus surgery for inverting papilloma. Laryngoscope 1993;103:711.

39. Ogusthorpe JD, Weisman RA. Medial maxillectomy for lateral nasal wall neoplasms. Arch Otolaryngol Head Neck Surg 1991;117:751–756.

40. Lund VJ, Howard DJ, Lloyd GA, Cheesman AD. Magnetic resonance imaging of paranasal sinus tumors for craniofacial resection. Head Neck Surg 1989;11:279–283.

41. Perry Ch, Levine P, Williamson BR, Cantrell RW. Preservation of the eye in paranasal sinus cancer surgery. Arch Otolaryngol Head Neck Surg 1988;114:632–634.

42. Anniko M, Franzen L, Löfroth PO. Long term survival of patients with paranasal sinus carcinoma. O.R.L. 1990;52: 187–193.

43. Smith PR, Clopp CT, Williams MM. Surgical treatment of cancer of the frontal sinus and adjacent areas. Cancer 1954;7:991–995.

44. Malecki J. New trends in frontal sinus surgery. Acta Otolaryngol (Stock) 1959;50:137–141.

45. Ketcham AS, Wilkins RH, Van Buren JM, Smith RR. A combined intracranial facial approach to the paranasal sinuses. Am J Surgery 1963;106:698–704.

46. Shah JP, Kraus D, Arbit E, Galicich JH, Strong EW. Craniofacial resection for tumours involving the anterior skull base. Otolaryngol Head Neck Surg 1992; 106:387–393.

47. Schramm VJ. Anterior craniofacial resection. In: Jackson CG, ed., Surgery of Skull Base Tumours. New York: Churchill Livingstone, 1991; pp. 67–86.

48. Cheesman AD, Lund VJ, Howard DJ. Craniofacial resection for tumours of the nasal cavity and paranasal sinuses. Head Neck Surg 1986;8:429–435.

49. Ketcham AS, Chretien PB, Van Buren JM, Smith RR. The ethmoid sinuses: a re-evaluation of surgical resection. Am J Surg 1973;126:469–473.

50. Lund VJ, Harrison DFN. Craniofacial resection for tumours of the nasal cavity and paranasal sinuses. Am J Surg 1988;156:187–190.

51. Van Tuyl R, Gussack GS. Prognostic factors in craniofacial surgery. Laryngoscope 1991;101:240–244.

52. Hordijk GJ, Brons EN. Carcinomas of the maxillary sinus: a retrospective study. Clin Otolaryngol 1985;10:285–288.

53. Kraus DH, Sterman B, Levin HL, Wood BG, Tucker H, Lavertu P. Factors influencing survival in ethmoid sinus cancer. Arch Otolaryngol Head Neck Surg 1992;118: 367–372.

54. Knegt PP, Dejong PC, Van Andel JG, De Boer MF, Eikenboom W, Van Der Schans E. Carcinoma of the paranasal sinuses: results of a prospective pilot study. Cancer 1985;56:57–62.

55. Sisson GA, Toriumi DM, Atiyah RA. Paranasal sinus malignancy: a comprehensive update. Laryngoscope 1989;99:143–148.

56. Lee F, Ogura JH. Maxillary sinus carcinoma. Laryngoscope 1981;91:133–139.

57. Rosenfeld DJ, Berenholz L, Glosgold M, Rao V, Spiegel J. Malignant neoplasms of the sphenoid sinus. Trans Pa Acad Ophtalmol Otolaryngol 1987;39:618–621.

29

Functional Endoscopic Sinus Surgery

Dean M. Clerico, MD, *David W. Kennedy,* MD,
and David Henick, MD

INTRODUCTION

Sinus surgery has undergone a dramatic change within the last 10 years owing in large part to the introduction of the nasal telescope. This device, along with the instrumentation developed to use with it, has permitted highly accurate diagnosis and effective treatment of chronic sinus disease. The key to diagnosing chronic or recurrent sinusitis is adequate visualization of the ostiomeatal complex (OMC). The importance of limited disease in the OMC as a cause of chronic and recurrent sinusitis has only recently gained widespread acceptance.

The nose faces the task of filtering inspired air, and the OMC becomes involved because the brunt of nasal air flow passes adjacent to this area *(1,2)*. A variety of particles, microbes, allergens, and tox-

ins found in ambient air are deposited near the narrow channels of the OMC with nasal breathing. It is not surprising, therefore, that inflammatory sinus disease frequently originates in the OMC. Goblet cell and glandular hyperplasia are seen in the mucosa of subjects with chronic sinusitis *(3),* resulting in mucosal thickening, ostial obstruction, and retention of secretions. A vicious cycle ensues in which these pathologic changes progress and clinical sinusitis results.

THEORY OF THE PATHOGENESIS OF CHRONIC SINUSITIS

Several early investigators remarked on the importance of the ethmoid area in triggering disease in the frontal and maxillary sinuses *(4–6)*. Despite these reports, sinus surgery focused mainly on the larger "dependent" sinuses (frontal and maxillary), from where symptoms appeared to

From: *Diseases of the Sinuses* (M. E. Gershwin and G. A. Incaudo, eds.), ©1996 Humana Press Inc., Totowa, NJ.

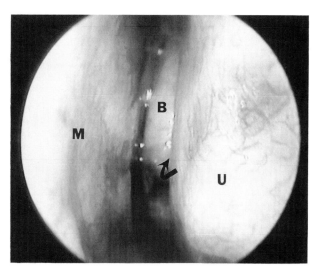

Fig. 1. Endoscopic view into the left middle meatus; M, middle turbinate; U, uncinate process; B, ethmoid bulla; curved arrow, ethmoid infundibulum.

Table 1
Range of Indications for Endoscopic Sinonasal Surgery

Inflammatory disease
    Chronic sinus disease
    Recurrent acute sinusitis
    Acute sinusitis with complications
    Sinonasal polyposis
    Sinus mucoceles
    Allergic fungal sinusitis
    Antrochoanal polyp
    Adenoid hypertrophy
Neurorhinologic disorders
    Rhinopathic headaches refractory to medical therapy
    Vasomotor rhinitis (vidian neurectomy)
Neoplastic disease
    Inverting papilloma
    Skull base tumors
    Pituitary tumors
    Paranasal sinus osteoma
    Sinonasal neoplasms
Orbital indications
    Dysthyroid ophthalmopathy
    Optic nerve compression
    Nasolacrimal duct obstruction
Reparative/restorative indications
    Cerebrospinal fluid rhinorrhea
    Epistaxis
    Submucus resection/septal spur resection (*see* Fig. 3)
    Choanal atresia/stenosis
    Intranasal foreign body

originate and where standard roentgenograms usually identified disease.

In the 1970s, Messerklinger *(7)* performed nasal endoscopic studies of mucociliary clearance that have formed the basis for modern endoscopic sinus surgery. He observed that where two opposing mucosal surfaces contact each other, disruption of normal mucociliary transport occurs at that point, leading to mucous stasis. He further identified the narrow channels of the ethmoid infundibulum and middle meatus as the primary sites of involvement in sinusitis (*see* Fig. 1). Earlier, Naumann had recognized the importance of this area and termed it the ostiomeatal unit *(8)*. More recent studies have confirmed that a small maxillary os (cross-sectional area below 5 mm^2) is a risk factor for the development of sinusitis *(9)*. OMC obstruction, with consequent blockage of both sinus ventilation and mucociliary drainage, is thus the final common pathway in the development of sinusitis in the majority of cases. Rarely, dental disease will cause persistent inflammation and sinus infection in the presence of a patent OMC.

Therapeutic intervention, whether medical or surgical, must therefore be aimed at relieving ostial obstruction. The trend away from radical extirpation of reversibly diseased sinus mucosa began in 1985 with Kennedy's reports on functional endoscopic sinus surgery (FESS) *(10,11)*. The primary goal of the surgery is to restore normal sinus ventilation, drainage, and ultimately function with minimal removal of reversibly diseased mucosa. FESS should also be distinguished from other endoscopic approaches that routinely sacrifice normal mucosa and structures (such as the middle turbinate).

INDICATIONS

The primary indication for FESS is chronic or recurrent acute sinusitis that is refractory to medical therapy. There is an evolving role for FESS in the management of acute sinusitis with orbital complications (such as subperiosteal abscess and orbital abscess), but this should be undertaken only by an experienced and skilled endoscopic surgeon. Extended indications for FESS include mucoceles and mucopyoceles, certain headache symptoms, sinus and skull base tumors, cerebrospinal fluid (CSF) leaks, orbital decompression, optic nerve decompression, and others (*see* Table 1).

Surgery is indicated for patients with chronic sinusitis who fail to improve significantly despite optimal medical therapy. Chronic sinusitis is defined as persistent mucosal disease that has not resolved with medical therapy and involves radiographic mucosal thickening of the sinuses, lasting a minimum of 8 wk in adults and 12 wk in children *(12)*. Optimal medical management should include prolonged courses of broad-spectrum oral antibiotics, nasal and/or oral steroids, and possibly antihistamines (in patients with proven atopy) or decongestants. The duration of such therapy should be at least 3 or 4 wk, with several such courses usually initiated. Recurrent acute sinusitis is defined as at least four episodes per year of acute sinusitis, with each episode lasting at least 10 d, in association with persistent mucosal abnormalities on CT 4 wk after medical therapy *(12)*. In cases of recurrent sinusitis, the CT may sometimes be "normal" (no mucosal disease) if it is obtained after optimal medical therapy, but surgery may still be indicated if there is significant evidence that bony variations or abnormalities of the OMC are predisposing the patient to recurrent symptoms. Conversely, mucosal abnormalities may be found in areas unrelated to symptomatology, so it is important to comment that CT findings alone should not dictate operative intervention.

With accurate diagnosis of OMC pathology by nasal endoscopy and coronal CT scanning, the minimally invasive approach afforded by FESS offers a legitimate option to constant or recurrent antibiotic use in the setting of recurrent acute sinusitis.

Sinonasal polyposis (*see* Fig. 2) frequently requires both medical and surgical treatment to achieve clinical improvement. The goal of FESS in these cases is to remove the polyp mass, and re-establish sinus drainage and ventilation. Complete surgical cure of polyposis, particularly when extensive disease is present, is unlikely. This is because many polyp patients appear to have an underlying mucosal hyperreactivity and tendency to reform polyps. Although polyps tend to recur after sinus surgery, redevelopment of symptomatic disease can be avoided by careful long-term endoscopic follow-up in the office setting. Local debridement and cleaning, long-term medical management with topical corticosteroids, intermittent courses of antibiotics, and occasional use of oral corticosteroids all play key roles in abating symptomatic disease in the polyp patient. Serial office endoscopy is essential in providing objective assessment of patients' responses to medical therapy.

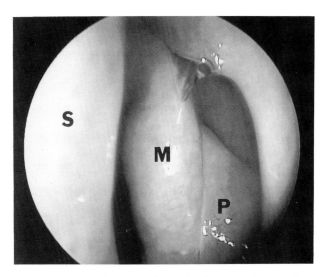

Fig. 2. Patient with a normal anterior rhinoscopic exam but who on diagnostic nasal endoscopy was found to have a polyp (P) emanating from the lateral surface of the middle turbinate (M). S, septum.

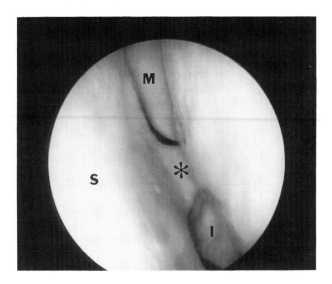

Fig. 3. Endoscopic view of a left septal spur (asterisk) impinging on the lateral nasal wall between the inferior (I) and middle (M) turbinates. S, septum.

The endoscopic approach is being utilized increasingly in the management of acute frontal sinusitis refractory to medical therapy *(13,14)*, a situation in which the external trephination procedure has traditionally been employed. Advantages of endoscopic management include a more physiologic and long-lasting treatment, which is less invasive and disfiguring than trephination, with less potential for recurrence.

In cases of acute sinusitis with periorbital or intraorbital complications, FESS can address the sinus infection as well as provide access to the medial orbital wall (lamina papyracea). Resecting the lamina will expose the periorbital fascia, which can be incised either to decompress orbital cellulitis or drain an orbital abscess. It should be emphasized that this procedure is not considered routine, and should be attempted only by skilled and experienced endoscopists. The traditional approach (external ethmoidectomy with orbital decompression and drainage) to the surgical management of orbital complications with acute sinus disease is still recommended for the vast majority of otorhinolaryngologists.

Frontal and ethmoid mucoceles are best managed, at least initially, with endoscopic surgery (15). Frequently, mucoceles erode bone, and intracranial extension can occur. The mucocele membrane typically is firmly adherent to the underlying dura and difficult to detach. In such cases, endoscopic marsupialization from below is both safe and effective. In addition, the patient is spared the morbidity associated with craniotomy.

The diagnosis of allergic fungal sinusitis should be considered in patients who do not respond to conventional medical therapy. The diagnosis is suspected on the basis of the presence of thick, brown (peanut-butter consistency) nasal secretions, the presence of fungal elements on stains or positive identification of organisms on culture, areas of increased (on computed tomography [CT]) or decreased (on magnetic resonance imaging [MRI]) signal intensity on imaging studies, and history of hypersensitivity to fungal antigens. Optimal therapy for allergic fungal sinusitis requires endoscopic surgical debridement (16) and careful, long-term endoscopic follow-up, along with oral corticosteroids and occasionally oral antifungal therapy.

Endoscopic sinus surgery has been employed rather successfully in the management of refractory headache syndromes (see Chapter 21 and refs. 17–19) in some cases, even when the initial diagnosis was a primary vascular or tension-type headache. Such patients may have either bony anatomical variations/abnormalities, or occult mucosal disease evident on CT of the sinuses. In all cases of headache with limited sinus symptomatology, surgery must be considered the treatment of last resort, and the risks of FESS weighed against the possible benefits.

Small neoplasms of the ethmoid roof, anterior skull base, medial orbital wall, or any accessible

sinus are amenable to endoscopic resection. Perhaps more importantly, office nasal endoscopy permits excellent visualization of the operative site, allowing for earlier detection of recurrent tumor growth in lesions, such as inverting papilloma, which has a high recurrence rate. In the management of skull base lesions, the endoscopic approach may spare the patient a craniotomy and/or more radical extirpative procedures.

CSF rhinorrhea may be idiopathic, iatrogenic, or posttraumatic. If a CSF leak results from prior endoscopic surgery, the most common site of injury is along the vertical lamella of the cribriform plate proximate to the anterior ethmoid artery. The bone is exceptionally thin in this area and the dura tightly adherent. Because of the anatomic orientation of the right-handed surgeon, this complication most commonly occurs on the patient's right side. The dural defect in these cases tends to be limited, and repair of the defect with a free tissue graft (septal mucoperichondrium or temporalis fascia) via the endoscopic approach is usually sufficient. Blunt trauma typically causes a more extensive dural defect, and closure may require several layers of support, perhaps with a free bone or cartilage graft along with a local pedicled mucosal flap. Craniotomy may be required for larger defects. The endoscopic management of skull base defects avoids the significant morbidity associated with a craniotomy.

In the surgical treatment of dysthyroid ophthalmopathy, endoscopic orbital decompression compares favorably with traditional techniques. Warren et al. (20), in a review of 305 patients undergoing traditional Walsh-Ogura decompression, noted an average ocular recession of 4 mm. Desanto (21) reported an average recession of 5.5 mm in 200 patients in whom transantral decompression was performed. Kennedy et al. (22), in their initial series, achieved a 4.7-mm recession with endoscopic decompression alone and a 5.7-mm recession with the endoscopic approach combined with lateral orbitotomy.

The nasal telescope permits superior visualization of the orbital apex via the posterior ethmoid sinuses, an area often not fully accessible by the external or transantral routes. This allows for optimal posterior orbit and optic nerve decompression in cases of traumatic optic neuropathy.

Dacryocystitis and lacrimal obstruction requiring surgical intervention can also be managed

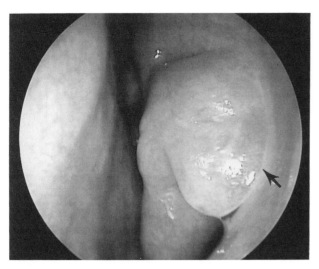

Fig. 4. Demonstration of a polyp growing from the anterior face of the left middle turbinate where it is in contact with the lateral nasal wall (arrow).

endoscopically, and encouraging preliminary results have been reported *(23)*.

A variety of other conditions can be addressed with the endoscopic approach (listed in Table 1).

DIAGNOSTIC NASAL ENDOSCOPY

Perhaps the chief benefit gained from the use of nasal telescopes is the ability to diagnose ethmoid disease and follow the course and/or resolution of sinus disease in the office setting (*see* Fig. 4). On initial patient presentation, a thorough and careful history is obtained. Since chronic sinusitis can masquerade as a variety of other disorders, specific inquiry is made not only about nasal congestion, discharge, and recurrent infection, but also about headaches, visual disturbance, fatigue, cough, halitosis, ear and dental pain, smell and taste disorder, allergy, immune dysfunction, asthma, bronchitis, and systemic disease. A complete otolaryngologic—head and neck—exam should precede the endoscopic examination.

Diagnostic nasal endoscopy is then performed with the patient in the upright or semisitting position. Each nasal cavity is sprayed with a topical decongestant and anesthetic. The 30°, 4.0-mm scope is most commonly employed, but occasionally an extremely narrow nasal cavity may necessitate using the 2.7-mm scope. The "three-pass" technique is advocated (*see* Fig. 5). The scope is first introduced into the nasal cavity along the floor

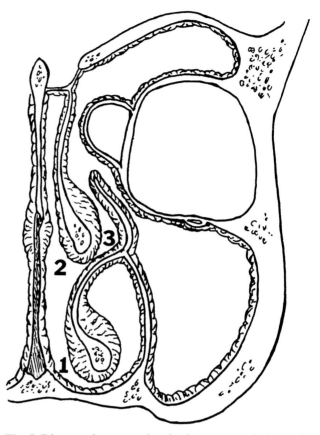

Fig. 5. Diagram demonstrating the three-pass technique of diagnostic nasal endoscopy. 1, the first pass of the telescope is along the floor of the nose between the septum and the inferior turbinate; 2, the second pass of the scope is below and medial to the middle turbinate; 3, the third pass is lateral to the middle turbinate into the middle meatus.

of the nose, medial to and below the inferior turbinate, and gradually advanced back to the nasopharynx. The examiner should note any inferior turbinate mucosal abnormality, the presence and character of secretions, the adenoids, and Eustachian tube. A second pass of the scope is then made between the middle and inferior turbinates. The middle meatus (anteriorly) and sphenoethmoid recess (posteriorly) can thus be noted. Frequently the sphenoid ostium can be seen above the posterior nasal choana within the sphenoethmoid recess, and isolated sphenoid or posterior ethmoid disease may be identified in this manner. The third pass of the scope is lateral to the middle turbinate into the middle meatus. This manipulation is frequently more uncomfortable for the patient, so additional anesthesia (4% cocaine solution of a cotton-tipped applicator) may be required. Within the middle meatus, the components of the OMC (uncinate process, ethmoid infundibulum, ethmoid bulla) can be visualized, and pathologic changes, such as hypertrophic mucosa, polyps, and purulent secretions, can be noted.

On the basis of clinical history and nasal endoscopic findings, the physician typically prescribes a course of therapy. A prolonged regimen of antibiotic therapy (usually 3–4 wk or longer) with topical nasal steroids is commonly recommended for patients with signs and symptoms of chronic or recurrent sinusitis. Oral systemic steroids may be prescribed if polyps are identified or if mucosal edema is excessive. Antihistamines are reserved for patients with proven atopy. On return visit, nasal endoscopy is again performed at which time the physician assesses the patient's response to therapy. Nasal endoscopy thus proves more sensitive than plain films and more cost-effective than repeat CT scanning in the diagnosis of ethmoid/OMC disease.

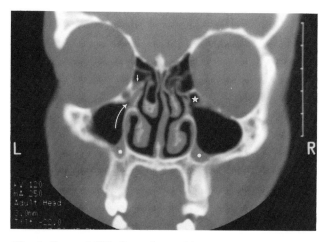

Fig. 6. Coronal CT of a patient with recurrent acute sinusitis demonstrating bimaxillary fluid (asterisks), with OMC opacification on the left (curved arrow), most likely secondary to an air–fluid level in the ethmoid bulla (small arrow). A small Haller cell (star) is most likely responsible for the OMC obstruction on the right.

RADIOGRAPHIC EVALUATION

Patients are selected for radiographic evaluation based on their response to medical therapy. Medical responders typically return to the office for periodic endoscopic exams, and the need for CT imaging is avoided. Patients whose symptoms recur following cessation of medical therapy and patients who do not respond to medical therapy are selected for CT evaluation. Patients may have normal endoscopic examinations, but if symptoms are persistent, CT is indicated. The role of imaging is therefore to define the paranasal sinus anatomy and identify regional disease in medical nonresponders. CT evaluation is reserved primarily for patients who are considered surgical candidates based on their clinical course and nasal endoscopic findings.

Plain films may be of some benefit in evaluating acute sinusitis, but since they fail to reveal the anatomic detail in the anterior ethmoid/OMC region, they are not useful in diagnosing chronic sinusitis. Coronal CT scanning (without contrast) with window width/length ratios to optimize bony detail is the imaging modality of choice (24). Axial views are occasionally useful in planning revision surgery, especially in the frontal and sphenoid regions. MRI does not define the fine bony architecture of the ethmoid labyrinth well, but is useful in evaluating paranasal sinus neoplasms. MRI should also be performed prior to surgery in all cases where sinus opacification occurs in an area adjacent to a skull base

defect. In this situation, MRI is helpful in distinguishing the nature of the soft tissue, and helps to exclude the possibility of a meningocele or encephalocele.

With rare exceptions, sinus CT should be obtained only after a prolonged course of medical therapy, so that abnormal radiographic findings have surgical significance. Debate continues over what constitutes "maximal medical therapy," but a minimum of 3 wk is reasonable in patients with recurrent sinusitis, and several such courses may be required in patients with chronic disease. These guidelines are modified for patients who develop complications of sinusitis while on medical therapy or intolerable side effects of the medications themselves. Antibiotic prophylaxis may have some value in patients with chronic and recurrent sinusitis (25). The CT will define areas of mucosal thickening, ostial obstruction, anatomic variations or abnormalities, and air–fluid levels that may indicate persistent or recurrent inflammatory disease (see Fig. 6). Care must be taken when interpreting sinus CTs, since 24–39% of the asympotomatic general public will display mucosal changes on CT (26). No patient is considered a surgical candidate on the basis of CT findings alone, but rather based on the combined information gathered from careful history, nasal endoscopic examination, response to medical therapy, and CT. A review of the radiographic anatomy of this region is warranted before further discussion of surgical technique.

RADIOGRAPHIC ANATOMY
OF THE LATERAL NASAL WALL
AND ETHMOID LABYRINTH

The coronal sinus CT is read in an anterior-to-posterior direction, starting with the frontal sinus. Complete absence of the frontal sinus is common and should be considered a variation of normal. The frontal recess is the drainage pathway of secretions that exit the frontal sinus through the frontal ostium and communicates with the ethmoid infundibulum inferiorly. The former term, "frontonasal duct," is no longer accepted terminology, since, in most cases, the anatomy of the area resembles a recess more than an actual tubular structure. Although the agger nasi and dome of ethmoid (defined later) form its anterior and posterior borders, the medial limit of the frontal recess is the superior-most attachment of the middle turbinate. This anatomical arrangement may explain why there is a tendency toward frontal recess stenosis after middle turbinate resection (27).

The frontal os has been described as the waist of an hourglass (28), with the dilated chambers of the frontal sinus above and frontal recess below the os. Mucociliary transport in the frontal sinus is unique in that the mucus recirculates within the sinus before exiting, and secretions at the frontal recess can even be transported into the sinus (29).

The agger nasi is defined as the eminence on the lateral wall of the nose just anterosuperior to the superior attachment of the middle turbinate. It is usually pneumatized, in which case an agger nasi cell(s) is present. This cell is the most anterior and superior of the anterior ethmoid cells. Its position near the ostium and floor of the frontal sinus gives it considerable significance in frontal sinus disease.

The OMC consists of bony structures (uncinate process, ethmoid bulla, middle turbinate) and air spaces (frontal recess, infundibulum, middle meatus, and the ostia of the anterior ethmoid, maxillary, and frontal sinuses). The uncinate articulates with the lacrimal bone anteriorly and occasionally with the inferior turbinate bone inferiorly. The uncinate usually is confluent with the agger nasi superiorly, often ascending superomedially to form the medial wall of an agger nasi cell. The uncinate courses posteriorly at its inferior portion, attaching to the membranous tissue of the posterior fontanelle. This fontanelle forms most of the medial wall of the maxillary sinus.

The ethmoid bulla is the largest, most consistently found anterior ethmoid cell(s). The bulla lies immediately posterior to the uncinate process, separated only by the three-dimensional, funnel-shaped space known as the ethmoid infundibulum. The two-dimensional distance between the uncinate anteriorly and the ethmoid bulla posteriorly is known as the hiatus semilunaris, which leads into the infundibulum situated more anterolaterally. The bulla is attached to the medial orbital wall (lamina papyracea) and occasionally to the skull base superiorly.

The middle turbinate forms the medial border of the ethmoid sinus system. Its superior bony attachment is with the lateral edge of the cribriform plate, whereas it has mucosal connections with the lateral nasal wall via the medial aspect of the agger nasi. Various anatomic variations of the middle turbinate have been described, including paradoxic curvature, partial or superior pneumatization (interlamellar cell), complete or inferior pneumatization (concha bullosa), and others. These variations in middle turbinate anatomy probably have pathologic significance (30).

Posterior to the ethmoid bulla is the basal lamella, the posterolateral attachment of the middle turbinate. This structure is usually a single partition of bone, but can occasionally be pneumatized and thus have an anterior and posterior wall. It articulates laterally with the medial orbital wall and with the ascending process of the palatine bone, which forms the posterolateral wall of the maxillary sinus. The lamella has an oblique vertical orientation, so that it lies more anteriorly at its superior aspect and more posteriorly at its inferior aspect. It usually does not articulate fully with the skull base. The basal lamella is the partition separating the anterior from the posterior ethmoid chambers.

The posterior ethmoid cells are larger and fewer in number than the anterior ethmoids. They are bounded medially by the superior turbinate, posteriorly by the anterior sphenoid wall, superiorly by the skull base, and laterally by the orbital wall. The superior turbinate may have a lamella by which it attaches to the medial orbital wall. The medial wall of the orbit courses more medially in this posterior region, and occasionally the bony canal housing the optic nerve can be identified in the posterior ethmoid. If a posterior ethmoid cell pneumatizes posteriorly into the sphenoid bone or lateral to the optic nerve, an Onodi cell is said to exist. The most posterolateral ethmoid cell typically is a pyramid-shaped sinus, with the wider base anterior and the apex posterior. The anterior face of the sphenoid sinus and sphenoid os are usually medial and somewhat inferior to this cell. The anterior wall of the sphenoid typically is convex and bulges forward anteriorly in this area.

The natural ostium of the sphenoid sinus is located medial to the superior turbinate and thus lies outside the ethmoid labyrinth. The floor of the sphenoid sinus lies at a level considerably below the ostium, so that drainage of secretions is not passive or gravity-dependent, but depends on active mucociliary clearance. Sphenoid sinus pneumatization patterns have been described as either presellar (or conchal), sellar, or postsellar *(31)*, depending on the relation of the back wall of the sinus to the sella turcica. The lateral walls of the sphenoid contain the indentations of the carotid artery and optic nerve.

The natural ostium of the maxillary sinus is located within the ethmoid infundibulum. It usually cannot be seen without removing the uncinate process. Accessory ostia, probably indicative of previous sinus disease, typically can be seen endoscopically, and occasionally radiographically, within the fontanelle posterior to the natural ostium. The medial wall of the maxillary sinus is largely devoid of bone, being comprised mostly of membranous tissue known as the posterior fontanelle. The small portion of membranous wall located anterior to the natural ostium is termed the anterior fontanelle. Mucus in the maxillary sinus is propelled by active mucociliary activity out through the natural ostium, which has a superior location along the medial wall of the sinus. If an ethmoid cell is located along the roof of the maxillary sinus within the antrum, a Haller cell is said to exist.

The anterior ethmoidal neurovascular bundle traverses the skull base in a horizontal direction and is an important landmark during endoscopic surgery. The point at which the anterior ethmoid artery enters the cranial cavity through the vertical (or lateral) lamella of the cribriform plate is the thinnest area of the entire skull base *(32)*. Posterior to this point, the skull base has a horizontal-oblique orientation (when viewed sagittally). Anterior to the anterior ethmoid nerve and artery, the skull base slopes upward in a vertical-oblique course. The bone of the skull base in this area is known as the dome of the ethmoid. The space between the

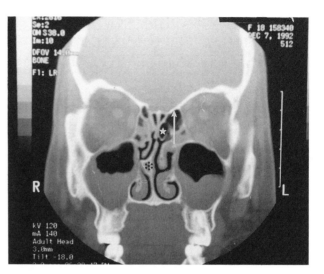

Fig. 7. CT of a patient with bilateral ethmoid and maxillary sinusitis and septal spur (asterisk). The left superior turbinate is pneumatized (star). The arrow indicates the height of the posterior ethmoid chamber as determined from the roof of the maxillary sinus.

dome of the ethmoid posteriorly and the agger nasi cell anteriorly is the frontal recess.

There are a number of key anatomical features on CT that the endoscopic surgeon must review in each patient undergoing FESS, including:

1. The shape and slope of the skull base, especially the angle that the lateral lamella of the cribriform makes with the horizontal portion of the cribriform plate;
2. The thickness of the skull base, including the presence of congenital or iatrogenic dehiscences of the skull base and medial orbital wall;
3. The vertical height of the posterior ethmoid labyrinth relative to the roof of the maxillary sinus in its medial portion (*see* Fig. 7), and whether an Onodi cell is present. An Onodi cell is a posterior ethmoid cell that has pneumatized into the sphenoid bone and/or sinus, in close relation to the optic nerve;
4. The relationship of the sphenoid intersinus septum to the lateral wall structures of the sphenoid (carotid artery and optic nerve);
5. The presence of atelectasis of the infundibulum or hypoplasia of the maxillary sinus, which would make inadvertent orbital entry more likely;
6. The drainage and ventilation pathway of the frontal sinus, which in most cases is immediately lateral to the attachment of the middle turbinate; and

7. The presence of a Haller cell, the partitions of which may need to be excised to ensure adequate drainage of the maxillary sinus.

It should be emphasized that this is not an exhaustive listing, and the surgeon should thoroughly and carefully examine the patient's CT scan before commencing the procedure. The CT scan should also be present in the operating room during the surgery in the event the surgeon needs to refer back to it.

FESS

FESS aims to remove the source of sinus disease while preserving mucosa and restoring normal physiology to the sinonasal tract. Accordingly, FESS addresses primarily ethmoid disease. Other forms of functional ethmoid surgery may be performed without the aid of endoscopes (i.e., intranasal ethmoidectomy), and other forms of endoscopic surgery may be performed although not necessarily functional. The technique of FESS will be discussed below.

Preceding the case, the patient's CT scan should be in the operating room on the view box, and the surgeon should thoroughly familiarize him/herself with the radiographic findings. The CT should be reviewed not only for the extent of mucosal disease, but for areas of bone erosion, varying tissue density indicating possible fungal disease, and anatomical landmarks. Anatomical variations, such as concha bullosa, Haller cells, and Onodi cells, must be noted in order to gain access to diseased areas effectively and safely. If the patient has had previous sinus surgery, the integrity of the skull base and orbital wall must be noted to avoid a potential complication. Two additional areas of importance are the lateral lamella of the cribriform plate and the vertical height of the posterior ethmoid sinus. The lateral lamella of the cribriform varies both in its vertical height and the angle at which it meets the horizontal lamella of the cribriform plate. Surgical trauma to this area is more likely if this angle exceeds 90°. Another common area where the skull base may be interrupted and CSF leak may occur is in the posterior ethmoid. This is probably because the skull base slopes slightly downward (inferiorly) in this region. For this reason, the surgeon should note the height of the posterior ethmoid before surgery. This is the distance on the CT from the roof of the maxillary sinus at its posterior wall (where the basal lamella inserts) to the roof of the posterior ethmoid sinus.

FESS can be performed under either local or general anesthesia. Local anesthesia with iv sedation and anesthesia monitoring is preferred by the authors in most cases, since this maximizes the safety of the procedure. The periorbita and skull base are generally more pain-sensitive structures, and verbal feedback from the patient during the procedure may be valuable. Additionally, should the patient develop an intraorbital hemorrhage during the surgery, avoiding general anesthesia allows the monitoring of the patient's vision on a minute-by-minute basis. Slight hypotension is helpful in minimizing troublesome bleeding during the procedure. The awake patient typically is fitted with earphones and listens to relaxing music during the procedure. This often will effectively divert attention away from the sound of ethmoid partitions being removed, which many patients report as the most unpleasant aspect of the whole surgical experience.

The nasal cavities are first decongested with a topical spray and then anesthetized with topical anesthetic (cocaine powder) using cotton applicators under endoscopic visualization. Three or four applicators are placed in the areas where injection of local anesthetic will be administered (see below and Fig. 8). Although the applicators are left in the nasal cavity for 5–10 min, a transpalatal sphenopalatine block via the greater palatine foramen is performed. This is more easily accomplished with the patient awake and lightly sedated, since an orotracheal tube will make this procedure more difficult. The applicators are then removed, and the lateral nasal wall is injected with local anesthetic (1 or 2% lidocaine with epinephrine 1:100,000). Injection sites are placed out of the direct path of the scope, so bleeding onto the scope lens will be minimized. Typical injection sites include:

1. The agger nasi (above the anterosuperior attachment of middle turbinate);
2. Just anterior to the uncinate process at the superior attachment of the inferior turbinate;
3. Through the basal lamella of the middle turbinate along the lateral wall in the region of the sphenopalatine ganglion; and
4. In the posterior aspect of the septum at its junction with the face of the sphenoid.

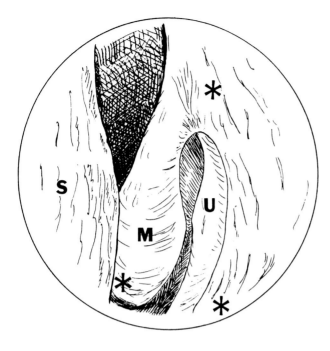

Fig. 8. Injection points for local anesthesia indicated by asterisks. S, septum; M, middle turbinate; U, uncinate.

If resection of any portion of the middle turbinate is planned, it is then injected in its anteromedial and inferior region. Waiting 5–10 min at this point will result in improved hemostasis for the rest of the case. An absorbent packing (Kennedy Intranasal Sinus Sponge, Merocel Corporation, Mystic, CT) is placed in the choana/nasopharynx to prevent aspiration of blood or tissue during the dissection.

The 0° telescope is used at the outset and for as much of the dissection as possible, since there is less distortion than with angled scopes. Initially, the procedure is performed in an anterior-to-posterior direction. In revision cases where normal landmarks are missing, starting posteriorly at the sphenoid os region and working forward anteriorly, may facilitate safe dissection in some instances. It may be necessary first to medialize the middle turbinate gently with a Freer or Cottle elevator to expose the uncinate process. If a concha bullosa is present, a vertical incision down the anterior face of middle turbinate is made, and the lateral lamella of the concha is resected. If either purulent secretions or suspicious-looking tissue is seen at any time throughout the operation, appropriate cultures or biopsies are taken.

The uncinectomy is then performed with a sickle knife, starting superiorly in the groove where the uncinate joins the lateral nasal wall. Care

should be taken not to make this incision too anteriorly, since the erectile tissue on the lateral nasal wall in this region will bleed excessively, and there is a somewhat greater risk of injuring the nasolacrimal duct. As the incision is carried inferiorly, the surgeon should attempt to deflect the uncinate bone medially with the knife, bringing it away from the lateral wall and making its removal with a straight forceps easier to accomplish. Since the uncinate is a crescent-shaped structure that curves posteriorly in its inferior aspect, the uncinectomy incision must be carried more posteriorly in this region. The uncinate process is then removed with a Blakesly-Weil forceps. It should be grasped superiorly and the forceps rotated so that the remnant of superior uncinate mucosa will not be pulled away from the lateral nasal wall (clockwise on the left side, counterclockwise on the right). If the incision is made too far laterally, orbital fat may be exposed. Should this occur, the surgeon must not traumatize the fat, since this could lead to bleeding within the orbit and possibly orbital hematoma. The surgeon should briefly discontinue the dissection and examine the patient's eye. If no orbital complication is apparent, the surgeon may proceed with further dissection posterior to the herniated orbital fat, taking great care not to induce further trauma to that region.

The uncinectomy exposes the ethmoid infundibulum and ethmoid bulla. The natural ostium of the maxillary sinus is usually not visible with a 0° scope at this point, so the middle meatal antrostomy is deferred until later in the case after changing to a 30° scope. The ethmoid bulla is penetrated with the straight forceps, and its entire bony wall removed. Dissection should extend to the medial orbital wall along the lateral aspect of the ethmoid cavity. Other smaller and less consistently found cells may be present, and their partitions are taken down to reveal the basal lamella. The basal lamella can be most easily identified by following the inferior margin of the middle turbinate posteriorly. The basal lamella should be penetrated at a sufficiently high level to leave an adequate inferior strut (thus preventing collapse of the middle turbinate against the medial orbital wall), but at a level sufficiently low to avoid traumatizing the skull base. This level roughly corresponds to the roof of the maxillary sinus. Septations and diseased mucosa in the posterior ethmoid are removed, while attempting to leave the mucosa on the skull base and orbital wall intact. Through-biting or cutting instruments can facilitate this, so that less healthy mucosa is inadvertently pulled away than with traditional ethmoid forceps. Care must be exercised when dissected along the lateral aspect of the posterior ethmoid, since the bony canal housing the optic nerve may be dehiscent in this area. The last (most posterior) posterior ethmoid cell typically has a pyramidal configuration, with the apex pointing posteriorly. In contrast to the relative concavity of this posterior ethmoid cell, the anterior wall of the sphenoid sinus typically is convex and bulges somewhat anteriorly.

The superior turbinate is located medially within the posterior ethmoid cavity. It may have one of three configurations:

1. Existing as a free-standing turbinate separate from the true posterior ethmoid cells;
2. Pneumatized similar to a concha bullosa; or
3. Existing as a single lamella of bone, but forming the medial wall of a posterior ethmoid cell.

In this latter case, the superior turbinate will have a horizontal lamella, situated just posterior to the basal lamella, which articulates with the medial orbital wall. Identifying the anterior face of the superior turbinate is useful at this point, since it ultimately attaches to the anterior face of the sphenoid sinus. The natural ostium of the sphenoid is located medial to the superior turbinate, between the turbinate and the septum. The sphenoid is safely entered once the os is identified. The anterior sphenoid wall is removed, usually with a rotating sphenoid punch, being careful that the mucosa on the inner aspect of the wall does not prolapse back into the sinus. The size of the sphenoidostomy depends in part on the presence and extent of disease. The surgeon should keep in mind that even when there is no overt sphenoid disease, blood and secretions will accumulate in the sinus postoperatively. The sphenoidostomy should therefore be large enough for the surgeon to gain access for suctioning and debridement in the postoperative period and should communicate with the sphenoid natural ostium. The lateral wall of the sphenoid sinus should never be manipulated so as to avoid injury to the optic nerve and carotid artery.

The skull base is easiest to identify at its junction with the anterior wall of the sphenoid sinus. From this point, the dissection is carried forward (anteriorly) along the skull base, with either the 0° or 30° scope. Although the posterior ethmoid neuro-

vascular bundle is not reliably seen, the anterior ethmoid artery and nerve can usually be seen in a bony canal coursing across the skull base more anteriorly. Dissection in this superomedial aspect of the ethmoid cavity must be performed with the utmost caution, since the skull base is thinnest and risk of CSF leak greatest in this region. Dissection is performed with the 45° upbiting forceps and punches.

Just anterior to the anterior ethmoid artery, the skull base turns upward where it is known as the dome of the ethmoid. Anterior to the bone that forms the dome of the ethmoid are the septations and spaces of the frontal recess. The mucosa in this area should be maximally preserved to prevent frontal recess stenosis. However, some dissection is usually necessary to visualize adequately the true ostium of the frontal sinus. The Kuhn-Bolger frontal recess curet and various through-cutting giraffe-style forceps are used in this area. The frontal os is usually located medial and anterior in the superior-most reaches of the frontal recess. Openings located more laterally toward the lamina papyracea usually correspond to supraorbital ethmoid cells. Every attempt is made to avoid traumatizing the mucosa around the frontal os. Grossly diseased mucosa in this area will often normalize once ethmoid disease is eradicated. If the frontal os cannot be visualized, an attempt to cannulate it with a curved suction tip or similar instrument should be made.

The 30° scope is then rotated to look laterally and inferiorly in the area of the natural ostium of the maxillary sinus. Any residual uncinate process that remains will prevent adequate visualization of the os and requires removal, usually with a back-biting forceps. The true os of the antrum is located far anteriorly, so that other more easily visualized openings along the medial wall of the sinus most likely represent accessory ostia. The tissue posterior to the natural ostium is the posterior fontanelle, which can be cut with endoscopic scissors at its junction with both the orbital wall and inferior turbinate. The posterior extent of these cuts is the back wall of the maxillary sinus, formed by the ascending process of the palatine bone. The size of the antrostomy should permit passage of a curved suction tip for postoperative care. The size of the antrostomy is probably secondary in importance to ensuring that it communicates with the natural ostium. Care must be taken not to injure the nasolacrimal duct, situated anterior to the natural ostium of the maxillary sinus. In general, the bone overlying the duct is thicker and less easily traumatized.

A powered rotary shaving device ("Hummer" Micro-debrider, Stryker Endoscopy, San Jose, CA) has recently been developed for endoscopic surgery that can facilitate dissection in many cases. The "Hummer" is most helpful in cases of polyps, but if the partitions of ethmoid bone are not too thick, a significant portion of the dissection can be performed with this device. The advantages of this instrument are that the oscillating blade is recessed so that it poses less risk to vital structures, there is continuous suction through the shaft so that the operative field can be cleared of blood while dissecting, and the cutting action removes tissue without damage to adjacent mucosa. Disadvantages include the lack of angulation to the cutting tips so that frontal recess dissection (where mucosal preservation is paramount) is not possible, the inability to palpate behind bony partitions to ensure safety, and the rather frequent clogging of the suction apparatus, which can delay the procedure.

The dissection is considered complete after the antrostomy is performed. A last look with the 0° scope to suction blood and perform a final inspection of the ethmoid cavity is suggested. The choanal sponge is removed, and the nasopharynx is suctioned. Packing is avoided unless persistent bleeding warrants it. In this case, an absorbent sponge coated with antibiotic ointment is usually placed in the ethmoid cavity overnight.

COMPLICATIONS

Because of the close proximity of the ethmoid sinuses to the eye and brain, injury to these structures during FESS is eminently possible. Fortunately, catastrophic complications involving these structures are rare and appear related to the severity of disease and experience of the surgeon (33). Minor complications are more common and include synechia formation, hemorrhage, epiphora, periorbital ecchymosis, and exacerbation of asthma.

Major complications include orbital hematoma, medial rectus injury, CSF leak with or without meningitis, carotid artery rupture, optic nerve injury, and death. In experienced hands, the complication rate from endoscopic surgery is comparable to or lower than that of traditional ethmoidectomy (34–37).

CSF leak is one of the most feared complications of FESS, but is often quite manageable at the time of the incident. If the surgeon notes a break in the skull base, CSF will often appear as a "black swirl" (the effect of any clear fluid when it intermingles with blood). If the defect is small, it can be repaired with a one-layer closure consisting of septal mucoperichondrium (most common) or temporalis fascia. Larger defects may require bone or cartilage to support prolapsing dura and brain. Most importantly, the surgeon must not simply pack the nose and hope the area will close spontaneously. This will only predispose the patient to meningitis or pneumocephalus (if the patient blows the nose). The first step in the endoscopic repair of a CSF leak is to ensure a clean, flat surface for the free graft by freeing mucosa from the perimeter of the bony defect. This will often require a bipolar cautery for meticulous hemostasis. A graft is then harvested, usually mucoperichondrium from the contralateral side of the nasal septum. The graft should be several times larger than the defect itself to ensure that the defect will not become exposed when the graft contracts during the postoperative healing phase. The graft is brought over the defect, with perichondrium contacting dura and the mucosal side toward the ethmoid cavity. Layers of microfibrillar collagen (Avitene™), absorbable cellulose (Gelfoam™), and sponge packing (Merocel™ sinus pack) are then placed below the graft for mild compression. Placement of a spinal drain should be considered to lower CSF pressure. Postoperatively, strict bed rest, stool softeners, and head-of-bed elevation should be ordered. The patient should undergo early postoperative CT evaluation if any possibility of an intracranial bleed exists.

There is no substitute for experience and thorough familiarity with anatomic landmarks to minimize the operative risk. Attendance at courses that feature cadaver dissection is a necessary prerequisite before performing FESS on patients. Initially, the novice surgeon should select less difficult cases (i.e., where minimal disease is present). In addition, the procedure should be aborted if the surgeon loses orientation or is uncertain of landmarks. Leaving disease untreated is preferable to causing a potentially catastrophic complication.

POSTOPERATIVE CARE

Postoperative debridement usually begins on the first postoperative day when the ethmoid sponge is

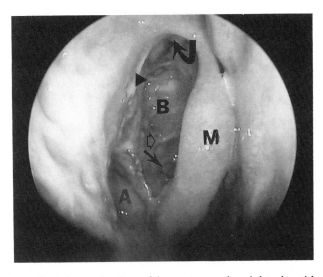

Fig. 9. Endoscopic view of the postoperative right ethmoid cavity with a 30° scope. M, middle turbinate; A, antrostomy; B, base of skull (ethmoid roof); straight arrow, sphenoid opening; open arrow, posterior ethmoid neurovascular bundle; arrowhead, anterior ethmoid neurovascular bundle; curved arrow, frontal recess.

removed. During the early postoperative period (the first 4–6 wk), the patient returns on a weekly basis for endoscopic examination and debridement of the ethmoid cavity. This is performed in the office setting under topical anesthesia only. Typically blood, mucus, clot, and fibrinous material are suctioned from the ethmoid cavity, sphenoid, and maxillary sinuses for the first 2–3 wk. Occasionally, loose pieces of ethmoid bone become apparent that may have been overlooked during surgery and should be removed with a forceps. This is especially important in the frontal recess, where such bony chips can become osteitic and promote inflammation and stenosis. Eschar, persistently inflamed mucosa and new scar are removed when present. Careful attention to the surgically created sinusotomies is mandated to prevent stenosis and ensure an optimal long-term result (*see* Fig. 9).

Further along in the postoperative period, the patient returns intermittently for routine examination. Since significant ethmoid disease can be present well before it causes symptoms *(35)*, minor manipulations in the office aimed at removing minimal disease can spare the patient major revision surgery.

The patient typically is kept on medical therapy in the early postoperative period until mucosal healing is complete, granulation tissue resolves,

Table 2
Staging for Chronic Sinusitis

Stage 1	Anatomic abnormalities
	All unilateral sinus disease
	Bilateral disease limited to ethmoid sinuses
Stage 2	Bilateral ethmoid disease with involvement of one dependent sinus
Stage 3	Bilateral ethmoid disease with involvement of two or more dependent sinuses on each side
Stage 4	Diffuse sinonasal polyposis

and no blood or mucus can be suctioned from any of the sinuses. Serial endoscopic examinations enable the physician to respond to objective disease and tailor appropriate medical therapy to the patient.

The need for long-term endoscopic follow-up cannot be overemphasized. Since FESS removes disease without changing the underlying inciting or precipitating factors, patients suffering from chronic sinus disease are at risk for developing recurrences with exposure to viruses, allergens, pollutants, and so on. Mucosal disease within the ethmoid cavity and dependent sinuses can be identified early and managed in the office under topical anesthesia in the majority of cases. Long-term endoscopic follow-up should therefore prove cost-effective in managing the chronic sinus patient, reducing the need for prescription medications and further surgery, decreasing morbidity from the disease, increasing patient productivity, and improving quality of life.

RESULTS

In capable hands, FESS is a highly effective surgical treatment for inflammatory sinus disease. Results indicate an 83–97.5% symptomatic improvement rate with 1–2 yr follow-up *(35,38–40)*. However, patient symptom improvement does not correlate well with resolution of mucosal disease. Kennedy found approx 45% of patients exhibited some evidence of mucosal disease at a mean of 18 mo after FESS, despite excellent subjective results *(35)*. The frontal recess was the most common site of persistent disease. The only significant factor that was found to be predictive of surgical prognosis was the preoperative extent of disease determined by CT scan *(see* Table 2).

Kennedy's findings highlight the importance of close endoscopic follow-up in the postoperative period. Postsurgical evaluation of results based only on patient symptomatology and anterior rhinoscopy is unreliable and should be abandoned. If late symptomatic recurrence is to be minimized, meticulous postoperative endoscopic evaluation to identify and treat objective disease is mandatory.

SUMMARY

FESS is a safe and effective means of managing surgical sinus disease. Perhaps more importantly, the use of the nasal telescope allows the physician to identify disease and monitor patient response objectively to medical and surgical therapy in the office setting. Visualization of the OMC is critical to the diagnosis of sinusitis. Coronal CT scanning greatly aids in determining the extent of disease and is useful for staging and prognostic purposes. Thorough familiarity with normal and abnormal sinus anatomy is a must for safe surgery.

REFERENCES

1. Cole P. Upper respiratory airflow. In: Proctor DF, Andersen I, eds. The Nose: Upper Airway Physiology and the Atmospheric Environment. Amsterdam: Elsevier Biomedical, 1982; pp. 163–189.
2. Wolfstorf J, Swift DL, Avery ME. Mist therapy reconsidered: an evaluation of the respiratory deposition of labelled water aerosols produced by jet and ultrasonic nebulizers. Pediatrics 1969;43:799–808.
3. Stammberger H. Endoscopic endonasal surgery—concepts in treatment of recurring rhinosinusitis. Part I. Anatomic and pathophysiological considerations. Otolaryngol Head Neck Surg 1986;94:143–147.
4. Hilding AC. Physiologic basis of nasal operations. Calif Med J 1950;94:147–156.
5. Messerklinger W. On the drainage of the normal frontal sinus of man. Acta Otolaryngol 1967;643:176–181.
6. Drettner B. The obstructed maxillary ostium. Rhinology 1967;5:100.
7. Messerklinger W. Endoscopy of the Nose. Baltimore, Urban and Schwarzenberg, 1978.
8. Naumann H. Pathologische anatoie der chronischen rhinitis und sinusitis. In: Proceedings VIII International Congress of Otorhinolaryngology. Amsterdam: Excerpta Medica, 1965; p. 80.
9. Aust R, Stierna P, Drettner B. Basic experimental studies of ostial patency and local metabolic environment of the maxillary sinus. Acta Otolaryngol (Stockh) 1994; Suppl. 515:7–11.
10. Kennedy DW, Zinreich SJ, Rosenbaum AE, Johns ME. Functional endoscopic sinus surgery: theory and diagnostic evaluation. Arch Otolaryngol 1985;111:576–582.
11. Kennedy DW. Functional endoscopic sinus surgery: technique. Arch Otolaryngol 1985;111:643–649.
12. Kennedy DW, ed. Sinus Disease: guide to First-Line Management. Darien, CT: Health Communications, 1994, p. 12.
13. Perkins JA, Morris MR. Treatment of acute frontal sinusitis: a survey of current therapeutic practices among members of the Northwest Academy of Otolaryngology. Am J Rhinol 1993;7:67–70.
14. Schaefer SK, Close LG. Endoscopic management of frontal sinus disease. Laryngoscope 1990;100:155–160.
15. Kennedy DW, Josephson JS, Zinreich SJ, Mattox DE, Goldsmith MM. Endoscopic sinus surgery for mucoceles: a viable alternative. Laryngoscope 1989;99:885–895.
16. Goldstein MF, Dunsky EH, Dvorin DJ, Lesser RW. Allergic fungal sinusitis: a review with four illustrated cases. Am J Rhinol 1994;8:13–18.
17. Clerico DM, Fieldman R. Referred headache of rhinogenic origin in the absence of sinusitis. Headache 1994;34:226–229.
18. Clerico DM. "Sinus headaches" reconsidered: referred cephalgia of rhinologic origin masquerading as refractory primary headaches. Headache 1995;35:185–192.
19. Chow J. Rhinologic headaches. Otolaryngol Head Neck Surg 1994;111:211–218.
20. Warren JD, Spector JG, Burde R. Long-term follow up and recent observations on 305 cases of orbital decompression for dysthyroid orbitopathy. Laryngoscope 1989;99:35–40.
21. Desanto LW. The total rehabilitation of Graves' ophthalmopathy. Laryngoscope 1980;90:1652–1678.
22. Kennedy DW, Goodstein ML, Miller NR, Zinreich SJ. Endoscopic transnasal orbital decompression. Arch Otolaryngol Head Neck Surg 1990;116:275–282.
23. Metson R. The endoscopic approach for revision dacryocystorhinostomy. Laryngoscope 1990;100:1344–1347.
24. Zinreich SJ, Kennedy DW, Rosenbaum AE, et al. Paranasal sinuses: CT imaging requirements for endoscopic surgery. Radiology 1987;163:769–775.
25. Gandhi A, Brodsky L, Ballow M. Benefits of antibiotic prophylaxis in children with chronic sinusitis: assessment of outcome predictors. Allergy Proc 1993;14:37–43.
26. Havas TE, Motbey JA, Gullane PJ. Prevalence of incidental abnormalities on computerized tomographic scans of the paranasal sinuses. Arch Otolaryngol 1988;114:856–859.
27. Swanson P. Lanza DC, Kennedy DW, Vining EM. The effect of middle turbinate resection upon the frontal sinus. Presented at the American Rhinologic Society, Palm Beach, May 1994.
28. Stammberger H. Functional Endoscopic Sinus Surgery. Philadelphia: B. C. Decker, 1991; p. 35.
29. Stammberger H. Functional Endoscopic Sinus Surgery. Philadelphia: B. C. Decker, 1991; p. 31.
30. Bolger WE, Butzin C, Parsons DS. CT analysis of bony and mucosal abnormalities for endoscopic sinus surgery. Laryngoscope 1991;101:56–71.
31. Lang J. Clinical Anatomy of the Nose, Nasal Cavity and Paranasal Sinuses. New York: Thieme Medical Publishers, 1989; p. 85.
32. Kainz J, Stammberger H. The roof of the anterior ethmoid—a place of least resistance in the skull base. Am J Rhinol 1990;4:191–199.
33. Stankiewicz JA. Complications of endoscopic intranasal ethmoidectomy. Laryngoscope 1987;97:1270.

34. Stammberger H. Endoscopic endonasal surgery—concepts in treatment of recurring rhinosinusitis. II. Surgical technique. Otolaryngol Head Neck Surg 1986;94:147–156.

35. Kennedy DW. Prognostic factors, outcomes and staging in ethmoid sinus surgery. Laryngoscope 1992;102(Suppl. 57):1–18.

36. Friedman WH, Katsantonis GP, Rosenblum BN, Cooper MH, Slavin R. Sphenoethmoidectomy: the case for ethmoid marsupialization. Laryngoscope 1986; 96:473–479.

37. Lawson W. The intranasal ethmoidectomy: evolution and an assessment of the procedure. Laryngoscope 1994;104 (Suppl. 64):1–49.

38. Hoffmann DF, May M, Mester RTR. Functional endoscopic sinus surgery—experience with the initial 100 patients. Am J Rhinol 1990;4:129–132.

39. Levine HL. Functional endoscopic sinus surgery: evaluation, surgery, and follow-up of 250 patients. Laryngoscope 1990;100:79–83.

40. Rice D. Endoscopic sinus surgery results at 2 year follow-up. Otolaryngol Head Neck Surg 1989;101:476–479.

30 Complications and Long-Term Sequelae of Functional Endoscopic Sinus Surgery in Children and Adults

Ian S. Mackay, FRCS
and Vincent L. Cumberworth, MB, CHB, BSC, FRCS

CONTENTS

INTRODUCTION

In 1929, Mosher (1) wrote,

If the ethmoidal labyrinth was placed in any other part of the body it would be an insignificant and harmless collection of bony cells. Placed where Nature put it, it has a number of major relationships so that the diseases and surgery of the labyrinth often lead to tragedy. It has been said that the ethmoidal operation is the easiest in surgery. So it is to the operator who lacks a surgical conscience. Theoretically, the operation is easy. In practice, however, it has proved one of the easiest operations with which to kill a patient.

From: *Diseases of the Sinuses* (M. E. Gershwin and G. A. Incaudo, eds.),
©1996 Humana Press Inc., Totowa, NJ.

Functional endoscopic sinus surgery (FESS) is an increasingly popular technique for the management of rhinosinusitis and nasal polyposis. Danielsen (2) described the most commonly encountered peroperative complications from FESS as ethmoidal artery injury (causing bleeding or increased intraorbital pressure risking optic nerve damage), penetration of the ethmoid roof or lamina papyracea, nasolacrimal duct damage on anterior widening of the middle meatal antrostomy, or optic nerve damage when operating in the posterior ethmoids or sphenoid.

Stankiewitz (3,4) has described a "learning curve" phenomenon, reporting a 5% incidence of major complications for his first 90 cases, which reduced to 0.7% for the subsequent 90. Many authors emphasize the importance of experienced course instruction and cadaver training to reduce the risk of complications. Rivron and Maran (5) described an FESS trainer to facilitate cadaver training in the technique, and Stanley (6) has suggested establishing endoscopic sinus laboratories akin to temporal bone laboratories. The importance of video facilities in teaching and monitoring junior staff cannot be overemphasized.

MINOR FESS COMPLICATIONS

May et al. (7), reported a 6.9% incidence of minor complications from a combined series of 2108 cases; a consecutive series of 461 patients at Charing Cross followed prospectively over 2 yr revealed a minor complication rate of 9.3%.

Synechiae

Kane (8) circulated a questionnaire to 100 otolaryngologists in Australia with a known interest in endoscopic nasal surgery: Most respondents reported adhesions as a common sequelae, some claiming benefit from stenting or from suturing the middle turbinate to the septum. Stammberger (9) observed synechiae between the head of the middle turbinate and the lateral nasal wall in 8% of 500 patients, but found that only 20% of these were actually symptomatic from their adhesions. Synechiae follow the creation of opposing wound surfaces and are particularly likely if anatomical variations narrow the entrance to the middle meatus. The adhesions were manageable endoscopically, and the insertion of a stent of silastic or other material usually eliminated them. He advocated scrupulous attention to atraumatic surgery and avoidance of injury to the mucosa of the middle turbinate rather than resecting it, which he felt could still lead to synechiae forming medially to obstruct the olfactory cleft as well as removing anatomical landmarks for future surgery.

From a review of 298 patients undergoing FESS, La Mear et al. (10) found that partial middle turbinectomy significantly reduced the rate of formation of synechiae and increased middle meatal antrostomy patency rates for patients with chronic sinusitis from 72 to 93%; differences for patients with polyposis were not statistically significant (83 and 89%, respectively). The absence of apparent complications from middle turbinectomy was attributed to the resection being subtotal with preservation of intranasal landmarks, only a small area

of loss of the ciliary epithelium, and the fact that the middle turbinate may be of less physiological significance than the inferior turbinate.

Symptomatic adhesions in the above series reported by May et al. (7) were principally attributed to lateralization of the middle turbinate and less commonly to stenosis of a surgically enlarged maxillary antrostomy.

A silicone stent designed to be inserted lateral to the middle turbinate has been reported by Salman (11) specifically to reduce the risk of adhesions or stenosis of the middle meatal antrostomy.

Nasolacrimal Duct

The nasolacrimal duct lies 3–6 mm anterior to the maxillary ostium in its course to the opening beneath the inferior turbinate at the Valve of Hasner. Serdahl et al. (12) reported eight cases of nasolacrimal duct obstruction requiring dacryocystorhinostomy after FESS; six were evident immediately and all within 2 wk. They suggested that anterior enlargement of the ostium should be limited to the thin lamellar bone of the anterior wall of the middle meatus and not continued anteriorly into the thick cortical bone surrounding the duct.

Kennedy et al. (13) reported 2 cases of epiphora from 117 middle meatal antrostomies and also advised limiting anterior bone removal with backbiting forceps. He reiterated that this complication can also follow inferior meatal antrostomy; Lund (14) quoted a 0.6% incidence of nasolacrimal duct damage from 320 external ethmoidectomies.

Intraoperative testing with fluorescein irrigation through a lacrimal catheter during 46 FESS procedures in 24 patients indicated occult injury (intranasal view of yellow dye at the middle meatus) in 7 (15%) of "lacrimal drainage systems." Injury occurred in 6 (25%) of the 24 patients, with bilateral injury in 1 case. However, postoperatively no patient had epiphora or dacryocystitis and later dye testing of 5 of these 6 patients showed that in only 2 did dye drain into the middle rather than the inferior meatus. Hence, although lacrimal apparatus injury may occur more commonly than expected, actual postoperative epiphora is rare (15).

In the event of epiphora following paranasal sinus surgery, CT dacryocystography with contrast injection of the lacrimal system may provide concurrent information about nasolacrimal duct obstruction and recurrent or persistent sinus disease (16).

Epistaxis

Of the Charing Cross series, 3.9% developed a minor primary bleed necessitating packing; it is our practice to place Merocel™ sponges in the middle meatuses at the end of surgery and for these to be removed in the recovery room after 15 min if the nose is dry. We feel that this does not lead to an increased rate of complications, but spares the patient the associated discomfort of packs in addition to specific complications of nasal packing, such as myospherulosis (if the dressing is impregnated with a petroleum-based ointment) (17) and toxic shock syndrome (18).

Anosmia and Hyposmia

A 0.4% incidence of anosmia occurred in our series, with all cases resolving. These cases may have represented an idiosyncratic reaction to the 10% cocaine nasal preparation used prior to surgery.

Pain

FESS may be associated with postoperative discomfort, which is perhaps underestimated: We observed that a small proportion of patients experience moderate frontal and facial discomfort between 2 and 5 d postoperatively, which may represent mild sinusitis secondary to edema in the region of the middle meatal antrostomy or frontal recess or osteitis.

Asthma

On contrasting their personal series of 1165 and 943 cases, respectively, May et al. (7) suggested that perioperative bronchospasm may occur more frequently with use of local anesthesia, possibly because of secretions triggering bronchospasm, and it is now their practice to use general anesthesia for patients with hyperreactive airways disease. Three instances of exacerbation of asthma postoperatively were observed at Charing Cross, all following general anesthesia (0.4%).

From a retrospective review of 232 patients, Gittelman et al. (19) suggested that the use of general anesthesia was associated with increased blood loss and operative time, but despite the fact that this group of patients were less well and had more extensive disease, the overall complication rate did not increase.

Dry Eyes

This phenomenon developed in one of our cases and settled spontaneously, probably because of a disturbance of the sphenopalatine ganglion akin to a postganglionic vidian neurectomy.

Transient Pupillary Dilatation or Ocular Motility Changes

Singh (20) reported 2 episodes of transient dilatation of a pupil following preoperative infiltration of 1% xylocaine with 1:100,000 adrenaline into the middle turbinates and lateral middle meatal wall, and topical peroperative phenylephrine packing. There was no penetration of the lamina papyracea, and surgery was terminated after anterior ethmoidectomy and middle meatal antrostomy; pupillary responses returned to normal 45 min later without any ocular sequelae. He postulated possible mechanisms, such as retrograde venous drainage from the area of infiltration of the lateral nasal wall or drainage of the topical phenylephrine to the ophthalmic veins, reflux of phenylephrine through the nasolacrimal duct, or conjunctival contamination from the surgeon's gloves. In response to this, Schaefer (21) referred to similar phenomena experienced elsewhere, including a case of transient blindness after xylocaine infiltration into the middle turbinate, probably owing to retrograde diffusion into the ophthalmic circulation. He described personal experience of transient mydriasis in a patient with widely dehiscent optic nerves in the sphenoid sinus, which recovered completely within hours. He suggested four procedures to minimize such problems, namely: preliminary placement of a vasoconstrictive agent against the mucosal surface to be injected, minimizing or avoiding injection into the middle turbinate, aspirating mucosal sites prior to injection, and allowing the eyes to be monitored throughout the procedure, whether performed under general or local anesthesia. One case of the senior author also experienced mild difficulty focusing in the first 24 h after FESS, without any other signs, which settled spontaneously.

MAJOR FESS COMPLICATIONS

Fatality

Wigand and Hosemann (22) reported a fatality after FESS after damage to the internal carotid artery in the sphenoid sinus led to demise from cerebral edema after a few days despite rapid hemostasis. Reinhart and Anderson (23) reported death following likely intracerebral injection of local anesthetic containing epinephrine in a patient with a history of previous sinus surgery that may have exposed brain tissue. Despite an emergency craniotomy for a large subdural hematoma and clipping of an avulsed branch of the anterior cerebral artery, the patient died after 12 d. Maniglia *(24)* also reported a death after anterior cerebral artery damage during endoscopic sinus surgery to biopsy a mass of the left sphenoid sinus and skull base, which was shown to be squamous carcinoma at autopsy.

Internal Carotid Artery Injury

Internal carotid artery injury during FESS is described above by Wigand and Hosemann *(22)* and also by Hudgkins *(25)*. In the latter case, nasal packing controlled the hemorrhage, and emergency angiography indicated a pseudoaneurysm of the cavernous carotid artery. Balloon occlusion was successfully performed, and there were no residual neurological deficits.

Stammberger *(9)* highlighted the potential danger to the internal carotid artery and optic nerve when removing bony septa in the sphenoid sinus. In the unfortunate event of carotid artery puncture, he suggested application of Oxycel sponge under pressure, tight packing, compression of the common carotid artery in the neck against the cervical vertebrae, and possible neurosurgical exploration.

From a study of the neurovascular relationships of the sphenoid sinus in 25 cadavers, Fujii et al. *(26)* found that the carotid artery produced a significant bulge into the sphenoid sinus in all except one side of one specimen, and in 8% there was no bony covering at all in the sinus. Kennedy et al. *(27)* found an apparent dehiscence of bone over the carotid artery in 22% and exposure in the posterior ethmoid sinus in 1.6%.

Brain Injury

Maniglia *(24)* described 2 cases of cribriform plate damage with frontal lobe injury and hematomata—one of which exhibited no neurological sequelae despite intracranial passage of the endoscope through the cribriform plate for 7 cm. This case required an external ethmoidectomy approach to repair the cribriform plate defect with a nasal septal flap, whereas the accompanying intracerebral hematoma was managed conservatively. The other case he described required an anterior frontal craniectomy and fascia lata repair.

A CT scan and neurosurgical review are mandatory; sudden changes in vital signs, such as bradycardia and hypotension, may indicate intracranial hemorrhage *(7)*.

Blindness

The two mechanisms for blindness following intranasal surgery are direct injury to the optic nerve and retrobulbar hematoma, which compromises the vascular supply and drainage of the eye by increased orbital pressure *(28)*.

The cadaver study of Fujii et al. *(26)* revealed protrusion of the optic canals into the superolateral part of the sphenoid sinus in all except one side of one specimen from a series of 25; in 78% the bony covering was <0.5 mm thick, and in 4% only the optic sheath and sinus mucosa covered the nerve. The thickness of the bony covering over the maximum area of bulging of the optic canal averages 0.28 mm, and in 12% there is bony dehiscence *(29)*. Three percent of optic nerves may traverse a posterior ethmoid air cell, with 23% having a significant projection into the sphenoid sinus *(30)*. Laterally pneumatized posterior ethmoid cells (Onodi cells) occur in 10% of patients *(31)*, and although it is unusual for them to encase the optic nerve completely, there is potential for damage if they do. Yeoh has recently reported that, among Asians, the optic nerve was present in the posterior ethmoid in 65% of 51 cadavers examined *(32)*. In 15% of these, the relationship was not apparent when viewed endoscopically, increasing the risk of accidental injury in Asians. Figure 1 illustrates pneumatization around the optic nerve.

The anterior ethmoidal artery is potentially at risk where it leaves the dome of the ethmoid sinus medially to enter the ethmoidal sulcus in the olfactory fossa, because the bone in the latter area is up to 10 times thinner than the neighboring ethmoidal roof. Furthermore, the dura is tightly adherent to bone at the entry and exit points of the anterior ethmoidal artery, and the lateral lamella of the cribriform plate easily breaks into sharp fragments, which can pierce dura *(33)*.

We have not included exposure of orbital fat as a major complication. From their combined series, May et al. *(7)* found that orbital complications of FESS were more likely to occur on removal of a very lateral uncinate process, close to the lamina papyracea, but that only 21 of 33 patients in whom orbital fat was noted developed any signs of orbital

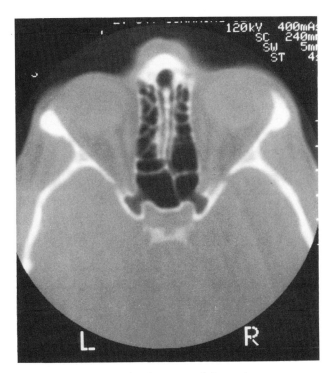

Fig. 1. Pneumatization around the optic nerves.

penetration. Certainly if orbital fat is exposed, further surgery should only proceed with extreme care; if doubt exists about the nature of the material removed, a flotation test may indicate whether the specimen is fat (floats—as does brain) or polypoid (sinks slowly).

Freedman and Kern *(34)* emphasized that a right-handed surgeon operating from the right side of the patient is more likely to encounter difficulty when operating on the right ethmoid than on the left. They reported 13 right-sided and 2 left-sided complications. The ophthalmological complications following bilateral ethmoid surgery were reported by Maniglia et al. *(35,36)* as two bilateral complications (one case owing to optic chiasm damage and the other owing to bilateral retrobulbar hematoma), seven patients with blindness of the right eye (five after hematoma and two unspecified), and three with left-sided blindness (all after hematoma). All eight intracranial and orbital complications from a series of 1077 intranasal ethmoidectomies occurred on the right side (36). Dessi et al. *(38)* similarly established that operation by a right-handed surgeon standing on the right side of the patient was an added risk factor from a review of 1192 intranasal sinus procedures performed under endoscopic control with video assistance.

Post-FESS blindness has been described, including one case of bilateral optic nerve transection in the orbits *(9,24)*, three cases of unilateral visual loss after hematoma despite decompression—although delayed in one case *(4)*—and another after unilateral bleeding *(31)*. Permanent medial rectus damage and diplopia after FESS were recorded by Maniglia *(24)*.

Stankiewitz *(28)* also reported three of his own cases, illustrating that prompt medical management can prevent blindness: In one case a patient experienced eye pain during a local anesthetic FESS procedure, and visual loss was reversed by orbital massage and iv mannitol; ecchymosis and eye pain with adduction settled conservatively in another patient. In a third case, under general anesthesia, rapid chemosis, proptosis, and mydriasis developed, which settled without sequelae after removal of packing, orbital massage, and iv mannitol.

An ethmoidal artery hemorrhage producing intraorbital hemorrhage, which threatens retinal perfusion, is an absolute emergency; experiments with central retinal artery occlusion indicated that the retina of the monkey can tolerate up to 100 min of ischemia, but after this irreparable damage ensues *(39)*. Management should include attempted hemostasis and decompression medially via an external ethmoidectomy approach or endoscopic decompression of the medial wall (lamina papyracea) or by a lateral canthotomy. Sacks et al. *(40)* considered that medical therapy, lateral canthotomy, and anterior chamber paracentesis may not provide adequate decompression after a significant retro-bulbar hemorrhage; they reported three cases of external ethmoid decompression removing the medial and inferior orbital wall, and a further case of transantral orbital decompression, all with successful recovery of vision and ocular motility. Thompson et al. *(41)* suggested an algorithm for treatment of intraoperative orbital hemorrhage during ethmoid surgery with the surgical steps commencing with medial orbitotomy, proceeding to lateral canthotomy and inferior cantholysis if there is no drainage and tension remains, and transantral inferior decompression if this fails to relieve pressure. The following have also been suggested: systemic corticosteroids, mannitol, acetazolamide, timolol eye drops, and orbital massage in addition to ophthalmological review *(3,42)*. Increasing intraorbital pressure can be assessed by serial measurements of proptosis, visual acuity, pupil size, extraocular muscle motion, tonometry, and fundoscopy *(43)*.

CSF Leak

The cribriform plate is lower than the fovea ethmoidalis, from which it is separated by the middle turbinate; furthermore, the dura is very adherent at this site such that bone penetration easily leads to a CSF fistula. Surgery medial to the middle turbinate is dangerous, but so is the area immediately superior and medial in the fovea ethmoidalis particularly near the anterior ethmoidal artery where the bone is thin and prone to shatter, as described above *(33,44)*.

CSF leak was the most commonly reported complication from the UK questionnaire and from the major series of May et al. *(7)*. They advocated entering the basal lamella posteriorly rather than anteriorly and a conservative approach for managing mucosa over the roof of the ethmoid sinus, citing a personal communication from Wigand, who attributed an early high incidence of CSF leak to "aggressive" removal of polypi from the ethmoid roof. If a "washout sign" is seen with leakage of clear fluid from a dural defect that washes away blood from the ethmoidal roof, then an immediate repair should be undertaken, typically with an endonasal-free or rotational mucoperichondrial flap. If CSF drainage continues for >3–5 d post-repair, an intrathecal drain may be considered, although the risks of intracranial infection and pneumatocephalus are increased. Alternatively, or should the drainage become heavy, then re-exploration of the site of the dural tear should be undertaken *(7)*. Hosemann and Wigand *(45)* found complete success with endoscopic endonasal repair of a circumscribed CSF leak using an autogenous mucosal graft in 18 patients over an average follow-up of 17 mo.

Kane *(8)* suggests that the more rapid diagnosis of such a CSF leak when viewing endoscopically rather than nonendoscopically increases the reporting of this complication for FESS compared to standard intranasal surgery.

In a prospective study of 150 CT scans, Dessi et al. *(46)* reported that the right ethmoidal roof was lower than the left in 8.6% of cases, whereas the reverse was present in only 1.2% and questioned whether this accounted for the higher incidence of endocranial complications and CSF leaks associated with right ethmoidectomy.

Table 1
Reported Major UK Complications
from 1992 Questionnaire

CSF leak	24
Orbital decompression required	4
Arterial ligation required	2
Temporary blindness	2
Permanent blindness	1
Transient diplopia	1
Pneumatocele	1
Dural tear	1

INCIDENCE OF MAJOR POST-FESS COMPLICATIONS

From his 1993 questionnaire, Kane *(8)* estimated that over 10,000 FESS procedures had been performed in Australia since the mid-1980s. Seventy-two surgeons responded, and the major complications reported were 8 intraorbital bleeds (2 requiring anterior ethmoidal artery ligation and 1 a lateral canthotomy) and 22 CSF leaks. Of the three orbital complications requiring surgical intervention, two have persistent medial rectus tethering and one has permanent optic nerve damage. Fourteen of the CSF leaks were repaired primarily with no sequelae, five underwent subsequent repair, and three closed with conservative management, although one of these developed meningitis. Minor complications included 15 hemorrhages not requiring surgery or transfusion and 15 cases with postoperative lacrimal problems, of which 3 needed dacryocystorhinostomy. His estimate of a 0.12% ocular complication rate and a 0.22% CSF leak rate are comparable with other estimates.

In 1992, we circulated a confidential questionnaire to the 653 members of the British Association of Otolaryngologists (BAOL), inquiring about experience, complications, and training for FESS *(47)*. The response rate was 60%, and 146 responders indicated that they perform FESS. Twenty-three had experienced a major complication of which CSF leak was by far the most common (Table 1). No serious complications occurred in the group of responders who had neither attended a course nor performed cadaver dissection. Conversely, of the 23 surgeons who did report major complications, all had either attended a course or performed cadaver dissection. Furthermore, the major complications appeared to affect the more experienced surgeons, since this group had performed an esti-

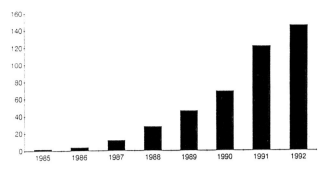

Fig. 2. Exponential increase in FESS performed in the UK.

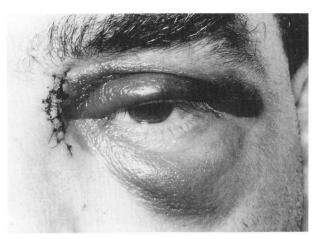

Fig. 3. Periorbital hematoma after decompression.

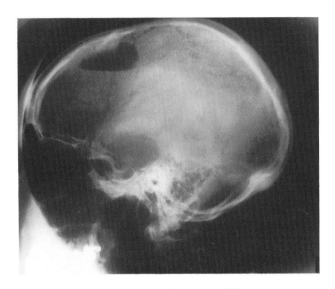

Fig. 4. Aerocele on lateral skull X-ray.

mated 345 procedures each, whereas those without major complications estimated their experience of FESS to be 62 cases each. The results indicated an approximate major complication rate of 0.23% from an estimated 15,399 procedures, and CSF leak was the most common serious complication cited, accounting for 24 of the 36 reports. Vleming et al. *(48)* similarly reported a 0.3% incidence of major FESS complications from a series of 1235 operations on 593 patients. May et al. *(7)* reported a 0.85% overall incidence of major complications from a combined series of 2108 FESS cases and Dessi et al. *(46)* a 1.3% rate.

The results of the survey did not support Stankiewitz's experience of a "learning curve" phenomenon. Furthermore, comments from some responders suggested that serious complications began to occur with more ambitious surgery and with increasing complacency. Nevertheless, the hazards to the novice are illustrated by Wigand *(31)*, who reported no major complications from a personal series of 220 patients, whereas a series of similar size from trainees in his clinic included complications, such as meningitis and brain abscess with subsequent death and blindness owing to intraorbital bleeding.

Data concerning the duration of practice of FESS were used to compile a histogram that indicates a near-exponential increase in the UK over the last 6 yr (Fig. 2). Undoubtedly, there is a similar growth worldwide, but it is salutary that Hosemann and Wigand *(45)* have been asked to provide expert opinions on nine life-threatening post-FESS complications in Germany over the last 3 yr.

Three major complications have occurred from a consecutive series of 675 cases over the last 4 years at Charing Cross Hospital. An orbital hematoma required immediate orbital decompression owing to rapidly increasing proptosis, but

resolved with no ocular complications (Fig. 3). A dural tear was repaired immediately with a free mucoperichondrial flap without apparent sequelae until an aerocele was seen on a plain skull X-ray 1 mo later (Fig. 4). Exploration by a right fronto-ethmoidectomy revealed only a small area of granulation tissue immediately posterior to the frontoethmoid recess; after repair by rotation of a mucoperichondrial septal flap, this settled uneventfully. Four days after bilateral FESS for massive nasal polyposis, a 60-yr-old man developed right CSF rhinorrhea following a violent sneeze. Endoscopic exploration located the leak to the right ethmoidal roof, which was repaired with a free septal mucoperichondrial graft with no subsequent problems.

DISCUSSION OF MAJOR POST-FESS COMPLICATIONS

Sinus surgery—either endoscopic or non-endoscopic—can be associated with major complications, including blindness, death, diplopia, intracranial hemorrhage, brain abscess, brain injury, meningitis, and CSF leaks *(35,36,42,49)*. However, the risks of such surgery have to be balanced against the fact that untreated acute or chronic sinus disease can also lead to fatal or major complications *(50)*.

Ohnishi et al. *(51)* identified five high-risk areas in FESS: the lamina papyracea, which is thin and has a convex bulge toward the ethmoid sinus; the ethmoidal sinus roof, where the bony canal of the anterior ethmoidal artery protrudes and the dura adheres closely to the sinus walls; the lateral lamella of the cribriform plate, which is the lateral wall of the olfactory bulb and can bulge into the medial wall of the anterior ethmoid sinus below the level of its roof; the posterior ethmoid sinus roof, where the posterior ethmoidal artery usually travels in a bony canal, but may lie below the roof; and the area between the sphenoid and posterior ethmoid sinuses, where the optic nerve may be damaged. They highlighted the risk of the Onodi cell (as above) where the optic canal bulges into the posterior ethmoid sinus and also that the internal carotid artery may produce a bulge into the sinus cavity where it courses along the lateral surface of the sphenoid bone within the cavernous sinus.

CT scanning including axial views at the level of the frontal sinuses and orbits may also reduce the risk by visualizing potentially dangerous anatomical abnormalities, such as in Fig. 1. We feel that although coronal scans are of the most help in terms of appreciation of the surgical anatomy—particularly at the level of the ostiomeatal complex—at least two axial views should be included (one at the level of the optic nerve and another at the level of the narrowest anteroposterior diameter of the frontoethmoid recess). Pan-sinus opacification is potentially more dangerous since diseased mucosa continues up to the lamina papyracea and cribriform plate, which may then be egg-shell-thin and more easily breached than if disease is localized to the ostiomeatal complex (giving the appearance of a "black halo") —*see* Figs. 5 and 6, respectively. All three serious complications in the personal series occurred in patients with pan-sinus opaci-

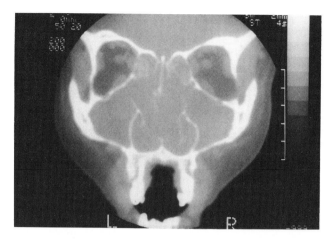

Fig. 5. Pan-sinus opacification on coronal CT scan.

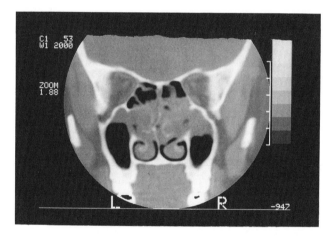

Fig. 6. "Black halo" on coronal CT scan.

fication. Enhanced anatomical localization by CT should increase in the future with the development of Computer-Assisted Surgery (CAS) *(52)*. Mosges and Klimek *(53)* reported use of CAS in 103 cases of endonasal surgery, finding a significant reduction in the duration of surgery and highlighting its ability to identify topographic landmarks even when the view is obscured by bleeding or pathology. Hudgkins *(25)* highlighted the role of the radiologist in identifying potentially dangerous anatomical variations on preoperative scans in addition to reporting any pathological changes evident.

RISK/BENEFIT RATIO

The efficacy of FESS has been confirmed in an objective prospective assessment in chronic rhinosinusitis with significant improvement in ciliary beat frequency and visual analog scores for nasal obstruction, headache, facial pain, anosmia, rhinor-rhea, and postnasal drip—particularly in the first three categories (54). The focal management permitted by FESS minimizes morbidity and is associated with success rates of 80–90%, even in patients with such predisposing factors as asthma, allergy, or the "ASA triad" of asthma, polyposis, and aspirin sensitivity, although the latter group were more likely to require additional medical or surgical treatment (55). However, one needs to consider whether the increased potential for risks and the time involved are justified by better results. Few trials to date have compared conventional sinus surgery with FESS.

The majority of series report results simply as comparisons of percentages of parameters of success, often based on retrospective questionnaires. The lack of a standardized classification system for subject types and for recording results subjectively and objectively on regular prospective long-term follow-up renders assessment and comparison of results difficult. Comparison with results of non-endoscopic surgery is important; May et al. (55) found that the reported success rates for both traditional and endoscopic sinus surgery are generally high and within similar ranges. They identified several factors important to the accurate reporting of results, including preoperative conditions, type of sinus pathology, imaging modalities used to assess the extent of disease, the number of revision procedures represented, length of follow-up, the reporting of number of patients or number of procedures, and the use of subjective or objective assessment of outcome.

Lund and Mackay (56) reported a combined series of 650 patients, 331 with chronic rhinosinusitis, 305 cases of gross polyposis, and 14 cases of recurrent acute sinusitis. After 6 mo, 87% considered themselves improved (78%) or cured (9%), 11% clinically unchanged, and 2% felt worse. There was no apparent difference in the results of the patients with chronic rhinosinusitis and diffuse polyposis; even patients with asthma and aspirin sensitivity exhibited good results: 94% were improved, 6% unchanged, and none worse. A comparison was made with a previous prospective study by the first author of 65 patients undergoing inferior meatal antrostomy for chronic rhinosinusitis (57) in which the success rate for improvement was comparable (84%), but scores for no improvement or worsening were higher for dis-

charge, blockage, headache, and facial pain. The authors comment that endoscopic surgery is more likely to benefit the sensation of obstruction owing to inflammatory ostiomeatal complex disease. Using a similar classification, Danielsen (2) reported post-FESS symptoms in 100 patients as asymptomatic (69%), improved (26%), and unchanged (5%); none were worse.

Schaitkin et al. (58) retrospectively reviewed 100 cases of FESS by one surgeon by classifying subjective postoperative symptoms, and also classified preoperative disease into anatomical variations, hyperplastic disease, suppurative disease, polyps, and the ASA triad. The overall success of the procedure in relieving sinus symptoms decreased from 98% at an average follow-up of 9 mo to 91% at 4 yr, with late failure principally occurring because of recurrent nasal polypi. Twelve percent of the group had triad symptoms: None of these achieved a complete surgical cure (in comparison to 25, 17, 80, and 35%, respectively, for anatomical variations, hyperplastic disease, suppurative disease, and polypi) and 82% achieved benefit in contrast to 100, 92, 100, and 90%, respectively. Surgery for anatomical variations and for suppurative infection produced at least improvement with medical therapy in all cases, but 8% of patients with hyperplastic disease and 10% with polypi had no benefit or were worse after surgery.

Kennedy (59) assessed 120 patients by symptom questionnaires and objectively by endoscopic follow-up. Marked subjective improvement occurred in excess of 80% of all disease groups, but objective assessment over a mean period of 18 mo revealed differences in the three disease categories of nonpolyposis, middle meatal polyposis, and diffuse polyposis: Well-healed cavities without evidence of scarring or pathology resulted in 77, 58, and 24%, respectively. Middle meatal antrostomies had an overall patency rate of 97% with the highest rate of stenosis in the diffuse polyposis group; frontal recess stenosis ensued in 12% of cases in which this area was dissected, also developing most frequently in patients with diffuse polyposis (27%). The only significant prognostic factor for the surgical outcome was the extent of disease.

From a symptom questionnaire of 234 patients who underwent endoscopic antral surgery, 91% were asymptomatic or greatly improved and only 9% were worse. Comparison of 117 inferior and

142 middle meatal antrostomies over a 3-yr period revealed a "wide window" in 71 and 87%, respectively; 19% of the former group stenosed compared to 9% of the latter, whereas 10 and 4% reclosed. Eighty-two percent of 220 patients who underwent complete endoscopic ethmoidectomy considered their disease healed or improved, but a poorer subjective result occurred in those with asthma, bronchitis, or sensitivity to nonsteroidal anti-inflammatory agents (31).

Stammberger (9) surveyed 500 patients up to 10 yr after FESS: 85% had "good or very good" results, 6% were "fair," 4% "moderate," and 5% no improvement or "bad." The best results from FESS occurred in anatomical variations causing stenoses, cephalgia, mycoses, initial procedure, allergy if good response to medical treatment, and mucoceles. The worst results were obtained in patients with diffuse polypoid rhinosinopathy, particularly in combination with aspirin sensitivity and asthma.

Antrochoanal polyps have commonly required Caldwell-Luc surgery previously, but Vleming and De Vries (60) reported complete success without complications in five cases; endoscopic surgery avoids potential damage to maxillary bone growth centers and developing dentition, which is a particular benefit in the younger age group who can present with this pathology. Cook et al. (61) reported successful endoscopic treatment of 32 patients with antrochoanal polyps with no recurrence over a 4–5 yr follow-up.

Hosemann et al. (62) reported an 86% cure and improvement in 9% of 56 patients who underwent endoscopic dacryocystorhinostomy; revision surgery was successful in 82% of cases.

The indications for endoscopic endonasal surgery are now becoming extended: The majority (69%) of inverted papillomas at Erlangen-Nurembourg are now managed endonasally (62). Seventeen percent of their patients required revision surgery, which was actually lower than that for external approaches (19%). They advocated the benefits of endoscopic surgery permitting retention of the normal paranasal bony framework, preservation of mucosa, and cosmesis (63). However, Myers and Petruzzelli (64) disputed this and believed that lateral rhinotomy, en bloc excision, and complete stripping of the sinus mucosa should be employed, particularly for advanced stage inverting papilloma of the sinonasal tract.

Furthermore, Hosemann et al. (62) now use an endoscopic approach for selected cases of endonasal malignancies: Approx 5% of malignant tumors of the nasal cavity, septum, and paranasal sinuses presenting were considered suitable.

FESS IN CHILDREN

Lazar et al. (65) evaluated the results of FESS in 210 children aged between 14 mo and 16 yr to reveal that 80% were improved, including the 8% who had previously undergone FESS. Of the children with asthma, 80% reported an improvement in their asthma postoperatively. There were no serious complications; the most common problems noted on follow-up endoscopy were adhesions and granulation tissue. Some had a minimal return of symptoms in the first 6 wk after FESS owing to edema and unhealed tissues. They suggested that children in whom sinusitis fails to improve after FESS should undergo evaluation for systemic disorders, such as cystic fibrosis, ciliary dyskinesia, immunodeficiency, and comprehensive assessment of allergies.

Haltom and Cannon (66) reported an 86% improvement following FESS in 44 children aged between 14 mo and 13 yr, without major complications. Parsons and Phillips (67) reviewed 52 children, of mean age 7.4 yr and at a mean follow-up period of 21.8 mo. The overall percentage improved with respect to nasal blockage, purulent nasal discharge, postnasal drip, chronic cough, halitosis, and headaches were 81, 88, 61, 84, 75, and 96%. Two-thirds of the patient group had preoperative allergic symptomatology and 19% no longer needed medication for their allergies. Of the 46% who suffered from asthma, 88% considered their symptoms less severe after FESS and none were worse, reinforcing the findings of Lazar et al. (65). They highlighted the exacting surgical requirements in children, and that the thin and tiny bony anatomy may be more easily damaged, particularly below the age of 6.

Traditional sinus procedures are also associated with risks in children: Caldwell-Luc procedures may affect facial growth, whereas inferior meatal antrostomies may damage tooth buds in the spongiotic bone beneath the sinus floor (68). They concluded that anatomical landmarks are already well developed even in the newborn, but advised caution during the resection of the uncinate process and enlargement of the natural ostium, since the inferior turbinate is located higher on the lateral nasal wall so that the anterior margin of the unci- nate is closer to the lamina papyracea and may even be attached, increasing the risk of orbital injury.

The study of Lund and Mackay (56) showed that patients with cystic fibrosis did worse than other groups with only 54% improved after 6 mo, owing to aggressive diffuse polyposis. There were no major complications. Cuyler (69) reported similar results of FESS in seven children with cystic fibro- sis, but we would concur with his conclusion that although FESS can only improve the anatomical drainage pathways and not cure the mucovis- cidosis, it is of value for the symptomatic relief of nasal disease.

Two cases of unilateral choanal atresia and one of unilateral choanal stenosis have been managed endoscopically here, all in young adults. These three patients required only overnight postop- erative stay, stenting was unnecessary, and all have an excellent surgical result after a mean period of 18 mo.

POTENTIAL LONG-TERM SEQUELAE

Mucoceles

These generally require so many years to develop that there are currently no longitudinal studies of sufficient duration to corroborate the imputation that they may be a long-term conse- quence of FESS, although scarring within the frontal recess, particularly in childhood, may result in this complication (Lund—personal communication).

From a review of 80 frontoethmoidal mucoceles, Lund (70) identified etiological factors in 71%; 27% had undergone previous surgery, although the time interval between etiology and presentation was significantly longer in both the "polyp" and "infection" group for surgery rather than nonsurgi- cal management. Their pathogenesis probably involves dynamic bone resorption and formation rather than pressure erosion, with interleukin-1 release from the epithelial cells causing bone erosion (71,72).

Moriyama et al. (73) concluded that postopera- tive mucoceles tend to develop 15–24 yr after ini- tial surgery and identified that performance of nasal surgery at a young age is a factor in the develop- ment of a mucocele. Three cases from the 47 oper- ated on over the 10-yr review period had only been treated by endonasal surgery. They advocated sufficient resection of the ground lamella and ethmoidal sinus lamellae at primary paranasal sinus surgery to prevent postoperative mucocele formation.

Facial Growth

Rhys-Evans and Brain (74) found that although septal surgery in the rabbit nose greatly retarded subsequent nasal and maxillary development, osteotomies did not affect growth. Similarly, Brain and Rock (75) found that childhood nasal trauma was associated with impaired eventual maxillary growth, despite the fact that none had sustained any loss of septal cartilage from the original injury. In midfacial degloving surgery, no significant cos- metic sequelae appeared to ensue if the integrity of the cartilaginous septum was preserved (76). Nei- ther is there evidence that craniofacial resection, lateral rhinotomy, or external ethmoidectomy causes significant distortion of facial growth other than that resulting from the original lesion, which often remodels, and hence, it is unlikely that lim- ited endoscopic surgery on the lateral nasal wall in the pediatric population should have any long-term detrimental affect (Lund—personal communication).

CONCLUSION

FESS is one of the most exciting recent develop- ments in otolaryngology. With adequate training and cadaver dissection, FESS should be associated with no higher incidence of complications than other approaches to the ethmoid while permitting more accurate removal of diseased mucosa to restore normal function. This is borne out by an overall review of the major complications reported from consecutive series shown in Table 2. This indicates a 0.41% major complication rate for FESS compared to a 1.2% figure for nonendoscopic intranasal ethmoidectomy and minor complication rates of 6.2 (almost half owing to adhesions) and 2.1%, respectively. Three major complications have been encountered from a consecutive series of 675 cases over the last 4 yr at Charing Cross—an incidence of 0.44%.

Complications should be minimized by adequate training, preoperative assessment, and CT scan- ning. A good field of vision in the operation is nec- essary with satisfactory hemostasis; operating with the 0° endoscope is safest, and caution is required

Table 2
Complications Reported in Major Series

Author	Op	No. pts	CSF leak	i/c Infection	Major orbital cx	Major hem.	Death	Adhesion
Stankiewitz (3)	FESS	90	1	—	1	2	—	6
Stankiewitz (4)	FESS	90	1	—	—	—	—	
Wigand and Hosemann (22)	FESS	1000+	10	2	—	1	1	No details of minor complications
Stammberger (9)	FESS	6000+	3	—	—	2	—	43
Lazar et al. (77)	FESS	773	2	1	—	—	—	191
May et al. (55)	FESS	2108	10	—	1	4	—	35
Vleming et al. (48)	FESS	593	2	—	—	—	—	15
Freedman and Kern (34)	INE	1000	1	1	—	12	—	—
Friedman and Katsantonis (78)	INE	584	4	—	—	3	—	—
Lawson (37)	INE	600	3	—	2	—	—	—
Lund (14)	EE	320	—	—	—	—	—	—

Author	Minor orbital cx	Minor hem.	Lacrimal	Asthma	Infection	Facial	Other
Stankiewitz (3)	8	3	—	—	—	—	—
Stankiewitz (4)	1	—	—	—	—	—	—
Wigand and Hosemann (22)							
Stammberger (9)	5	11	—	—	—	5	1 Pneumatocephalus
Lazar et al. (77)	34	48	10	—	—	56	13 Otalgia
May et al. (55)	36	13	3	28	—	—	—
Vleming et al. (48)	2	11	1	1	2	—	2 Pneumatocephalus, 1 mucocele
Freedman and Kern (34)	4	—	1	3	—	1	1 Anosmia
Friedman and Katsantonis (78)	3	4	—	17	—	—	2 Frontal mucoceles
Lawson (37)	3	2	2	—	—	—	2 Atrophic rhinitis
Lund (14)	—	2	—	—	—	—	—

with use of 30 and 70° endoscopes when it is easier to become disoriented.

One of the benefits of the FESS "philosophy" is the careful follow-up with regular nasal toilet under local anesthesia with endoscopic control. It is at this stage that the last polyp may be removed or the final cell opened rather than taking any unnecessary risk during primary surgery—particularly if the field should be at all bloody.

REFERENCES

1. Mosher E. The surgical anatomy of the ethmoidal labyrinth. Ann Otol, Rhinol Laryngol 1929;38: 869–901.
2. Danielsen A. Functional endoscopic sinus surgery on a day case out-patient basis. Clin Otolaryngol 1992;17:473–477.
3. Stankiewitz JA. Complications of endoscopic intranasal ethmoidectomy. Laryngoscope 1987;97:1270–1273.
4. Stankiewitz JA. Complications in endoscopic intranasal ethmoidectomy: an update. Laryngoscope 1989;99:686–690.
5. Rivron RP, Maran AGD. The Edinburgh FESS trainer: a cadaver-based bench-top practice system for endoscopic ethmoidal surgery. Clin Otolaryngol 1991;16:426–429.
6. Stanley RE. Letter. Singapore Med J 1992;33:532,533.
7. May M, Levine HL, Schaitkin B, Mester SJ. Complications of endoscopic sinus surgery. In: Levine HL, May M, eds., Endoscopic Sinus Surgery. New York: Thieme, 1993; pp. 193–243.
8. Kane K. Australian experience with functional endoscopic sinus surgery and its complications. Ann Otol, Rhinol Laryngol 1993;102:613–615.

9. Stammberger H. Functional Endoscopic Sinus Surgery. Philadelphia: B. C. Decker, 1991.

10. La Mear WR, Davis WE, Templer JW, McKinsey JP, Del Porto H. Partial endoscopic middle turbinectomy augmenting functional endoscopic sinus surgery. Otolaryngol, Head Neck Surg 1992;107:382–389.

11. Salman SD. A new stent for endoscopic sinus surgery. Otolaryngol, Head Neck Surg 1993;109:780,781.

12. Serdahl CL, Berris CE, Chole RA. Nasolacrimal duct obstruction after endoscopic sinus surgery. Arch Ophthalmol 1990;108:392.

13. Kennedy DW, Zinreich SJ, Shaalan H, Kuhn F, Naclerio R, Loch E. Endoscopic middle meatal antrostomy: theory, technique and patency. Laryngoscope 1987;97(Suppl. 43):8 pt 3:1–9.

14. Lund VJ. Surgery of the ethmoids—past, present and future: a review. J Royal Soc Med 1990;83:451–455.

15. Bolger WE, Parsons DS, Mair EA, Kuhn FA. Lacrimal drainage system injury in functional endoscopic sinus surgery. Arch Otolaryngol, Head Neck Surg 1992;118: 1179–1184.

16. Massoud TF, Whittet HB, Anslow P. CT-dacryocystography for nasolacrimal duct obstruction following paranasal sinus surgery. Br J Radiol 1993;66:223–227.

17. Paugh DR, Sullivan MJ. Myospherulosis of the paranasal sinuses. Otolaryngol, Head Neck Surg 1990;103: 117–119.

18. De Vries N, Van der Baan S. Toxic shock syndrome after nasal surgery: is prevention possible? Rhinology 1989; 27:125–128.

19. Gittelman PD, Jacobs JB, Skorina J. Comparison of functional endoscopic sinus surgery under local and general anaesthesia. Ann Otol, Rhinol Laryngol 1993; 102:289–293.

20. Singh J. Endoscopic sinus surgery (letter). Arch Otolaryngol, Head Neck Surg 1992;118:105.

21. Schaefer SD. Endoscopic sinus surgery (reply). Arch Otolaryngol, Head Neck Surg 1992;118:105.

22. Wigand ME, Hosemann WG. Results of endoscopic surgery of the paranasal sinuses and anterior skull base. J Otolaryngol 1991;20:385–390.

23. Reinhart DJ, Anderson JS. Fatal outcome during endoscopic sinus surgery: anaesthetic manifestations. Anaesth Analg 1993;77:188–190.

24. Maniglia AJ. Fatal and other major complications of endoscopic sinus surgery. Laryngoscope 1991;101: 349–354.

25. Hudgkins PA. Complications of endoscopic sinus surgery. The role of the radiologist in prevention. Radiol Clin North Am 1993;31:21–32.

26. Fujii K, Chambers SM, Rhoton AL. Neurovascular relationships of the sphenoid sinus. J Neurosurg 1979; 50:31–39.

27. Kennedy DW, Zinreich SJ, Hassab MH. The internal carotid artery as it relates to sphenoethmoidectomy. Am J Rhinol 1990;4:7–12.

28. Stankiewitz JA. Blindness and intranasal endoscopic ethmoidectomy: prevention and management. Otolaryngol, Head Neck Surg 1989;101:320–329.

29. Kainz J, Stammberger H. Danger areas of the posterior rhinobasis. An endoscopic and histo-anatomical study. Laryngol-Rhinol-Otol 1991;70:479–486.

30. Bansberg SF, Harner SG, Forbes G. Relationship of the optic nerve to the paranasal sinuses as shown by computed tomography. Otolaryngol, Head Neck Surg 1987; 96:331–335.

31. Wigand ME. Endoscopic Surgery of the Paranasal Sinuses and Anterior Skull Base. Stuttgart: Georg Thieme Verlag. New York: Thieme Medical Publishers, 1990.

32. Yeoh H. Anatomic variations and sinusitis (abst.) XV Congress of European Rhinological Society 1994, 169.

33. Kainz J, Stammberger H. The roof of the anterior ethmoid—a place of least resistance in the skull base. Am J Rhinol 1989;3:191–199.

34. Freedman HM, Kern EB. Complications of intranasal ethmoidectomy: a review of 1000 consecutive operations. Laryngoscope 1979;89:421–434.

35. Maniglia AJ, Chandler JR, Goodwin WJ, Flynn J. Rare complications following ethmoidectomies: a report of 11 cases. Laryngoscope 1981;91:1234–1242.

36. Maniglia AJ. Fatal and major complications secondary to nasal and sinus surgery. Laryngoscope 1989;99:276–283.

37. Lawson W. The intranasal ethmoidectomy: an experience with 1077 procedures. Laryngoscope 1991;101: 367–371.

38. Dessi P, Castro F, Triglia JM, Zanaret M, Cannoni M. Major complications of sinus surgery: a review of 1192 procedures. J Laryngol Otol 1994;108:212–215.

39. Hayreh SS, Kolder HE, Weingeist TA. Central retinal artery occlusion and retinal tolerance time. Ophthalmology 1980;87:75–78.

40. Sacks SH, Lawson W, Edelstein D, Green RP. Surgical treatment of blindness secondary to intraorbital haemorrhage. Arch Otolaryngol, Head Neck Surg 1988;114: 801–803.

41. Thompson RF, Gluckman JL, Kulwin D, Savoury L. Orbital haemorrhage during ethmoid sinus surgery. Otolaryngol, Head Neck Surg 1990;102:45–50.

42. Buus DR, Tse DT, Ferris BK. Ophthalmologic complications of sinus surgery. Ophthalmology 1990;97:612–619.

43. May M, Hillsamer P, Hoffman DF. Management of orbital hematoma following functional endoscopic sinus surgery. Am J Rhinol 1991;5:47–49.

44. Stankiewitz JA. Cerebrospinal fluid fistula and endoscopic sinus surgery. Laryngoscope 1991;101:250–256.

45. Hosemann W, Wigand ME. Merit and demerit of endoscopic surgery. Rhinology 1992; Supplement 14:141–145.

46. Dessi P, Moulin G, Triglia JM, Zanaret M, Cannoni M. Difference in height of the right and left ethmoidal roofs: a possible risk factor for ethmoidal surgery. Prospective study of 150 CT scans. J Laryngol Otol 1994;108: 261,262.

47. Cumberworth VL, Sudderick RM, Mackay IS. Major complications of FESS. Clin Otolaryngol 1994;19:248–253.

48. Vleming M, Middelweerd MJ, De Vries N. Complications of endoscopic sinus surgery. Arch Otolaryngol, Head Neck Surg 1992;118:617–623.

49. Wayoff M, Jankowski R. Medicolegal aspects in sinus surgery. Rhinology 1991;29:257–261.

50. Maniglia AJ. Letter. Laryngoscope 1989;99:871.

51. Ohnishi T, Tachibana T, Kaneko Y, Esaki S. High risk areas in endoscopic sinus surgery and prevention of complications. Laryngoscope 1993;103:1181–1185.

52. Schlondorff G, Mosges R, Meyer-Ebrecht D, Krybus W, Adams L. CAS (computer assisted surgery). A new procedure in head and neck surgery. HNO 1989;37:187–190.

53. Mosges R, Klimek L. Computer assisted surgery of the paranasal sinuses. J Otolaryngol 1993;22:69–71.

54. Lund VJ, Holmstrom M, Scadding GK. Functional endoscopic sinus surgery in the management of chronic rhinosinusitis. An objective assessment. J Laryngol Otol 1991;105:832–835.

55. May M, Levine HL, Schaitkin B, Mester SJ. Results of surgery. In: Levine HL, May M, eds., Endoscopic Sinus Surgery. New York: Thieme Medical Publishers, 1993.

56. Lund VJ, Mackay IS. Outcome assessment of endoscopic sinus surgery. J Royal Soc Med 1994;70–72.

57. Lund VJ. Inferior meatal antrostomy. J Laryngol Otol 1988;102(Suppl. 15):1–18.

58. Schaitkin B, May M, Shapiro A, Fucci M, Mester SJ. Endoscopic sinus surgery: 4 year follow up on the first 100 patients. Laryngoscope 1993;103:1117–1120.

59. Kennedy DW. Prognostic factors, outcomes and staging in ethmoid sinus surgery. Laryngoscope 1992;102(Suppl. 57):1–18.

60. Vleming M, De Vries N. Endoscopic sinus surgery for antrochoanal polyps. Rhinology 1991;29:77,78.

61. Cook PR, Davis WE, McDonald R, McKinsey JP. Antrochoanal polyposis: a review of 33 cases. ENT J 1993;72:401–410.

62. Hosemann W, Gode U, Wigand ME. Indications, technique and results of endonasal endoscopic ethmoidectomy. Acta Oto-Rhinol-Laryngolog 1993;47:73–83.

63. Waitz G, Wigand ME. Results of endoscopic sinus surgery for the treatment of inverted papillomas. Laryngoscope 1992;102:917–922.

64. Myers EN, Petruzzelli GJ. Endoscopic sinus surgery for inverting papillomas (letter). Laryngoscope 1993;103:711.

65. Lazar RH, Younis RT, Gurucharri MJ. Endoscopic sinus surgery in children. In: Levine HL, May M, eds., Endoscopic Sinus Surgery. New York: Thieme Medical Publishers, 1993.

66. Haltom JR, Cannon CR. Functional endoscopic sinus surgery in children. J Miss State Med Assoc 1993;34:1–6.

67. Parsons DS, Phillips SE. Functional endoscopic sinus surgery in children: a retrospective analysis of results. Laryngoscope 1993;103:899–903.

68. Wolf G, Anderhuber W, Kuhn F. Development of the paranasal sinuses in children: implications for paranasal sinus surgery. Ann Otol, Rhinol Laryngol 1993;102:705–711.

69. Cuyler JP. Follow-up of endoscopic sinus surgery on children with cystic fibrosis. Arch Otolaryngol, Head Neck Surg 1992;118:505,506.

70. Lund VJ. Anatomical considerations in the aetiology of fronto-ethmoidal mucocoeles. Rhinology 1987;25:83–88.

71. Lund VJ, Milroy CM. Fronto-ethmoidal mucocoeles: a histopathological analysis. J Laryngol Otol 1991;105:921–923.

72. Lund VJ, Henderson B, Song Y. Involvement of cytokines and vascular adhesion receptors in the pathology of fronto-ethmoidal mucocoeles. Acta Oto-Laryngol 1993;113:540–546.

73. Moriyama H, Nakajima T, Honda Y. Studies on mucocoeles of the ethmoid and sphenoid sinuses: analysis of 47 cases. J Laryngol Otol 1992;106:23–27.

74. Rhys-Evans PH, Brain DJ. The influence of nasal osteotomies and septum surgery on the growth of the rabbit snout. J Laryngol Otol 1981;95:1109–1119.

75. Brain DJ, Rock WP. The influence of nasal trauma during childhood on growth of the facial skeleton. J Laryngol Otol 1983;97:917–923.

76. Howard DJ, Lund VJ. The midfacial degloving approach to sinonasal disease. J Laryngol Otol 1992;106:1059–1062.

77. Lazar RH, Younis RT, Long TE. Functional endonasal sinus surgery in adults and children. Laryngoscope 1993;103:1–5.

78. Friedman WH, Katsantonis GP. Intranasal and transantral ethmoidectomy: a 20 year experience. Laryngoscope 1990;100:343–348.

Index